Textbook of Surgery of Larynx and Trachea

Marc Remacle • Hans Edmund Eckel
Editors

Textbook of Surgery of Larynx and Trachea

Second Edition

Springer

Editors
Marc Remacle
Department of Oto-Rhino-Laryngology
Centre Hospitalier de Luxembourg
(CHL)
Luxembourg, Luxembourg

Hans Edmund Eckel
Department of Oto-Rhino-Laryngology
A.ö. Landeskrankenhaus
Klagenfurt, HNO
Klagenfurt, Austria

ISBN 978-3-031-09620-4 ISBN 978-3-031-09621-1 (eBook)
https://doi.org/10.1007/978-3-031-09621-1

This Springer imprint is published by the registered company Springer Nature Switzerland AG
The registered company address is: Gewerbestrasse 11, 6330 Cham, Switzerland

Foreword

I began my career in laryngology in 1992 with my Fellowship at the Vanderbilt Voice Center under the direction of Robert Ossoff. Early that year, I had the privilege and pleasure to meet Professor Marc Remacle when he came to our institution as a visiting lecturer. Marc's humility, candor, and insight into laryngology and surgical techniques were immediately intriguing. Little did I suspect that that brief meeting would develop into a lifelong friendship between colleagues. A year or 2 later, I had the opportunity to get to know Marc when we both traveled through Brazil at the request of our friends Denilson Fomin and Jose Antonio Pinto. They kept us busy that week with 14 lectures each and live surgery in between lectures. The Brazilians know how to work and how to have fun after. While Marc and I were kept busy with teaching and surgery, in between at social events, I had the opportunity to exchange ideas and learn from Professor Remacle. His love for and skill in surgery were inspirational. During that trip, we identified in each other kindred spirits or brothers from different mothers. The trip was exhausting but glorious.

Over the years since, Marc and I have watched our careers and families grow. I have learned from Marc innumerable surgical nuances, skills in organizing meetings, and how to be friend. With his love and skill for surgery, it is fitting that Marc co-edits a text on laryngeal surgical techniques. His vast experience over the years, and yes that is reference to the length of his career, provides him with insight that only comes from practice. This enables Marc to identify value and nuances that create excellent outcomes. Marc teaches from his heart. It is his sincere desire to shape others into the best physician and surgeon they can be. In editing this text, Marc furthers his goals.

I know Professor Hans Eckel primarily through reputation and chance meetings over the years. Professor Eckel is recognized by his colleagues through his accomplishments in laryngology and laryngeal surgery. Having authored or co-authored over 150 scientific manuscripts on laryngology and head and neck surgery, Dr. Eckel has developed a vast knowledge of our field. He is a thoughtful clinician scientist whose work over the years has helped to shape the practice of modern laryngology. His works educate and inform the practice of both the novice and experienced laryngeal surgeon. Hans Eckel is a collaborative physician/surgeon who serves as a role model for the team approach to understanding laryngeal disease. It is also fitting that Hans applies his knowledge developed over years of practice to editing a text on laryngeal diseases.

Surgery of Larynx and Trachea is a balanced text targeted for both the novice and experienced laryngeal surgeon. The topics cover our field in a broad manner and still provide nuanced information of value to all practitioners. Regarding the value of this, the second edition of the text, Drs. Remacle and Eckel have chosen their contributors wisely from colleagues who are known as experts in the field and on the topics which they have been asked to write about. The second edition updates all the existing chapters with current knowledge and adds additional chapters on currently relevant topics such as robotic laryngeal surgery; office-based laryngeal procedures; endoscopic approaches for early and advanced laryngeal neoplasia; laryngeal papillomatosis and a current understanding of the role HPV may have in the development of laryngeal cancer; as well as current concepts on reconstruction of laryngeal and pharyngeal defects. The text is edited for relevance to both the novice and experienced laryngeal surgeon. The topics are complete, and I hope you will find this as informative as I have. I would like to express my thanks to Drs. Eckel and Remacle for putting this work together.

Mark S. Courey

Department of Otolaryngology-
Head and Neck Surgery
Icahn School of Medicine
at Mount Sinai
New York, USA

Division of Laryngology-
Mount Sinai Health System
Eugen Grabscheid Voice Center
New York, USA
mark.courey@mountsinai.org

Preface

Laryngology in Europe is as diverse as possible, a consequence of different traditions, schools, national protagonists, and languages throughout Europe. While in some countries, e.g., Germany, otology was clearly the prevailing subspecialty for decades, others, like France, Italy, or Spain, traditionally have a stronger focus on laryngology. The scientific output of these countries witnesses these long-lasting traditions.

After the World War II, the USA has clearly taken the lead in practically all fields of experimental and clinical medicine. For me personally, friendship with laryngologists in France, Belgium, the Netherlands, the UK, Spain, Italy, and the USA was the key to discover the many faces of laryngology. For those who aspire to become laryngologists in Europe, the consequences are evident: *"The world is a book and those who do not travel read only one page"* (Augustine of Hippo).

Laryngology and laryngeal surgery reach out into neighboring medical fields and are constantly inspired by their advances: surgical and medical oncology, radiotherapy, speech and voice disorders, pathology, respiratory medicine, immunology, and virology are some examples of fields for fruitful exchange of knowledge and experience.

Over time, some head and neck surgeons have discovered a specific interest in the communicative, social, and emotional consequences of their occupation, and they joined the laryngological community. Some phoniatricians have eventually been bored by the permanent pedagogic approach to their patients' discomforts and wished to incorporate surgical and medical approaches to disorders of voice, airway, and swallowing. Yet others find it tempting to permanently deal with urgent and life-threatening conditions in the head and neck and decided to become airway specialists, a highly focused subset of laryngologists.

In recent years, research into laryngeal anatomy and physiology, technical advances, and pharmacological progress have provided the laryngological community with an abundance of new insights into the basic laryngeal functions—protection of the lower airway during deglutition, respiration, and voice production—and therapeutic options. Consequently, our attitude toward health and medical care has changed considerably. While cure was the only ambition of most medical and surgical interventions in the past, the preservation and improvement of physical function are now equally important issues. Individuals in today's developed societies depend on communicative skills rather than on physical work, and laryngology has become a major medical subspecialty dealing with communication disorders.

The European Laryngological Society has been seminal in uniting forces in the pursuit of laryngeal research and education throughout Europe. It has maintained close, friendly, and inspiring relations to fellows in North America and worldwide. The society brings together those who joined forces in compiling the texts for this book, both from Europe and the USA.

The book is designed to serve as an introduction to some of the most relevant clinical aspects of laryngology. We encourage readers to seek stimulation in the chapters we provide and to use them as a starting point for a journey into the world of contemporary voice disorder management, swallowing rehabilitation, central airway compromise, and laryngeal tumors.

The editors hope that this textbook may serve as a basis for future research and for discussion among laryngologists and as a source of inspiration to our readers.

We express our gratitude to Springer editors who made this book possible, to the contributors to this project, and to our fellows, students, and families.

Luxembourg, Luxembourg — Marc Remacle
Klagenfurt, Austria — Hans Edmund Eckel
March 2022

Contents

Physiology of the Larynx

1

Aude Lagier and Antoine Giovanni

1.1 Introduction

The larynx is a small organ located at the anterior part of the neck, in a very critical place: it is both the aerial exit of the aerodigestive crossroads and the inlet of the lower respiratory tract. The human larynx is a complex structure of several cartilages mobilized by small muscles called intrinsic laryngeal muscles. It participates in very important functions in humans. Two functions are necessary for life: breathing and protecting the airway during swallowing or with protective reflexes like cough. The third one is the phonation. It is more specific to humans and very important as the voice is our most effective way of communication. Phylogenetically, the larynx is present in lungfish as a sphincter at the entry of the lungs. In lower mammals, swallowing and breathing pathways are separated by the overlapping of uvula and epiglottis [1]. This configuration is still present in some mammals like deers and in newborns who are exclusive nasal breathers. As the infant grows, the larynx moves downward along with the growth of the pharynx, which allows the creation of resonance cavities and then the arising of the function of articulation [2].

Key Points
The functions of the larynx are:

- Breathing
- Protection the lower respiratory tract
  - During swallowing
  - With protective reflexes
- Phonation

1.2 Larynx and Breathing (Quietly)

1.2.1 Quiet Spontaneous Breathing

The larynx is a duct made of cartilages and is supposed to remain opened during the two phases of breathing (i.e., inspiration and expiration). Remaining opened during inspiration is challenging because the negative pressure inside the airway may lead the inlet of the larynx to collapse. The first role, static, of the

A. Lagier (✉)
Service d'ORL, CHU de Liège, Liège, Belgium
e-mail: aude.lagier@chuliege.be

A. Giovanni
Service d'ORL, CHU La Conception, Assistance Publique-Hôpitaux de Marseille, Marseille, France
e-mail: antoine.giovanni@ap-hm.fr

M. Remacle, H. E. Eckel (eds.), *Textbook of Surgery of Larynx and Trachea*,
https://doi.org/10.1007/978-3-031-09621-1_1

cartilages of the larynx is to prevent this collapse, and it is mainly the role of the cricoid cartilage, which is the only complete ring of the respiratory tract. Surgeons avoid removing part of the cricoid without reconstruction because of it (literature about the question of reconstruction is important; as an example, see Rovo [3]). Conversely, the geometry of complete ring leads to the impossibility of extension, and an intraluminal tumor in the subglottal space is more likely to be responsible of dyspnea.

The subglottal level (inside the cricoid cartilage) and trachea are considered as a whole organ so-called subglottal tract which is devoted to breathing and can be compared to a single tube 16.0–19.5 cm length in women and men, respectively [4].

The larynx is the location of an important respiratory resistance due to the glottis which is a level of narrowing in the airway and responsible of 25–60% of the overall resistance [5]. Contrary to the subglottal tract, the glottis is dynamic during breathing. During normal, quiet, and slow breathing, about 50% of the subjects progressively open their glottis during inspiration, and it progressively narrows during expiration [6, 7]. The glottal opening begins with the inspiration, and there are electromyographic evidence of activation of the posterior cricoarytenoid muscle (PCA muscle) prior to the activation of the diaphragm [8]. The thyroarytenoid (TA) and the cricothyroid (CT) muscles are also active during inspiration, antidromically to the PCA during quiet breathing, and also during hyperventilation [9, 10]. On the other hand, the narrowing begins before the onset of expiration, and the TA muscle is still activated during this phase. This finding is more frequent in men than in women where the glottis remains more stable along the breathing cycle. Intrinsic laryngeal muscles are activated with both tonic and phasic motor units firing during breathing.

There is a general agreement to explain that widening the glottis area during inspiration helps air intake and that narrowing the glottis during expiration slows down the passive expiratory flow and enables to control the end-expiratory lung volume. This motion is also an energy-saving model which reduces the loss of energy of the airflow.

1.2.2 Breath Modulation Maneuvers

Voluntary sniff provides the maximal glottal opening with rapid phasic recruitment of both PCA and CT muscles [9].

During voluntary tachypnea, the glottal area is larger during the whole cycle compared to normal breathing, with 44% of dynamic changes only, in both men and women [7].

1.2.3 Breath-Hold Maneuvers

Breath-hold maneuvers are associated with arytenoid adduction and glottis closure in most subjects, completed by vestibular folds adduction and anterior arytenoid tilt during effortful breath-hold maneuvers. High inter- and intra-individual variability is observed for the presence and degree of closure of the larynx during that task [11].

1.2.4 Effect of Capnia Variations on the Glottal Geometry

In the case of pathological increase or decrease of capnia, the larynx resistance varies in order to facilitate the normalization of the capnia: the glottis enlarges in case of hypercapnia and narrows in case of hypocapnia [5, 6]. Interestingly, this adaptation is inhibited during phonation, and the laryngeal resistance during phonation remains stable whatever the level of the capnia [5]. In case of hypercapnia, the PCA activity increases, but so does the activity of the TA during expiration, which consequently reduces the airflow and maintains alveolar expansion [9].

Key Points
Two laryngeal areas are specifically involved in the breathing function:

- The glottis is the narrower area and responsible for the laryngeal resistance to airflow. It is dynamically controlled during breathing.
- The subglottal space is responsible for permanent opening of the larynx, due to its static properties.

1.3 Larynx and Cough

Cough is a protective response that leads to ejection of mucus or foreign bodies from the lungs thanks to the generation of high-velocity airflow. It is most often a reflex, but it can also be voluntarily controlled. The larynx and the tracheobronchial tree are the main reflexogenic zones for cough. Three phases are occurring during cough: inspiratory, compressive, and expulsive. The inspiratory phase is present during voluntary cough and cough reflex due to trachea-bronchial stimulation but may be absent in response to stimuli at the vocal fold or upper level leading to a so-called expiration reflex [12]. During the inspiratory phase, the PCA and CT muscles co-contract along with the diaphragm, and the larynx abducts promoting the inspiratory flow. During the compressive phase, the adductor muscles (i.e., TA, lateral cricoarytenoid, LCA, and inter-arytenoid, IA) contract while minimal activity is present in PCA and CT. Consequently, the glottis closes while the expiratory muscles contract. During this phase, the larynx should be sealed in order to increase the subglottal pressure and to make the cough efficient. During the last phase, the expulsive phase, the larynx suddenly opens due to the activation of the PCA and inhibition of the adductor muscles, while the expiratory muscles are still contracting [13].

Key Point
- Cough is an airway protective reflex which necessitates the sealing of the larynx.

1.4 Larynx and Swallowing

Swallowing relies on a rapid, complex, and sequential neuromuscular activity of the oral cavity, tongue, pharynx, larynx, and esophagus. In this function, the larynx has to seal in order to prevent inhalation. Swallowing requires that the larynx closes rapidly and completely. Two levels are involved in the laryngeal closure during swallowing: the vocal folds and the vestibule (including the vestibular folds, the arytenoid cartilages, and the epiglottis).

1.4.1 Swallowing and Breathing

Swallowing interrupts the respiratory cycle with an apneic period during the pharyngeal phase, when the larynx is closed and the bolus is moved through the pharynx. Most of the swallows (80% or greater) begin during the expiratory phase, but it is possible to swallow during the inspiratory phase. The duration of the inspiration and of the expiration is prolonged when a swallow occurs [14]. Thus swallowing disturbs the respiratory cycle, and, conversely, swallowing function can be disturbed by dyspnea.

1.4.2 Laryngeal Closure During Swallowing

The arytenoid adduction and tilting movement are the first events of the pharyngeal phase. It precedes the laryngeal elevation of approximately 340 ms, so it can be observed during the fiber-endoscopic evaluation of swallowing. It is linked to the inhibition of the PCA muscle while there is minimal activity in the TA, and it is not associated with the glottis closure [15].

The epiglottal inversion leads to sealing with the arytenoid cartilages that are tilted at that time. Epiglottal inversion is the result of several factors. It relies on the activation of the suprahyoid muscles to pull the hyoid bone upward and forward, the thyrohyoid muscle and the vertical muscles of the pharynx pull the larynx toward the hyoid, and the tongue root moves backward. All these mechanisms, associated with the pharyngeal peristaltism, lead to the epiglottal inversion [9]. The aryepiglottic folds direct the bolus around the larynx, in the laryngopharynx [16].

The compression of the vestibule, dependent on the relative positions of the arytenoids and the epiglottis, occurs from bottom to top on videofluoroscopic studies [16, 17].

Several adductor muscles are activated for the laryngeal closure, including TA, LCA, and IA. Temporal activation and magnitude of activity in the TA and IA are highly correlated [18]. The activity in the TA muscles is synchronous of the laryngeal elevation (endoscopic white-out during swallowing) [15]. The vocal folds begin to close at the midway of laryngeal elevation, approximatively 500 ms after the first event of the pharyngeal phase, i.e., the arytenoid approximation [15], and completely close at the peak of elevation; vocal fold reopening occurs at the midway of larynx descent at the end of the pharyngeal phase [19]. This glottal closure occurs before the ventricular closure [20].

It is noteworthy that there are high variability inter-studies and inter-individuals [21]. For example, the viscosity of the bolus significantly alters the sequence of laryngeal closure as related to hyoid movement: glottal closure occurs earlier with thin liquids than with thick liquids [20]. The volume of the bolus also has consequences on the timing of swallowing events: higher volumes lead to longer UES opening, longer laryngeal closure duration, and longer pharyngeal transit but do not impact the duration of hyoid excursion [21]. These variations may explain the long-lasting controversies about the sequence of action during swallowing. The above paragraph describes the latest available data. In pathology, patients can compensate any failure of these mechanisms and are trained to with speech therapy. As an example, some patients with epiglottectomy [22] or partial laryngectomy [23] can swallow safely.

Key Points

Swallowing necessitates rapid, complex, and sequential neuromuscular activity.

Typically, the closing sequences are as follows:

- Arytenoids anterior tilt
- Epiglottis inversion
- Glottal closure
- Vestibular closure from bottom to top

1.5 Larynx and Phonation

Key Point

- Phonation results from the transformation of an aerodynamic energy into an acoustic energy thanks to the oscillation of the vocal folds.

Phonation is important in animals and even more in humans who use it as the substratum for speech and language. Phonation is the result of the transformation of an aerodynamic energy into an acoustic energy thanks to the oscillation of the vocal folds. The larynx is mandatory for the production of a natural speech, and restoring the voice after total laryngectomy is a remaining challenge. But the vocal sound is only a component of speech. The sound created at the level of the larynx is very different from the sound issued by the mouth. It is selectively filtered and amplified mainly by the upper airway. As the geometry of the upper airway varies, the resonances also vary. The morphology of these organs also explains not only the proximity of speech between members of a family but also the persistence of regional accents after laryngectomies. The control and modulation of the geometry of the upper respiratory tract are the basis of articulation and allow creating the different phonemes.

The vocal folds attach anteriorly on the posterior aspect of the angle between the thyroid lamina and posteriorly on the vocal process of the arytenoid cartilages. They can be divided into three parts: the anterior two thirds are the membranous part of the vocal folds, and the posterior third is their cartilaginous part. The membranous part is the one responsible for phonation.

The vocal folds oscillate passively, as the result of the interaction between the airstream and the structures of the vocal folds. It is the basis of the myoelastic theory described by Van De Berg in 1958 which is still commonly accepted [24].

Key Points

Some physical parameters are critical for phonation:

- Expiratory airstream
- Vocal folds apposition (i.e., control of the prephonatory and phonatory geometry of the glottis)
- Control of the physical properties of the vocal folds (length, tension)
- Vibratory capacity of the vocal folds

1.5.1 Expiratory Airstream

The driving force of phonation is typically the expiratory airflow. Phonation is possible with inspiratory airflow, and this is occasionally used by healthy subjects for the expression of some emotions like surprise. The use of inspiratory airstream for phonation, so-called reverse phonation, is considered pathological when it is the main way of phonation. These vocal fold oscillations secondary to inspiration airflow are also responsible for the sound of stridor in bilateral vocal fold paralysis.

The expiratory airflow during phonation is subsequent to a prephonatory air intake, shorter than quiet inspiration, which is due to the activation of the diaphragm. The expiration is controlled to be longer and also to make the airflow and subsequently the air pressure rather constant. The passive forces of elastic recoil are involved, counterbalanced by diaphragm activation at the beginning of the phase. Sometimes, the energy necessary for the phonation has to increase in intensity or duration: during singing or vocal effort, or when the vocal folds are pathologic. In these cases, accessory inspiratory muscles (external intercostal muscles, scalene muscles, sternocleidomastoid muscles) may participate to the prephonatory inspiration, and the expiration is further dynamically controlled by the activation of the expiratory muscles (all abdominal muscles and internal intercostal muscles) [25].

1.5.2 Vocal Folds Apposition and Control of Their Physical Properties

The optimal adduction configuration is a critical issue in phonation. If the vocal folds are not close enough, the voice is weak and of poor quality. Conversely, excessive contact leads to vocal straining, resulting in a tight, pressed voice quality. The ideal configuration appears to occur when the vocal folds are almost in contact before phonation [26] (decreased prephonatory glottis width). A slight posterior gap may be established by balancing the activity of the adductor (IA and LCA) and abductor muscles (PCA).

The movements of the vocal folds mainly result of the mobilization of a set of two complex joints (i.e., the cricoarytenoid joints), under the action of the intrinsic laryngeal muscles. The adduction of the vocal process of the arytenoid cartilages (in order to close the glottis) is a complex movement combining anterior tilt, supero-medial shift, and a lesser degree of internal rotation of the cricoarytenoid joint [27]. Understanding the role of the intrinsic muscles in vocal fold movements is of interest in physiological and clinical fields.

Currently, three groups of intrinsic laryngeal muscles are defined: adductors for vocal fold closing, which can be divided into arytenoid adductors and membranous vocal fold adductors [28], abductors for vocal fold opening, and lengtheners for increasing vocal folds length. These latter also induce vocal fold tension, especially when they contract simultaneously with muscles that shorten the vocal folds [29]. During phonation, EMG studies showed that all adductor muscles (TA, LCA, and IA) are active. CT and TA have a sequential contraction during pitch elevation, most likely stiffening the vocal fold due to their opposite actions of lengthening and shortening the vocal fold [29, 30].

The prephonatory glottal configuration is determined by the degree of adduction of the folds and by the viscoelasticity of the vocal folds tissues. The three viscoelastic-related physical properties are mass, stiffness, and viscosity [31]. Adduction and viscoelasticity of the vocal folds are very important in the voice quality, in the control of the fundamental frequency, and in the relationship between fundamental frequency and subglottal pressure [32]. Glottal configuration may differ with the phonetic context [29] but also with the expressive intention or with the different singing modes [33, 34]. Improving the prephonatory glottal configuration is the main objective in the surgery of unilateral laryngeal paralysis: the better the adduction, the better the voice [35].

1.5.3 Vibratory Capacity of the Vocal Folds

The membranous part of the vocal folds (i.e., their anterior two thirds) is a multilayered structure, and each layer has specific viscoelastic properties. From surface to depth, the layers are epithelium, lamina propria, and vocal muscle [36] (Fig. 1.1).

1.5.3.1 Epithelium

The vibrating free edge is covered with squamous non-keratinizing epithelium, which is more resistant to the mechanical constraints produced by vibration and contact than the pseudo-stratified respiratory mucosa that lines the rest of the larynx. The thickness of the epithelium is 0.05 à 0.1 mm; the thicker part is the mid-third of the vocal fold. This epithelium shows no mucus gland at the free edge of the vocal fold [37], but the mucus produced by the nearby glands creates a mucus layer that prevents from dehydration and participates to the voice quality, probably because it promotes the synchronization of the vocal fold oscillations [38]. The basement membrane is attached to the underlying lamina propria by interlacing fibers [39].

1.5.3.2 Lamina Propria

The lamina propria is the most important structure conferring to the vocal folds their oscillating

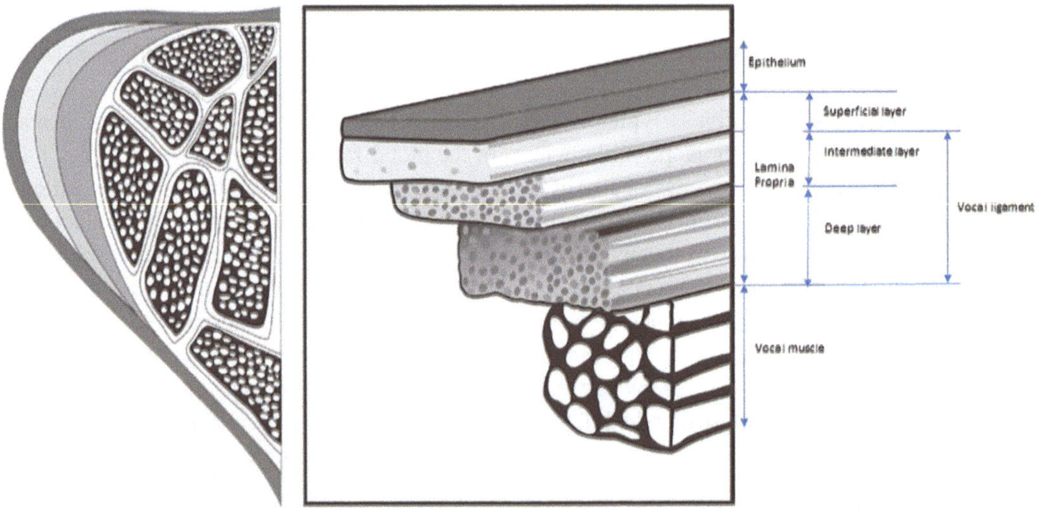

Fig. 1.1 Frontal section showing the multilayered structure of the vocal fold. (From Hirano [36])

properties. As described by Hirano [36], it is traditionally divided into three layers according to the histological composition regarding elastin and collagen fibers.

The superficial layer, so-called Reinke's space (thickness: 100–200 μm), is loose with few fibers and high rate of proteoglycans such as hyaluronic acid [40, 41]. The intermediate and deep layers, corresponding to the vocal ligament, have higher density of fibers. In the intermediate layer, fibers are mainly elastin fibers, with an intermediate concentration. It is noteworthy that the intermediate layer is not constant and is present only in the mid-third of the vocal folds. In the deep layer, fibers are more concentrated and thick, and they are mainly collagen [41, 42]. Interstitial proteins regulate vocal fold viscosity, which is an essential physical factor in vibration. Proteins also contribute to absorption of mechanical shocks caused by vibration. Collagen fibers are mainly orientated longitudinally, with little divergence anteroposteriorly and mediolaterally. They are wavy which has a potential to stretch [42]. The distribution of fibrous and interstitial proteins probably depends on the mechanical stress to which the vocal folds are subjected and may be genetically determined.

Two of the most important cells of the lamina propria are fibroblasts and myofibroblasts [43]. Fibroblasts play a key role in maintaining the integrity of the lamina propria. They allow replacement of proteins. Myofibroblasts are present only after trauma or damage requiring regeneration or repair of the extracellular matrix. Most of the synthesis and turn over of the proteins and cells of the vocal fold takes place in the maculae flavae which are located at the anterior and posterior extremities of the vocal folds [44].

1.5.3.3 Vocal Muscle

The vocal muscle is the deeper part of the vocal fold; it is the medial belly of the thyroarytenoid muscle. It inserts anteriorly on the posterior aspect of the thyroid angle and posteriorly on the basis of the arytenoid cartilage, from the vocal process to the muscular process. The superior fibers insert on the lateral and inferior area of the vocal process and run horizontally. The inferior fibers insert laterally to the vocal process and on the basis of the muscular process. The medial fibers run parallel to the vocal ligament. Anteriorly, the muscle structure results from a torsion of the muscular fibers when the vocal fold is adducted. The vocal muscle is composed of a high percentage of slow-tonic muscle fibers, in opposition to the lateral belly of the thyroarytenoid muscle which has more rapid muscle fibers [45].

1.5.4 Vocal Fold Vibration

All current theories and models of vocal fold vibration are based to some extent on the myoelastic-aerodynamic theory formulated by Van Den Berg [24]. When the vocal folds are contacting each other with appropriate force on either side of the midline of the glottis (prephonatory position), airflow from the trachea is blocked and subglottal pressure increases. Vibration begins when subglottal pressure below the vocal folds exceeds their resistance (phonation threshold pressure) and some air is released into the supraglottal region. As soon as the vocal folds separate, allowing some air to rush out, subglottal pressure decreases and the folds close back as a result of the elastic recoil and the Bernoulli effect. Cyclic repetition of these closing and opening movements results in vibration [46] (Fig. 1.2).

Even the healthy normal vocal folds are not perfectly symmetric so each oscillator could oscillate at its own frequency. The contact of the vocal folds during each cycle has the effect of synchronizing the vibrating masses [47]. It is promoted by the presence of mucus at the surface of the vocal folds [38]. This process is effective as long as differences between the two vocal folds stay within a certain range. For example, this mechanism is impaired in unilateral vocal fold paralysis, and the difference can be heard. The biphonation that we can sometimes hear results from the alternance of synchronization/desynchronization of the two vocal folds [48]. Another factor promoting synchronization is the Bernoulli effect, which applies equally to the two

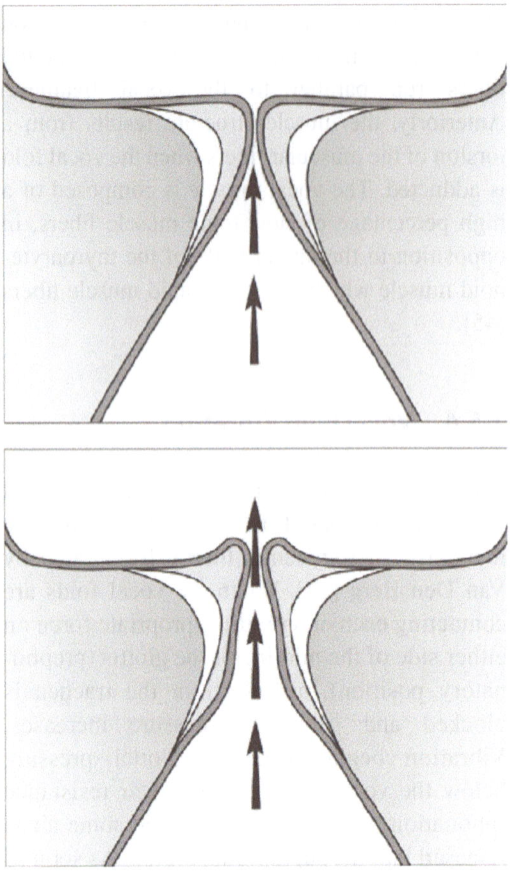

Fig. 1.2 Frontal section of the vocal folds shows resolution of the elastic conflict between subglottal air (opening force) and muscle and the elastic fold (closing force)

vocal folds and so tends to have the same effects as a function of glottal configuration.

Another, more complex phenomenon is reciprocal modulation of the folds characterized by the presence of subharmonics and bifurcations (i.e., sudden state changes). This problem is frequently observed in patients with unilateral laryngeal paralysis, which is often associated with sudden voice shifts [49]. A healthy example of bifurcation is the change of vibratory mechanisms of the larynx in singing voice. Vibratory mechanisms are the different configurations that the laryngeal vibrator can take throughout the human voice frequency range, as detected by the analysis of vocal fold contact area at the cycle level (electroglottography). The question of the depth of the vibration is still controversial and depends on the laryngeal mechanism. The reduction in amplitude of the EGG signal in mechanism 2 (roughly "head mechanism") compared to mechanism 1 (roughly "chest mechanism") may result from a reduction of the contact surface area between the vocal folds, which could be related to a reduction in the thickness of the vibrating part of the fold. Based on the multilayered structure of the vocal fold, it is possible to infer that when a critical point is reached, the heterogeneity in the mechanical properties of the structures may induce a decoupling between these layers. During the transition from mechanism M1 to mechanism M2, the cover may decouple from the deep layer. The latter is no longer or minimal part of the vibration, and this leads to an abrupt reduction of the vibrating mass [50].

Key Points

The phonatory threshold pressure depends on several parameters [51]:

- Stiffness of the vibrating portion of the vocal fold
- Viscosity of the vocal fold
- Thickness of the free edge of the vocal fold
- Width of the glottal opening prior to phonation
- Transglottal pressure gradient

Normal subglottal pressure at the phonatory threshold is between 2 and 4 hPa, and it is around 7 hPa in conversational speech. However, higher pressures may be necessary when a louder voice is required; over 200 hPa can be observed during a shout [52]. Higher pitch is often associated to higher phonation threshold pressure, but the vowel has no impact on the phonatory threshold pressure [53]. In pathological conditions involving vocal fold lesions, mucosal stiffness leads to an increase in phonatory threshold pressure. In the case of unilateral laryngeal paralysis, the prephonatory glottal gap is too wide, and the speaker

Table 1.1 Voice fundamental frequency as a function of age and sex [54, 55]

Subject	Weight (kg)	Height (m)	Fold length (mm)	Arytenoid length	F0 (Hz)
Newborn	3.5	0.50	2	2	500
8-year-old	30	1.20	6	3	300
Adult woman	60	1.60	10	4	200
Adult man	75	1.80	16	4	125

must compensate by increasing the subglottal pressure. Increased phonatory threshold pressure is a fairly accurate indicator of voice strain in disease states.

1.5.5 Control of the Fundamental Frequency

The pitch of the human voice is related to the fundamental frequency (F0) of vocal fold vibration. As shown in Table 1.1, pitch depends on the length of the vocal folds and the sex, age, and weight of the person. Vocal fold thickness has also been shown to affect pitch, which increases with thickness in both men and women.

Pitch control depends on adjusting the F0 of vibration. This adjustment can involve regulation of mass or tension, which can be done actively by contracting the intralaryngeal muscles or passively by contraction of the perilaryngeal muscles. Basically, pitch control involves the combined actions of two muscles: the CT muscle, which acts on vocal fold length, and the TA muscle, which acts on the muscle mass of the fold [28]. This adjustment mechanism can be viewed as bipolar, according to the "body-cover" theory described by Hirano and Titze. If the CT muscle is contracted and the TA muscle is relaxed, the total length of the vocal fold and the overall stiffness of all layers increase, so the F0 increases. The action of the TA on the F0 is more complex: at low intensity, when F0 is high, the activation of TA leads to lowering the F0, and at low F0, the contraction of the TA leads to increasing F0 [30]. It is related to differences in tension and biomechanical properties of the tissue layers. According to Hirano, contraction of the TA muscle should be associated with an increase in body tension and a decrease in cover tension. If the vibrating tissue is composed only of superficial layers (mucosa and lamina propria), then contraction of the TA muscle leads to lowering of the F0. Conversely, if the vibrating tissue is composed mainly of muscle, contraction of the TA muscle leads to a rise in the F0. Correlation between the F0 and TA activity becomes more and more positive as the depth of vibration increases. Each layer of the vocal fold has distinct biomechanical properties, depending on what is known as the length–tension ratio (i.e., tension induced in the material by changes in length, known as the stress–strain curve). In this regard, it has been shown that collagen fibers are more resistant to elongation than elastin fibers. Variations in the concentration of collagen and elastin in each layer of the lamina propria explain differences in behavior during elongation. A stress–strain curve can be obtained for the whole vocal fold. Total fold strain (tensile strain) corresponds to a combination of various active and passive actions that occur during tensioning.

Another mechanism that can be used for pitch control relies on the use of mechanism 2 (see above) [50]. The airstream can also be modulated to control the frequency: the higher the subglottal pressure, the higher the F0 [32]. Finally, strong correlation between the hyolaryngeal elevation and the increasing F0 has been described [56].

1.5.6 Control of Vocal Intensity

Intensity is controlled by combined regulation of subglottal pressure and glottal configuration. Higher intensity is achieved by simultaneously increasing vocal fold adduction and subglottal pressure. Because increased vocal fold adduction leads to longer contact time between the vocal folds, higher intensity is accompanied by a shortened open phase of the vocal folds cycle [57]. Glottal resistance is adjusted to ensure the best possible yield from the conversion of aerodynamic to acoustical energy with minimal effect on vocal fold vibration. To increase the intensity, the glottis operates on a more "open–shut" than "wave" basis. However, glottal efficiency decreases, and a large amount of energy is dissipated at the vocal fold level in the form of friction, which can cause local inflammation and even fold lesions [58].

We can infer that the mechanism underlying "voice straining," used to increase loudness, is similar to the mechanism used to compensate for abnormalities in laryngeal vibration.

1.6 Nervous System Control

1.6.1 Peripheral Nervous System

The innervation of the larynx is totally due to the vagus nerve (X), which provides two nerve trunks to the larynx: superior and inferior laryngeal nerves, responsible for the motor control and the sensibility of the larynx.

1.6.1.1 Sensitive Innervation

The larynx produces many vital protective reflexes; its sensitive innervation is very important in triggering these reflexes. The main sensitive innervation of the larynx is the upper laryngeal nerve, branch of the vagus nerve (X). Other cranial nerves (trigeminal nerve and glossopharyngeal nerve) may also play a role, at least in animals [59]. The myelinated and non-myelinated terminal nerve branches of these nerves form a plexus in the submucosa that sends nerve endings into the epithelium [59].

Sensitive Receptors in the Larynx

Superficial receptors are in very high density on the laryngeal face of the epiglottis, the aryepiglottic fold, and the posterolateral and internal side of the arytenoid. At the level of the vocal fold, the receptors are denser in the posterior part than in the anterior part.

Histological studies have revealed so-called free nerve endings (nociceptive or thermal fibers), corpuscular endings, Merkel cells, and Meissner corpuscles, which are all mechanoreceptors, located in the larynx and on the epiglottis. Certain fibers of the upper laryngeal nerve respond to the pressure stimulus. These receptors are divided into two groups: superficial receptors close to the mucosa and deep receptors in the laryngeal muscles and joints. These receptors seem to be stimulated not only during normal breathing but also during laryngeal movements [59].

Neuromuscular spindle-type muscle receptors (similar to the "Golgi tendon organ") may be found near the insertions of the muscle fibers of the vocalis muscle on the vocal ligament where the fibers cross in the upper part of the vocalis muscle [60] and on the vocal process of the arytenoid cartilage. The former would be sensitive to the muscle tension of the vocalis muscle; the latter would be sensitive to the adduction pressure of the arytenoids [61]. However, these are pseudo-spindles, with a different myosin composition from that of the usual spindles [62].

The larynx also contains chemoreceptors similar to the taste receptors on the tongue, but unlike the tongue, they are not joined together in the form of papillae. They are mainly located at the entrance of the larynx, at the epiglottis and the aryepiglottic folds. These receptors respond to stimuli that deviate from the saline composition for the saline concentration (154 mmol/L NaCl), or its pH (<4.5 or >8.7). Water in particular is a powerful stimulus [59].

The Superior Laryngeal Nerve, the Main Sensory Nerve of the Larynx

The upper laryngeal nerve detaches from the vagus nerve (X) at the lower end of the nodal ganglion and then runs downward, inward, and forward toward the pharyngeal wall. It runs backward and then inward to the internal carotid artery and then down along the lateral pharyngeal wall and crosses the inner side of the external carotid below the lingual artery. After a path of 3–20 mm, in the vicinity of the lingual artery and the great horn of the hyoid bone, it divides into an internal and an external branch.

The internal branch [59, 63] of the upper laryngeal nerve enters the larynx by perforating either the thyrohyoid membrane or the thyroid cartilage. Inside the larynx, it runs rostrally and divides into anterior (or upper), middle, and posterior (or lower) branches. The posterior (or lower or descending) branch has the largest diameter and the longest path and innervates the posterior part of the aryepiglottic fold, the tip of the arytenoid cartilage, its posterior and internal surfaces, the mucosa of the posterior laryngeal wall, the posterior part of the subglottal mucosa, bilaterally with ipsilateral predominance, and the lateral and anterior wall of the laryngopharynx. The innervation of the inter-arytenoid muscle thus appears to be mixed: by each of the two laryngeal nerves. The communicating branch, formed by Galen's anastomosis, joins the posterior branch of the inferior laryngeal nerve. The sensory fibers of the posterior branch of the inferior laryngeal nerve run rostrally in the submucosa of the anterior wall of the hypopharynx and divide into two branches. One branch forms the Galen's anastomosis. The other penetrates the larynx between the cricoarytenoid and thyroarytenoid muscles, innervating the caudal side of the vocal cord and the subglottis along with the internal branch of the superior laryngeal nerve.

1.6.1.2 Motor Innervation

The External Branch of the Superior Laryngeal Nerve

The external branch of the superior laryngeal nerve is the thinnest branch of division of the superior laryngeal nerve (0.2 mm diameter). It crosses the common carotid artery on its posterior aspect and then follows the superior thyroid artery on its deep (posterior) aspect. Its relationship with the inferior constrictor muscle of the pharynx is variable: it can be superficial or deep. The deep position in relation to this muscle is the most frequent [64]. If it is superficial, it remains outside the thyroid capsule but may adhere to the upper thyroid artery. The point at which the nerve branch crosses the upper thyroid artery determines the level of risk of intraoperative nerve damage during thyroidectomy [65]. It then runs into the cricothyroid space (Reeves space), before entering the cricothyroid muscle. Dissection of this space during a thyroidectomy must be done with caution.

It carries the motor nerve impulse to the cricothyroid muscle. Some authors have also attributed a branch to the thyroid gland [66, 67], the cricothyroid membrane, and connections with the pharyngeal plexus and the lower constrictor muscle of the pharynx [68]. A branch communicating with the inferior laryngeal nerve is inconstant (20–50%) [69, 70]. This branch crosses the CT muscle and enters the larynx under the lower edge of the thyroid cartilage, thus reaching the lateral cricoarytenoid muscle to enter the thyroarytenoid muscle. This branch has a motor function with fibers that anastomose within the TA muscle with the fibers of the inferior laryngeal nerve or terminate directly on the muscle fibers of the TA and a sensory function for the capsule of the cricothyroid joint or subglottal mucosa.

The Inferior Laryngeal Nerve

The origin and path of the inferior laryngeal nerve (or recurrent laryngeal nerve) differ depending on the side. The right inferior laryngeal nerve detaches from the vagus nerve in front of the subclavian artery and then bypasses this artery from below and passes behind it. The laryngeal nerve then travels upward and inward into the groove formed by the trachea and esophagus.

The left inferior laryngeal nerve detaches from the vagus nerve opposite to the inferior aspect of the aortic arch, and then it goes around this artery from below, close to the arterial ligament. It then runs upward, toward the larynx, in the dihedral angle formed by the trachea and esophagus.

The trunk of the inferior laryngeal nerve divides, on each side before entering the larynx, into an anterior branch for the intrinsic musculature of the larynx and a posterior branch which represents the lower part of the ramus communicans.

There are many variations on the inferior laryngeal nerve branching [71]. The first branch innervates the PCA muscle. There are anastomoses with the branch intended for the IA muscle [72]. The next branch is intended for the interarytenoid muscle. Then the branch has a genu above the cricothyroid joint and enters the larynx. The terminal branches of the nerve innervate the LCA and the TA. These two muscles appear almost as a single unit during dissections. The LCA is innervated by a single branch that forms a dense anastomotic plexus in the center of the muscle.

The inferior laryngeal nerve terminates in the TA muscle. Just before its entry, the nerve branch separates into numerous fascicles which are distributed through the vocal and vestibular folds. The innervation of the TA is by far the densest anastomotic network of all the laryngeal muscles, especially on the medial edge of the muscle near the vocal ligament.

1.6.1.3 Brain Stem Nuclei

The Nodal Ganglion, the Nucleus of the Solitary Tract

The cell bodies of sensory neurons of superior laryngeal nerve are located at the rostral part of the ipsilateral nodal ganglion; their number is on average 340. Those that make up the inferior laryngeal nerve average 125 and occupy the rostral and middle parts of the ganglion. They are unipolar neurons about 60 μm in diameter. The central endings of these neurons are located in the brain stem, in the ipsilateral nucleus tractus solitarii.

The Nucleus Ambiguus

The cell bodies of motor neurons dedicated to the larynx are located in the ipsilateral nucleus ambiguus, from the rostral end for the cricothyroid muscle to the posterior caudal region for the other muscles [73].

Key Points

Peripheral neurologic supply of the larynx:

- All originates in the vagus nerves (X)
- Two nerves on each side:
  - Superior laryngeal nerve: mainly sensitive and motor for the CT muscle
  - Inferior (recurrent) laryngeal nerve: motor for all intrinsic laryngeal muscles except CT and secondary sensitive function
- Distribution of branches to the muscles is very variable
- Lots of anastomoses do exist and are the substratum of spontaneous reinnervation in laryngeal paralysis

1.6.2 Central Nervous Control of the Larynx

Central nervous system control includes both relatively automatic behaviors, present at birth, and volitional control acquired with development for all the functions of the larynx [74]. Automatic controls are located in brain stem and midbrain.

1.6.2.1 Cortical Centers

Cortical control of the larynx is bilateral within each hemisphere. The brain areas responsible for motor control of the pharynx and larynx are located in the lower part of the precentral gyrus (i.e., primary motor cortex) of both hemispheres. This area is responsible for voluntary laryngeal control for speech, breathing, and swallowing [75].

There are many connections in the brain, particularly with auditory cortex (e.g., the superior temporal gyrus) and language-related centers (e.g., the gyrus supramarginalis). The associative pathways between pharyngolaryngeal motor regions and cortical and subcortical auditory zones are especially noteworthy.

1.6.2.2 Breathing

Breathing pacing is automatic and processed at the brain stem level. Both the pre-Bötzinger complex for inspiratory pacing and the retrotrapezoid nucleus–parafacial respiratory group in the medulla have inputs to the laryngeal motoneurons for inspiratory and expiratory outputs, respectively [9, 76].

The apnea during the pharyngeal phase of swallowing is also centrally controlled [77]. Laryngeal motoneurons in the nucleus ambiguous, the ventral swallowing group, were shown to be active in swallowing and breathing [78]. The same neurons are involved in the central pattern generator for breathing and swallowing, and, depending on the inputs from the superior laryngeal nerve, the firing patterns of these neurons can change, creating cough, breathing, or swallowing [78, 79].

1.6.2.3 Swallowing

The cortical control of swallowing may be involved in volitional control of the oral phase of swallowing involving bolus manipulation, chewing, and the initiation of the pharyngeal phase. The cortical area dedicated to swallowing is bilateral and quite large including the regions for facial musculature (primary motor and sensitive cortex). Integrity of these areas is required to initiate swallowing.

The control of the pharyngeal phase is more intricate. Classically, brain stem control involves the patterning of the pharyngeal phase and the premotor inputs to the pharyngeal and laryngeal motoneurons on both sides. Contrary to phonation, there are evidence of the integration of laryngeal motoneurons in swallowing function at the brain stem level, modulated by sensory and cortical inputs. The sensory inputs for triggering and modulating swallowing are conveyed by superior laryngeal nerve and glossopharyngeal nerve. Cortical modulation is dependent on the activation of the lateral pre- and post-central region, the anterior right insula, the inferior parietal area, and the bilateral anterior cingulate [80] (Fig. 1.3). Thus, the initiation and patterning of pharyngeal phase are under active cortical control for both spontaneous and volitional swallowing [74]. Brain stem integration triggers the swallow action and synchronizes oropharyngeal and laryngeal movements with UES relaxation [79].

Two groups of neurons involved in swallowing are described: the dorsal and ventral groups. Neurons in the ventral swallowing group, located in the nucleus ambiguus, give inputs to the laryngeal motoneurons [9, 79].

Internal Schema

Some recent studies showed evidence of an internal sensorimotor scaling system to achieve laryngeal vestibule closure and upper esophageal sphincter opening while adapting the hyolaryngeal excursion to the airway configuration [81].

Afferent input to the swallowing system is shown in dashed lines and comes from the glossopharyngeal (IX) and superior laryngeal nerves (SLN) into the nucleus tractus solitarius (NTS) and to the dorsal swallowing group of neurons (DSG).

The sensory inputs in the NTS are relayed to the pons and interact with the taste inputs in the pons and then have input to the ventral posterior nucleus in the thalamus (Th) which has input to the oral facial regions in the sensory cortex adjacent to the central swallowing area (CSA) in the pericentral lateral motor and sensory cortex.

Inputs to the CSA are also from the supplementary motor area (SMA) and the anterior insula.

Output from the CSA is via the corticobulbar pathway to the dorsal swallowing group (DSG) which provides patterning for the pharyngeal phase of swallowing and has inputs to premotor neurons to activate motoneurons on both sides of the brain stem as shown for the nucleus ambiguus to control the laryngeal muscles during swallowing. This system also connects to many other

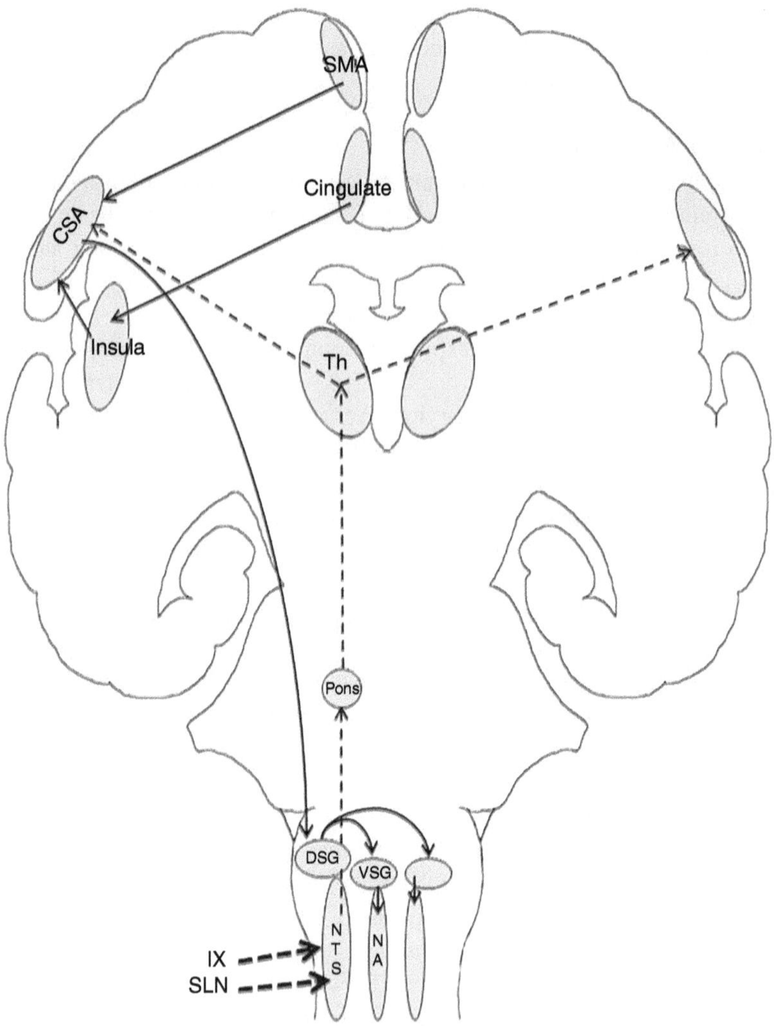

Fig. 1.3 Schematic diagram of central nervous system control of the human swallowing (following Ludlow [74]). Connections are only shown on one side, but the same system is present and simultaneously activates on both the left and right sides

motoneurons for the facial, tongue, jaw, lips, and pharynx to control the patterning of multiple muscles during swallowing.

1.6.2.4 Phonation

Voice production depends on neuromotor coordination of all muscles involved in phonation, ranging from posture and respiratory muscles to the muscles of the larynx, pharynx, and buccolabial articulatory apparatus. Dissociating voice and speech control is not easy. The lateral hypothalamus, parietal operculum, amygdala, and cerebellum are involved in non-speech and non-volitional vocalization (such as laugh [82]). Voluntary non-speech vocalization involves, in addition to the motor primary cortex and pre-motor area, the auditory cortex, a part of the limbic system (anterior cingulate) and periaqueductal gray, bilaterally. Voluntary speech vocalization is associated with activation of the sensorimotor cortex bilaterally but considerably more in the left side [83]. The left superior temporal gyrus is also activated, even when the participant cannot hear his own voice, suggesting that auditory areas containing the targets of voice for speech are activated during the production of learned laryngeal control tasks [83]. There is no evidence of some integration at the brain stem level for phonation [74] (Fig. 1.4).

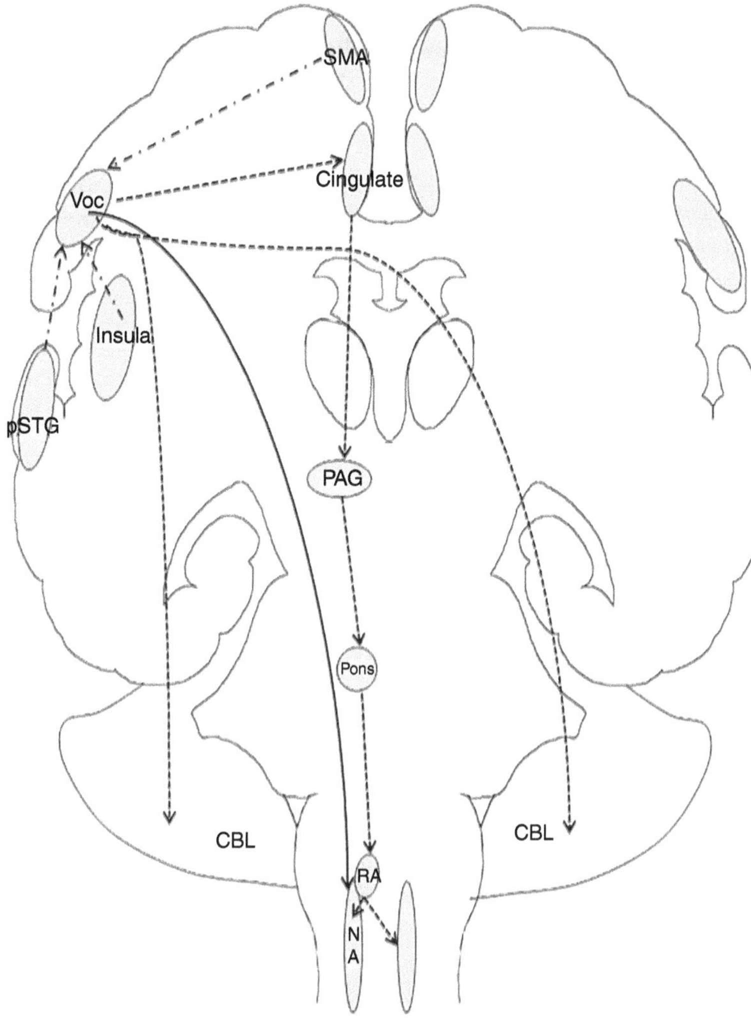

Fig. 1.4 Schematic diagram of central nervous system control of human voice (following Ludlow [74]). Connections are only shown on one side, but the same system is present on both the left and right sides

Audio-Phonatory Control (Feedback Control) and Internal Schema (Feedforward Control)

Auditory feedback is a necessary component of voice control. The functional relationship between the auditory cortical areas and the areas dedicated to phonation is the substratum of this audio-phonatory control. Audio-phonatory control depends on commands produced by corticobulbar pathways in response to acoustic input arriving in the auditory cortex as well as a range of acoustic–laryngeal reflexes. Per example, some studies observed the adaptation of frequency when the speaker is exposed to a manipulated auditory feedback of his own voice [84, 85]. Interestingly, when the manipulation of the feedback stops, the speaker maintains the adaptations learned during the experience. This is evidence of a feedforward control based on the auditory target of the speaker. Feedforward control during phonation takes place during the prephonatory period and during the sound production. Prephonatory adjustment explains how singers produce sounds at a predetermined pitch and intensity. Prephonatory regulation in the cortex depends on the adequacy of the input supplied by laryngeal mechanoreceptors concerning tension and position of the various muscles and articulations and the internal schemas of the sound target.

Input to the primary integrative vocalization center (Voc) and ongoing modulation is from the posterior superior temporal gyrus (pSTG) as well as inputs from the supplementary motor area (SMA) and the insula (irregular hatched lines).

Output from the primary integrative vocalization center is shown by solid lines for the direct pathway via the corticobulbar pathway. Dotted lines show outputs to the cerebellum bilaterally and the pathway from the primary integrative vocalization center to the cingulate, the periaqueductal gray (PAG), the pons, and the reticular area in the medulla (RA) which then has input to the nucleus ambiguus (NA) on the ipsilateral and contralateral sides.

Key Points

- Cortical laryngeal areas are located in the lower part of the precentral gyrus (i.e., primary motor cortex) of both hemispheres.
- Breathing is mainly involuntary and controlled at the brain stem level. Voluntary breathing activates the cortical laryngeal areas on both sides.
- Swallowing involves brain stem integration, with cortical modulation, from both hemispheres but with a predominant side.
- Phonation involves cortical activation, with predominance on the same side as the language areas (left side). There is no brain stem integration.
- Several structures modulate the activation of the brain stem, mainly other cortexes, subcortical gray structures, and the cerebellum.

References

1. Negus V. The comparative anatomy and physiology of the larynx. London: W. Heinemann Medical Books; 1949.
2. Woodson GE. Laryngeal neurophysiology and its clinical uses. Head Neck. 1996;18:78–86.
3. Rovó L, Bach Á, Sztanó B, Matievics V, Szegesdi I, Castellanos PF. Rotational thyrotracheopexy after cricoidectomy for low-grade laryngeal chrondrosarcoma. Laryngoscope. 2017;127:1109–15.
4. Hanna N, Smith J, Wolfe J. How the acoustic resonances of the subglottal tract affect the impedance spectrum measured through the lips. J Acoust Soc Am. 2018;143:2639.
5. Gillespie AI, Slivka W, Atwood CW Jr, Verdolini Abbott K. The effects of hyper- and hypocapnia on phonatory laryngeal airway resistance in women. J Speech Lang Hear Res. 2015;58:638–52.
6. England SJ, Bartlett D Jr, Daubenspeck JA. Influence of human vocal cord movements on airflow and resistance during eupnea. J Appl Physiol Respir Environ Exerc Physiol. 1982;52:773–9.
7. Scheinherr A, Bailly L, Boiron O, Lagier A, Legou T, Pichelin M, Caillibotte G, Giovanni A. Realistic glottal motion and airflow rate during human breathing. Med Eng Phys. 2015;37:829–39.
8. Brancatisano TP, Dodd DS, Engel LA. Respiratory activity of posterior cricoarytenoid muscle and vocal cords in humans. J Appl Physiol Respir Environ Exerc Physiol. 1984;57:1143–9.
9. Fregosi RF, Ludlow CL. Activation of upper airway muscles during breathing and swallowing. J Appl Physiol. 1985;2014(116):291–301.
10. Sun QJ, Berkowitz RG, Pilowsky PM. Response of laryngeal motoneurons to hyperventilation induced apnea in the rat. Respir Physiol Neurobiol. 2005;146:155–63.
11. Martin BJ, Logemann JA, Shaker R, Dodds WJ. Normal laryngeal valving patterns during three breath-hold maneuvers: a pilot investigation. Dysphagia. 1993;8:11–20.
12. Magni C, Chellini E, Lavorini F, Fontana GA, Widdicombe J. Voluntary and reflex cough: similarities and differences. Pulm Pharmacol Ther. 2011;24:308–11.
13. Fontana GA, Lavorini F. Cough motor mechanisms. Respir Physiol Neurobiol. 2006;152:266–81.
14. Uysal H, Kızılay F, Ünal A, Güngör HA, Ertekin C. The interaction between breathing and swallowing in healthy individuals. J Electromyogr Kinesiol. 2013;23:659–63.
15. Van Daele DJ, McCulloch TM, Palmer PM, Langmore SE. Timing of glottal closure during swallowing: a combined electromyographic and endoscopic analysis. Ann Otol Rhinol Laryngol. 2005;114:478–87.
16. Vose A, Humbert I. "Hidden in plain sight": a descriptive review of laryngeal vestibule closure. Dysphagia. 2019;34:281–9.
17. Ekberg O. Closure of the laryngeal vestibule during deglutition. Acta Otolaryngol. 1982;93:123–9.
18. McCulloch TM, Perlman AL, Palmer PM, Van Daele DJ. Laryngeal activity during swallow, phonation, and the Valsalva maneuver: an electromyographic analysis. Laryngoscope. 1996;106:1351–8.
19. Flaherty RF, Seltzer S, Campbell T, Weisskoff RM, Gilbert RJ. Dynamic magnetic resonance imaging of vocal cord closure during deglutition. Gastroenterology. 1995;109:843–9.

20. Inamoto Y, Saitoh E, Okada S, Kagaya H, Shibata S, Ota K, Baba M, Fujii N, Katada K, Wattanapan P, Palmer JB. The effect of bolus viscosity on laryngeal closure in swallowing: kinematic analysis using 320-row area detector CT. Dysphagia. 2013; 28:33–42.
21. Molfenter SM, Steele CM. Physiological variability in the deglutition literature: hyoid and laryngeal kinematics. Dysphagia. 2011;26:67–74.
22. Leder SB, Burrell MI, Van Daele DJ. Epiglottis is not essential for successful swallowing in humans. Ann Otol Rhinol Laryngol. 2010;119:795–8.
23. Pizzorni N, Schindler A, Castellari M, Fantini M, Crosetti E, Succo G. Swallowing safety and efficiency after open partial horizontal laryngectomy: a videofluoroscopic study. Cancers (Basel). 2019;11:549.
24. Van Den Berg J. Myoelastic theory of voice production. J Speech Hearing Res. 1958;1:227.
25. Pettersen V. Muscular patterns and activation levels of auxiliary breathing muscles and thorax movement in classical singing. Folia Phoniatr Logop. 2005;57:255–77.
26. Berry DA, Verdolini K, Montequin DW, Hess MM, Chan RW, Titze IR. A quantitative output-cost ratio in voice production. J Speech Lang Hear Res. 2001;44:29–37.
27. Prades JM, Dumollard JM, Timoshenko AP, Durand M, Martin C. Descriptive anatomy of the cricoarytenoid articulation: application to articular dynamics in carcinology. Surg Radiol Anat. 2000;22:277–82.
28. Lagier A, Guenoun D, Legou T, Espesser R, Giovanni A, Champsaur P. Control of the glottal configuration in ex vivo human models: quantitative anatomy for clinical and experimental practices. Surg Radiol Anat. 2017;39:257–62.
29. Poletto CJ, Verdun LP, Strominger R, Ludlow CL. Correspondence between laryngeal vocal fold movement and muscle activity during speech and nonspeech gestures. J Appl Physiol (1985). 2004;97:858–66.
30. Titze IR, Luschei ES, Hirano M. Role of the thyroarytenoid muscle in regulation of fundamental frequency. J Voice. 1989;3:213–24.
31. Jiang J, Lin E, Hanson DG. Vocal fold physiology. Otolaryngol Clin N Am. 2000;33:699–718.
32. Alipour F, Scherer RC. On pressure-frequency relations in the excised larynx. J Acoust Soc Am. 2007;122:2296–305.
33. Freeman E, Woo P, Saxman JH, Murry T. A comparison of sung and spoken phonation onset gestures using high-speed digital imaging. J Voice. 2012;26:226–38.
34. Herbst CT, Ternström S, Svec JG. Investigation of four distinct glottal configurations in classical singing—a pilot study. J Acoust Soc Am. 2009;125:EL104–9.
35. Hoffman MR, Witt RE, Chapin WJ, McCulloch TM, Jiang JJ. Multiparameter comparison of injection laryngoplasty, medialization laryngoplasty, and arytenoid adduction in an excised larynx model. Laryngoscope. 2010;120:769–76.
36. Hirano M. Morphological structure of the vocal cord as a vibrator and its variations. Folia Phoniatr (Basel). 1974;26:89–94.
37. El-Hifnawi H, El-Hifnawi E. Light and electron microscopical studies of the anatomical and functional distribution of glands in human vocal cords. Arch Otorhinolaryngol. 1984;240:277–85.
38. Ayache S, Ouaknine M, Dejonkere P, Prindere P, Giovanni A. Experimental study of the effects of surface mucus viscosity on the glottic cycle. J Voice. 2004;18:107–15.
39. Gray SD, Pignatari SS, Harding P. Morphologic ultrastructure of anchoring fibers in normal vocal fold basement membrane zone. J Voice. 1994;8:48–52.
40. Gray SD, Hammond E, Hanson DF. Benign pathologic responses of the larynx. Ann Otol Rhinol Laryngol. 1995;104:13–8.
41. Gray SD. Cellular physiology of the vocal folds. Otolaryngol Clin N Am. 2000;33:679–98.
42. Bailly L, Cochereau T, Orgéas L, Henrich Bernardoni N, Rolland du Roscoat S, McLeer-Florin A, Robert Y, Laval X, Laurencin T, Chaffanjon P, Fayard B, Boller E. 3D multiscale imaging of human vocal folds using synchrotron X-ray microtomography in phase retrieval mode. Sci Rep. 2018;8(1):14003.
43. Hirano M, Sato K, Nakashima T. Fibroblasts in human vocal fold mucosa. Acta Otolaryngol. 1999;119:271–6.
44. Sato K, Hirano M, Nakashima T. 3D structure of the macula flava in the human vocal fold. Acta Otolaryngol. 2003;123:269–73.
45. Han Y, Wang J, Fischman DA, Biller HF, Sanders I. Slow tonic muscle fibers in the thyroarytenoid muscles of human vocal folds; a possible specialization for speech. Anat Rec. 1999;256:146–57.
46. Berke GS, Moore DM, Hantke DR, Hanson DG, Gerratt BR, Burstein F. Laryngeal modeling: theoretical, in vitro, in vivo. Laryngoscope. 1987;97:871–81.
47. Ouaknine M, Garrel R, Giovanni A. Separate detection of vocal fold vibration by optoreflectometry: a study of biphonation on excised porcine larynges. Folia Phoniatr Logop. 2003;55(1):28–38. https://doi.org/10.1159/000068058.
48. Giovanni A, Ouaknine M, Guelfucci R, Yu T, Zanaret M, Triglia JM. Nonlinear behavior of vocal fold vibration: the role of coupling between the vocal folds. J Voice. 1999;13:465–76.
49. Herzel H, Berry D, Titze IR, Saleh M. Analysis of vocal disorders with methods from nonlinear dynamics. J Speech Hear Res. 1994;37:1008–19.
50. Roubeau B, Henrich N, Castellengo M. Laryngeal vibratory mechanisms: the notion of vocal register revisited. J Voice. 2009;23:425–38.
51. Titze IR, Schmidt SS, Titze MR. Phonation threshold pressure in a physical model of the vocal fold mucosa. J Acoust Soc Am. 1995;97:3080–4.
52. Lagier A, Legou T, Galant C, Amy de La Bretèque B, Meynadier Y, Giovanni A. The shouted voice: a

pilot study of laryngeal physiology under extreme aerodynamic pressure. Logoped Phoniatr Vocol. 2017;42:141–5.
53. Plexico LW, Sandage MJ. Influence of vowel selection on determination of phonation threshold pressure. J Voice. 2012;26:673.e7–12.
54. Baken RJ. Clinical measurement of speech and voice. London: Taylor and Francis; 1987.
55. Nicollas R, Garrel R, Ouaknine M, Giovanni A, Nazarian B, Triglia JM. Normal voice in children between 6 and 12 years of age: database and nonlinear analysis. J Voice. 2008;22:671–5.
56. Hong YT, Hong KH, Jun JP, Hwang PH. The effects of dynamic laryngeal movements on pitch control. Am J Otolaryngol. 2015;36:660–5.
57. Ishizaka K, Isshiki N. Computer simulation of pathological vocal-fold vibration. J Acoust Soc Am. 1976;60:1193–8.
58. Dikkers FG, Nikkels PG. Benign lesions of the vocal folds: histopathology and phonotrauma. Ann Otol Rhinol Laryngol. 1995;104:698–703.
59. Bradley RM. Sensory receptors of the larynx. Am J Med. 2000;108:47S–50S.
60. Sanders I, Han Y, Wang J, Biller H. Muscle spindles are concentrated in the superior vocalis subcompartment of the human thyroarytenoid muscle. J Voice. 1998;12:7–16.
61. Nagai T. Encapsulated nerve structures in the human vocal cord. An electronmicroscopic study. Acta Otolaryngol. 1987;104:363–9.
62. Brandon CA, Rosen C, Georgelis G, Horton MJ, Mooney MP, Sciote JJ. Staining of human thyroarytenoid muscle with myosin antibodies reveals some unique extrafusal fibers, but no muscle spindles. J Voice. 2003;17:245–54.
63. Sanders I, Mu L. Anatomy of the human internal superior laryngeal nerve. Anat Rec. 1998;252:646–56.
64. Friedman M, LoSavio P, Ibrahim H. Superior laryngeal nerve identification and preservation in thyroidectomy. Arch Otolaryngol Head Neck Surg. 2002;128:296–303.
65. Dionigi G, Kim HY, Randolph GW, Wu CW, Sun H, Liu X, Barczynski M, Chiang FY. Prospective validation study of Cernea classification for predicting EMG alterations of the external branch of the superior laryngeal nerve. Surg Today. 2016;46: 785–91.
66. Morton RP, Whitfield P, Al-Ali S. Anatomical and surgical considerations of the external branch of the superior laryngeal nerve: a systematic review. Clin Otolaryngol. 2006;31:368–74.
67. Page C, Laude M, Legars D, Foulon P, Strunski V. The external laryngeal nerve: surgical and anatomic considerations. Report of 50 total thyroidectomies. Surg Radiol Anat. 2004;26:182–5.
68. Kierner AC, Aigner M, Burian M. The external branch of the superior laryngeal nerve: its topographical anatomy as related to surgery of the neck. Arch Otolaryngol Head Neck Surg. 1998;124:301–3.
69. Henry M, Pekala PA, Sanna B, Vikse J, Sanna S, Saganiak K, Tomaszewska IM, Tubbs RS, Tomaszewski KA. The anastomoses of the recurrent laryngeal nerve in the larynx: a meta-analysis and systematic review. J Voice. 2017;31:495–503.
70. Wu BL, Sanders I, Mu L, Biller HF. The human communicating nerve. An extension of the external superior laryngeal nerve that innervates the vocal cord. Arch Otolaryngol Head Neck Surg. 1994;120:1321–8.
71. Maranillo E, León X, Ibañez M, Orús C, Quer M, Sañudo JR. Variability of the nerve supply patterns of the human posterior cricoarytenoid muscle. Laryngoscope. 2003;113:602–6.
72. Sanders I, Wu BL, Mu L, Li Y, Biller HF. The innervation of the human larynx. Arch Otolaryngol Head Neck Surg. 1993;119:934–9.
73. Davis PJ, Nail BS. On the location and size of laryngeal motoneurons in the cat and rabbit. J Comp Neurol. 1984;230:13–32.
74. Ludlow CL. Central nervous system control of voice and swallowing. J Clin Neurophysiol. 2015;32:294–303.
75. Simonyan K, Horwitz B. Laryngeal motor cortex and control of speech in humans. Neuroscientist. 2011;17:197–208.
76. Feldman JL, Mitchell GS, Nattie EE. Breathing: rhythmicity, plasticity, chemosensitivity. Annu Rev Neurosci. 2003;26:239–66.
77. Paydarfar D, Gilbert RJ, Poppel CS, Nassab PF. Respiratory phase resetting and airflow changes induced by swallowing in humans. J Physiol. 1995;483:273–88.
78. Gestreau C, Grélot L, Bianchi AL. Activity of respiratory laryngeal motoneurons during fictive coughing and swallowing. Exp Brain Res. 2000;130:27–34.
79. Jean A. Brain stem control of swallowing: neuronal network and cellular mechanisms. Physiol Rev. 2001;81:929–69.
80. Sörös P, Inamoto Y, Martin RE. Functional brain imaging of swallowing: an activation likelihood estimation meta-analysis. Hum Brain Mapp. 2009;30:2426–39.
81. Wong SM, Domangue RJ, Fels S, Ludlow CL. Evidence that an internal schema adapts swallowing to upper airway requirements. J Physiol. 2017;595:1793–814.
82. Wattendorf E, Westermann B, Fiedler K, Kaza E, Lotze M, Celio MR. Exploration of the neural correlates of ticklish laughter by functional magnetic resonance imaging. Cereb Cortex. 2013;23:1280–9.
83. Loucks TM, Poletto CJ, Simonyan K, Reynolds CL, Ludlow CL. Human brain activation during phonation and exhalation: common volitional control for two upper airway functions. NeuroImage. 2007;36:131–43.
84. Jones JA, Munhall KG. Remapping auditory-motor representations in voice production. Curr Biol. 2005;15:1768–72.
85. Larson CR, Burnett TA, Kiran S, Hain TC. Effects of pitch-shift velocity on voice Fo responses. J Acoust Soc Am. 2000;107:559–64.

Assessment of Voice and Respiratory Function

2

Liang Ker

Key Points

- The four most common methods of assessing the voice includes (1) auditory perceptual assessment of voice quality, (2) endoscopic imaging of vocal fold vibration, (3) acoustic assessment of voiced sound production, and (4) aerodynamic assessment of airflow rates during voicing. As the lungs are the power source for voice production, assessment of the respiratory function is important too.

2.1 Introduction

We use our voice daily; it is a window to many functions in our lives. In the most primitive form, we use our voice for survival—a baby cries as an expression of hunger and pain. Our voices do not simply communicate the spoken words plainly; we use our voice to express our emotions and personality. A number of professions rely on their voices as a primary tool of trade; this includes teachers, singers, coaches, lawyers, etc. A mild voice disorder may be tolerated by non-professional voice users, but the same may significantly reduce the professional voice user's capacity at work. A well-functioning voice enables us to play our roles in society.

In this chapter, we will discuss practical methods to assess the voice and respiratory function.

2.2 Inspection and Auditory Assessment

The assessment of the voice and respiratory function begins immediately as the patient comes through the door. A well-built gentleman who walks in comfortably gives us a hint of his health and fitness, as compared to an elderly gentleman who enters the consult room in a wheelchair and with supplementary oxygen.

History-taking from the patient gives us an opportunity to listen and assess the patient's voice. A detailed history allows us to understand his voice problem, the severity of voice impairment, duration of illness, triggering events, etc., while a keen pair of ears allows us to perform a perceptive assessment of his voice.

The assessment may be carried out during conversational speech, or the patient may be given a passage to read. A standard reading passage should be used. "The Rainbow Passage" is a classic passage for English-speaking persons as it is a phonetically balanced passage, with all speech sounds of the English language included [1].

L. Ker (✉)
Department of Otolaryngology, Head and Neck Surgery, National University Hospital, Singapore, Singapore
e-mail: liang_ker@nuhs.edu.sg

M. Remacle, H. E. Eckel (eds.), *Textbook of Surgery of Larynx and Trachea*,
https://doi.org/10.1007/978-3-031-09621-1_2

During the reading of the passage, attention is paid to the effort of breathing. Is the patient able to read the passage out loudly and clearly? Or does he struggle with his breath and manages a few phrases at a time. This may signify lung function insufficiency. How is his articulation? Can the words be heard clearly and distinctly? Challenges with articulation often points to issues within the resonating chambers of the airway.

2.2.1 GRBAS Scale

A commonly used vocal assessment tool is the GRBAS scale. It is a scale that grades the components of speech on a four-point scale, from 0 to 3. With 0 = normal voice, no deviance, 1 = mild deviance, 2 = moderate deviance, and 3 = severe deviance. G is for Grade, a global score for the patient's voice in general, R for Roughness, B for Breathiness, A for Asthenia, and S for Strain. The GRBAS scale gives us a hint to the diagnosis of the patient's voice disorder. Roughness and breathiness generally suggest a vocal fold issue. Roughness, or harshness of the voice, is typically produced when there is vocal fold irregularity. This vocal fold pathology causes irregular glottis pulses and abnormal fluctuation in fundamental frequency, leading to vocal fry, diplophonia, and register breaks. Breathiness develops when there is glottis insufficiency during phonation, leading to turbulence and air leakage through the glottis gap during adduction of the vocal folds. Asthenia and strain usually reflect a neuromuscular disorder of the larynx [2, 3]. GRBAS is a popular assessment tool as it is sufficiently reliable, with good inter- and intra-rater reproducibility [4, 5].

Recording the patient's voice helps with vocal assessment and analysis. Ideally, the vocal recordings should be performed in a sound-treated room. A quiet room with ambient noise less than 45 dB is an acceptable alternative. Recording position and distance between the mouth and microphone should be kept constant. The patient should be recorded at his comfortable speaking pitch, and then further assessment can be made at different pitch range, at different loudness, and at singing voice to assess the change in voice quality [1, 6]. If specific pathologies are to be ruled out, the patient may be given specific passages to read, in order to elucidate the disorder, e.g., reading the adductor vs. abductor phrases and sentences in patients with spasmodic dysphonia.

2.2.2 IINFVo Perceptual Rating Scale

The IINFVo perceptual rating scale is an alternative voice grading assessment tool for patients with substitution voicing and spasmodic dysphonia. The IINFVo rating scale is scored based on five parameters, namely, impression, intelligibility, noise, fluency, and voicing. Each parameter is scored between 0 (very good substitution voicing) and 10 (very deviant substitution voicing) on a visual analogue scale [7–10].

- I—Impression of overall voice quality, acceptability, and adequacy for daily use.
- I–Intelligibility.
- N—Noise, which stands for unintended, additive noise. It reflects the amount of annoyance caused by the audibility of all sorts of uncontrollable noise produced during speech (i.e., clicks, air turbulence, bubbly speech).
- F—Fluency, which reflects the perceived smoothness of the sound production and accounts for any undesirable interruptions.
- Vo—Voicing, which means that speech are heard as voiced or voiceless correctly.

The perceptual rating scale has been found to have consistent inter-rater reproducibility, comparable to the GRBAS scale [9].

Finally, a self-evaluation by the patient, on the perception of his own vocal function, is imperative. While it may be subjective in nature, the self-evaluation of the patients acts as an adjunct to clinical practice. It allows us to determine the level of disability the patient experience in terms of his daily living, professional life, and emotional state. Using the patient's self-evaluation scores, with our objective assessment, we would be able to formulate a treatment goal for the patient that is acceptable and motivating.

2.2.3 Voice Handicap Index (VHI)

The Voice Handicap Index (VHI) is a commonly used scale. It attempts to quantify the psychosocial consequence of a voice disorder. Its survey consists of 30 self-assessment questions, based on three parameters: functional, physical, and emotional. The statements are scored on a five-point scale, from 0 to 4 (with 0 = never and 4 = always), and allows for a maximum score of 120. The survey allows for grading of severity of vocal dysfunction, 0–30 = minimal handicap, 31–60 = moderate handicap, and 61–120 = severe handicap [11]. A validated shortened version of the Voice Handicap Index, the VHI-10, may be used in a busy clinic. It has 10 questions examining the same 3 parameters, and with 40 as the maximum point. The VHI is useful when comparing the vocal function before and after a therapeutic intervention [12–15].

2.3 Examination and Vocal Fold Imaging

Physical examination of the patient's head and neck is important. The nasal cavity, oral cavity, oropharynx, and hypopharynx function as the resonating chamber for voice production. Pathologies in these areas affect its function and will in turn affect the quality of the voice. Pathology in the neck, especially the infrahyoid muscles, may contribute to insufficiency in movement and excursion of the larynx during speech.

2.3.1 Videolaryngostroboscopy

Videolaryngostroboscopy is the main clinical tool used to examine the larynx. It is used to diagnose vocal disorders, as well as to evaluate the effectiveness of a therapeutic intervention. The videolaryngoscope may be introduced as a rigid 70-degrees telescope through the mouth, or as a flexible endoscopy via the nares. Both devices have their strengths and weaknesses. The rigid telescope provides clear and magnified images of the vocal fold; however, it is less well tolerated, and with the patient's tongue protruded, certain vocal task becomes difficult (Fig. 2.1a, b).

The videolaryngoscope uses the theory of persistence of vision and Talbot's law to allow visualization and assessment of the vocal fold movement. The human eye has a physiological limitation of picking up an image at a speed of

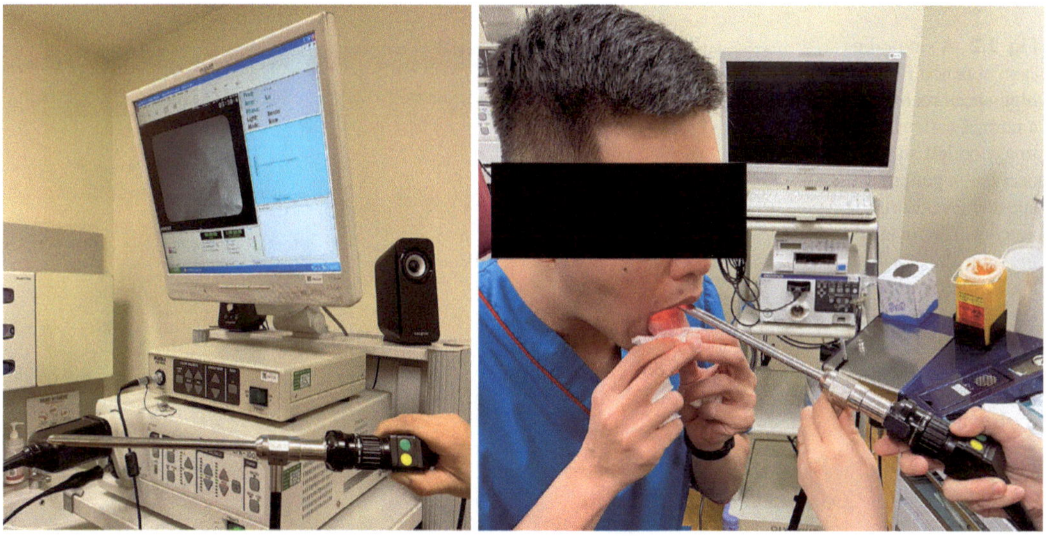

Fig. 2.1 (**Left**) Picture of a rigid stroboscope system (Kay System, KayPENTAX) used in the Ng Teng Fong General Hospital (NTFGH) voice clinic, Singapore. (**Right**) The patient is tasked to open his mouth and have his tongue pulled forward in order to have clear visualization of the larynx via the rigid stroboscope

0.2 s; any image presented more quickly than that would become a blur. The videolaryngoscope senses the frequency of the vocal sample and then synchronizes the image capture rate to the flash rate of the strobe lights accordingly. It uses Talbot's law to reduce flicker and blurring of images, to create an apparent slow-motion view of the periodic vocal fold movement by effectively sampling successive phases of the movement across successive vocal fold cycles [16].

The images are captured on video format; this allows for playback and analysis, as well as to compare pre- and post-intervention changes. Four basic parameters are used for analysis: glottic closure, regularity, mucosal wave, and symmetry. These findings can be rated on a four-point scale, 0 = normal, no deviance, 3 = severe deviance) [2, 17–19].

1. Glottic closure

   Glottic closure insufficient is observed when the vocal folds adduct during phonation.

   The types of closure insufficiency can be categorized as such:

   (a) Longitudinal. This may be seen 60% of healthy, middle-age women with normal voice.
   (b) Ventral.
   (c) Irregular.
   (d) Oval.
   (e) Hour-glass shape.

2. Regularity

   This reflects the movement transition between each successive vocal fold cycle.

3. Mucosal wave

   A smooth mucosal waveform is produced when a healthy vocal fold moves. Aberration usually signifies a pathology affecting the structures and layers within the vocal folds.

4. Symmetry

   Symmetry refers to the mirroring motion of vocal cords with each other. Asymmetry is usually caused by a pathology in the vocal cord, limiting its movement and vibratory qualities.

2.3.2 High-Speed Videokymography (SHVK)

This high-speed system uses a video camera that can capture up to 8000 images/s. The camera selects one horizontal plane, transverse to the glottis, from the whole laryngeal image. The successive line images are presented in real time on a monitor (Fig. 2.2). The device allows us to

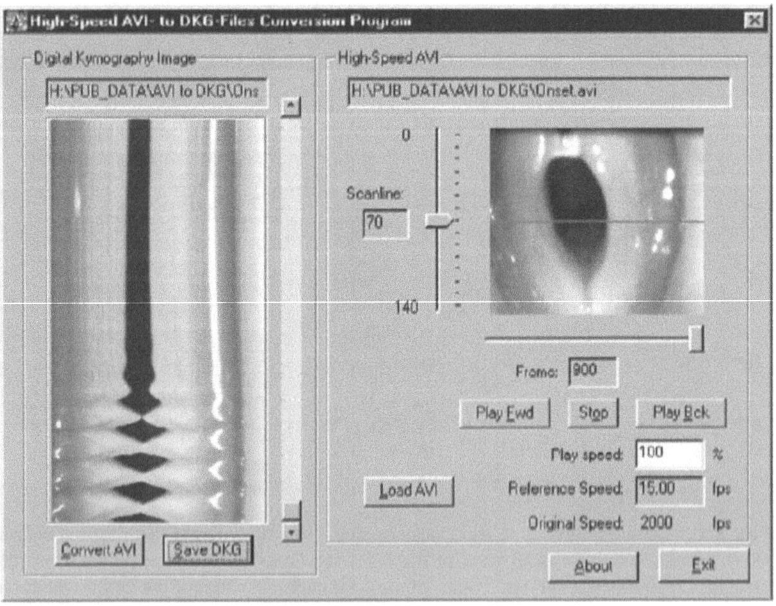

Fig. 2.2 A single-line scan obtained from a high-speed recording in a normal patient. The image on left shows oscillation pattern at a specific level during voicing. The image on the right shows vibrating vocal folds and the single line that was selected for examination. Study was performed on the Kay System, KayPENTAX. *Source:* Surgery of Larynx and Trachea

observe left-right asymmetries, open quotient, propagation of mucosal waves, movement of the upper and lower margins of the vocal folds in closing phase, etc. [20, 21].

2.4 Respiratory Function Assessment in Clinic

2.4.1 Maximum Phonation Time (MPT)

This is the simplest and most commonly used examination technique in clinics worldwide. The patient is tasked to take a deep breath and say /a:/ in his comfortable pitch range and loudness, for the longest possible time. The duration of his phonation is measured in seconds, and the best of three attempts is taken [22, 23].

This test assesses the patient's lung capacity based on an assumption of a normal functioning voice box. A normal female MPT is between 15 and 25 s, while a normal male's MPT is between 25 and 35 s. The normative range for MPT in a child is lower owning to their smaller lung volume [24].

Expectedly, this simple test has its limitations. It is prone to learning and fatigue effect, which affects the patient's performance and resultant MPT. Also, a patient with a significant glottic insufficiency during phonation would have a short MPT, and this is not because of poor lung capacity.

2.4.2 Pulmonary Function Tests: Spirometry

This is noninvasive test that allows us to examine the pulmonary capacity. A spirometer is a device with a mouthpiece hooked up to a small electronic machine. The patient's nose is clipped to prevent nose breathing; the mouthpiece is inserted, and he forms a tight seal on the mouthpiece using his lips and will be instructed to inhale and exhale in different ways. The spirometer collects the various pulmonary information and plots it onto a graph.

Various information can be obtained from these simple tests: tidal volume (VT), the amount of air inhaled or exhaled during normal breathing; minute volume (MV), the total amount of air exhaled per minute; vital capacity (VC), the total volume of air that can be exhaled after inhaling maximally; functional residual capacity (FRC), the amount of air left in the lungs after exhaling normally; residual volume, the amount of air left in the lungs after exhaling maximally; total lung capacity, the total volume of the lungs when filled with as much air as possible; forced vital capacity (FVC), the amount of air exhaled forcefully and quickly after inhaling maximally; forced expiratory volume (FEV), the amount of air expired during the first, second, and third seconds of the FVC test; forced expiratory flow (FEF), the average rate of flow during the middle half of the FVC test; and peak expiratory flow rate (PEFR), the fastest rate that one can force air out of your lungs (Fig. 2.3).

The normal values for these pulmonary function tests vary from person to person, and these results can be compared to the normative values of the population; it may be adjusted according to age, height, sex, and race. The results can be used to compare pre- and post-therapeutic performance [25–27].

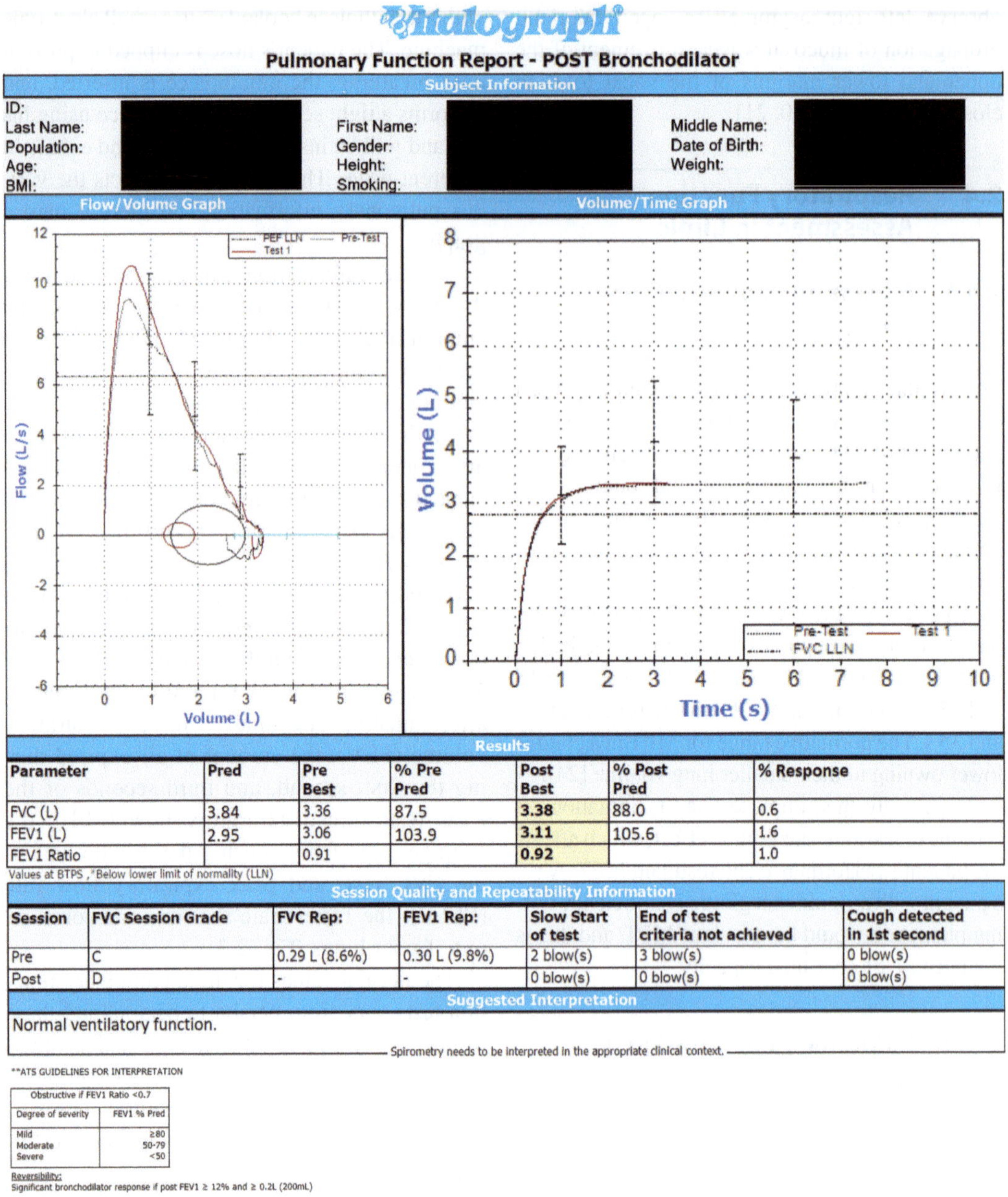

Results

Parameter	Pred	Pre Best	% Pre Pred	Post Best	% Post Pred	% Response
FVC (L)	3.84	3.36	87.5	**3.38**	88.0	0.6
FEV1 (L)	2.95	3.06	103.9	**3.11**	105.6	1.6
FEV1 Ratio		0.91		**0.92**		1.0

Values at BTPS ,*Below lower limit of normality (LLN)

Session Quality and Repeatability Information

Session	FVC Session Grade	FVC Rep:	FEV1 Rep:	Slow Start of test	End of test criteria not achieved	Cough detected in 1st second
Pre	C	0.29 L (8.6%)	0.30 L (9.8%)	2 blow(s)	3 blow(s)	0 blow(s)
Post	D	-	-	0 blow(s)	0 blow(s)	0 blow(s)

Suggested Interpretation

Normal ventilatory function.

Spirometry needs to be interpreted in the appropriate clinical context.

**ATS GUIDELINES FOR INTERPRETATION

Obstructive if FEV1 Ratio <0.7	
Degree of severity	FEV1 % Pred
Mild	≥80
Moderate	50-79
Severe	<50

Reversibility:
Significant bronchodilator response if post FEV1 ≥ 12% and ≥ 0.2L (200mL)

Fig. 2.3 An example of a spirometry report generated for a patient with normal pulmonary function. In this case, the patient's respiratory performance was tested pre- and post-bronchodilator

2.5 Other Types of Vocal and Respiratory Function Tests

These tests are adjunct assessment tests to give us further information about the patient's vocal and respiratory functions. They focus mainly on the acoustic assessment of the voiced sound quality and the aerodynamic of airflow through the larynx.

Acoustic assessment is an objective and non-invasive method of assessing the voice. Acoustical analysis provides a numerical value for each vocal parameters, and this is valuable. With the existence of normative databases characterizing voice quality, and using intelligent tools to combine the various parameters, it is possible to distinguish between normal and pathological voice, and the vocal pathology may even be elucidated. These tools can monitor pre- and post-intervention outcomes, and these numerical values are useful for academic research.

The patient is tasked to produce a sustained (/a:/) at his comfortable frequency and intensity. The voice is recorded and the acoustic parameters analyzed [5].

Acoustical parameters include:

- Short-term fundamental frequency perturbation
- Short or medium-term amplitude perturbation and voiceless segments
- Harmonics-to-noise ratio (HNR)
- Long-term frequency and amplitude modulation
- Very long-term amplitude variation
- Sub-harmonics
- Tremor

The fundamental frequency (Fo), measured in Hertz, is defined as the periodic waveform produced by the vocal fold movements in a second. Measurements of Fo disturbance, jitter, and shimmer are useful in describing the vocal characteristics. Jitter is defined as the parameter of frequency variation from cycle to cycle, and shimmer relates to the amplitude variation of the sound wave. The harmonics-to-noise ratio is an assessment of the ratio between periodic components and non-periodic component comprising a segment of voiced speech.

The jitter is affected mainly by the lack of control of vibration of the vocal folds; the voices of patients with pathologies often have a higher percentage of jitter. It is normal to vary between 0.5% and 1.0% of the normal value during sustained phonation.

Shimmer changes with the reduction of glottal resistance and mass lesions on the vocal cords and is correlated with the presence of noise emission and breathiness. It is considered pathological voice for values less than 3% for adults and around 0.4% and 1% for children.

A voice with a high HNR is considered sonorant and harmonic voice. A low HNR denotes asthenic voice and dysphonia. A HNR value of less than 7 dB is considered pathological [28].

2.5.1 Phonetogram or Voice Range Profile (VRP)

The phonetogram or voice range profile (VRP) is a quantitative voice assessment that describes the acoustic characteristics with respect to fundamental frequency and sound intensity. VRP is obtained by asking the patient to produce a sustained vowel at both minimal and maximal intensity, across his own maximum frequency range. VRP helps the clinician diagnose pathologies and assess pre- and post-therapeutic outcomes. However, the reliability and validity of these results are limited [29].

2.5.2 Subglottic Air Pressure Measurement

Subglottic air pressure measurement is useful as a test for the pulmonary function. It also assesses the swallowing function. This is an invasive test; it is measured either by insertion of an esophageal transducer or by direct puncture of the airway at the cricothyroid membrane. Various pulmonary characteristics are measured: total lung capacity, tidal volume, functional residual capacity (FRC), and residual volume. This test is usually performed for academic purposes [30].

2.6 Adjunct Tests for Vocal Assessments

2.6.1 Electromyography

This is an electrophysiological investigation, to examine the neuromuscular function of the larynx. It is useful in conditions where there is vocal fold immobility; it allows the clinician to differentiate between nerve palsy, paresis, and joint fixation. It is also useful for monitoring the laryngeal muscles in botulinum injection. The procedure is performed with the patient supine and neck extended; a fine needle electrode is inserted into the thyroarytenoid muscle through the cricothyroid membrane at 45° cranially, 20° laterally, and a depth of 1.5–2 cm. The cricothyroid muscle is reached by inserting the electrode off the midline, close to the inferior border of the thyroid cartilage [31–34].

References

1. Sataloff RT. Professional voice. San Diego: Singular Publishing Group; 1997.
2. Hirano M. Clinical examination of voice. New York: Springer; 1981.
3. Dejonckere PH, Lebacq J. Acoustic, perceptual, aerodynamic and anatomical correlations in voice pathology. ORL J Otorhinolaryngol Relat Spec. 1996;58:326–32.
4. De Bodt M, Wuyts F, Van de Heyning P, Croeckx C. Test re-test study of GRBAS-scale. J Voice. 1997;11:74–80.
5. Dejonckere PH, Remacle M, Fresnel-Elbaz E, Woisard V, Crevier Buchman L, Millet B. Differentiated perceptual evaluation of pathological voice quality: reliability and correlations with acoustic measurements. Rev Laryngol Otol Rhinol. 1996;117: 219–24.
6. Watson C. Database management of the voice clinic and laboratory. J Voice. 1994;3:99–106.
7. Moerman M, Martens JP, Dejonckere PH. Application of the voice handicap index in 45 patients with substitution voicing after total laryngectomy. Eur Arch Otorhinolaryngol. 2004;261:423–8.
8. Moerman M, Pieters G, Martens JP, Van Der Borgt MJ, Dejonckere PH. Objective evaluation of the quality of substitution voices. Eur Arch Otorhinolaryngol. 2004;261:541–7.
9. Moerman M, Martens JP, Crevier Buchman L, de Haan E, Grand S, Tessier C, Woisard V, Dejonckere PH. The INFVO perceptual rating scale for substitution voicing: development and reliability. Eur Arch Otorhinolaryngol. 2006;263(5):435–9.
10. Moerman M, Martens JP, Van Der Borgt MJ, Pelemans M, Gillis M, Dejonckere PH. Perceptual evaluation of the (I)INFVO rating scale. Eur Arch Otorhinolaryngol. 2006;263:183–7.
11. Jocobson BH, Johnson A, Grywalski C, Silbergleit A, Jacobson G, Benninger MS, Newman CW. The Voice Handicap Index (VHI): development and validation. Am J Speech Lang Pathol. 1997;6:66–70.
12. Rosen CA, Lee AS, Osborn J, Zullo T, Murry T. Development and validation of the voice handicap index – 10. Laryngoscope. 2004;114:1549–56.
13. Speyer R, Wieneke GH, Dejonckere PH. The use of acoustic parameters for the evaluation of voice therapy for dysphonic patients. Acta Acustica United Acustica. 2004;90:520–7.
14. Speyer R, Wieneke GH, Dejonckere PH. Documentation of progress in voice therapy: perceptual, acoustic and laryngostroboscopic findings pretherapy and posttherapy. J Voice. 2004;18:325–39.
15. Speyer R, Wieneke GH, Dejonckere PH. Self-assessment of voice therapy for chronic dysphonia. Clin Otolaryngol. 2004;29:66–74.
16. Mehta DD, Deliyski DD, Hillman RE. Why laryngeal stroboscopy really works: clarifying misconceptions surrounding Talbot's law and the persistence of vision. J Speech Lang Hear Res. 2010;53(5):1263–7.
17. Dejonckere PH, Wieneke GH, Lebacq J. Laryngostroboscopy and glottis dysrhythmias. Acta Otorhinolaryngol Belg. 1989;43:19–29.
18. Hirano M, Bless DM. Videostroboscopic examination of the larynx. San Diego: Singular Publishing; 1993.
19. Dejonckere PH, Crevier L, Elbaz E, Marraco M, Millet B, Remacle M, Woisard V. Quantitative rating of videolaryngostroboscopy: factor analysis of the vibratory characteristics in communication and its disorders: a science in progress. Nijmegen: Nijmegen University Press; 1999. p. 170–1.
20. Neubauer J, Mergell P, Eysholdt U, Herzl H. Spatiotemporal analysis of irregular vocal fold oscillations: biphonation due to desynchronization of spatial modes. J Acoust Soc Am. 2001;110:3179–92.
21. Svec JG, Schutte HK. Videokymography: high-speed linescanning of vocal fold vibration. J Voice. 1996;10:201–5.
22. Hirano M. Objective evaluation of the human voice: clinical aspects. Folia Phoniatr. 1989;41:89–144.
23. Neiman GS, Edeson B. Procedural aspect of eliciting maximum phonation time. Folia Phoniatr. 1981;33:285–93.
24. Kent RD, Kent JF, Rosenbek JC. Maximum performance tests of speech production. J Speech Hear Res. 1987;52:367–87.
25. Hyatt RE, Black LF. The flow-volume curve: a current perspective. Am Rev Respir Dis. 1973;107:191.
26. Robin ED. Respiratory medicine. In: Medicine, vol. III. New York: Scientific American; 1982. p. 1–7.
27. Salvit DH. Role of the pulmonary junction in voice assessment. In: Rubin JS, Sataloff RT, Korovin GS, Gould WJ, editors. Diagnosis and treatment of voice disorders. New York: Igaku-Shoin; 1995. p. 327–40.
28. Teixeira JP, Oliveira C, Lopes C. Vocal acoustic analysis – jitter, shimmer and HNR parameters. Proc Technol. 2013;9(2013):1112–22.
29. D'alatri L, Marchese MR. The speech range profile (SRP): an easy and useful tool to assess vocal limits. Acta Otorhinolaryngol Ital. 2014;34(4):253–8.
30. Rothenburg M. Interpolating subglottic pressure from oral pressure. J Speech Hear Disord. 1982;47:218–24.
31. Blitzer A. Laryngeal electromyography. In: Rubin JS, Sataloff RT, Korovin GS, Gould WJ, editors. Diagnosis and treatment of voice disorders. New York: Igaku-Shoin; 1995. p. 316–26.
32. Dejonckere PH. EMG of the larynx. Liege: Press Production; 1987.
33. Dejonckere PH, Knoops P, Lebacq J. Evoked muscular potential in laryngeal muscles. Acta Otolaryngol Belg. 1988;42:494–501.
34. Munin MC, Murry T, Rosen CA. Laryngeal electromyography. Otolaryngol Clin N Am. 2000;33:759–70.

3 Anatomy and Microanatomy of the Larynx

Defining Molecular Laryngology

Markus Gugatschka, David Hortobagyi, and Liang Ker

Key Points

Anatomy and Microanatomy of the Larynx

- The human larynx is the crucial organ at the intersection of phonation, respiration, and swallowing.
- The vocal folds are the core structure of the larynx, embedded in the laryngeal framework. Phonation requires the integrity of all layers of the vocal fold, namely, the mucosa (which is further subdivided into epithelium, basement membrane zone, and the trilaminar lamina propria) and the vocal fold muscle.
- The underlying mechanism of phonation bases on the combination of two theories: the body-cover theory and the myoelastic-aerodynamic theory.
- Pathologies of one or more layers of the vocal folds, such as Reinke's edema, carcinoma, or vocal fold scars, lead to oscillatory irregularities and subsequently to dysphonia.
- Most benign lesions of the vocal folds are located in the lamina propria. Laryngeal papillomatosis and carcinoma originate from the vocal fold epithelium.

Regenerative Medicine

- Regenerative medicine is a causal therapy approach that aims to restore organ integrity including function. As such this approach is rather rare, as most established therapies in the realm of laryngology are symptomatic only.
- Regenerative medicine bases on the following elements: cell therapy, material-based approaches, application of cytokines or growth factors, and, according to newer classifications, gene therapy.
- Tissue engineering can be seen as a subclass of regenerative medicine, combining the previously mentioned elements, with the purpose of replacing pathological tissue with an in vitro fabricated fragment of healthy tissue.

M. Gugatschka (✉) · D. Hortobagyi
Division of Phoniatrics, ENT University Hospital Graz, Medical University Graz, Graz, Austria
e-mail: markus.gugatschka@medunigraz.at; david.hortobagyi@medunigraz.at

L. Ker
Department of Otolaryngology, Head and Neck Surgery, National University Hospital, Singapore, Singapore
e-mail: liang_ker@nuhs.edu.sg

M. Remacle, H. E. Eckel (eds.), *Textbook of Surgery of Larynx and Trachea*,
https://doi.org/10.1007/978-3-031-09621-1_3

3.1 Introduction

The human larynx is a highly complex anatomical structure at the intersection between respiratory and digestive tract and serves as an organ for swallowing and voice production. The anatomical and physiological requirements to meet these goals are unique in the human body.

In order to fully comprehend physiology and pathophysiology of the larynx, it is mandatory to understand the specific anatomical and micro-anatomical structures. Minoru Hirano's body-cover model [1] and the myoelastic-aerodynamic theory of phonation [2] are proof of that.

However, research in the realm of laryngology and phoniatrics is hampered by the highly sensitive structures of the larynx, especially the human vocal folds (VF) and their small sizes, which makes it virtually impossible to study biological processes and mechanisms in vivo as every intervention (biopsy, injection of drugs, etc.) carries the unbearable risk of scarring and hence permanent dysphonia. Likewise, the status of reinnervation following an injury of the recurrent laryngeal nerve can only be followed indirectly via endoscopy or directly by electromyography, but the delivery of drugs to the site of the process (including the follow-up) remains insecure.

Therefore, many basic questions remain unanswered in laryngology including the underlying pathophysiology of diseases such as Reinke's edema, the impact of allergies on the VF, or the causal treatment of diseases such as VF scarring. It is also unclear and could not be proven on a cellular level so far, if vocal activation following VF surgery or injury has detrimental or beneficial effects on wound healing and functional recovery.

In the following chapter, we seek to give an overview on both gross anatomy and microanatomy of the involved structures and aim to delineate the consequences on the physiological level, including selected laryngeal diseases.

3.2 Gross Anatomy

The larynx develops from the endodermal lining and the mesoderm of the fourth to sixth branchial arches. At birth, the tip of the epiglottis reaches the level of the first cervical vertebra and may come in contact with the soft palate. Due to further development, the larynx descends and is found at the height between the third to fifth cervical vertebrae. During puberty, the descent and growth of the larynx progress and finally extend from the third to sixth cervical vertebrae.

The larynx can be divided into three levels. The glottis is the intermediate level and is located between the vocal folds. The region above the glottis is referred to as supraglottis. The space below is called subglottis and merges inferiorly into the trachea.

3.2.1 Laryngeal Framework

The laryngeal framework consists of nine cartilages, three unpaired (thyroid, cricoid, and epiglottis) and three paired (arytenoid, cuneiform, and cornicula larynges). The most prominent cartilage, from an exterior view on the neck, is the thyroid, particularly its laryngeal prominence, also known as Adam's apple. Caudally to it lies a signet-shaped cartilage called the cricoid, representing an essential landmark for tracheostomy. Between these two cartilages, a depression is palpable, where the cricothyroid membrane is located. This membrane is sectioned in coniotomy for an emergency airway access.

During endoscopy, the larynx can be observed from superior (Fig. 3.1). From this point of view, the epiglottis becomes clearly visible. It is a leaf-shaped structure, consisting of elastic cartilage. Its function, to avoid aspiration during swallowing, has been controversially discussed since the nineteenth century. A more recent study examined the deglutition of three patients after epiglottectomy. They could show that all individuals fully regained their ability to swallow, assuming

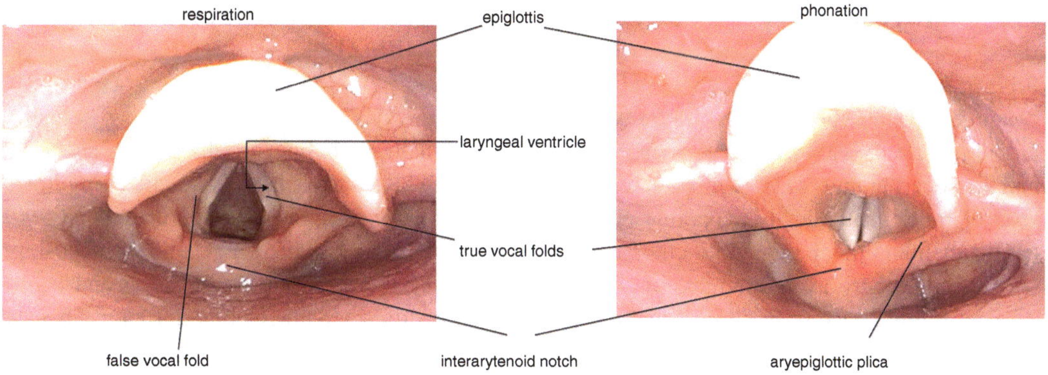

Fig. 3.1 Anatomical structures of the larynx during endoscopy

that the epiglottis is, at least in adults, only a vestigial [3].

Via a mucosal fold, namely, the aryepiglottic plica, the epiglottis is posteriorly and caudally on both sides linked to the arytenoid cartilages. Each arytenoid cartilage has a base, three processes, and three surfaces. The base of the cartilage is concave and provides a smooth surface for the articulation with the cricoid cartilage. There are two processes that arise from the base of the arytenoid cartilage—the vocal and muscular processes. The long vocal process projects anteriorly, gives attachment to the vocal ligament, and corresponds to the cartilage part of the vocal fold. The muscular process shows posterolaterally and gives attachment to the posterior and the lateral cricoarytenoid muscle. The former muscle is the only one, which is able to open the glottis, whereas the latter and the other intrinsic laryngeal muscles are responsible for narrowing the space between the vocal folds, which is also known as rima glottidis. Therefore, the intrinsic muscles are important for an immaculate phonation as well as respiration. The extrinsic muscles, on the other hand, elevate or depress the larynx and consequently play a pivotal role during swallowing [4].

Cranially to the glottis, a mucosal protrusion can be seen, which looks similar to the true vocal fold and is therefore often referred to as false vocal fold. Between these, an oblong cavity extends, the laryngeal ventricle, ending into a caecal pouch. The laryngeal ventricle consists of dozens of mucous glands, lubricating the true vocal folds. Additionally, the false vocal folds are assumed to play a major role in the vocal tract resonance [5, 6].

3.2.2 Innervation

The motoric as well as the sensory laryngeal innervation is provided by the tenth cranial nerve, the vagal nerve. The superior laryngeal nerve divides into an internal branch, which penetrates, accompanied by the superior laryngeal artery, the thyrohyoid membrane and supplies the mucosa of the supraglottis. The external branch innervates the cricothyroid muscle.

The remaining intrinsic laryngeal muscles, as well as the rest of the laryngeal cavity, are supplied by the recurrent laryngeal nerve. This nerve has an asymmetrical course on either side of the neck. On the right side, it arises anteriorly to the subclavian artery, winds posteromedially around the artery, and ascends in or adjacent to the tracheoesophageal groove posterior to the thyroid gland. It enters the larynx posteriorly to the cricothyroid joint. On the left side, the nerve arises ventrally to the aortic arch and winds posteromedially around the ligamentum arteriosum. The ascent to the larynx follows a similar course as the right recurrent nerve [4].

3.3 Microanatomy

From a histological point of view, the VF are composed of the superficial part of the thyroarytenoid muscle also referred to as vocalis muscle and the covering mucosa. The mucosa itself consists of three anatomically separable elements: the epithelium, the basement membrane zone (BMZ), and the tri-layered lamina propria (LP). This is of importance from a functional perspective and the basis for the body-cover model presented in 1974 by Minoru Hirano [1].

3.3.1 Epithelium

The larynx is an intersection of two very diversely functioning systems, namely, the respiratory system and parts of the digestive tract [7]. This is reflected by the laryngeal epithelium as the VF are covered by a stratified squamous epithelium, like the digestive tract, whereas the other parts of the larynx consist of a pseudostratified respiratory epithelium. This structure is important in order to withstand the mechanical forces the VF are exposed to during phonation. To ensure further stability, cells are connected to each other and the BMZ via adherent junctions called desmosomes (cell-to-cell) and hemidesmosomes (cell-to-basement membrane). Furthermore, communication pathways and tight junctions between cells have been described. The integrity, especially of the latter, is essential for impeccable secretion and absorption of ions and hence for the composition of the laryngeal secrete. Since the VF are the narrowest part of the upper respiratory tract, the VF epithelium is in particular subjected to noxae. Consequently, the laryngeal secrete has important functions, acting as a barrier against biological and chemical pollutants. Providing humification to the VF ensures furthermore undisturbed VF vibration.

Macroscopically, the VF epithelium appears to have an even surface. But magnification reveals that there are wrinkles and grooves which facilitate the adhesion of the laryngeal secrete and the movement of the mucosal wave during phonation [8–11].

3.3.2 Basement Membrane Zone (BMZ)

The BMZ is a narrow stabilizing structure between the epithelium and the LP. It connects the adjacent layers to each other via anchoring fibers, consisting predominantly of collagen type IV. Previous studies suggest a genetic predisposition regarding the density of these fibers and consequently differing vulnerability during mechanical stress. Furthermore, it plays an important role in VF dysplasia/carcinoma. Whereas in carcinoma in situ the BMZ remains intact, it is disrupted in case of invasive carcinoma [12]. In case of VF lesions, an unaffected and therefore smooth oscillation indicates that the pathology has not exceeded the epithelium [13].

3.3.3 Lamina Propria

According to the concentration of extracellular fibers, the LP is subdivided into three sections (superficial, intermediate, deep), smoothly merging into one another. The consistency and stiffness increase towards the deeper layers. While the superficial part, also known as Reinke's space, consists of loose connective tissue, the deepest layer has a high proportion of collagen fibers, resembling macroscopically a ligament, therefore better known as the vocal ligament. The intermediate layer is distinguished from the deeper layer by a higher concentration of elastin fibers. Besides collagen and elastin, the LP contains a plethora of other macromolecules. Hyaluronic acid is seen as a kind of counterpart to collagen, since it is the main factor responsible for the pliability. Also, fibronectin, the most abundant glycoprotein in the LP, is an important component and supports the interaction between cells and ECM. An equilibrium of all these molecules is essential for an undisturbed phonation.

Vocal fold fibroblasts (VFF) are the major cellular representatives in the LP and are responsible for its metabolism (see Fig. 3.2a, b). In vivo studies showed that at the time of birth the LP is a unilayered structure. It is presumed that the mechanical stimulation during phonation con-

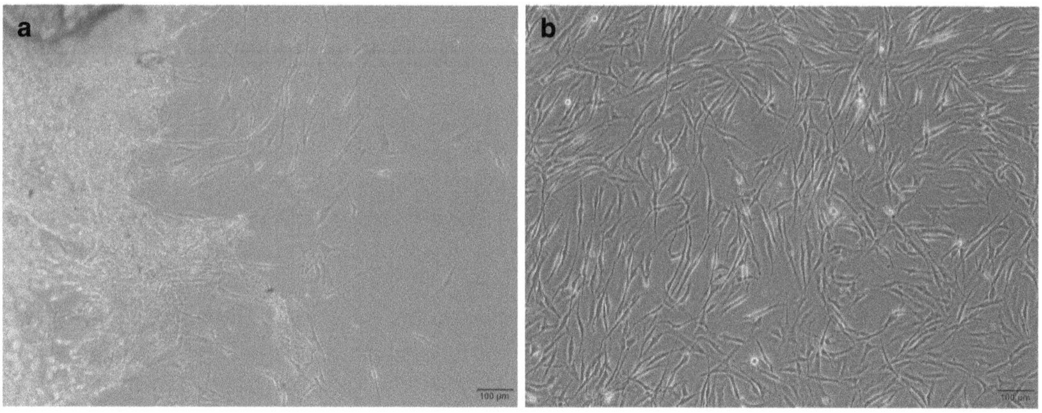

Fig. 3.2 (**a**) Vocal fold fibroblasts growing out of human vocal fold mucosa (© Tanja Grossmann). (**b**) Human vocal fold fibroblasts in cell culture (© Tanja Grossmann)

tributes tremendously to the development of a trilamination. This indicates that VFF are susceptible to mechanical stimuli. Since VFF are anchored in the ECM via transmembrane receptors, conformational changes of the tissue generate intracellular signals. In further consequence, this leads to epigenetic changes and therefore has an impact on ECM- as well as on inflammation-related protein production. This conversion of a mechanical impulse into a biochemical signal is called mechanotransduction. Besides the development of the LP, mechanotransduction is also attributed to other essential physiological and pathophysiological processes. To get a deeper knowledge of these, different phonomimetic bioreactors were developed, enabling the study of the effect of mechanical forces on cells in vitro.

The anterior and posterior ends of the VF, also known as maculae flavae, are especially exposed to tensional stresses during phonation. These regions are populated by a particular kind of VF fibroblasts, called stellate cells. It has been proposed that stellate cells are stem cells, playing an important role during inflammatory reactions [14–17].

3.3.4 Vocal Fold Muscles

The vocalis muscle can be seen as the superficial part of the thyroarytenoid muscle. A high density of stretch receptors, called muscle spindles, supports the assumption that it is particularly important for the fine-tuning of the VF tension and consequently for the pitch. Moreover, compared to limb skeletal muscles, laryngeal muscles possess a particularly high density of mitochondria per fiber volume, reflecting the high demands of energy required for respiration and phonation [18].

Cell lineage tracing enables a visualization of different cell markers and consequently determines the origin and migration of cells. Studies using this method suggest that the intrinsic laryngeal muscles derive from the same origin as the extraocular head muscles and substantially differ from skeletal muscles. This knowledge might influence future voice therapy [19, 20].

3.4 Physiology and Pathophysiology

The VF are the core structure of the larynx and the primary source of voice production. The underlying mechanism of phonation can be explained by the combination of two theories: (1) the body-cover theory and (2) the myoelastic-aerodynamic theory of phonation which will be explained in short in the following paragraphs.

3.4.1 Body-Cover Theory

The VF are not uniform solid structures but rather composed of different layers. Minoru Hirano postulated the so-called body-cover theory, where he differentiated between three functional units, each with different biomechanical properties. The deepest layer is the body which consists of the vocalis muscle and the deep layer of the lamina propria. The transition zone includes the intermediate layer. The deep and the intermediate layer can be summarized as vocal ligament [5]. The cover compromises the superficial portion of the lamina propria, the BMZ, and the epithelium and is the oscillating part in response to the contraction of the stiff body layer. During phonation, the "cover" smoothly slides on the "body" as air passes the VF. Therefore, he described the VF as at least a "double-structured oscillator." This perspective elucidates the intertwining of the different layers [21].

3.4.2 Myoelastic-Aerodynamic Theory

During voice production, the glottis opens and closes cyclically. One such cycle is described below: The air pressure below the glottis created by the lungs is referred to as subglottal pressure. Once the pressure below the closed glottis has exceeded the pressure above, the air displaces the loosely attached mucosa, which enables the release of a small amount of air. The minimum of air pressure that drives the vocal folds apart is referred to as phonation threshold pressure. This is followed by a closure of the glottis, which is driven by several factors, described by the myoelastic-aerodynamic theory. The suction effect, caused by the fast airflow (Bernoulli effect) and the elastic components of the vocal folds, achieves a vocal fold closure. Titze expanded the theory and demonstrated that these factors only contribute minimally to the initiation of the vocal fold oscillation. Owing to the inherent physical and geometric properties of the vocal folds, energy is transferred continuously from the air stream to the glottal tissue leading to a self-sustained oscillation, thereby overcoming frictional energy losses [22, 23].

3.4.3 Pathophysiology: Voice Production in a Pathological State

The integrity of all VF layers is of utmost importance for an optimal oscillation and consequently voice production. This becomes especially apparent in pathological states, of which a small selection will be discussed below. Due to ethical reasons as well as a difficult accessibility of healthy human VF tissue, many (patho-)physiological processes are barely understood. As a consequence, many therapies are based on symptomatic approaches.

Various models have been developed to study VF biology and pathology. Animal trials play a particularly important role in this context. Efforts are made to reduce them, since cell cultures provide a good alternative. However, for a long time, it was not possible to study mechanotransductive processes in vitro. In order to overcome this problem, bioreactors were developed in the recent years. A recently published device was engineered evaluated by Kirsch et al. [24]. This particular system enables the exposure of VF cell types (VFF and VF epithelial cells) to vibratory stimulation with frequencies similar to the human voice. Studies based on this approach explored the pathophysiology of VF diseases such as Reinke's edema [25], or voice rest following VF inflammation (due to surgery or infection) [26].

3.5 Selected VF Diseases

3.5.1 Vocal Fold Scars

One of the unsolved problems in laryngology is VF scarring. Scar tissue formation can be, depending on its expansion, accompanied by significant deterioration of oscillatory functions of the VF and consequently cause dysphonia. At a cellular aspect, VF scarring is associated with a differentiation of the VFF into myofibroblasts

[27]. These differ not only phenotypically but also in their expression profile. As a result, this scar tissue contains a higher amount of collagen fibers. In a healthy LP, these are aligned in parallel to the VF edge, whereas histological examinations have shown that collagen fibers follow a disordered pattern in scar tissue. Additionally, lower concentrations of hyaluronic acid (HA) and elastin were described [28]. Consequently, the viscoelastic properties are impaired, leading to irregular oscillation.

According to in vivo studies on rats, age may play an essential role in VF wound healing. Myofibroblasts in younger rodents produced higher amounts of (scar protective) HA than the older ones. Furthermore, younger laboratory animals showed a superior response to the antifibrotic hepatocyte growth factor (HGF).

In the past years, researchers were investigating the effects of stem cells on wound healing and mature VF scar by injecting them into animal and human VF. The idea behind is that stem cells secrete a cocktail of different cytokines which might achieve a complete or partial recovery of the scar. However, the results were highly variable, and objective parameters were not always measured [29, 30]. Further differentiation needs to be done between a freshly injured VF and a mature VF scar, as they respond differently to any kind of treatment.

3.5.2 Reinke's Edema

Reinke's edema is, in most cases, simple to diagnose by laryngoscopy. It is usually found in smoking women pursuing a talkative profession (e.g., teacher). Clinically they are characterized by a pronounced low frequency of the voice. The VF appear swollen with dilated vessels which shine through the epithelium. Even if this disease was already described in the late nineteenth century, the underlying pathophysiological process is still not fully understood. Considerable progress has been achieved in the past years. Nicotine abuse seems to play a major role in the development of Reinke's edema [31]. However, due to an overrepresentation of women in most studies, an involvement of specific hormones is assumed as well.

A thorough examination of the vessels under electron microscopy showed a leaky endothelium. Recent molecular studies revealed an upregulation of pro-angiogenetic factors in Reinke's edema. During in vitro experiments, the combination of mechanical stimulation and exposure of VFF to cigarette smoke extract confirmed these results. These studies support the assumption that talkative persons are at higher risk. Simultaneously, elevated levels pro-inflammatory of COX-2 induced by cigarette smoke were only suppressed after mechanical stimulation.

Other in vitro studies showed that genes associated with collagen expression were downregulated, whereas the HA-related genes were significantly increased. The combined effect of increased leaky vessels, higher HA concentration, and simultaneously reduced amount of collagen may lead to the typical clinical appearance [4, 32–35].

3.5.3 Vocal Fold Lesions

There is obviously a plethora of other different benign as well as malignant VF lesions which can affect all layers. Benign ones, such as nodules and granuloma, are preferably treated by voice therapy to avoid postoperative scarring and an impairment of phonation. However, benign lesions with an extended manifestation and malignant lesions are removed by chordectomy or, as an ultima ratio, by total laryngectomy. This of course is associated with a significant deterioration of functionality and quality of life. A more profound knowledge of biomolecular processes in these pathologies is desirable to improve diagnostics and prognosis as well as to expand therapeutic options or even provide a causal therapy [12].

Take-Home Messages

- The human larynx is an overly complex organ at the intersection between respiratory and digestive tract. Despite recent progress in understanding the physiology and pathophysiology of many of its functions, a lot of fundamental questions remain unanswered due to the difficult accessibility of the laryngeal structures. Most of the laryngeal muscles cannot be displayed during endoscopy, as they are either covered by mucosa or hidden by overlying structures.
- The VF themselves are highly complex structures, and a detailed knowledge of its (micro-)anatomy and pathophysiological processes are essential to enhance diagnosis, therapy, and prognosis. Progress during the last few years led to unprecedented insights in VF biology, as well as VF pathophysiology. For the first time, cellular changes leading to macroscopical changes could be observed. Understanding these processes may lead to a paradigm shift and the development of new treatment strategies. A very recent study showed that an early mechanical activation of human VF fibroblasts in an inflammatory state led to decreased levels of certain pro-inflammatory and pro-fibrogenic cytokines, indicating that early voice use following VF surgery may be beneficial to the healing process [26]. These studies aim to provide a sound basis for subsequent clinical trials.

References

1. Hirano M. Morphological structure of the vocal cord as a vibrator and its variations. Folia Phoniatr (Basel). 1974;26(2):89–94.
2. Titze IR. Comments on the myoelastic - aerodynamic theory of phonation. J Speech Hear Res. 1980;23(3):495–510.
3. Leder SB, Burrell MI, Van Daele DJ. Epiglottis is not essential for successful swallowing in humans. Ann Otol Rhinol Laryngol. 2010;119(12):795–8.
4. Sato K, Hirano M, Nakashima T. Electron microscopic and immunohistochemical investigation of Reinke's edema. Ann Otol Rhinol Laryngol. 1999;108(11 Pt 1):1068–72.
5. Noordzij JP, Ossoff RH. Anatomy and physiology of the larynx. Otolaryngol Clin N Am. 2006;39(1): 1–10.
6. Sataloff RT, Heman-Ackah YD, Hawkshaw MJ. Clinical anatomy and physiology of the voice. Otolaryngol Clin N Am. 2007;40(5):909–29, v.
7. Perin S, McCann CJ, Borrelli O, De Coppi P, Thapar N. Update on foregut molecular embryology and role of regenerative medicine therapies. Front Pediatr. 2017;5:91.
8. Gray SD, Titze IR, Alipour F, Hammond TH. Biomechanical and histologic observations of vocal fold fibrous proteins. Ann Otol Rhinol Laryngol. 2000;109(1):77–85.
9. Gray SD, Titze IR, Chan R, Hammond TH. Vocal fold proteoglycans and their influence on biomechanics. Laryngoscope. 1999;109(6):845–54.
10. Catten M, Gray SD, Hammond TH, Zhou R, Hammond E. Analysis of cellular location and concentration in vocal fold lamina propria. Otolaryngol Head Neck Surg. 1998;118(5):663–7.
11. Levendoski EE, Leydon C, Thibeault SL. Vocal fold epithelial barrier in health and injury: a research review. J Speech Lang Hear Res. 2014;57(5): 1679–91.
12. Schultz P. Vocal fold cancer. Eur Ann Otorhinolaryngol Head Neck Dis. 2011;128(6):301–8.
13. Gray SD, Pignatari SS, Harding P. Morphologic ultrastructure of anchoring fibers in normal vocal fold basement membrane zone. J Voice. 1994;8(1): 48–52.
14. Sato K, Hirano M, Nakashima T. Comparative histology of the maculae flavae of the vocal folds. Ann Otol Rhinol Laryngol. 2000;109(2):136–40.
15. Sato K, Hirano M, Nakashima T. 3D structure of the macula flava in the human vocal fold. Acta Otolaryngol. 2003;123(2):269–73.
16. Gugatschka M, Kojima T, Ohno S, Kanemaru S, Hirano S. Recruitment patterns of side population cells during wound healing in rat vocal folds. Laryngoscope. 2011;121(8):1662–7.
17. Li NY, Heris HK, Mongeau L. Current understanding and future directions for vocal fold mechanobiology. J Cytol Mol Biol. 2013;1(1):001-4653.1000001.
18. Thomas LB, Harrison AL, Stemple JC. Aging thyroarytenoid and limb skeletal muscle: lessons in contrast. J Voice. 2008;22(4):430–50.
19. Sanders I, Rai S, Han Y, Biller HF. Human vocalis contains distinct superior and inferior subcompartments: possible candidates for the two masses of vocal fold vibration. Ann Otol Rhinol Laryngol. 1998;107(10 Pt 1):826–33.
20. Martins RH, Benito Pessin AB, Nassib DJ, Branco A, Rodrigues SA, Matheus SM. Aging voice and the laryngeal muscle atrophy. Laryngoscope. 2015;125(11):2518–21.

21. Vahabzadeh-Hagh AM, Zhang Z, Chhetri DK. Hirano's cover-body model and its unique laryngeal postures revisited. Laryngoscope. 2018;128(6):1412–8.
22. Titze IR. The physics of small-amplitude oscillation of the vocal folds. J Acoust Soc Am. 1988;83(4):1536–52.
23. Van Den Berg J. Myoelastic-aerodynamic theory of voice production. J Speech Hear Res. 1958;1(3):227–44.
24. Kirsch A, Hortobagyi D, Stachl T, Karbiener M, Grossmann T, Gerstenberger C, et al. Development and validation of a novel phonomimetic bioreactor. PLoS One. 2019;14(3):e0213788.
25. Grossmann T, Steffan B, Kirsch A, Grill M, Gerstenberger C, Gugatschka M. Exploring the pathophysiology of Reinke's edema: the cellular impact of cigarette smoke and vibration. Laryngoscope. 2021;131(2):E547–54.
26. Hortobagyi D, Grossmann T, Tschernitz M, Grill M, Kirsch A, Gerstenberger C, et al. In vitro mechanical vibration down-regulates pro-inflammatory and pro-fibrotic signaling in human vocal fold fibroblasts. PLoS One. 2020;15(11):e0241901.
27. Vyas B, Ishikawa K, Duflo S, Chen X, Thibeault SL. Inhibitory effects of hepatocyte growth factor and interleukin-6 on transforming growth factor-beta1 mediated vocal fold fibroblast-myofibroblast differentiation. Ann Otol Rhinol Laryngol. 2010;119(5):350–7.
28. Allen J. Cause of vocal fold scar. Curr Opin Otolaryngol Head Neck Surg. 2010;18(6):475–80.
29. Hertegard S, Nagubothu SR, Malmstrom E, LeBlanc K. Treatment of vocal fold scarring with autologous bone marrow-derived human mesenchymal stromal cells-first phase I/II human clinical study. Stem Cell Res Ther. 2020;11(1):128.
30. Mattei A, Magalon J, Bertrand B, Grimaud F, Revis J, Velier M, et al. Autologous adipose-derived stromal vascular fraction and scarred vocal folds: first clinical case report. Stem Cell Res Ther. 2018;9(1):202.
31. Branski RC, Saltman B, Sulica L, Szeto H, Duflo S, Felsen D, et al. Cigarette smoke and reactive oxygen species metabolism: implications for the pathophysiology of Reinke's edema. Laryngoscope. 2009;119(10):2014–8.
32. Kravos A, Hocevar-Boltezar I, Gersak K. Serum levels of sex hormones in males with Reinke's edema. Eur Arch Otorhinolaryngol. 2013;270(1): 233–8.
33. Marcotullio D, Magliulo G, Pezone T. Reinke's edema and risk factors: clinical and histopathologic aspects. Am J Otolaryngol. 2002;23(2):81–4.
34. Duflo SM, Thibeault SL, Li W, Smith ME, Schade G, Hess MM. Differential gene expression profiling of vocal fold polyps and Reinke's edema by complementary DNA microarray. Ann Otol Rhinol Laryngol. 2006;115(9):703–14.
35. Gugatschka M, Darnhofer B, Grossmann T, Schittmayer-Schantl M, Hortobagyi D, Kirsch A, et al. Proteomic analysis of vocal fold fibroblasts exposed to cigarette smoke extract: exploring the pathophysiology of Reinke's edema. Mol Cell Proteomics. 2019;18(8):1511–25.

4 Fundamentals of Laryngeal Surgery: Approaches, Instrumentation, and Basic Microlaryngoscopic Techniques

Hans Edmund Eckel and Marc Remacle

Key Points

- The majority of laryngeal lesions are located in the mucosa or submucosal space making them easily accessible to endoscopic surgery.
- Advantages of the endoscopic approach include the avoidance of skin incisions, division of the thyroid cartilage, and tracheotomy.
- Open laryngeal surgery is required for the cartilaginous structures of the larynx, if the position of the larynx is to be altered or if the anatomical situation prevents adequate endoscopic visualisation.
- CO_2 laser systems are frequently used in laryngeal surgery, particularly in phonosurgery, stenosis surgery, and the resection of most laryngeal tumours.
- Complications of laryngeal surgery include airway fires during surgical laser use: mucosal lesions of the lips, oral cavity, and oropharynx; dental injuries; intraoperative and postoperative bleeding; and oedema.

H. E. Eckel (✉)
Department of Oto-Rhino-Laryngology, A.ö. Landeskrankenhaus Klagenfurt, HNO, Klagenfurt, Austria
e-mail: hans.eckel@kabeg.at

M. Remacle
Department of Oto-Rhino-Laryngology, Centre Hospitalier de Luxembourg – Eich, Luxembourg, Luxembourg
e-mail: remacle.marc@chl.lu

4.1 Introduction

Laryngeal surgery aims at the improvement or restoration of laryngeal function (i.e., phonation, airway protection during deglutition, and airway patency) and at the removal of neoplastic alteration of benign or malignant growths.

Essentially, laryngeal surgery can be done transorally or via an external approach. In recent years, transoral endoscopic surgery has seen enormous progress, while open surgery is now usually restricted to ablative or reconstructive surgery at the cartilaginous framework of the larynx. Adequate endoscopy, functional evaluation of voice, swallowing and respiration as needed, and imaging provide the prerequisites for indicating, planning, and performing surgery of the larynx.

4.1.1 Basic Techniques for Laryngeal Endoscopy

Laryngeal endoscopy is the mainstay of all diagnostic procedures in laryngology. It is done by transnasal flexible endoscopy, allowing for a

M. Remacle, H. E. Eckel (eds.), *Textbook of Surgery of Larynx and Trachea*,
https://doi.org/10.1007/978-3-031-09621-1_4

better evaluation of laryngeal function during phonation and swallowing, or transorally by rigid endoscopes allowing for a higher optical resolution. Rigid endoscopes are preferred for many office routine examinations because their processing after use is easier and faster as compared to flexible endoscopes. Stroboscopy may be included into the process of laryngeal endoscopy to visualise vibrating patterns of the vocal cords. Videostroboscopy is the standard in assessing voice or swallowing disorders. Fiberoptic endoscopic evaluation of swallowing has become the standard procedure in swallowing disorders [1]. High-speed digital imaging is frequency-independent and can show very short or aperiodic mucosal vibration. Enhanced endoscopy such as narrow band imaging is designed to visualise the mucosal vasculature and typical vascular patterns in neoplasia.

Direct laryngoscopy under general anaesthesia is indicated for all laryngeal diseases in which the larynx cannot be examined in the conscious patient (children) or in which mirror laryngoscopy, telescopic laryngoscopy, or flexible endoscopy has revealed findings in the larynx, hypopharynx, or trachea that require further investigation. Suspension laryngoscopy uses an identical approach but fixes the laryngoscope by means of a chest support. The surgeon's hands are free for bimanual manipulation. Using an operating microscope additionally provides a three-dimensional view of the endolaryngeal anatomy. Besides inspection of the mucosal surface with the operating microscope and introduction of rigid endoscopes, this technique allows selective excisional biopsies, even enabling the surgeon to take large samples if required. In addition, visual inspection can be supplemented by tactile examination (e.g., to assess the mobility of an ankylosed arytenoid cartilage). Currently, the CO_2 laser can be used for excisional biopsies, completely resecting smaller mucosal lesions of indeterminate nature in a procedure that is both diagnostic and therapeutic. Intraoperative rigid endoscopy with NBI has a very high sensitivity of 100% and a specificity of 95% in the distinction of severe dysplasia, CIS, or invasive cancer. Piazza et al. found a significantly higher sensitivity of intraoperative vs. preoperative endoscopy with NBI (sensitivity 98% vs. 61%) [2].

4.2 Fundamentals of Endolaryngeal Surgery and Equipment

Endolaryngeal surgery is done using Kleinsasser's microlaryngoscopy technique [3]. The patient is positioned in a supine position. A rigid laryngoscope of appropriate size is inserted through the oral cavity and the oropharynx and held in place using a chest support. The use of an operating microscope allows for three-dimensional visualisation of the endolaryngeal structures and for bimanual surgical handling of instruments inside the larynx. The basic setup is shown in Figs. 4.1 and 4.2.

Other important prerequisites are preoperative assessment of dental status, adequate mouth protection during the procedure to prevent dental injuries, and a trained, proficient surgeon. Suitable options for ventilation during general anaesthesia are the use of an endotracheal tube (using a laser-safe ventilation tube for laser-assisted procedures), jet ventilation, or mask ventilation with intermittent apnoea. The

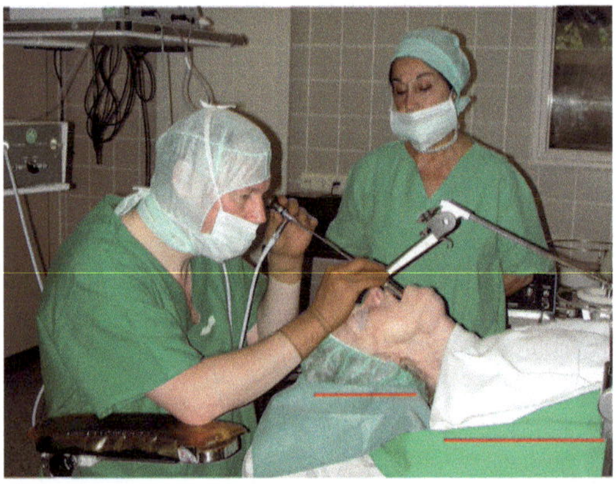

Fig. 4.1 Basic setup for direct laryngoscopy. A rigid endoscope is used to visualise the anatomical structures of larynx and trachea. Positioning of the head and body are indicated by red lines

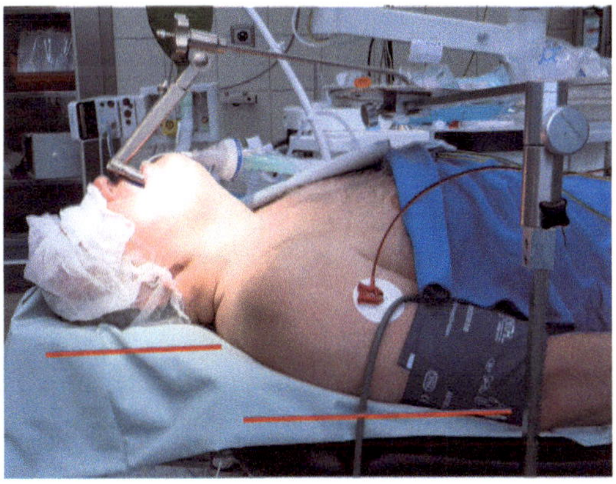

Fig. 4.2 Basic setup for microlaryngoscopic surgery

necessary equipment includes an assortment of laryngoscopes and stands, an operating microscope, micro-instruments, the CO_2 laser, monopolar cautery probes, rigid telescopes, and suction. Some procedures also require implants and their corresponding application instruments (collagen, fat, cartilage, dispersed silicone) and photographic or video equipment. The essential problems in any minimally invasive procedure, regardless of whether it is in the abdominal cavity, knee joint, or larynx, are obtaining an adequate view of the operative field and the ability to use the necessary instruments at the surgical site. In laryngeal surgery, operating laryngoscopes are employed for this purpose. Since no laryngoscope can satisfy all requirements, the laryngeal surgeon should have an assortment of different models on hand. The most important are listed below:

- Kleinsasser-type laryngoscopes (different sizes, Fig. 4.3) are still valid for microsurgery of benign laryngeal lesions. Recent modifications have been proposed by major companies for better exposition of the anterior commissure or for laser-assisted microsurgeries. Laryngoscopes are now equipped with wall-integrated channels for smoke evacuation and light guide. The inner part of the scopes should be ebonised or sandblasted to prevent laser beam reflection and to favour maximum dispersion of the beam.

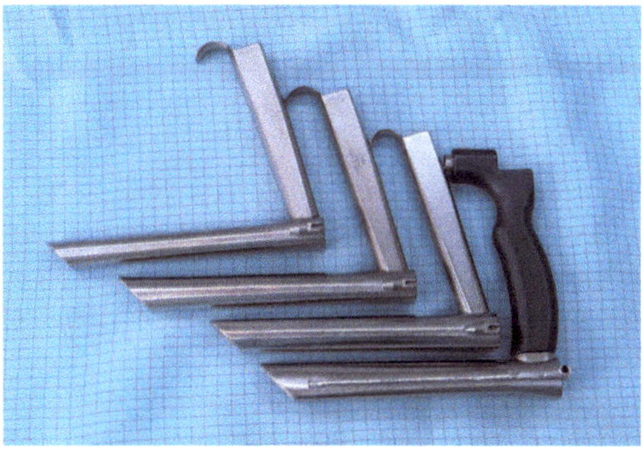

Fig. 4.3 Kleinsasser-type laryngoscopes of different sizes

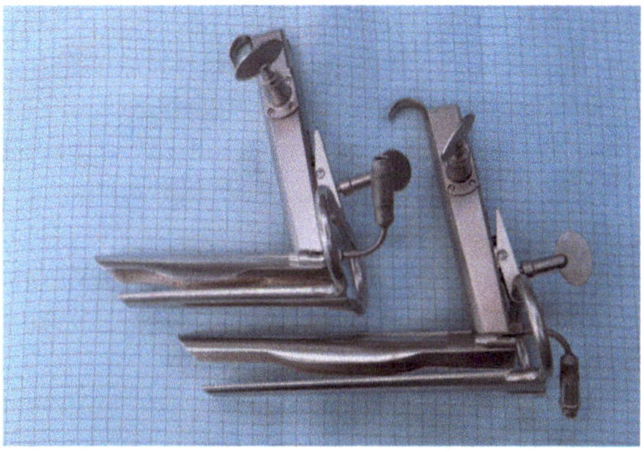

Fig. 4.4 Bivalved laryngoscope

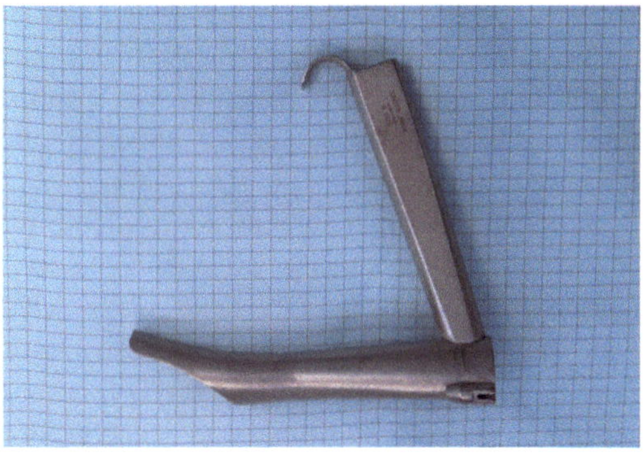

Fig. 4.5 Lindholm laryngoscope

- Bivalved laryngoscopes in various sizes are necessary for approaching the supraglottic larynx and the hypopharynx (Fig. 4.4).
- Lindholm laryngoscope, when inserted into the vallecula epiglottica, affords an excellent view of supraglottic structures (ideally of the entire larynx, Fig. 4.5).

- Diverticuloscope for endoscopic cricopharyngeal myotomy.
- Paediatric laryngoscopes (various models).

Instrumentation for endolaryngeal surgery was originally designed for cold steel microsurgery. Many of these instruments have been adapted for laser-assisted surgery with a channel for smoke evacuation.

The micro-instruments are usually all 22 cm in length, and most are paired symmetrical sets with a right and a left directed working end. The basic box should have the instruments designed originally by Kleinsasser with the thin curved forceps with serrated teeth and the cup forceps for biopsies. The Bouchayer "heart-shaped" forceps are ideal for microsurgery of the vocal fold. The head of the forceps is directed 45° to the left or right sides and 45° to the top, allowing a perfect and gentle holding of the vocal fold. Microscissors, sickle knives, and flap elevators, straight or curved, are of course mandatory for cold steel surgery.

Three to four suction tubes with different diameters are also necessary.

A monopolar electrocautery is needed for bleeding control. Electrocautery connected to a suction tube or forceps is available and can be recommended. Many surgeons just realise the coagulation by contact between a basic electrocautery blade and the suction tube or the forceps.

Stronger and larger forceps are available for endoscopic cancer surgery when bigger specimens have to be handled. The table is completed with wet towels for protection of the patient's face in case of laser-assisted surgery, swabs soaked in adrenaline solution (1:100,000) for controlling oozing and for protecting the cuff of the ventilation tube in case of laser surgery, and a silicone tooth guard or folded gauze sponge for teeth protection.

Other instruments can be necessary according to some specific surgeries like the Brünings syringe or the Ford injection device for fat, collagen, or other substances injection. These are also related to the surgeon's own preferences and experience. They are presented in the next following chapters.

4.3 Laser Systems Used in Laryngeal Endoscopic Surgery

The CO_2 laser is the undisputed workhorse of laser surgery in laryngology. Owing to its frequent use in tumour surgery, nowadays it is available in the ENT departments of most larger hospitals. Designed for surgery, its wavelength is 10,600 nm with absorption by water inducing minor peripheral thermal effects in the surrounding tissues. The CO_2 laser meets the requirements for most benign and malignant laryngeal lesions, particularly in phonosurgery, stenosis surgery, swallowing rehabilitation, and the resection of most laryngeal tumours.

The initial CO_2 laser microwave was a continuous wave (CW). At a given power, it provided continuous output. The continuous exposure resulted in much heating of collateral, non-target tissue by conduction. In order to minimise the thermal effect, pulsed mode was developed for the CO_2 laser (Sharpulse®). The thermal reduction is even more important with SuperPulse or UltraPulse waves. SuperPulse and UltraPulse are pulsed waves with high peak of power delivered in millisecond pulses or less. The resultant average pulse power, pre-set during programming, usually ranges between 1 and 10 W. The interpulse pause of approximately 1 ms, called thermal relaxing time, permits the tissue to cool. This reduces significantly the thermal effect and consequent coagulation of the area surrounding the impact. SuperPulse has higher peak power (400–500 W) than UltraPulse (200 W) but less energy because its delivering time is shorter. This pulse energy determines tissue impact and must reach the necessary threshold for ablation. Energy below ablation threshold leads to stronger thermal impact. UltraPulse adjusts its pulse energy automatically such that it is always above ablation threshold. This is not the case with SuperPulse. The SuperPulse shape is cone shaped which means that some part (the rising and falling parts) is below ablation threshold which means this part of the energy goes into tissue and heats it up more. UltraPulse is very rectangular, so one may have slightly more thermal damage with SuperPulse as compared to UltraPulse.

Besides the laser unit itself, accessories are available for the optimum delivery of laser energy to the operative site.

The micromanipulator, which is attached to the operating microscope and connected to the laser arm, yields the smallest possible beam diameter presently available, i.e., 250 µm for a focal length of 400 mm. This micromanipulator makes possible the accurate tissue incision and dissection required for phonosurgery. By means of a computer-guided system of rotating mirrors, the scanner allows the beam to sweep a given surface with extreme rapidity. This feature makes it a very effective tool when macroscopic vaporisation is required. A "shaving" effect a few microns deep is achieved during each beam sweep with very little in-depth thermal penetration. The usual shape chosen for the surface is the circle. This mode of laser use is suitable for the selective, superficial removal of mucosal lesions in cases where histologic examination is not required, and the main aim is to achieve uniform tissue ablation with the least possible collateral injury. An example is the removal of papillomas or patchy areas of leukoplakia, which can be histologically confirmed prior to actual laser ablation. The result of this procedure is a superficial mucosal wound with no thermal alteration of the underlying tissue. This type of wound undergoes rapid secondary epithelialisation and can heal to an excellent functional result.

The AcuBlade is a scanner software modification that allows the beam to travel across the target as a straight or curved incision line instead of "shaving" a given surface. Various lengths (range 0.5–3.5 mm) and penetration depths (range 0.2–2 mm) are programmable. The operator can, at all times, modify the parameters proposed by the laser-controlling software. This incision line can be rotated to the left or right thanks to a driving belt articulated with the scanner. This belt is moved with a joystick-controlled electrical motor.

The software-calculated penetration depth is based on the average absorption of the CO_2 laser by living soft tissues. Depending on the desired length and penetration, the software calculates the required power and pulse duration for the single pulse mode. The AcuBlade was designed for SuperPulse and continuous modes which can originate from the same optical cavity [4]. The AcuBlade is now available with the UltraPulse technology. The guiding system of the incision line is fully electronic and integrated in the scanner.

Incisions are sharper with UltraPulse, making the dissection more comfortable, mainly when approaching major vocal fold structure as the vocal ligament. This difference in efficiency is interesting for delicate phonosurgery of the vocal fold in single pulse mode, but this is not an advantage for other procedures as cordectomy when the shooting is usually in continuous mode. On the opposite, more coagulation along the incision line can be looked for.

The differences between SuperPulse and UltraPulse in their use for AcuBlade are only perceptible during surgery. That doesn't affect the postoperative period and the functional results.

For the selection of suitable laser parameters (pulse shape and duration, power output, etc.), the reader is referred to selected publications and to Chaps. 1, 2, and 6 of this volume.

In the treatment of laryngeal haemangioma, especially when dealing with large tumours, the neodymium-doped yttrium aluminium garnet (Nd:YAG) laser or other fibre-guided lasers with good absorption in the red like KTP or diode have the advantage of a greater penetration depth in tissue, producing deeper coagulation of the haemangioma. Nd:YAG laser emits at 1064 nm. Its frequency is doubled by passing the light through potassium titanic phosphate (KTP) to produce KTP laser, which then emits at 532 nm.

Diode laser, has a wavelength of 805 nm, which situated it between CO_2 and Nd:YAG. As a result, the tissue effects of the KTP and diode are altogether different from those of the Nd:YAG laser, mainly from the thermal effects point of view. It must be remembered that the thermal diffusion of Nd:YAG is on more than 4 mm in the surrounding tissues.

However, circumscribed haemangiomas can be successfully carefully shrunken by coagulation or excised locally with the CO_2 laser.

Argon lasers can also be used to treat vascular neoplasms owing to the absorption of the light by red blood pigment. A special laser treatment modality is photodynamic therapy (tissue lasing following the selective uptake of a photosensitizing agent). The efficacy of photodynamic therapy or PDT has been documented for a number of benign, preneoplastic, and neoplastic mucosal lesions. On the other hand, the costs of the procedure and concerns about unpredictable mucosal scarring still limit its application in the treatment of benign lesions of the larynx and trachea. PDT is more frequently used for palliative treatment of head and neck cancer untreatable anymore by surgery, radiotherapy, and/or chemotherapy.

A hollow fibre transmitting the CO_2 laser is also commercially available. So far only rough ablations or incisions are only possible.

Pulsed dye laser (PDL) which was originally developed to treat skin conditions, such as birthmarks that involve blood vessels, has been used transnasally in the office for the treatment of angiectatic polyp or Reinke's oedema. Long-term results are pending.

4.4 Robotic Surgery

Transoral robotic surgery (TORS) has shown expedited patient recovery while maintaining excellent outcomes following oropharyngectomy. The application of TORS to supraglottic laryngectomy and hypopharyngectomy has repeatedly been reported with promising initial data. The combination of the two procedures, supraglottic and hypopharyngeal TORS resection, has been adapted to successfully perform a TORS total laryngectomy [5]. A separate chapter in this book will focus in detail on current advancements of TORS in laryngeal surgery.

4.5 Endolaryngeal Versus Extralaryngeal Approach to the Larynx

The vast majority of all benign laryngeal lesions are located in the mucosa or submucosal space of the larynx, making them easily accessible to endoscopic inspection. Advantages of the endoscopic approach include the avoidance of skin incisions, division of the thyroid cartilage, or tracheotomy. Therefore, it causes less surgical trauma and related additional morbidity. As a consequence, open operations on the larynx are now considered obsolete unless surgery is required for the cartilaginous structures of the larynx, if the position of the larynx is to be altered, or if there are particular problems that prevent adequate endoscopic visualisation of the anatomic structures. In the great majority of cases, the surgical resection of benign laryngeal pathology is the only reasonable therapeutic option in cases where treatment is warranted. Except for oncological surgery, which aims at the removal of diseased structures, laryngeal surgery is driven by functional considerations, aiming at improvements of voice, deglutition, or airway patency. If doubt exists as to the nature of a given lesion, it may be prudent to leave some of the pathology behind and resect it in a later sitting if this will better preserve the functional integrity of the larynx.

For smaller glottic and supraglottic carcinomas, transoral laser-assisted surgery has become the treatment of choice at most institutions throughout Europe. The oncological results are excellent, and functional compromise is limited [4, 6].

In intermediate size glottic and supraglottic cancer, advanced concepts of open partial surgery still have a place [7]. However, these approaches may not be suitable for the vast majority of patients. In spite of their functionally excellent results in individual patients, it seems unlikely that these approaches will gain general impact on laryngeal cancer care on a larger scale.

For the treatment of advanced laryngeal and hypopharyngeal cancer, open surgery and particularly total laryngectomy with partial or circumferential pharyngectomy, along with uni- or bilateral neck dissection, have been the standard of care for most patients treated with surgery. In the vast majority of patients, this surgery can achieve local and regional control. However, the loss of normal speech and the need for a permanent tracheotomy have a deleterious impact on quality of life [8].

4.6 Anaesthesia, Perioperative Care, and Adjunctive Medical Therapy

Laryngeal surgery can be done under general endotracheal anaesthesia and using jet ventilation. Endotracheal intubation is generally preferred in operations where there is likely to be heavy bleeding (tumour resection, arytenoidectomy, laryngeal papillomatosis). Special laser-safe tubes should be used to protect against tube combustion and airway fires.

Routine intravenous administration of 250 mg methylprednisolone before endolaryngeal procedures may be considered to prevent laryngeal oedema in more extensive procedures. Antibiotic prophylaxis (e.g., 3 g ampicillin–sulbactam or 600 mg clindamycin i.v.) is also given for more extensive procedures, especially those involving the exposure of laryngeal cartilages. Patients generally require postoperative monitoring in an intensive care unit (ICU) following laser surgery for airway stenosis. For all other procedures, ICU monitoring is generally unnecessary from a surgical standpoint.

4.7 Office-Based Laryngeal Procedures

Office-based procedures have replaced endolaryngeal procedures under general anaesthesia for many indications in recent years. They will be covered separately in Chap. 12.

4.8 Complications of Endoscopic Laser Surgery

A number of authors have described complications of endoscopic laser surgery in the larynx, trachea, and hypopharynx [9, 10]. These mostly involve the combustion of ventilation tube materials and anaesthetic gas mixtures during surgical laser use in the larynx. The surgeon should consider the possibility of these complications in every laser operation and take appropriate precautions. Combustion of tube materials can be avoided by the use of laser-safe tubes. Ignition of anaesthetic gas mixtures during procedures using jet ventilation can be prevented by ventilating the patient with room air (rather than pure oxygen) and by operating in intermittent apnoea. Reports of airway fires in the current literature must be viewed more as a result of poorly trained operating room personnel than as inherent risks of laser surgery. Possible laser-associated complications are less important in endolaryngeal surgery than complications caused by the laryngoscope itself. In a study by Klussmann et al. [10], 75% of 339 consecutive microlaryngoscopy patients were found to have small mucosal lesions of the lips, oral cavity, and oropharynx. These lesions caused significant complaints for some time but resolved without squeals in a few days. Dental injuries occur in approximately 6% of all patients, but they predominantly affect patients who already have significant carious damage to the teeth, pre-existing loose teeth, periodontal disease, or a fixed denture. Figure 4.6 shows a typical avulsion of a maxillary anterior tooth during microlaryngoscopic surgery.

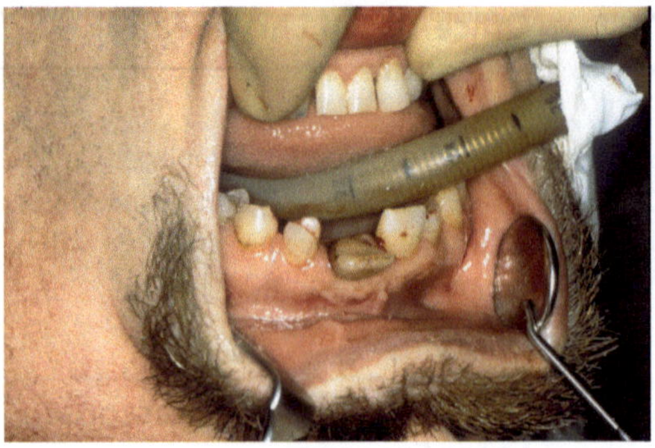

Fig. 4.6 Avulsion of a maxillary anterior tooth during microlaryngoscopic surgery

Patients with healthy dentitions did not sustain dental injuries in this study. The nature of the denture injuries ranged from simple loosening and enamel fractures to chipped teeth and complete dental displacement. No laser-associated complications were observed. Microlaryngoscopic procedures may be followed by transient functional impairment of the hypoglossal nerve and lingual nerve. By and large, this type of complication cannot be completely avoided in microlaryngoscopic surgery, but the range of complications is definitely more limited than in open laryngeal surgery. In summary, laser surgery of benign lesions of the larynx, pharynx, and trachea can be considered a minimally invasive surgical approach with a very low risk of complications.

4.9 Tips and Pearls to Avoid Complications

- Preoperative examination of patient's dental situation allows risk assessment with regard to dental injuries during microlaryngoscopic surgery.
- Different positions of the patient's head should be tried in cases of difficult laryngeal exposure.
- Comprehensive surgical equipment, including a variety of different laryngoscopes, CO_2 laser, electrocautery, microscope, and rigid endoscopes (0°, 30°, and 70°), should be available during laryngeal surgery.
- Endolaryngeal exposition of glottic and subglottic structures is best when jet ventilation is used in place of ventilation tubes.
- Special laser-safe tubes should be used to protect against tube combustion and airway fires.
- Intraoperative administration of 250 mg of methylprednisolone avoids laryngeal oedema.

References

1. Curtis JA, Seikaly ZN, Dakin AE, Troche MS. Detection of aspiration, penetration, and pharyngeal residue during flexible endoscopic evaluation of swallowing (FEES): comparing the effects of color, coating, and opacity. Dysphagia. 2020; https://doi.org/10.1007/s00455-020-10131-0.
2. Piazza C, Cocco D, De Benedetto L, Del Bon F, Nicolai P, Peretti G. Narrow band imaging and high definition television in the assessment of laryngeal cancer: a prospective study on 279 patients. Eur Arch Otorhinolaryngol. 2010;267(3):409–14. https://doi.org/10.1007/s00405-009-1121-6.
3. Kleinsasser O. Endolaryngeal microsurgery. J Otolaryngol Soc Aust. 1968;2(3):3–7.
4. Peretti G, Piazza C, Ansarin M, De Benedetto L, Cocco D, Cattaneo A, Nicolai P, Chiesa F. Transoral CO_2 laser microsurgery for Tis-T3 supraglottic squamous cell carcinomas. Eur Arch Otorhinolaryngol. 2010;267(11):1735–42. https://doi.org/10.1007/s00405-010-1284-1.
5. Lawson G, Mendelsohn AH, Van Der Vorst S, Bachy V, Remacle M. Transoral robotic surgery total laryngectomy. Laryngoscope. 2013;123(1):193–6. https://doi.org/10.1002/lary.23287.
6. Peretti G, Nicolai P, Redaelli De Zinis LO, Berlucchi M, Bazzana T, Bertoni F, Antonelli AR. Endoscopic CO_2 laser excision for tis, T1, and T2 glottic carcinomas: cure rate and prognostic factors. Otolaryngol Head Neck Surg. 2000;123(1 Pt 1):124–31.
7. Succo G, Crosetti E, Bertolin A, Piazza C, Molteni G, Cirillo S, Petracchini M, Tascone M, Sprio AE, Berta GN, Peretti G, Presutti L, Rizzotto G. Treatment

for T3 to T4a laryngeal cancer by open partial horizontal laryngectomies: prognostic impact of different pathologic tumor subcategories. Head Neck. 2018;40(9):1897–908. https://doi.org/10.1002/hed.25176.

8. Eckel HE, Bradley PJ. Treatment options for hypopharyngeal cancer. Adv Otorhinolaryngol. 2019;83:47–53. https://doi.org/10.1159/000492308.
9. Bernal-Sprekelsen M, Vilaseca-Gonzalez I, Blanch-Alejandro JL. Predictive values for aspiration after endoscopic laser resections of malignant tumors of the hypopharynx and larynx. Head Neck. 2004;26(2):103–10.
10. Klussmann JP, Knoedgen R, Wittekindt C, Damm M, Eckel HE. Complications of suspension laryngoscopy. Ann Otol Rhinol Laryngol. 2002;111(11):972–6.

Microphonosurgery Using Cold Steel

5

Declan Costello, Nicholas Gibbins, and Matthew Cherko

Key Points

- 'Cold steel' laryngeal surgery is the cornerstone of other per-oral laryngeal surgical techniques.
- Advances in instrumentation, optics and anatomical understanding have led to much more refined surgical procedures, with improved patient outcomes.
- Many laryngeal instruments are available; a core set of instruments should be available to any surgeon undertaking laryngeal surgery.

5.1 Introduction

Microphonosurgery is the bedrock of surgical management of vocal fold pathology. The vast majority of laryngeal surgery is performed using 'cold steel' instruments as a means of excising lesions, taking biopsies and altering the configuration of the vocal folds. It is important to understand and master cold steel laryngeal surgery before using other methods such as laser, powered instruments, etc. Learning the skills of handling the steel instruments will give the trainee surgeon a good appreciation of the mechanics of the larynx, along with the biomechanical properties of the vocal folds. In this way, the surgeon can learn how best to use a range of instruments to treat vocal fold pathology.

Palpation of the vocal folds under general anaesthetic gives the surgeon a good understanding of the nature of the epithelial surfaces and can help to uncover lesions that are sometimes not seen in the clinic. Furthermore, it is very important to develop the skills of correct placement of the laryngoscope in order to maximise exposure of the vocal folds for other forms of treatment such as laser surgery. As in all forms of surgery, access and exposure are the key to a successful ability to operate on the surgical target. In addition to correct placement of the laryngoscope, the choice of laryngoscope is a significant factor in successful surgical exposure of the vocal folds.

The fundamental pieces of equipment required for phonomicrosurgery are as follows:

- Laryngoscope—in general, this should be the largest laryngoscope that can be introduced into the patient's mouth (see below) to give

D. Costello (✉)
Wexham Park Hospital, Slough, UK
e-mail: d.costello@nhs.net

N. Gibbins
University Hospital Lewisham, London, UK
e-mail: Nicholas.gibbins@nhs.net

M. Cherko
National Centre for Airway Reconstruction, Charing Cross Hospital, Imperial College Healthcare NHS Trust, London, UK
e-mail: m.cherko@nhs.net

M. Remacle, H. E. Eckel (eds.), *Textbook of Surgery of Larynx and Trachea*,
https://doi.org/10.1007/978-3-031-09621-1_5

the best possible access. However, it is important to have a selection of laryngoscopes available for different situations.
- Mouth guard for protection of the teeth.
- Suspension arm.
- Microscope—with a lens of 400 mm working distance.
- Phonomicrosurgical instruments (palpators, scissors, forceps, blades, etc.).
- Endoscopes—0°, 30° and 45° are all very useful in different situations.

5.2 History of Phonomicrosurgery

The history of laryngology is vast, and many pioneers have made significant contributions to the field we now know, spanning well over 100 years. The focus of this section is to highlight some of the key milestones and contributions to the development of modern day phonomicrosurgery.

5.2.1 Development of Laryngoscopy

Breaking away from mirror laryngoscopy that had pre-dated his technique, Kirstein introduced direct laryngoscopy ('autoscopy') in 1895 [1] and described the removal of a vocal cord tumour with the intention to improve voice. He performed autoscopy with the patient in a sitting position, with the neck flexed in relation to the chest and the head extended at the atlantooccipital joint. In the early 1900s, Chevalier Jackson would adapt this technique to recreate the 'sniffing position' in a supine patient with an assistant elevating the head (the Boyce-Jackson position), providing optimal exposure of the vocal folds for phonosurgery [2].

Jackson adapted the use of a spatula to design his own laryngoscope adding a proximal tube and eventually incorporating distal illumination via a light carrier [3]. He also devised means to deliver suction capability distally, a feature which nowadays resides as a smoke extractor facility to enhance the use of laser. At the same time, Gustav Killian had described suspension laryngoscopy to allow the operator to free both hands for instrumentation [4]. The combination of optimal positioning and suspension is a cornerstone of current practice in laryngeal surgery.

Recognising the importance of magnification, Wilhelm Brünings and Jackson first used a monocular microscope in the 1950s to perform microlaryngeal surgery. This would soon be complemented by the invention of the binocular operating microscope which provided essential depth perception. Subsequently, Harold Hopkins' invention of the fibreoptic endoscope in 1954 hailed a new era in visualisation of the larynx and diagnosis of laryngeal pathology [5]. The additional element of stroboscopy that followed revealed the vibratory mucosal waveform—a key concept in understanding disorders of phonation.

5.2.2 Evolution of Phonosurgery

The term phonosurgery was eventually formally coined by Hans von Leden and Godfrey Arnold in the early 1960s [6]. It was in that decade that several major developments spurred on the practice of operating to improve or restore voice. Oskar Kleinsasser, professor of Otolaryngology at the University of Marburg, not only developed new instruments for microlaryngeal surgery but also collaborated with optical systems manufacturer Carl Zeiss to produce a 400 mm focal length lens operating microscope for laryngeal surgery [7]. The magnification and binocular vision provided allowed far greater precision in both assessing and instrumenting the larynx.

However, there was a limit to the surgical precision afforded when operating on an awake patient. General endotracheal anaesthesia with muscular paralysis paved the way for much more precise endolaryngeal surgery, releasing the limitation that local anaesthetic procedures were plagued with prior [8]. The rapidly progressing practice of direct laryngoscopy did not make its counterpart indirect laryngoscopy obsolete, as its role within the field was still being adapted. Karel

Sedlacek was a particular advocate, operating on a topicalised larynx in an awake patient to allow for real-time feedback of the voice [9].

Minoru Hirano, professor of otolaryngology in Japan, detailed the complex layered microstructure of the vocal folds and described the cover-body theory of vocal fold vibration [10]. He recognised that varying the tension and flexibility in the vocal fold was responsible for altering vocal register and intensity. This understanding led to an adaptation of the term phonosurgery to phono*micro*surgery—describing the technique of maximal preservation of the vocal fold microstructure [11]. The important principles of utilising the microflap approach to dissect within natural anatomical planes avoid injury to the underlying vocal ligament and preserve as much of the overlying vocal fold mucosa had gained recognition amongst experts in the field [12].

5.2.3 Voice Altering Surgery

In 1911, Wilhelm Brünings was the first to describe medialisation of the vocal fold with augmentation using an injection of paraffin [13]. This was later abandoned due to the unfortunate development of paraffinomas. Teflon as an alternative was popularised and then also plagued with foreign body reaction and granuloma formation and so the search for more inert material went on, eventually settling on the acceptability of calcium hydroxylapatite, autologous fat or hyaluronic acid that are used today. Laryngeal injection continued as a theme with the introduction of botulinum toxin as a treatment for spasmodic dysphonia, described by Andrew Blitzer as a less radical form of treatment compared to Herbert Dedo's recurrent laryngeal nerve section [14].

Whilst Nobuhiko Isshiki, a pioneer in laryngeal framework surgery, famously categorised thyroplasties in 1976 [15], Jurgen Wendler described a microscopic technique as an alternative to the type IV operation in the aim of voice feminisation, which he termed glottoplasty. The ability to laser ablate the epithelium of the anterior vocal folds and suture the edges together, to effectively shorten the vibrating length of the vocal folds, is a tribute to the development in the field of phonomicrosurgery, and many modern-day laryngologists have contributed to finessing the practice further including Robert Sataloff and Steven Zeitels, to name a couple.

5.2.4 Instruments and Devices

The introduction of lasers expanded the laryngologist's array of instruments. In the early 1970s, the CO_2 laser was integrated with the operating microscope via a micromanipulator, providing excellent control and precision [11]. As well as allowing excision of benign and malignant laryngeal lesions, laser was also being used to perform arytenoidectomy to restore the airway in patients with bilateral permanent vocal cord palsy. The KTP laser also gained credit in treating vascular lesions of the larynx due to its wavelength targeting absorption by haemoglobin.

Despite its expanding use, the caveat to the use of laser energy is collateral thermal damage, which risks scarring and subsequent disruption of the mucosal waveform [12]. For this reason, as well the tactile feedback provided, cold steel dissection has strongly maintained its place in phonomicrosurgery, particularly for benign avascular lesions where the aim is to preserve native mucosa and minimise collateral injury. The appreciation of cold steel surgery has been evident in the engineering and production of more refined specialist instruments, such as those contributed by Marc Bouchayer, who is also credited for expanding the understanding of benign vocal fold lesions such as epidermoid cysts and mucosal bridges.

The addition of modern powered tools and energy devices has further augmented the ability of the laryngologist in dealing with pathology. The laryngeal microdebrider (Medtronic, USA) and laryngeal wand coblator (Smith & Nephew, UK) are examples of more recent additions to the laryngologists' toolkit and have both been utilised to effectively debride laryngeal papilloma.

Together with the advances in imaging with more powerful endoscopes and image processing technology (see later sections in chapter), the ability to diagnose and treat lesions affecting the voice is now a hugely established and well-equipped practice, emanating from scientific discovery and visionary clinical innovation.

5.3 Operating Laryngoscopes

Over 50 different types of operating laryngoscope have been developed over the 125 years since Kirstein first described his autoscope in 1895 (Fig. 5.1), with some of the most commonly used being the Lindholm, Dedo-Pilling, Kleinsasser and Rhys-Evans laryngoscopes and the Zeitels glottiscope. Looking at all these, there are features that they have in common and that remain as important today as they did in 1895.

5.3.1 Basic Components

The laryngoscope must be a straight solid barrel shape and made of a solid material to prevent collapse. This stops the tongue from obscuring the view and allows easy suctioning. They are typically made from steel. There must be a way of passing adequate light through the scope. This can be by a light cable attachment integrated into the scope or a detachable light carrier to the side(s) or clipped to the underside of the scope. The proximal end of the scope is wider than the distal end to allow easier instrumentation. Lastly there must be a suitable handle with an attachment to allow suspension. This must be stable enough to hold the scope in position whilst operating.

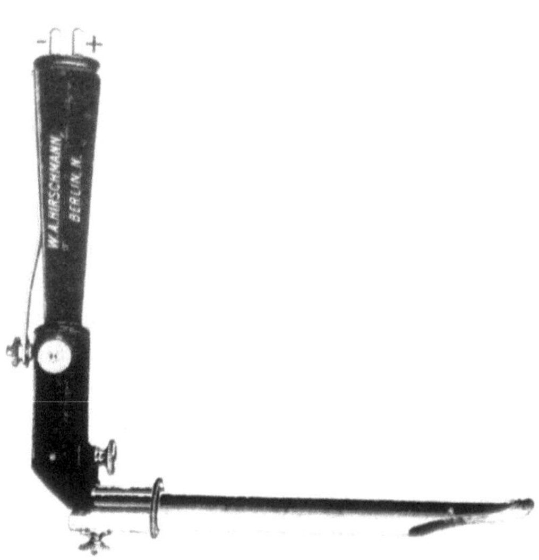

Fig. 5.1 Kirstein's original autoscope. Note how little has changed to the overall structure in 125 years. (Medical Historical Library, Harvey Cushing/John Hay Whitney Medical Library, Yale University—reprinted with permission)

There are many excellent operating laryngoscopes on the market to cater for every type of surgery and surgeon. This will not be an exhaustive review of all but will point out areas that might need to be looked at by surgeons when selecting their laryngoscope of choice. There is no one laryngoscope that is better than the others and that it is a personal choice. For example, the Lindholm laryngoscope has a wider anterior blade that is placed in the vallecula. Elevation of the laryngoscope anteriorly pushes the tongue forwards and the epiglottis retracted along with it. However, in some cases, the elastic cartilage of the epiglottis is so lax, or it is placed in such an extreme retroflexed position that it is impossible to view the whole larynx with this scope and the blade needs to be passed posterior to the epiglottis, or another style of laryngoscope used, to obtain a view. The majority of laryngoscopes are placed posterior to the epiglottis and, along with the tongue tissues, are elevated anteriorly in one movement.

All manufacturers of operating laryngoscopes offer a wide range; this includes variety in width to allow for any size of patient from neonate to adult and a variety of lengths to encompass the whole spectrum of human anatomy from the high larynx and short neck of a neonate to the very long neck and low laryngeal position of a tall adult.

The distal end of the laryngoscope is usually a rounded isosceles triangle, but for the anteriorly placed larynx, an anterior commissure scope can be used which has both a more acute anterior angle and extends more anteriorly.

This chapter will not be covering oesophagoscopes or bronchoscopes, both of which could merit a chapter. Often, these pieces of equipment are used at the same time as the operating laryngoscope and should be a part of the laryngologist's armamentarium.

5.3.2 Additional Components

Components have been added to the basic structure of the laryngoscope over the years as other technologies have been developed (e.g. laser). These usually come as standard with the laryngoscope and include a jet needle that can be attached to allow low-frequency (handheld) jet ventilation and a similar needle for suction of laser plume. Low-frequency jet ventilation was a very common practice but is slowly being replaced by high-frequency jet ventilation. This requires more specialist equipment discussed below.

5.3.3 Extended Components

5.3.3.1 Laser

Further adaptations include laryngoscopes with a matte finish for CO_2 laser use. The matte finish prevents reflection of the laser beam off the insides of the metal laryngoscope which causes unwanted tissue damage.

5.3.3.2 Distending

To obtain an improved view of the supraglottis, posterior glottis and post-cricoid space, a laryngoscope with distending capabilities can be used to give a wider field of view. The anterior and posterior blades of the scope function independently so that, once inserted, the blades can be distracted. Usually the blades come apart parallel to each other as there is one degree of movement. However, the Weerda bivalved pharyngoscope (most commonly used for the endoscopic approach to a Zenker's diverticulum) has two degrees of movement; the first is distraction of the blades parallel to each other, and the second is to separate the distal tips of the blades.

5.3.3.3 Distending with Laser

Using a distending laryngoscope, or laryngopharyngoscope, to approach the glottis or supraglottis gives an excellent view. However, as the blades separate, the barrel nature of the standard operating laryngoscope is lost. Using laser in this situation increases the risk of unwanted tissue damage so scopes with side flaps that cover the lateral spaces are available.

5.3.3.4 Angled Scopes

Occasionally the larynx is so anteriorly placed that no amount of manipulation or the use of different scopes will give an adequate view. In these instances, the use of a laryngoscope with a 'duckbill'-shaped anterior lip with a port to insert and hold an angled endoscope can be helpful.

5.3.3.5 High-Frequency Jet Ventilation

The use of high-frequency jet ventilation is particularly useful for subglottic stenosis and other airway work, having been developed specifically for laryngotracheal surgery. This requires specific laryngoscopes with various attachments for both high- and low-frequency jet gas, airway pressure and gas monitoring and humidification, as well as the essential illumination.

5.4 Operating Microscopes

Otolaryngology has always been at the forefront of the use of operating microscopes. The first surgeon to use the microscope to aid an operation was the Swedish otologist Carl-Olof Siggram Nylén in 1921 for inner ear surgery. Gynaecologists, especially in Germany, took up the use of the microscope for cervical visualisation with the colposcope with enthusiasm, but in ENT the next step forwards was by Dr. Horst Wullstein of the Würzburg Department of ENT. He used his microscope to mobilise the stapes, and it had some of the fundamental workings that one still finds today and that are the cornerstone of the operating microscope, a magnification changer, coaxial illumination and choice of working distances.

Further additions added over the following 60 years included camera attachments, double microscopes or sidearm observer tubes, motorised zoom (via controls on the handles or foot pedals), ceiling mounts and so on. Divergence of the working details of the operating microscope was introduced according to the specialty it was being used by; specifications for neurosurgery, ophthalmology, gynaecology, urology and neurosurgery have all been added and continue to improve the view and adaptability of its use. The operating microscope has now moved from being an option to a necessity.

However, the standard requirements for all operating microscopes have remained the same; binocular vision, a long working distance (to get one's hands and instruments into the operative field), stability, and adequate even light over the whole field. In the modern operating theatre and surgical practice, the ability to attach a camera, photo-document and record the procedure is now also considered mandatory. In the future, integration with image guidance technology and a variety of light filters or fluorescence will almost certainly become standard.

Zeiss can be said to have produced the first modern surgical operating microscope in 1953. However, other companies also make excellent microscopes including Leica Microsystems; smaller companies such as Visine Industries (dental and otolaryngology) and Topcon (ophthalmic and general use) produce microscopes with fewer features. Nikon and Olympus make a wide range of endoscopes but have not ventured into the microscope market, which will be discussed later in the chapter. There are also leasing companies that offer several models of the microscopes mentioned. In the authors' experience, applying for funds to buy a new microscope is easier if one is able to demonstrate that it can be used by a number of different specialities, spreading the cost.

5.4.1 Setup

Unless they are ceiling mounted, the operating microscope is a large piece of equipment, creating a sizeable footprint in the operating theatre. Along with the trays of equipment, recording stack system, anaesthetic equipment and all the staff, this means that ensuring everything has a dedicated space becomes very important. Having all the equipment on the same side of the patient means that space becomes cramped, movement through the theatre is less efficient, and reacting to an emergent situation is slower. Ensuring that there is an ordered approach to setting up the equipment is essential.

There are of course many ways of placing equipment in the operating theatre environment, but the following is suggested:

1. Anaesthetic equipment (inc. jet ventilation, thrive/optiflow, etc.) on the left-hand side at the foot of the patient.
2. If you are right-handed, the operating equipment/trays are to your immediate right with the scrub nurse.
3. The recording stack system stands just distal to the operating equipment on the same side. Most have a dual screen setup with a large screen for the main view (facing the surgeon) and a smaller screen with recording capability. Turn the smaller screen towards the anaesthetist so that they can see the airway; they feel reassured to be able to see what is going on, especially when ventilating with tubeless ventilation techniques (e.g. jet ventilation).
4. The operating microscope is placed on the left-hand side of the patient. If used, the laser would also be attached on the left-hand side with the microscope.

If you are left-handed, then swap the equipment around so that the equipment is on the left so that instruments are handed to your dominant hand.

5.4.2 Laser

Lasers and the safety aspects of using them will be discussed in another chapter. They must be mentioned briefly here as they are intimately related to the operating microscope setup. The most commonly used in the head and neck is the CO_2 laser that has both direct line-of-sight laser beam and handheld fibre devices. However, using the CO_2 laser beam requires the use of a micro-manipulator that is attached to the microscope. Without the laser, the operating microscope has a wide range of focal lengths, but using the laser mandates a fixed focal length of 400 mm to allow a sharp focussed laser point.

5.5 Rigid Endoscopes

5.5.1 A Brief History

The endoscope was first described by Philipp Bozzini in the early nineteenth century. His invention, the 'Lichtleiter', allowed illuminated visualisation of internal body cavities through delivery of candlelight via angled mirrors [16]. The term endoscopy (specifically l'endoscopie) was first coined in 1853 by French surgeon Antonin J. Desormeaux, lending him the title 'Father of endoscopy'. He produced and utilised an instrument to visualise internal body cavities, and his key concepts of passing a light source through a rigid tube with an internal lens system have been retained in the design of rigid endoscopes thereafter. A series of improvements by Kussmaul, Nitze and Fourestier followed [17, 18]. However, it was the coming together of Harold Hopkins, a professor of applied optics, with the precision medical instrument manufacturer, Karl Storz, in 1965 that really transformed the business of medical endoscopy [19, 20]. They engineered the revolutionary Hopkin's rod-lens system, reversing the traditional arrangement between glass and air within the scope (see Fig. 5.2) and producing an image with superior brilliance, image quality and viewing angles. Coupled with the invention of the video computer chip in the mid-1980s [21], it is now used ubiquitously in modern-day clinical practice worldwide. Although popularised in laparoscopic surgery, the endoluminal use of endoscopes in ENT soon after became established. This provided the laryngologist an alternative means of imaging the larynx both in the clinic setting and in the operating theatre—the latter will be a focus in this section.

5.5.2 Specification

Rigid endoscopes are produced by several manufacturers worldwide, with the leading five being Karl Storz, Olympus, Stryker, Richard Wolf and B. Braun. The main distinguishing criteria in a manufacturer's range are the length and calibre of the endoscope and the angulation of the distal lens. Generally, for use in operative laryngology, the calibre may range from 4 to 10 mm, the length from 20 to 30 cm and the angle between 0 and 70°. Advancements in the design of the rigid

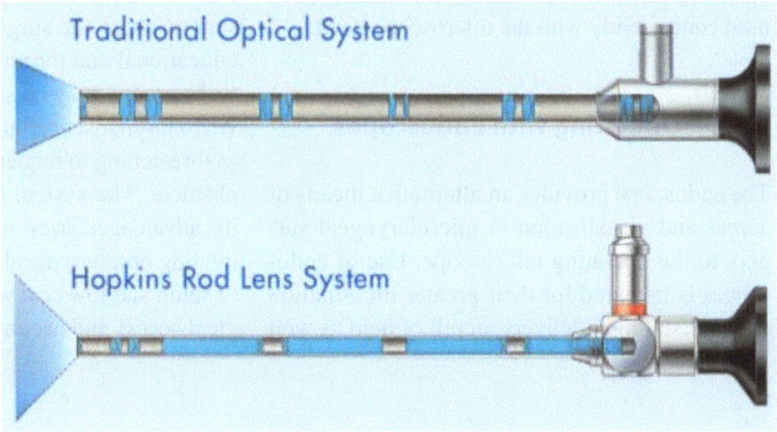

Fig. 5.2 The Hopkin's rod used longer glass rods, spaced with 'air lenses' to achieve better optics compared to the conventional configuration of long air spaces between thin glass lenses

endoscope (initially developed by Harold Hopkins, Fig. 5.2) have introduced both multi-angle scopes and 3D scopes, but their use has not of yet become mainstream in laryngology.

5.5.3 Setup

Although the endoscope in itself is a relatively small instrument, for its use in operative laryngoscopy, it should be coupled with a light delivery and video stack system. Portable light packs have been designed to attach to the light port of the rigid endoscope and may prove their weight in gold in urgent life-saving manoeuvres within an emergency airway pack with an endotracheal tube railroaded over the endoscope. However, to ensure high-quality and reliable light in the operating theatre, a cold light fountain is generally used. Traditional halogen light systems have been replaced by modern Xenon or LED light sources, producing higher brightness and more natural colour temperatures of 6000–6400 K.

Multiple video stack systems have been designed to relay the image from the camera to a display device. Although the quality of an HD system has proved more than ample to operate with for many years now, the more recent introduction of 4K and even 8K ultra high-definition systems on larger displays produces exceptional image quality and resolution—well suited to the delicacy involved in microphonosurgical procedures [22]. Overall, akin to the use of the operating microscope, this setup uses a fair amount of operating theatre real estate, especially when used concurrently with the microscope itself.

5.5.4 Operating with Endoscopes

The endoscope provides an alternative means of access and visualisation in microlaryngeal surgery to the operating microscope. Use of endoscopes is favoured for their greater illumination due to distal light delivery, depth of field as well as ability to enhance visualisation of microscopic 'blind zones' (such as the ventricles, anterior commissure and inferior border of vocal folds)—especially if angled scopes are utilised.

In order to combat the issue of single-handed operating whilst holding the endoscope, their use can be combined with video laryngoscopes whereby the endoscope is mounted in a channel within the specialist laryngoscope to allow hands-free access to the larynx. Examples of such scopes include the original Kantor-Berci scope, or the newer Havas operating laryngoscope (Karl Storz, Germany).

5.5.5 Exoscopy

Exoscopy, an emerging technique in surgery, describes the technique of extracorporeal imaging in contrast to the scope being placed within the body. The Vitom 3D Exoscopic System is a video telescope operating microscope (VITOM®) introduced by Karl Storz (Germany). Initially used in other surgical fields, the system has been adopted by ENT with its use in operative laryngology first described by Carlucci et al. in 2012 [23]. The benefits it may provide in laryngology are its compatibility with classical microlaryngeal operating instruments, integration with imaging techniques such as blue light and the integration of the CO_2 laser micromanipulator [24]. Unlike the limitation of the microscope to allowing only the primary operator the depth of field view, the exoscope setup allows all theatre staff to share the surgeon's view, improving the educational and training aspect of the surgery.

Exoscopy may be seen as the successor to the video laryngoscope but has been touted by some as threatening to render the operating microscope obsolete. The system has even been praised for its advantages over robotic-assisted surgery in treating oropharyngeal cancer in terms of its ease of setup and low cost whilst still maintaining surgical access and accuracy [25].

5.6 Instruments

When considering phonomicrosurgery (PMS) with cold steel instruments, one can be overwhelmed by the array of instruments on offer. A standard tray comes with several layers of instruments. As each tray is removed from the packaging and laid on the scrub table, they seem to spread, and due to their necessary long thin design, they can get mixed up very easily. Every set of instruments that one can purchase has a number of instruments that are essential and standard but also has a few instruments particular to that set. These specific pieces will not be discussed here as they only become useful if one has performed many hundreds of procedures and you deem that a specific pathology needs a specific instrument to help you.

However, there are a series of instruments that are fundamental in the practice of PMS that will be discussed here in generic terms. Each company will have their own version, and the authors do not prefer one over another. The discussion here will be around the minimum basic instrumentation that is needed to perform almost all procedures that you will encounter. These are the instruments that are used for the majority of cold steel operating.

5.6.1 Forceps

Heart-shaped forceps and 'crocodile' or micro-forceps to the right and left (Figs. 5.3 and 5.4).

Like any surgery, PMS relies on good lighting (covered under operating microscopes) and good retraction. These forceps are critical to good PMS. The heart-shaped forceps allow non-traumatic handling of the vocal fold and retraction of its epithelium towards the midline. The pressure of the forceps is spread along a wide front thereby reducing the trauma to the epithelium. The inner aspect of forceps is gently ridged, as opposed to smooth, to reduce the amount of force needed to grasp the tissue without it slipping through.

The 'crocodile' or micro-forceps are used when grasping a specific target (epidermoid

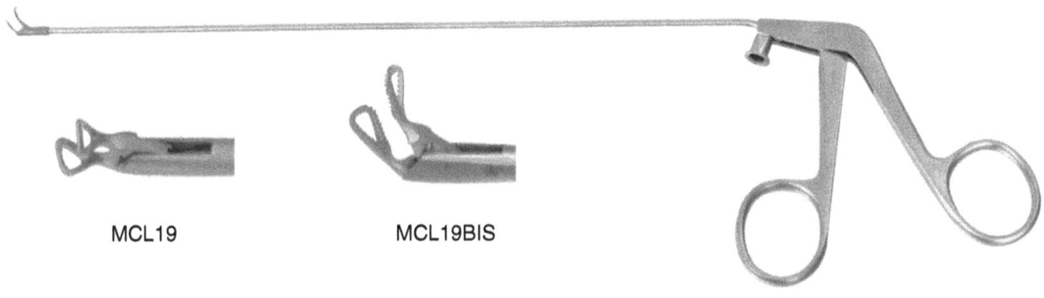

Fig. 5.3 Bouchayer 'heart-shaped' forceps

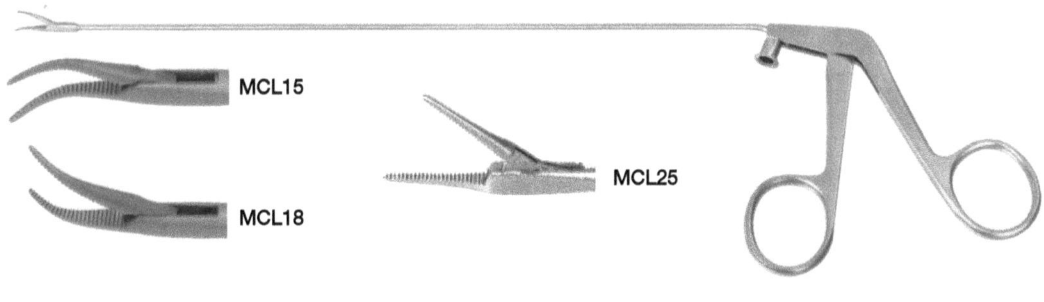

Fig. 5.4 Bouchayer 'crocodile' forceps

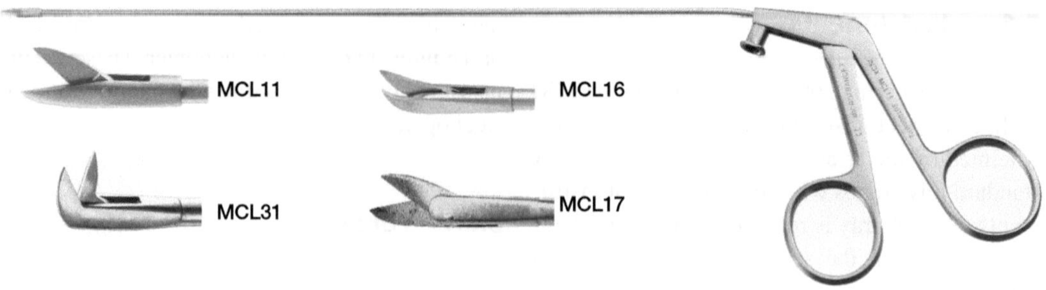

Fig. 5.5 Bouchayer scissors

Fig. 5.6 Lancet blade

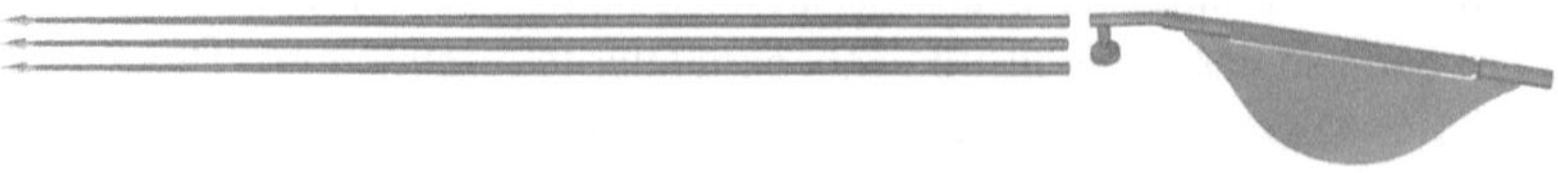

cyst once the cordotomy has been produced, scar tissue) rather than for retracting the whole vocal fold. They are more precise and targeted but subsequently need more closing pressure to ensure the tissue does not slip through the blades.

5.6.2 Scissors/Blades

Curved scissors to the right and left (Fig. 5.5).

Scissors can be curved or straight. Those pictured are curved and are used to cut through any tissue that the blunt dissectors (below) are unable to go through. If the dissector does not easily go through tissue, then it is important not to use force. This can indicate that the tissue is fibrous and needs to be cut. For example, epidermoid cysts are often tethered anteriorly and posteriorly. The medial and lateral edges of the cyst are cleared easily with the blunt dissectors, and it is tempting to try to excise the whole cyst with this instrument, but it is doomed to failure without using the scissors to cut these fibrous strands.

Blades come in many forms all of which have their pros and cons. Any blade used in the larynx needs to be very sharp and stay so. Many surgeons prefer disposable blades that can be used for one operation and discarded before they lose their sharpness (Fig. 5.6).

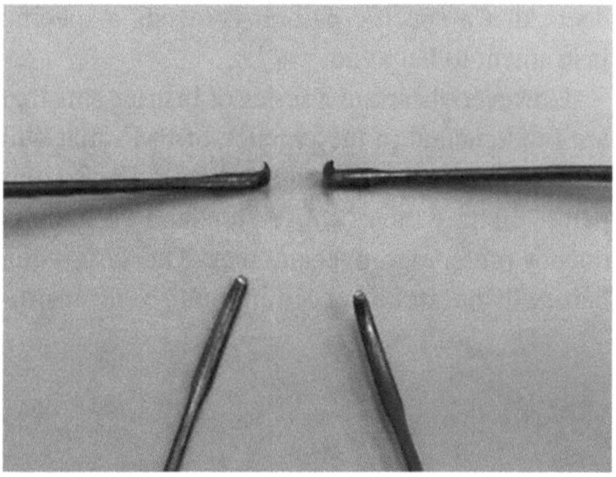

Fig. 5.7 Curved elevators

5.6.3 Blunt Dissectors/Elevators

Curved and 90° elevators to the right and left (Figs. 5.7 and 5.8).

Blunt dissectors are vital for the majority of dissection under the epithelium or within the SLP. Once the pathology has been retracted using the forceps described above, it is removed by isolating it using the retractors described above and the tissue around it peeled off using the dissector. This causes the minimum disruption to the SLP, and, with the dissection being blunt rather than sharp, the hypothesis is that less trauma to the layers of collagen fibres in the SLP occurs, less scarring occurs, and therefore it is more likely that the vocal fold vibration is maintained.

Fig. 5.8 Bouchayer palpator

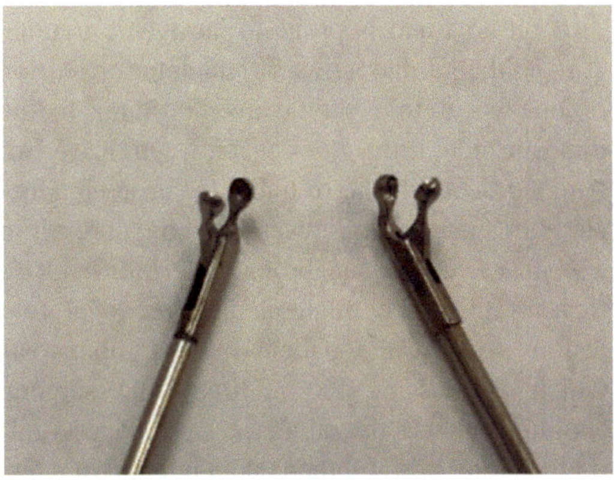

Fig. 5.9 Cupped biopsy forceps

5.6.4 Biopsy Forceps

Cupped biopsy forceps to the right and left (Fig. 5.9).

Cupped biopsy forceps are used when a pathology is unable to be removed in toto and a sample needs to be taken for histological analysis. It is the author's experience that using the biopsy forceps in the contralateral hand (i.e. forceps to the left are held in the right hand) and using the other hand to manipulate the larynx is the most controlled way to take a biopsy. The laryngeal pathology can be gently pushed into the forceps, reducing the tremor from the operating hand.

5.6.5 Microdebrider

A small microdebrider is a popular method of debulking laryngeal tumours or for the removal of laryngeal papillomatosis. The debrider has a rotating end with sharp edges to cut the tissue and is attached to suction so that tissue is sucked into and up the centre of the debrider. The standard technique is to suck the tissue into the open debrider, retract it away from the normal tissue and then press the pedal to activate the rotating end. The 2.9 mm diameter microdebrider, or laryngeal 'skimmer', is the standard equipment of choice for most paediatric ENT surgeons with laryngeal papillomatosis. Like all instruments, care must be taken not to cause damage to the underlying tissues, and laryngeal webs and granulomas have been reported following its use.

5.6.6 Monopolar Diathermy

Diathermy is used either to stem bleeding that is occurring or to prevent bleeding from happening by cauterising feeding vessels to a pathology.

5.7 Principles of Phonomicrosurgery

An understanding of the layered microstructure of the vocal folds is critical to successful phonomicrosurgery. Normal phonation relies on several factors, including vocal folds with straight edges, with good closure and with normal pliability (the so-called mucosal wave seen on stroboscopic examination). The principle of any operation on the vocal folds is to try to retain this layered microstructure, in order to allow normal pliability to be restored. In particular, the integrity and maintenance of the superficial lamina propria are vital in allowing the vocal fold to remain supple and pliable and hence for normal vibration to occur during phonation.

The importance of the **superficial lamina propria** (Reinke's space) cannot be overstated. If this anatomical space is disrupted or if there is extensive dissection, the healing epithelium can become tethered to the underlying ligament (intermediate and deep lamina propria)—this will result in a loss of pliability of the vocal fold—in other words, a scar. Resolving scarring of the vocal folds is an immensely challenging situation, so it is critical to minimise the risk of this occurring in the first place.

Some lesions are situated anatomically in the superficial lamina propria, so dissection in this plane is unavoidable. This is particularly true for vocal fold intracordal cysts.

The use of the **suction tube** should be done with the utmost care as it can cause significant trauma if misused. In particular, a selection of suction tubes should be available, and in general fine sucker should be used where possible. Some further factors should be considered when using suction:

1. The suction machine should be set to a low power so as to avoid excessive negative pressure at the tip of the suction tube.
2. If a superior cordotomy is made, and hence the superficial lamina propria is exposed, it is important not to suction directly into the subepithelial layer.
3. Covering the occlusion finger hole on the suction handpiece will increase the suction intensity; it should only be covered when the tip is not touching any critical tissues—for example, the vocal fold itself or any vascular areas. The occlusion hole can be safely covered when, for example, suctioning secretions in the subglottis or in the pharynx.

In general, it is important not to dissect too deeply in the vocal fold. In other words, dissection should be limited to the most superficial tissues possible so as to preserve the subepithelial tissues.

When removing epithelial lesions, it is inevitable that there will be an epithelial defect created; this should be as small an area as possible. Where feasible, any redundant epithelial tissue should be used to cover the subepithelial space. The initial healing of the vocal fold is relatively rapid: the epithelium will largely be reformed within 2 days of surgery (this is the basis of voice rest post-operatively).

If a large lesion is being removed (e.g. gross Reinke's oedema), this will leave a significant defect (and exposed superficial lamina propria) if the whole lesion is simply excised. In this situation, it is preferable to try to preserve some of the overlying mucosa so that the remaining defect can be covered.

The **anterior commissure** is a particularly difficult area and is prone to iatrogenic trauma. Any epithelial dissection on the anterior portion of one vocal fold should avoid trauma to the opposite side; if this does occur, it will leave two bare surfaces which are liable to cause an adhesion (an anterior glottic web) which can result in a poor voice and can be extremely difficult to treat. If there are bilateral anterior vocal fold lesions (e.g. if the patient has papillomatosis which is crossing the midline), the surgeon should consider operating in two stages—initially on one side and then (at an interval of a few weeks) on the other. This will minimise the risk of an anterior glottic web.

5.8 Setup for Cold Steel Microlaryngoscopy

The principles of the setup for cold steel microlaryngoscopy are described elsewhere (Chap. 4), but it is important to bear in mind a few elements when planning phonomicrosurgery.

5.8.1 Choice of Laryngoscope

Adequate exposure of the focal folds is critical in facilitating successful surgical treatment. In general, the largest laryngoscope possible will be the optimal choice. In the authors' practice, the **Lindholm** laryngoscope is an excellent option: with its wide proximal opening, it allows the surgeon a large degree of movement of the hands, which in turn results in easier manipulation and dissection of the vocal folds. If the patient's anatomy does not allow the use of a large laryngoscope, the surgeon can move through a choice of other scopes, including the Rhys-Evans, Kleinsasser, Dedo-Pilling or (in extremis) the anterior commissure laryngoscope.

5.8.2 Position of the Patient

Microlaryngeal surgery requires a straight line of sight down the middle of the laryngoscope to the vocal folds. It is important that the patient is positioned to gain the best possible view of the vocal folds. This is best achieved in a position of 'sniffing the morning air'—in other words, flexion at the thoracocervical junction and extension at the craniocervical junction. Extension of the whole neck is **not** helpful. In general, the patient's head should be supported on a head ring or may require no support at all. A shoulder support is not required.

5.8.3 Introducing the Laryngoscope

A suitable tooth shield is placed on the patient's upper incisors. The laryngoscope is placed in the patient's mouth, ensuring that the lips are not traumatised. The laryngoscope is advanced into the oropharynx and then directed towards the larynx. At all times, it is important to avoid pressure on the teeth. If the vocal folds are not easily seen, the head should be *lifted* (not, as is sometimes seen, lowered)—this exaggerates the flexion at the thoracocervical junction and extension at the craniocervical junction.

When an adequate view of the vocal folds has been achieved, the suspension arm is attached and tightened so that it is supported on a Mayo table (or similar) clamped to the operating table.

The choice of surgical technique to treat vocal fold lesions will depend on the position and nature of the lesion itself.

5.8.4 Position of the Surgeon

It is important that the surgeon is comfortable when performing microlaryngeal surgery and that he/she achieves stability of the arms and hands, with the microscope eye pieces at a comfortable height. The forearms should be resting on the chair for stability: some operating departments have chairs with specific arm rests; an alternative is to use a standard operating chair and to turn the seat around by 180° and simply rest the arms on the back of the chair.

If required, the patient's position can be changed to ensure that the surgeon sits in a reasonable position.

5.8.5 The 'Difficult' Laryngoscopy

A good view of the vocal folds is paramount for successful microlaryngeal surgery but can be difficult to achieve. Certain anatomical features can make it difficult to introduce the laryngoscope: the most common issues are limited mouth opening or neck stiffness. Mandibular retrusion and/or prominent incisors are also problematic. Macroglossia is rare but can impede laryngoscopy. In all of these cases, it is important to stick with the general principles outlined above and to use the largest laryngoscope that can safely be deployed. When encountering difficulty in accessing the vocal folds, the surgeon should (as always) lift the head to exaggerate the flexion at the thoracocervical junction and extension at the craniocervical junction. However, if it is still impossible to achieve an adequate view, a smaller laryngoscope should be used. Rarely, this means using the anterior commissure laryngoscope.

The laryngoscope is usually placed centrally in the mouth, but if it is proving difficult to view the vocal folds, a further technique to achieve a view is to approach the oropharynx from the side of the mouth. But if necessary, the laryngoscope can be placed laterally, in the corner of the mouth, and the tongue swept to the side. This is not usually possible with the larger laryngoscopes (e.g. the Lindholm) but is possible with smaller scopes.

5.9 Surgery for Various Lesions

When initially examining the vocal folds under the microscope, the first step is a careful palpation of the vocal folds. This is often best performed with a palpator (dissector/elevator).

5.9.1 Excision of Vocal Fold Polyp

Once adequate exposure and access have been achieved, carefully assess with probing which surface the polyp arises from (be it the superior or inferior lip of the vocal fold) and whether it is pedunculated or sessile.

A small, pedunculated lesion may be medially retracted using atraumatic heart-shaped 45-degree offset grasping micro-forceps and microscissors used to excise it from the healthy mucosa of the vocal fold. Any uneven mucosal edges should later be trimmed, again with microscissors.

Otherwise, a microflap can be utilised by incising the mucosa just adjacent and usually lateral to the underlying lesion with a lancet or sickle knife, before using a microflap elevator or microscissors to develop the flap submucosally and delineate the lateral margin of the polyp fully. Microlaryngeal forceps may be used to retract the flap mucosa and progress the dissection around the polyp accordingly. Haemostasis can be maintained using 1:10,000 adrenaline-soaked pledgets to avoid compromised accurate visualisation of tissue planes. Once the margins of the polyp are clearly visualised, the polyp should be excised either along with any adherent diseased mucosa using angled microscissors, or the gelatinous material may be extracted with a cupped forceps or microsuction, leaving the overlying mucosa intact. If the latter is performed, the remaining mucosa should be redraped and assessed, and either thickened or redundant mucosa is then excised to allow neat apposition of healthy mucosa for optimal healing.

5.9.2 Nodules

Confirmation of the diagnosis of vocal fold nodules is essential before deciding on management: bilateral lesions may often be mistaken for nodules but may represent a unilateral lesion (e.g. cyst or polyp) with contralateral oedema. Subtle differences in size, position on the vocal fold and colour may alert the clinician to the fact that the lesions are not nodules.

Once certain that soft nodules are present (soft nodules have some vibratory quality to them on stroboscopy compared to hard nodules that do not), the treatment is virtually always voice therapy. However, if voice therapy has not succeeded in resolving the issue, it may be that the nodules have matured and the subepithelial matrix cannot be reabsorbed. The histopathological appearances of a nodule and a polyp are the same; pathologists often arbitrarily classify nodules as those lesions under 3 mm and polyps as those greater than 3 mm. Hard nodules often do not respond to speech therapy and need to be excised.

Once in the operating theatre, both hard and persistent soft nodules can be excised using a microflap technique.

1. The nodule is held with non-traumatic graspers and pulled medially.
2. A small incision is made with scissors or ideally a sharp microblade just superior to the nodule.
3. The free superior edge of the incision is re-grasped and extended medially.
4. The nodule is rolled medially and is excised using scissors around the edge of the mature 'jelly'.
5. A tiny epithelial defect is left, and the SLP is left undisturbed. This defect will heal within 72 h.
6. Post-operative speech therapy is strongly recommended to prevent recurrence of the nodules if caused by vocal technique issues.

5.9.3 Vocal Fold Cyst

Vocal fold cysts are usually classified as either subepithelial or epidermoid. Subepithelial cysts (mucus retention cysts) lie either on or just under the epithelium. They can therefore be excised using the same technique as for nodules (see above). The only additional procedure would come after step 4. This would be as follows:

5. Always examine the site of cyst excision to look for a linear scar that can run very close to where the edge (superior usually but can be inferior) of the cyst is.

Very little epithelial defect remains, and this will heal in a matter of days.

Epidermoid cysts lie deeper within the superficial lamina propria and require a slightly more involved operation, and clear post-operative guidance should be given to the patient about vocal rest, therapy and a realistic length of time for full vocal recovery given.

1. Grasp the ipsilateral vocal fold with non-traumatic graspers and retract medially.
2. Make a linear superior cordotomy incision, anterior to posterior, using a microblade. If unavailable, then one can use the straight microscissors or those curved to the contralateral fold (i.e. curved to the right for the left fold and vice versa).
3. Re-grasp the superior medial edge of the incision and retract medially to expose the SLP.
4. Use a blunt dissector or elevator to separate the tissues.
5. Expose the cyst on all sides.
6. It is usually tethered either anteriorly or posteriorly, or it has ruptured out through the vocal fold free edge, creating a vergeture. In the former case, curved scissors will cut the tethers and release the cyst, and in the latter, excision of the vergeture is also required leaving an epithelial defect.
7. Removal of tissue from the SLP will leave a space that can be filled (e.g. with hyaluronic acid).
8. Post-operative vocal rest for 5 days is recommended followed by a graduated return to vocal use, led by an experienced speech therapist.

5.9.4 Papilloma

Laryngeal papillomatosis is covered elsewhere in this book, and surgical treatment is usually with powered instruments, laser or coblation. However, small lesions can be treated with cold steel excision.

5.9.5 Scar, Sulcus and Webbing

A full discussion of the management of vocal fold scar and sulcus can be found in Chap. 8 of this book. Anterior glottic webbing remains a difficult condition to treat: in general, the principle is to divide the web (often with the CO_2 laser) and then to place an implant between bare edges of the vocal folds; this is secured in place for a number of weeks and then removed. The author's experience is that using a thin silastic sheet is a good option, secured with a non-absorbable suture, which is passed out through the skin and tied outside the neck.

5.9.6 Granuloma

Vocal process granuloma arises as a consequence of exposure of the arytenoid cartilage. The diagnosis is usually made clinically rather than with a biopsy, and indeed biopsy can result in further exposure of cartilage and hence an exacerbation of the granuloma. The treatment of granuloma is almost universally non-surgical, by reducing irritation and ongoing trauma. Often, this entails comprehensive treatment of reflux and voice therapy to avoid abusive behaviours such as coughing, throat clearing and vocal abuse. Rarely, however, a very large granuloma can require surgical excision if there is airway compromise or significant voice dysfunction. The principle of surgery in this situation is to avoid exposing more cartilage at the base of the granuloma; hence, it is important when excising a granuloma to leave a small amount of tissue overlying the cartilage. Some surgeons will inject steroids into the remaining tissue.

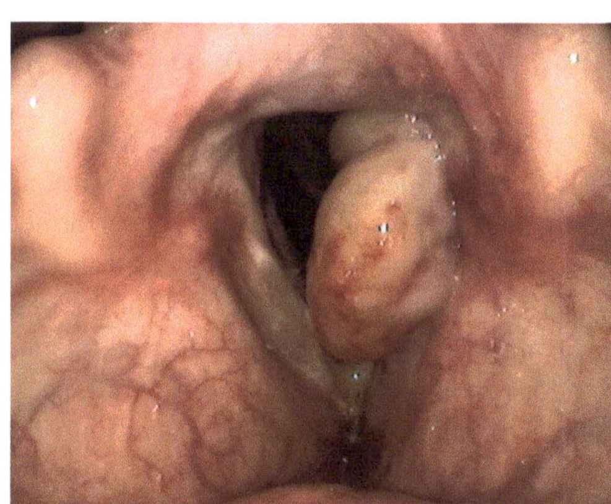

5.10 Microscopic Injection Techniques

In current clinical practice, many vocal fold injections are performed in the clinic in the awake patient: these include injection of botulinum toxin (for spasmodic dysphonia), injection of augmentation (filler) materials (for vocal fold paralysis/glottic insufficiency) and injection of steroids (for a variety of conditions). However, many patients still require injection under general anaesthesia.

The positioning and suspension of the laryngoscope proceed as usual to expose the vocal folds. The choice of needle will depend on the nature of the material being injected. Some injection materials (e.g. calcium hydroxylapatite) will be supplied with their own rigid needle.

5.10.1 Augmentation Injection

For injection of augmentation materials (e.g. calcium hydroxylapatite, hyaluronic acid), the needle tip should be placed in the vocal fold lateral to the vocal ligament—in other words, into the thyroarytenoid (TA) muscle. Depending on the degree of glottic insufficiency, augmentation material can be injected into two or three points in the TA muscle. A modest degree of 'overfilling' should be performed to allow for the fact that the carrier material will dissipate; ultimately, when this occurs, one hopes that the vocal fold will have a straight edge.

5.10.2 Botulinum Toxin Injection

The treatment of adductor spasmodic dysphonia usually entails injection of botulinum toxin into the TA muscle. This is almost always performed transcutaneously in the clinic using electromyography (EMG) to confirm the position of the needle in muscle. Rarely, patients do not tolerate injections in clinic and require a general anaesthetic. The injection material is placed into the TA muscle. A rigid needle may be used (as for augmentation injection). As an alternative, a butterfly needle can be modified by cutting off one of the wings and cutting off most of the other wing; the remnant of the wing can be gripped by crocodile forceps to advance the needle into the vocal fold (This technique was developed by Guri Sandhu, Charing Cross Hospital, London).

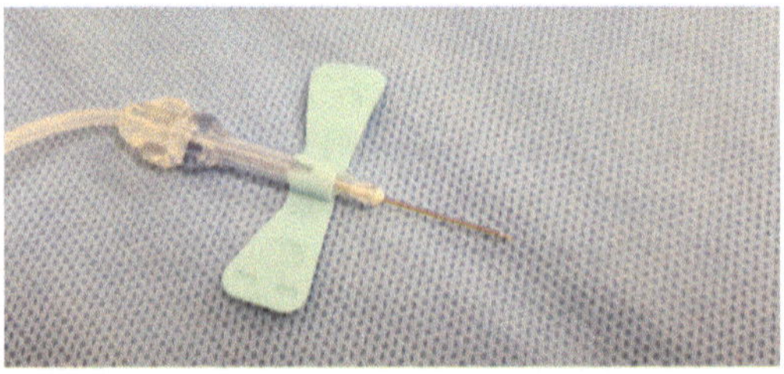

5.11 Training in Laryngology

5.11.1 Principles of Training

Microlaryngeal surgery is technically challenging, providing a test of skill in dexterity and fine instrument handling. This, together with the limited exposure junior medical trainees receive in the field, adds an emphasis to provide high-quality training to those wishing to develop microlaryngeal surgery as a sub-specialty interest.

One challenge is that of allowing adequate observation by a trainee. The addition of the 'sidearm' to the operating microscope in the 1960s had no doubt ameliorated this issue, but the lack of binocular vision for the observer manifests in lack of depth perception, which is critical in truly appreciating the surgical technique. Modern video stack systems however provide excellent display of the image gained either through rigid endoscopy or the operating microscope and extend the spectacle of surgery to multiple trainees and observers. This also allows for better supervision of the trainee by the trainer.

Most phonosurgical procedures are single operator, and therefore the need to recreate teaching of technical aspects through simulation has been explored. Within otolaryngology, the use of simulated temporal bone procedures with both animal and virtual models is commonplace.

Simulation in laryngology has not quite been as prevalent but in recent years has taken big strides forwards.

Due to the unique dynamics of microlaryngoscopy, it is not just important to teach tissue handling but also positioning, laryngoscope and suspension manipulation and use of the microscope or endoscope for visualisation. A variety of laryngeal mount holders have been developed for this reason [26, 27], and reproduction of the ergonomics of the theatre environment and use of actual operating microscopes have added to the realism [28]. Improving laryngoscopy technique with measurements of soft tissue manipulation through manikins with integrated pressure sensors has also been demonstrated [29].

5.11.2 Laryngeal Models

When considering the simulated larynx, studies have described the use of human, animal and synthetic larynges for procedural training. Human cadavers obviously provide the greatest anatomical accuracy, but their availability is limited, and the effect of formaldehyde can abolish any sense of realism when it comes to tissue handling and tactile feedback [30]. Mounted fresh cadaver larynges have been used to overcome this problem and provide excellent feedback in medialisation injection training [31], but again the human tissue logistics limit their utilisation on a wide scale.

The porcine model is economical and has been praised for its similarity to the human larynx, allowing useful teaching in laryngoscopy, biopsy, medialisation injection and submucosal flap elevation [32]. Ovine models have been favoured for simulating laryngotracheal reconstruction [33], and rabbit models lend themselves well to paediatric tracheostomy training [34]. Live-anaesthetised rabbit models in particular have been reported to simulate paediatric emergency airway procedures accurately with regard to bleeding, movement, physiological changes and the interplay between surgeon and anaesthetist.

When it comes to synthetic models, 3D printing has revolutionised the ability to recreate structurally accurate replicas. Although it is more cost-effective than silicone elastomer casting, using 3D printing alone to model the larynx has been shown to be inferior with regard to reproducing the tactile properties of real tissue [35]. However, when the rigidity of a 3D-printed laryngeal framework is combined with a silicone-based 'soft tissue' insert, this allows much more realistic laryngeal injection simulation ([36]? use pics). Higher-fidelity models in this class can further provide audible feedback to confirm successful needle placement for transcervical laryngeal injection [37].

5.11.3 Simulation Platforms

Since Chevalier Jackson's instructional videos on his choking doll, 'Michelle', simulating emergency airway management with manikins has come a long way. So-called 'low-fidelity' manikins are readily available and can be used to teach airway procedures such as rigid bronchoscopy and foreign body extraction, fibreoptic intubation, cricothyroidotomy or tracheostomy. Low-fidelity models should not necessarily be seen as inferior teaching adjuncts, as such models in bronchoscopy training have been credited for their ability to avoid unnecessary distraction whilst the focus of the task is on attaining a new psychomotor skill [38]. Of the manikins available, the AirSim (TruCorp Ltd.) has been rated highly for its resemblance of upper airway anatomic sites [39].

Technological advancements in simulation technology have led to the production of much more impressive, high-fidelity manikins. One such is a life-sized paediatric model which produces audible stridor and asymmetric chest wall movements for a more immersive experience in to the emergency scenario management [40]. Virtual reality platforms have increasingly been introduced in medical practice, and as bronchoscopy training has already benefited from this technology for over 20 years [41], it is likely that its development will lead to further training opportunities in laryngeal surgery in the future.

5.12 Optical Enhancement Techniques

The definition of images one can obtain of the larynx via the microscope or endoscope has improved dramatically over the last 30 years. Now it is possible to have 4K high-resolution and 3D images that will aid the surgeon in both diagnosis and treatment.

Although not strictly a part of this chapter, different imaging modalities are an important part of preoperative and intraoperative techniques.

5.12.1 Blue Light Imaging

Blue light imaging (BLI) is the most common alternative visualisation technique used in laryngoscopic surgery. Depending on the company, it is variably known as narrow band imaging (NBI, Olympus), iScan (Pentax), Piet (Xion) or Spectra (Storz). This list is not exhaustive, but the premise and basis remain the same throughout; haemoglobin absorbs light variably across the visible spectrum, with the peak absorption at 415 nm and a smaller peak at 540 nm. This corresponds to the wavelengths of blue and green light, respectively. When the correct light source or filter is applied, the majority light is filtered out except for blue and green light. The overall picture becomes blue/green and sharper as longer wavelengths are filtered out, so do not penetrate (and reflect) as deeply into the tissues as white light. The haemoglobin in the blood vessels of the epithelium and immediate sub-epithelium absorbs the light and does not reflect it—the blood vessels appear almost black—and the vasculature stands out.

Malignancies and papillomata in the upper aerodigestive tract have certain vascular patterns that can be recognised and categorised according to the intraepithelial papillary capillary loop classification of Ni et al. This technique has been used intraoperatively to identify tumours in the gastrointestinal, urogenital and respiratory tracts with success. The use of blue light imaging intraoperatively in the upper aerodigestive tract is rapidly on the rise but is currently not available as integrated into the operating microscopes. The filter must be available on the recording stack system. One of the authors currently uses a Storz stack system, and the Spectra imaging is used for every case. Rather than alternative imaging, it should be thought of as an added source of information to improve the overall clinical picture. The use of BLI has been likened to an 'optical biopsy' and appears to be better than white light imaging (WLI) at detecting malignancies (sensitivity and negative predictive value are high) and possibly at pre-malignant conditions.

As with any technique or novel piece of equipment, it should be used regularly to get an appreciation of how it works with normal tissue as well as with the abnormal. The authors would advocate using it on every patient in theatre. This will ensure the clinician becomes familiar with the appearance of normal tissues under BLI and then be able to ascertain how clearly abnormal tissues differ under BLI. Familiarity with the range of pathologies will lead to a greater understanding about intermediary stages (IPCL III, IV and possibly Va—Figs. 5.10 and 5.11).

5.12.2 Fluorescence

The use of fluorescence intraoperatively may be able to assist the surgeon in delineating dysplastic, malignant and papillomatous tissue from normal. Currently this is used in neurosurgery with fluorescence with 5-aminolevulinic acid (5-ALA) allowing differentiation of cancer such as a glioma from normal brain tissue. Before surgery, the patient drinks a 5-ALA solution that is selectively taken up by glioma cells. During surgery, the correct fluorescence mode is activated on the microscope, and the tumour cells shine up as red, with a background of blue normal tissue. This allows a much clearer differentiation of the different types of tissue. Although this is not currently available in ENT, the near future may allow cancer cells to be highlighted in this manner allowing for more accurate endoscopic resection.

Fluorescence imaging after systemic injection of cetuximab-IRDye800CW, and viewing with the near infrared spectral region for optical fluorescence imaging, has high sensitivity and

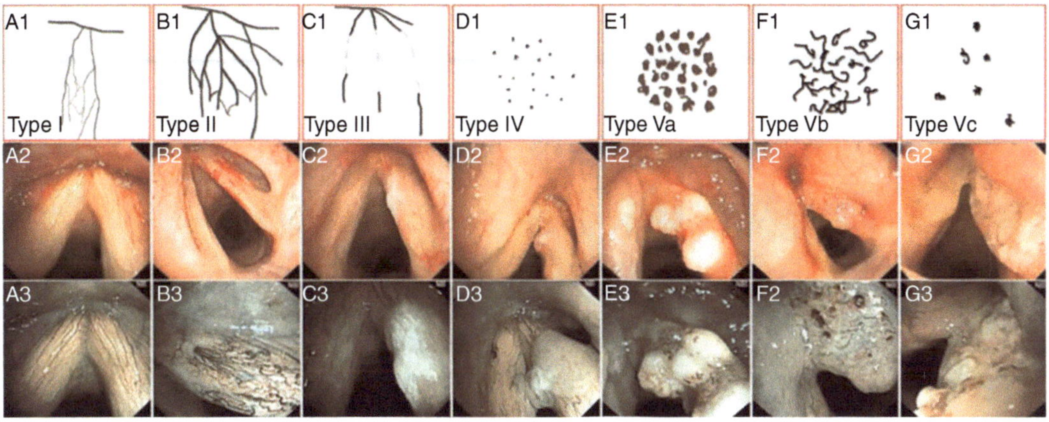

Fig. 5.10 IPCL classification from Ni et al. Diagrams of microvasculature and endoscopic views of vocal folds, illustrating classification of intraepithelial papillary capillary loop features using narrow band imaging. Type I (**a1**, **a2** and **a3**): thin, oblique and arborescent vessels are interconnected and intraepithelial papillary capillary loops are almost invisible. Type II (**b1**, **b2** and **b3**): diameter of oblique and arborescent vessels is enlarged, and intraepithelial papillary capillary loops are almost invisible. Type III (**c1**, **c2** and **c3**): intraepithelial papillary capillary loops are obscured by white mucosa. Type IV (**d1**, **d2** and **d3**): intraepithelial papillary capillary loops can be recognised as small dots. Type Va (**e1**, **e2** and **e3**): intraepithelial papillary capillary loops appear as solid or hollow, with a brownish, speckled pattern and various shapes. Type Vb (**f1**, **f2** and **f3**): intraepithelial papillary capillary loops appear as irregular, tortuous, line like shapes. Type Vc (**g1**, **g2** and **g3**): intraepithelial papillary capillary loops appear as brownish speckles or tortuous, line-like shapes with irregular distribution, scattered on the tumour surface

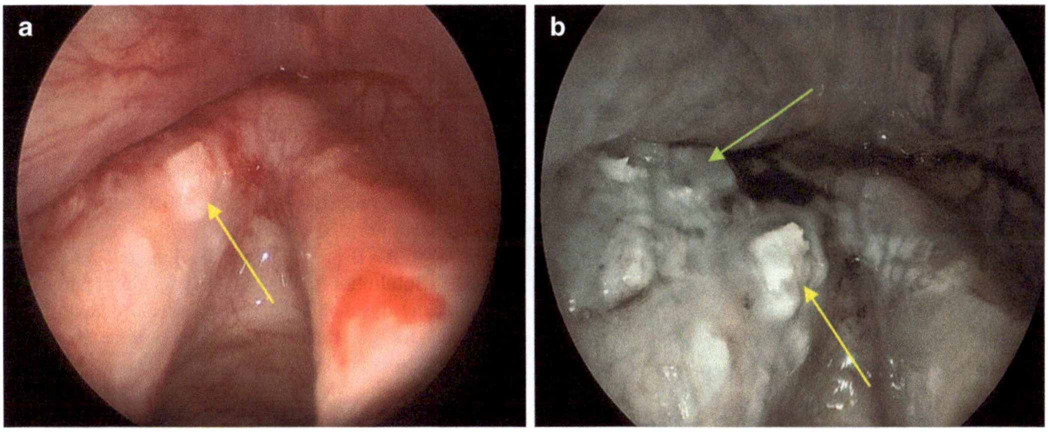

Fig. 5.11 (**a**, **b**) Patient taken to theatre for biopsy of leucoplakia patch on vocal fold (yellow arrow). BLI in theatre highlighted ventricular abnormality that was biopsied and found to be malignant (green arrow)

specificity in localising disease in surgical margins of malignant disease, with a negative predictive value of 87%. This was far greater than surgical or pathological assessment (58% and 66%, respectively) [42]. The ability of fluorescence in this study to identify tumour more accurately than current methods is encouraging for possible in vivo applications. If this becomes used, new filters on microscopes will be needed (Fig. 5.12).

Future integration of microscopes with virtual imaging modalities, navigation or augmented reality is all in the experimental stage. However, one thing is for certain—augmented and alternative visualisation of the upper aerodigestive tract will be a routine part of assessment and treatment.

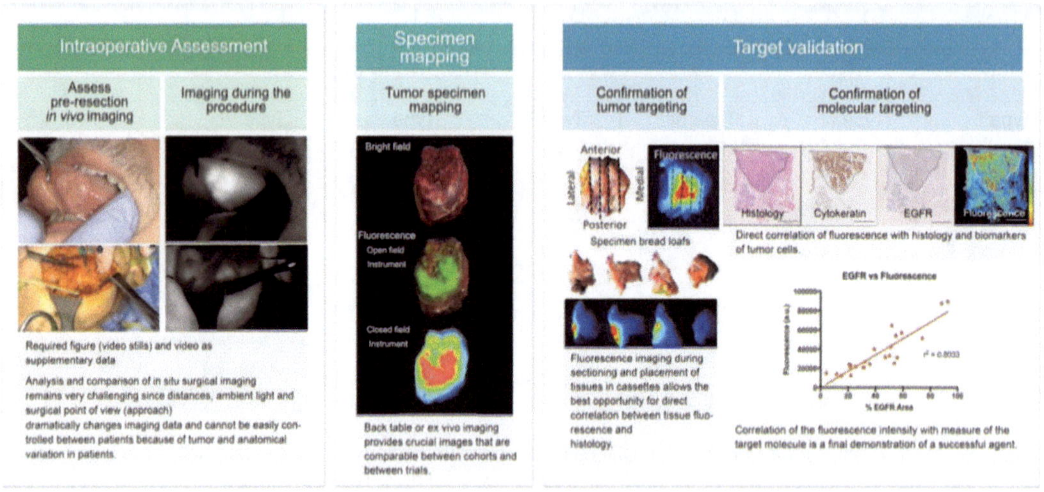

Fig. 5.12 Proposed standardised assessment for fluorescence localisation of malignant head and neck disease. Tumour mapping (middle picture) requires the correct light filter that may in future be integrated into the operating microscope. (Reproduced with permission from Prof Eben L Rosenthal, Department of Otolaryngology, Stanford University, Stanford, CA, 94305, USA)

References

1. Kirstein A, Thorner M. Autoscopy of the larynx and the trachea. (Direct examination without mirror.) (Authorised translation (altered, enlarged, and revised by the author) ed.). Philadelphia: F.A. Davis; 1897.
2. Hochman I, Zeitels S, Heaton J. Exposure and visualization of the glottis for phonomicrosurgery. Oper Tech Otolaryngol Head Neck Surg. 1998;9(4):192–5. https://doi.org/10.1016/S1043-1810(98)80003-1.
3. Zeitels SM. Chevalier Jackson's contributions to direct laryngoscopy. J Voice. 1998;12(1):1–6. https://doi.org/10.1016/s0892-1997(98)80069-6.
4. Killian G. Die Schwebelaryngoscopie. Eur Arch Oto Rhino Laryngol. 1912;26:277–317.
5. Nogueira JF Jr, Hermann DR, Américo Rdos R, Barauna Filho IS, Stamm AE, Pignatari SS. A brief history of otorhinolaryngolgy: otology, laryngology and rhinology. Braz J Otorhinolaryngol. 2007;73(5):693–703.
6. von Leden H. The history of phonosurgery. In: Gould WJ, Sataloff RT, Spiegel JR, editors. Voice surgery. USA: Mosby – Year Book Inc.; 1993. p. 65–95.
7. Kleinsasser O. Mikrolaryngoscopie und Endolaryngeale Mikrochirurgie. Stuttgart: Schattauer-Verlag; 1968.
8. Priest RE, Wesolowski S. Direct laryngoscopy under general anesthesia. Trans Am Acad Ophthalmol Otolaryngol. 1960;64:639–48.
9. Sedlacek K. Microlaryngoscopy. In: Cvejic D, Kosanovic M, editors. Phoniatrics. Belgrade, Zavod za udzbenike i nastavna sredstva; 1982. p. 77.
10. Hirano M. Vocal mechanisms in singing: laryngological and phoniatric aspects. J Voice. 1988;2(1):51–69.
11. Zeitels SM. Phonomicrosurgery I: principles and equipment. Otolaryngol Clin N Am. 2000;33(5):1047–62. https://doi.org/10.1016/s0030-6665(05)70263-2.
12. Garrett CG, Ossoff RH. Phonomicrosurgery II: surgical techniques. Otolaryngol Clin N Am. 2000;33(5):1063–70. https://doi.org/10.1016/s0030-6665(05)70264-4.
13. Sulica L, Rosen CA, Postma GN, et al. Current practice in injection augmentation of the vocal folds: indications, treatment principles, techniques, and complications. Laryngoscope. 2010;120(2):319–25. https://doi.org/10.1002/lary.20737.
14. Blitzer A, Brin MF, Fahn S, Lange D, Lovelace RE. Botulinum toxin (BOTOX) for the treatment of "spastic dysphonia" as part of a trial of toxin injections for the treatment of other cranial dystonias. Laryngoscope. 1986;96(11):1300–1.
15. Isshiki N, Morita H, Okamura H, Hiramoto M. Thyroplasty as a new phonosurgical technique. Acta Otolaryngol. 1974;78(5–6):451–7. https://doi.org/10.3109/00016487409126379.
16. Ramai D, Zakhia K, Etienne D, Reddy M. Philipp Bozzini (1773–1809): the earliest description of endoscopy. J Med Biogr. 2018;26(2):137–41. https://doi.org/10.1177/0967772018755587.
17. Cunningham LL Jr, Peterson GP. Historical development of endoscopy. Atlas Oral Maxillofac Surg Clin North Am. 2003;11(2):109–27. https://doi.org/10.1016/s1061-3315(03)00018-0.
18. Spaner SJ, Warnock GL. A brief history of endoscopy, laparoscopy, and laparoscopic surgery. J

Laparoendosc Adv Surg Tech. 1997;7(6):369–73. https://doi.org/10.1089/lap.1997.7.369.
19. Cockett WS, Cockett AT. The Hopkins rod-lens system and the Storz cold light illumination system. Urology. 1998;51(5A Suppl):1–2. https://doi.org/10.1016/s0090-4295(98)00060-0.
20. Ellis H. The Hopkins rod-lens system. J Perioper Pract. 2007;17(6):272–4. https://doi.org/10.1177/175045890701700605.
21. Berci G, Shulman AG, Morgenstern L, Paz-Partlow M, Cuschierei A, Wood RA. Television choledochoscopy. Surg Gynecol Obstet. 1985;160(2):176–7.
22. Yamashita H, Aoki H, Tanioka K, Mori T, Chiba T. Ultra-high definition (8K UHD) endoscope: our first clinical success. Springerplus. 2016;5(1):1445. https://doi.org/10.1186/s40064-016-3135-z.
23. Carlucci C, Fasanella L, Ricci Maccarini A. Exolaryngoscopy: a new technique for laryngeal surgery. Acta Otorhinolaryngol Ital. 2012;32(5):326–8.
24. Carobbio ALC, Missale F, Fragale M, Mora F, Guastini L, Parrinello G, Canevari FRM, Peretti G, Mattos LS. Transoral laser microsurgery: feasibility of a new exoscopic HD-3D system coupled with free beam or fiber laser. Lasers Med Sci. 2021; https://doi.org/10.1007/s10103-020-03221-w.
25. Crosetti E, Arrigoni G, Manca A, Caracciolo A, Bertotto I, Succo G. 3D exoscopic surgery (3Des) for transoral oropharyngectomy. Front Oncol. 2020;10:16. https://doi.org/10.3389/fonc.2020.00016.
26. Foulad A, Bui P, Dailey SH, Verma SP. VOCALSS: versatile optimally constructed aid for laryngeal surgery simulation. Laryngoscope. 2015;125(5):1169–71. https://doi.org/10.1002/lary.25091.
27. Holliday MA, Bones VM, Malekzadeh S, Grant NN. Low-cost modular phonosurgery training station: development and validation. Laryngoscope. 2015;125(6):1409–13. https://doi.org/10.1002/lary.25143.
28. Fleming J, Kapoor K, Sevdalis N, Harries M. Validation of an operating room immersive microlaryngoscopy simulator. Laryngoscope. 2012;122(5):1099–103. https://doi.org/10.1002/lary.23240.
29. Salud LH, Peniche AR, Salud JC, de Hoyos AL, Pugh CM. Toward a simulation and assessment method for the practice of camera-guided rigid bronchoscopy. Stud Health Technol Inform. 2011;163:535–41.
30. Bhalla S, Tolley N, Awad Z. Creating a validated simulation training curriculum in otolaryngology. Curr Otorhinolaryngol Rep. 2020;8:96–105. https://doi.org/10.1007/s40136-020-00275-w.
31. Amin M, Rosen CA, Simpson CB, Postma GN. Hands-on training methods for vocal fold injection education. Ann Otol Rhinol Laryngol. 2007;116(1):1–6. https://doi.org/10.1177/000348940711600101.
32. Awad Z, Patel B, Hayden L, Sandhu GS, Tolley NS. Simulation in laryngology training; what should we invest in? Our experience with 64 porcine larynges and a literature review. Clin Otolaryngol. 2015;40(3):269–73. https://doi.org/10.1111/coa.12360.
33. Okhovat S, Milner TD, Clement WA, Wynne DM, Kunanandam T. Validation of animal models for simulation training in pediatric laryngotracheal reconstruction. Ann Otol Rhinol Laryngol. 2020;129(1):46–54. https://doi.org/10.1177/0003489419870820.
34. Both CP, Diem B, Alonso E, Kemper M, Weiss M, Schmidt AR, Deisenberg M, Thomas J. Rabbit training model for establishing an emergency front of neck airway in children. Br J Anaesth. 2021;126(4):896–902. https://doi.org/10.1016/j.bja.2020.12.032.
35. Kavanagh KR, Cote V, Tsui Y, Kudernatsch S, Peterson DR, Valdez TA. Pediatric laryngeal simulator using 3D printed models: a novel technique. Laryngoscope. 2017;127(4):E132–7. https://doi.org/10.1002/lary.26326.
36. Lee M, Ang C, Andreadis K, Shin J, Rameau A. An open-source three-dimensionally printed laryngeal model for injection laryngoplasty training. Laryngoscope. 2021;131(3):E890–5. https://doi.org/10.1002/lary.28952.
37. Ainsworth TA, Kobler JB, Loan GJ, Burns JA. Simulation model for transcervical laryngeal injection providing real-time feedback. Ann Otol Rhinol Laryngol. 2014;123(12):881–6. https://doi.org/10.1177/0003489414539922.
38. Fielding DI, Maldonado F, Murgu S. Achieving competency in bronchoscopy: challenges and opportunities. Respirology. 2014;19(4):472–82. https://doi.org/10.1111/resp.12279.
39. Woo JA, Malekzadeh S, Malloy KM, Deutsch ES. Are all manikins created equal? A pilot study of simulator upper airway anatomic fidelity. Otolaryngol Head Neck Surg. 2017;156(6):1154–7. https://doi.org/10.1177/0194599816674658.
40. Deutsch ES, Dixit D, Curry J, et al. Management of aerodigestive tract foreign bodies: innovative teaching concepts. Ann Otol Rhinol Laryngol. 2007;116(5):319–23. https://doi.org/10.1177/000348940711600501.
41. Colt HG, Crawford SW, Galbraith O III. Virtual reality bronchoscopy simulation: a revolution in procedural training. Chest. 2001;120(4):1333–9. https://doi.org/10.1378/chest.120.4.1333.
42. Warram JM, de Boer E, van Dam GM, Moore LS, Bevans SL, Walsh EM, Young ES, Carroll WR, Stevens TM, Rosenthal EL. Fluorescence imaging to localize head and neck squamous cell carcinoma for enhanced pathological assessment. J Pathol Clin Res. 2016;2(2):104–12. https://doi.org/10.1002/cjp2.40. PMID: 27499920; PMCID: PMC4907060.

CO_2 Laser Surgery for the Larynx

6

Vyas M. N. Prasad and Marc Remacle

Key Points

- The CO_2 laser is primarily designed to cut and ablate by vapourisation of water within the cellular matrix. Spreading the beam of the laser by the micromanipulator can, in smaller vessel bleeds, stop them by creating enough heat to form a coagulum. Larger bleeds, seen more often near the arytenoids or in the thyroarytenoid muscles, require monopolar diathermy to successfully stop them.
- Superpulse or ultrapulse modes allow for very short peaks of less than 1 ms or less. It vaporises at depths of only 20–30 microns per pulse with residual thermal damage of only 100–150 microns. Beam sizes of 100–200 microns ablate tissue rapidly, vapourising them with little or no collateral thermal damage.
- The scanner is a device attached to the micromanipulator, between the distal end of the articulating arm of the laser and the micromanipulator. An electronic attachment from the laser console is connected to the scanner to provide straight or curved lines and circles of varying lengths and diameters, respectively. This is achieved by the rotation of a series of mirrors within the scanning device creating a beam 'sweep' across an area (i.e. circle or a line).
- Since the CO_2 laser is of a much longer wavelength, it is incapable of being used with conventional laser fibres. Advances in laser fibre development have led to the manufacture of several types of 'hollow' fibres. These fibres, called waveguides, allow for the reflection of light off the shiny inner ceramic material lining the fibre core and thereafter guided out to the external environment.
- The reliability of frozen section margins using dedicated and experienced histopathologists reduced the differences between it and routine histological examination (paraffin sections) to a concordance of 94.8%.
- The CO_2 laser has revolutionised transoral laryngeal surgery. It is used for both benign and oncological purposes

V. M. N. Prasad
Singapore Medical Centre and MWHE Medical Centre, Singapore, Singapore

M. Remacle (✉)
Department of Oto-Rhino-Laryngology-Head Neck Surgery, Centre Hospitalier de Luxembourg, Luxembourg, Luxembourg

M. Remacle, H. E. Eckel (eds.), *Textbook of Surgery of Larynx and Trachea*,
https://doi.org/10.1007/978-3-031-09621-1_6

with exceptional results when the technology is mastered and applied appropriately. It has the ability to be used in free beam, magnified directly and passed through flexible fibres to handle the multitude of laryngeal pathologies that require a reliable, precise and effective surgical tool.

6.1 Introduction

The CO_2 laser was developed by Kumar Patel from Bell Laboratories, USA, in 1963 [1]. Realising the potential for CO_2 laser application in the narrow, poorly illuminated confines of the larynx, Jako and Strong utilised the CO_2 laser in experimental animal studies followed by human beings with success in the 1970s and in so doing pioneered transoral laser laryngeal surgery [2–4]. The tool they had adopted has now become the workhorse in the laryngeal armamentarium when precision in cutting and ablation is required. Incorporating the fine beam with magnification and illumination, Kleinsasser's suspension microlaryngoscopy freed both hands enabling the surgeon to manipulate and resect/remove concurrently [5]. This landmark development paved the way for CO_2 laser laryngeal surgery to be an equal contender to open procedures and radiotherapy in the treatment of early laryngeal cancers and in time superseding both in many instances [6–17].

The aims of this chapter are not to dwell on the myriad scenarios where the CO_2 laser has been successfully used in MIS but to appraise the reader of the technology itself, the nuances of different energy pulse wave forms and their respective utilities, the strengths and weaknesses of the CO_2 laser in the larynx, scanning technology, fibre delivery and finally other potential uses using platforms that can help the surgeon in the often complex, curvilinear anatomy of the upper aerodigestive tract and its passage to the larynx.

6.2 Basics of Laser Physics

LASER is an acronym for light amplification by stimulated emission of radiation. The CO_2 laser is, by definition, an inert gas-based laser that is invisible. The laser unit consists of a main chamber (optical cavity) where light or electrical energy is utilised to 'pump' the lasing medium, i.e. CO_2, and using Einstein's postulate, the optical cavity in the chamber bounces the photons of light emitted across opposing mirrors (Fig. 6.1), amplifying the energy (resulting in gain) with every reflection [18]. This invisible light is coupled to another laser beam (Helium-Neon inert 'red' beam), which acts as the visible aiming beam when emitted from the laser chamber through a system of silver lined reflecting periscopic mirrors in the articulating arm and out either through an attachment to the operating microscope (micro-manipulator) or handheld carriers. This allows the CO_2 laser beam to be visualised. Like all lasers, the light is monochromatic—a single wavelength (10,600 nm), well into the infrared spectrum. It is coherent, collimated and selectively absorbed by water—the principal constituent in cells. The CO_2 laser has the capability to emit infrared light energy in pulses and continuously, a property not shared by all other lasers and can therefore deliver energy in pulses due to the varying nature of energy release and/or mechanism of delivery. Medical lasers have preferential and selective tissues that absorb their light. These tissues

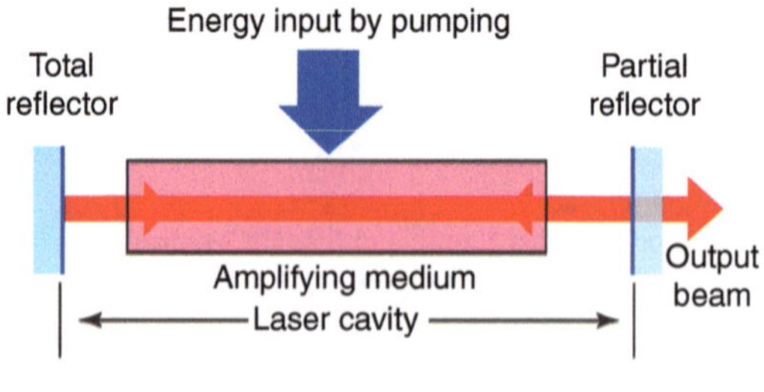

Fig. 6.1 Principle components of a laser

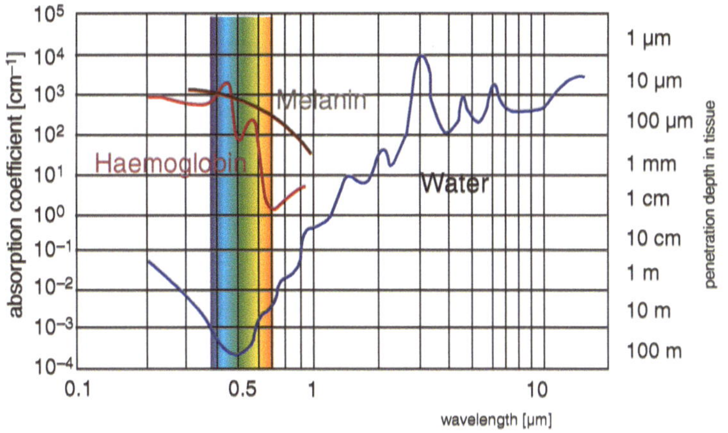

Fig. 6.2 Absorption and penetration depth in water and other biological tissue constituents for different wavelengths (IntechOpen)

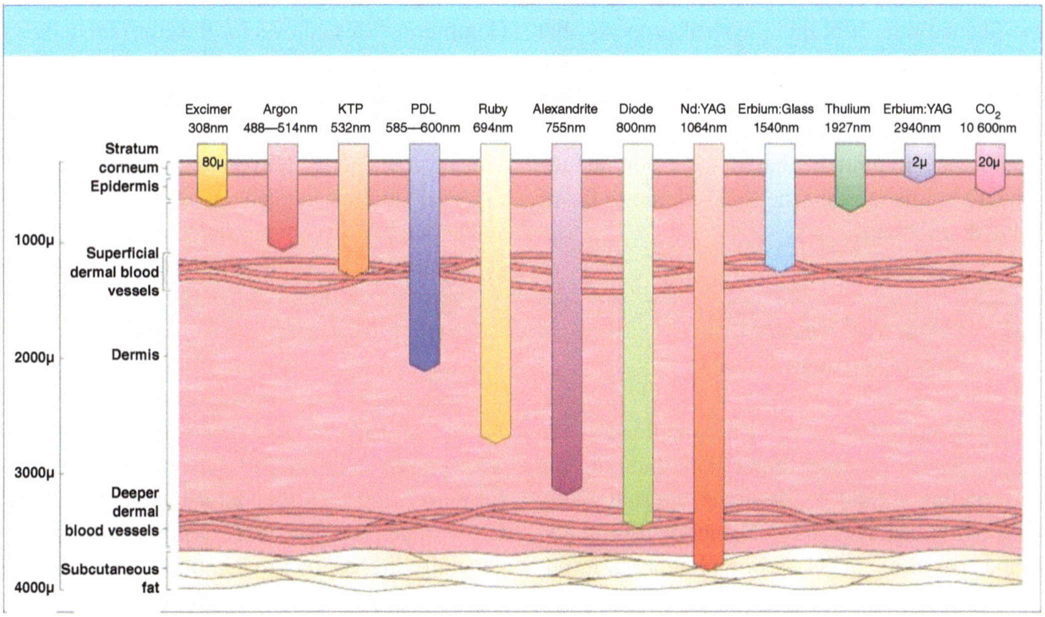

Fig. 6.3 Depth of optical penetration by various lasers

contain **chromophores** which may be pigmented such as blood (haemoglobin) and skin (melanin) or non-pigmented (water). These tissues selectively absorb, reflect and transmit or scatter the laser energy (Figs. 6.2 and 6.3). The absorbed energy alters the target tissue by mainly thermal but also by chemical and mechanical means.

6.3 Laser Flux, Fluence and Irradiance

Laser fluence is the time-integrated flux of any electromagnetic radiation or particle stream. Fluence in optics is analogous to radiant exposure and is defined as the energy of a laser pulse divided by the area it is illuminating. It-is therefore an optical energy density. Fluence is measured in J/cm^2, while fluence rate is in W/cm^2. An understanding of laser fluence is essential to fully appreciate the basis of photothermolysis—the central tenet of laser application. Selective photothermolysis is a concept used to localise thermal injury to a specific target based on its absorption characteristics, the wavelength of light used, the duration of the pulse and the amount of energy delivered. Anderson and Parrish described the selective and localised tissue damage with sparing of surrounding tissues [19]. This is possible when the threshold fluence is equalled and/or exceeded with resulting tissue destruction. The rate at which the energy is delivered to a tissue is the fluence rate. It is this physical property that has been central in the preferential use of the newer CO_2 lasers. Irradiance, although sharing the same unit of measurement as fluence rate, i.e. W/cm^2, is different in that it does not include scattered radiation into the said volume of tissue from all directions.

6.4 Thermal Relaxation and Damage Time

Thermal relaxation time (TRT) is defined as the time taken for the laser target alone (and not the surrounding tissue) to dissipate approximately 63% of the incidental thermal energy. It is related to the size of the target chromophore (e.g. laryngeal mucosa containing water for CO_2 laser). Thermal damage time is the time required for the entire target including the primary chromophore and surrounding tissue to cool by 63%.

Tissue damage depends on the selective absorption of laser energy by the appropriate chromophore depending on the properties of that particular laser. These properties include the laser wavelength specifically and the absorption coefficient of the chromophore. When the energy is delivered in a pulse duration that is less than or equal to the TRT, the tissue is damaged. If the pulse duration is longer than the TRT, the target tissue merely dissipates the energy to the surrounding tissue, damaging it. Besides the pulse duration, the fluence reaching the target should exceed the threshold fluence of the tissue to cause destruction. This target threshold fluence is the net fluence after subtracting that which was reflected and scattered or transmitted.

6.5 Continuous Wave vs. Pulsed Wave

Continuous wave allows for the constant delivery of low power and a long pulse duration resulting in a wide, ill-defined zone of thermal injury. It is useful when thermal relaxation is not a priority. This form of energy delivery requires the machine to be adequately 'cooled' as the heat generated when pumping is immense, often destroying a laser that cannot handle the overheating. Given the need for minimal collateral tissue injury in delicate phonosurgical cases, continuous wave CO_2 lasers were rarely if at all used. Newer technological advances improved the energy delivery of the CO_2 laser with the development of pulsed wave energy delivery. Pulsed wave releases optical power in pulses at an adjustable duration and rate of repetition. The level of power delivered is generally higher than its continuous wave counterpart, but pulsed waves can ablate effectively by concentrating power over a very short burst (pulse width). This feature reduces spread of heat to adjacent tissue which can cause damage and results in **not** ablating the intended area. Peak pulse power is another application where the laser uses a 'Q-switching' mechanism that allows for an extremely short burst of power for a given pulse energy. These modalities are available in the CO_2 laser and provide a variety of options to the surgeon.

6.6 Ultrapulse and Superpulse Modes

There are presently many CO_2 laser manufacturers globally focussing not just on ENT applications. Two of the original manufacturers who were responsible for the main types of CO_2 lasers that were used commonly for laryngeal surgery were Sharplan (from its designers Messrs., Sharon and Kaplan), producing the superpulse laser, and Coherent, the ultrapulse laser. They eventually merged to produce the Lumenis laser which was hybridised but retained either superpulse or ultrapulse modes. The ultrapulse laser allowed for very short peaks of less than 1 ms or less. It vaporises at depths of only 20–30 microns per pulse with residual thermal damage of only 100–150 microns. Beam sizes of 100–200 microns ablate tissue rapidly, vapourising them with little or no collateral thermal damage. The superpulse laser is like the ultrapulse with some differences in its energy waveform. Its peak is sharper and higher than the ultrapulse (which is rectangular), but the rising and falling parts of the waveform are below the ablation threshold giving it a disadvantage to the ultrapulse which produces more precise cuts with less collateral thermal injury (Figs. 6.4 and 6.5).

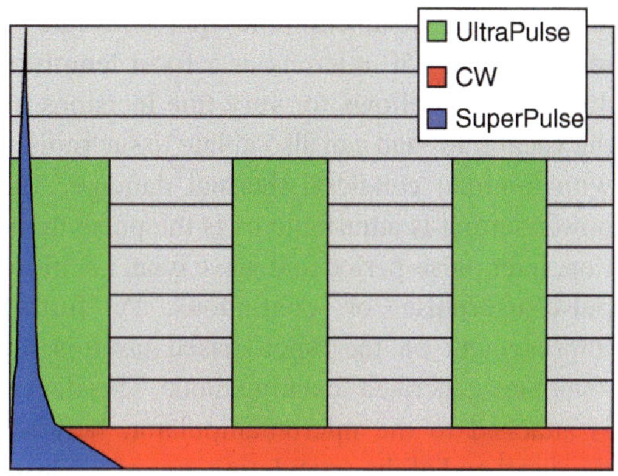

Fig. 6.4 Continuous, ultrapulse and superpulse modes for CO_2 laser

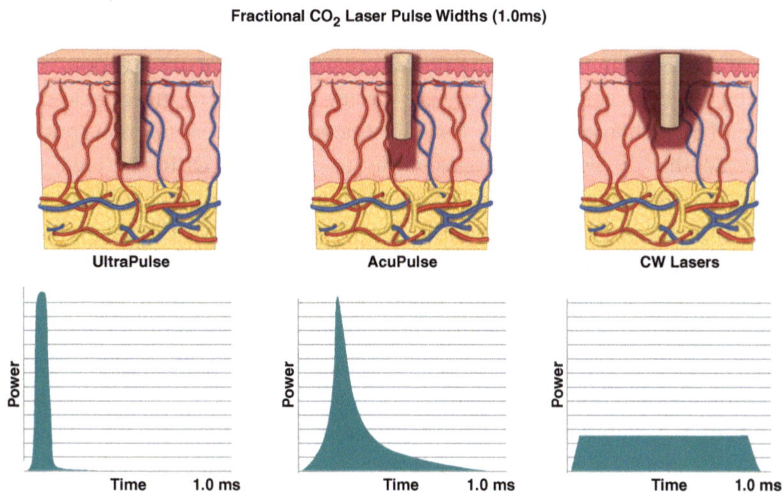

Fig. 6.5 Degree of tissue ablation depth with ultrapulse, superpulse (AcuPulse) and continuous wave (CW) lasers

6.7 Scanning Technology

The CO_2 laser can be attached to an operating microscope via a removable device called a micromanipulator which is essentially a collection of lenses focusable on a mirror with a joystick control that directs the laser beam to the target tissue under magnification with adjustable working distances. The spot size can be minimised to 250 microns at a focal length of 400 mm. This allows for very fine incisions on the vocal folds and can also ablate tissue rapidly with minimal collateral thermal damage. The power setting is adjustable as is the pulse duration, inter pulse-period and wave type, i.e. ultrapulse/superpulse or continuous. A further improvement on the 'spot'-based laser is the computer-generated scanning mode. This device is attached to the micromanipulator, between the distal end of the articulating arm of the laser and the micromanipulator. An electronic attachment from the laser console is connected to the scanner to provide straight or curved lines and circles of varying lengths and diameters, respectively. This is achieved by the rotation of a series of mirrors within the scanning device creating a beam 'sweep' across an area (i.e. circle) or a line. The technology allows for adjustments in the depths of penetration—as little as 100 microns with lengths and diameters as small as 0.7 mm upwards. Consequently, the surgeon does not need to adjust the power setting as the laser system will have already made the necessary adjustments automatically to provide the correct fluence for linear cutting or spot vapourisation and ablation (Fig. 6.5a–e). As described in Sect. 6.3, the fluence is a combination of the power, spot size and rate of firing (on-off period). The laser beam is configured to create these three shapes by such a rapid movement of the spot creating the appearance of lines and circles. No one point in the multitude of spots receives the total power that the laser setting displays, but rather, this power is equally distributed across the entire shape chosen thereby maximising fluence, creating an extremely regular incision and reducing collateral heat damage and charring [20, 21]. The after-effects are minimal with little charring or oedema obviating the need for a covering tracheostomy. Furthermore, given the minimal tissue necrosis, ablation of the laryngeal cartilages induces very little perichondritis. Given the dual modality of tissue interaction, i.e. vapourisation of water by the infrared wavelength creating steam and the denaturation of proteins forming a coagulum, there may be further tissue effects. These include the sealing of small blood vessels and lymphatics perhaps helping to reduce metastases from surgery. Finally, the use of continuous mode is not advocated when precision of cutting and ablation is desirable as this mode does not provide high enough power surges over extremely short spaces of time to deliver the requisite fluence for clean cuts and instant char-free vapourisation and ablation. This is even more relevant to finer work seen in phonomicrosurgery.

Different laser device manufacturers market their technology in different, unique proprietary ways. For example, Lumenis lasers describe their scanning technology as 'SurgiTouch' with the microspot called 'AcuSpot' and the scanning modality 'AcuBlade' (Figs. 6.6a–f and 6.7).

Attachments for operating rigid bronchoscopes and handpieces for skin resurfacing or other non-ENT uses (e.g. circumcision) are also available making the case for investment in the technology more economical when shared across several specialties.

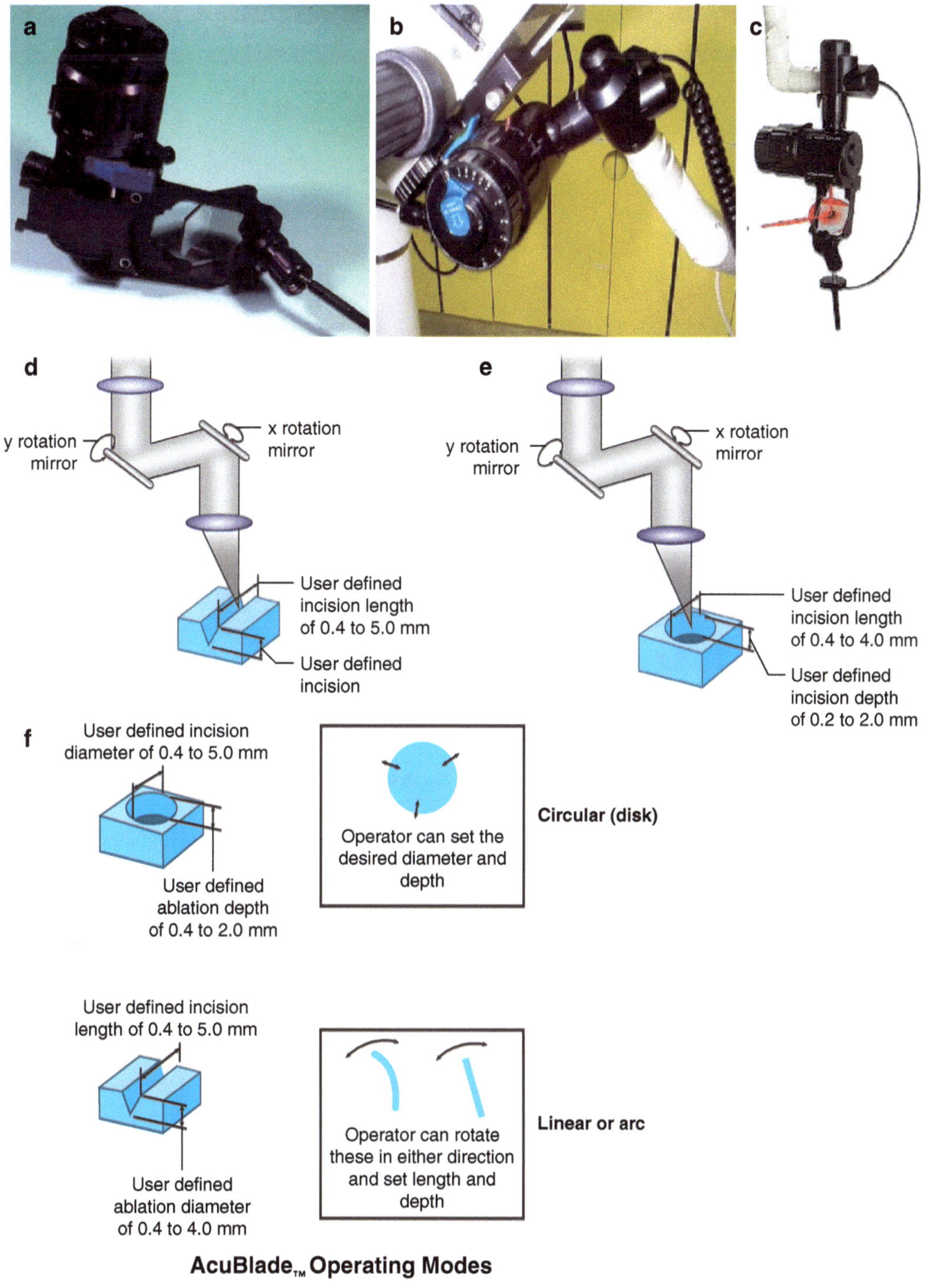

Fig. 6.6 (**a**–**e**) CO_2 laser technology. (**a**) Micromanipulator—AcuSpot®. (**b**) AcuBlade® Scanner. (**c**) Micromanipulator with laser beam. (**d**) Scanning mode linear cut. (**e**) Scanning mode—ablation circle. (**f**) AcuBlade® operating modes

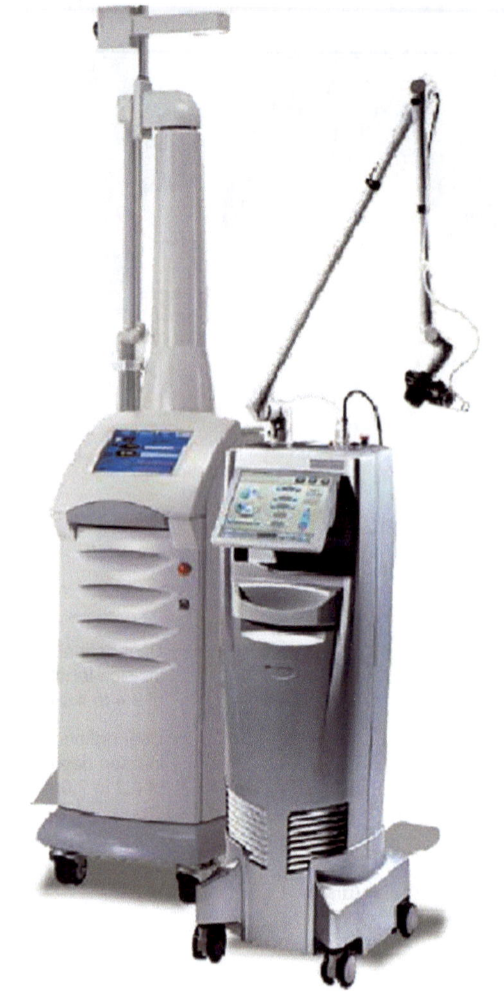

Fig. 6.7 Lumenis AcuPulse Duo CO_2 laser on right, ultrapulse on left

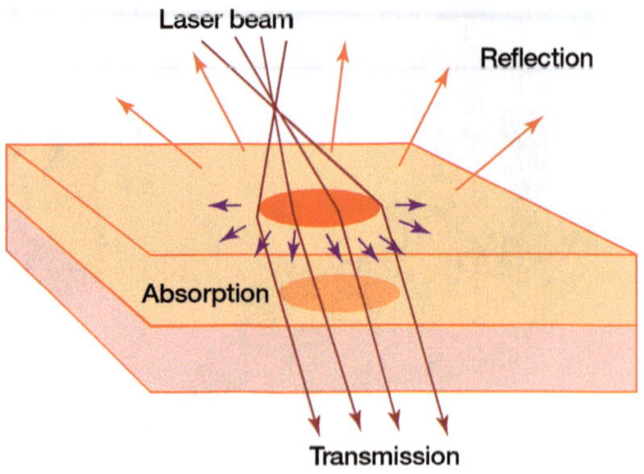

Fig. 6.8 Tissue interaction

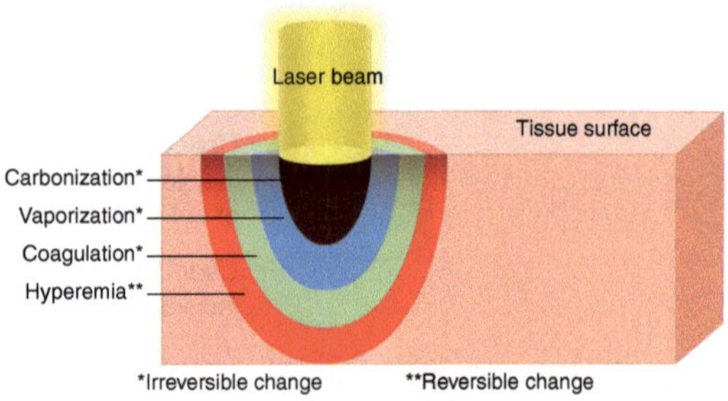

Fig. 6.9 CO_2 laser effects on a microspot

6.8 CO_2 Laser Effects on Tissue

When the electromagnetic wave energy of the CO_2 laser strikes tissue, it is either reflected, absorbed or scattered and/or conducted away. Being an invisible wavelength, it is preferentially absorbed by water which is the main component of human tissues besides bone (Fig. 6.8). The light energy has three main effects—photothermal, photochemical and photoacoustic. It is the photothermal effects that are most relevant to its application in laryngeal laser surgery. The laser energy heats the water up and, at approximately 55 °C, denatures the protein, creating a coagulum. If no further increase in temperature takes place, the tissue will necrose and slough off from the blister created. Raising the temperature to 99 °C results in charring but not vapourisation. At 100 °C, the water starts to boil; the tissue explodes with steam released along with any cellular debris. Further increase in temperature creates carbonisation, and solid particles released in the path of the beam start to glow like embers [9]. This incandescence is seen if the operator continues to fire the laser at carbonised tissue. Heat is transmitted to the surrounding tissue by conduction, but this is inefficient in that it does not ablate but merely damages the surrounding tissue, leaving necrotic areas which heal poorly, have a propensity to bleed and can become infected (Fig. 6.9).

Photoacoustic (photomechanical) effects are seen when very intense laser power is applied over an extremely small area over nanoseconds resulting in shock waves to the surrounding tissue. These effects are utilised in lithotripsy and ophthalmology with other laser types (Nd:YAG laser). Photochemical effects are seen in photodynamic therapy (PDT) [22]. They are associated with resonant matching of chemical bonds in proteins within malignant tissue that are sensitised with a photoactive drug and targeted by a specific (coloured) wavelength of light (pulse dyed or diode lasers).

6.9 Haemostasis

The CO_2 laser is primarily designed to cut and ablate by the rapid vapourisation of water within the cellular matrix. Unlike the KTP or Nd:YAG lasers which have greater tissue penetration of several millimetres, the CO_2 laser is haemostatically mediocre with depths of penetration of mere microns. The relatively clean field with minimal bleeding noticed is both a feature of the mild haemostatic properties of the CO_2 laser and the sparsely vascular tissue of the glottis. Although blood is predominantly water, the effects of the CO_2 laser are not mainly photoangiolytic, and a laser strike to a small arteriole results in the quick pulsating release of blood that within seconds obscures the narrow laryngoscopic field. The temptation to stop the bleeding with the CO_2 laser as a 'diathermy' is understandable, but increasing the diameter of the spot or power of the laser for vessels larger than 0.5 mm does little to arrest haemorrhage. Diffusing the beam of the laser at the micromanipulator dial can, in smaller vessel bleeds, stop them by creating enough heat to form a coagulum. Larger bleeds, seen more often near the arytenoids or in the thyroarytenoid muscles, require monopolar diathermy to successfully stop them.

6.10 Histopathological Considerations

Historically, laser resection of laryngeal cancers was fraught with difficulties and challenges in the interpretation of the margins of the specimen or the operative site. The thermal effects of the original CO_2 laser causing coagulation and carbonization of more than 100 micron made histological analysis unreliable. Frozen sections taken were even more unsafe to commit a diagnosis to. Over the subsequent 30 years, the development of pulsed waves (ultrapulse and superpulse), followed with the scanning technology (e.g. AcuBlade, SurgiTouch, Lumenis, USA), minimised the coagulation zone from 100 microns (AcuSpot) to a mere 20 microns (AcuBlade). The reliability of frozen section margins using dedicated and experienced histopathologists reduced the differences between it and routine histological examination (paraffin sections) to a concordance of 94.8% based on research published by our team [10] (Fig. 6.10). This high negative predictive value has limited the need, cost and emotional stress of a second look procedure. The histopathologist in our series followed a conventional regulation of not

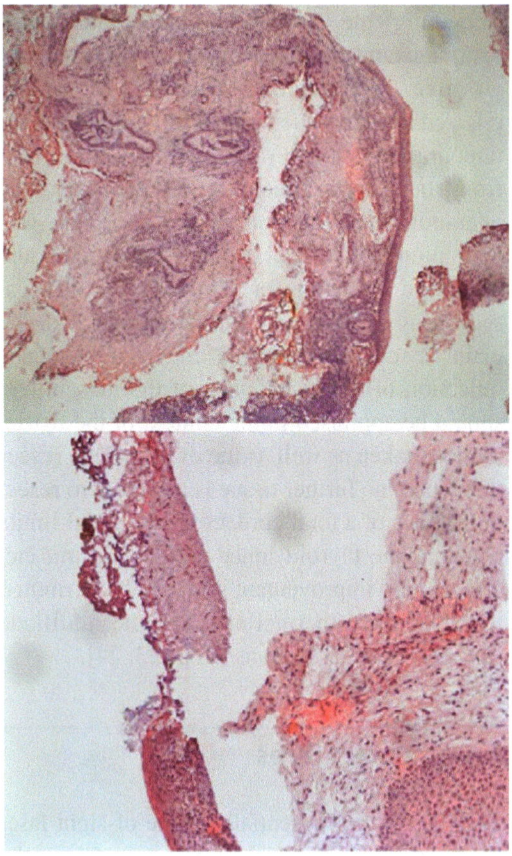

Fig. 6.10 Samples of frozen section analysis at light power field. Architecture and nucleocytoplasmic ratios can still be appreciated

examining the coagulated area and would restrict examination to the area adjacent that was free of coagulation. This adjacent area is referred to as the true margin and is assessed for tumoural invasion. Frozen sections were sent from the tumour specimen's margins and the operation site. The rest of the specimen was then pinned to a cork board, annotated and placed in formalin for definitive histological sectioning and staining. Tissue retraction of the main specimen's margins may give a false reflection of the inadequacy of the margin and should be appraised in the context of the frozen sections taken as well as the extent of the resection where no further tissue is available to resect in the case of a total cordectomy's lateral limits reaching the thyroid inner perichondrium, etc. The marked improvement seen can be attributed to the minimal thermal effect of the AcuBlade system—only 20 microns deep [23, 24].

6.11 Laser Fibres

The CO_2 laser is essentially a line-of-sight laser designed to fire a straight-free beam. Given the long wavelength (10,600 nm), the laser is transmitted through a series of reflective mirrors in the articulating arm from its optical unit to the surgical site. The laser is designed to work best when it strikes the surface of the surgical site at 90°. The upper aerodigestive tract is a curvilinear anatomical area with several obstacles in the path of the laryngeal surgeon including the lips, teeth, tongue, soft palate and epiglottis. The larynx can be difficult to visualise in normal patients with small chins, low-set larynges, crowded oropharynges, etc. Accessing the various areas of the larynx can also pose difficulties. The ventricles, subglottis and posterior commissure are some examples where straight line of sight optics can struggle to get a good view and instruments and lasers cannot access easily. Angle scopes and flexible scopes provide alternatives to the conventional operating microscope. Similarly so, the need to bend the laser light to access these areas is equally important.

Laser optical fibre delivery allows for the transmission of particular wavelengths of light energy. Most fibre delivery systems utilise solid-core laser fibres which are made of silica and are surrounded by a lower refractive index glass or polymer. The fibres are very fine with diameters ranging from 200 microns upwards which allow them to be passed through the instrument channels of flexible endoscopes. The wavelengths which are easily transmitted are between 250 and 2500 nm for powers up to 10 kW. The laser light passes through the core via a series of total internal reflections based on the differing refractive indices with minimal energy loss. These fibres are designed to be applied either directly on tissue (contact mode) or slightly away from tissue (near-contact mode). This allows for differing types of energy delivery, i.e. direct heat vs. selective absorption. Since the CO_2 laser is of a much longer wavelength, it is incapable of being used with conventional laser fibres. Advances in laser fibre development have led to the manufacture of several types of 'hollow' fibres. The original fibres were rigid by definition but had some flexibility to be passed through the side port of a flexible endoscope. Newer fibres are far more flexible and easily negotiate the contours of the upper airway. These fibres are called waveguides and, as their name implies, allow for the reflection of light off the shiny inner ceramic material lining the fibre core and thereafter guided out to the external environment. Two of the original waveguides are the OmniGuide BeamPath flexible CO_2 laser system and the FiberLase CO_2 fibre. Both these systems are used in the near-contact mode with a focal length of less than 1 cm from the surface of the tissue when the laser is applied at 90°. The FiberLase can be used five times but unlike the free beam laser cannot be attached to a scanner. It emits up to 40 W of continuous wave laser mode and up to 15 W when in superpulse wave form. Continuous wave produces the greatest thermal effect and is best for haemostasis, while superpulse produces the most precise cuts with the least haemostatic effect. Our experience with FiberLase is that it can safely seal vessels up to 0.5 mm, but bipolar or suction monopolar is required for vessels that are wider. The FiberLase is 2 m long with an outer diameter of 1.04 mm. The inner coating is metallic silver with silver iodide. The covering is made of biocompatible silica which adds to the flexibility and durability of the fibre. The power transmitted is approximately 60–70% of the initial power with an effective spot size of 320 microns. The beam divergence is low so the fibre can be used at working distances of up to 5 mm in non-contact mode. A fibre can be passed through a variety of rigid and malleable microsurgical handpieces with different lengths and bends for uses in the ear, nose and throat. Tip damage or carbonisation can be easily remedied with either simple wiping and cleaning for the latter or renewing it using a kit for stripping and cleaving provided by the manufacturers. Disposable sheets have been developed for narrower videoendoscopes to avoid damage to them, but the fibre can fit easily through the side channel of a flexible bronchoscope to access the trachea. The fibre is licensed to be used up to five times before disposal in Europe [25].

6.12 TORS and the CO_2 Laser

Transoral robotic surgery (TORS) has become more popular in the recent years in the treatment of a variety of oropharyngeal and tongue base conditions—benign and malignant. Although not designed specifically for laryngeal use, there are instances where surgical robots have been used to certain advantage. The authors have published their experience in two such TORS systems—the DaVinci and the Medrobotics Flex [26–30]. Both systems were designed to mainly use monopolar cautery for haemostasis and cutting tissue. One of the drawbacks is the high thermal effects of electrocautery including oedema and crusting. Our experience with the FiberLase laser wave guide combined with the DaVinci initially and thereafter the Flex systems was positive. The laser was applied at 7–15 W in continuous or superpulse modes for surgery in the tongue base, supraglottis and on palatine tumours. Similarly good results were obtained using the Flex system for the glottis at much lower power settings, i.e. 2–3 W in superpulse [31].

6.13 Pitfalls and Pearls in CO_2 Laryngeal Laser Surgery

The CO_2 laser is a tool and should be used in the capacity that allows it to assist the surgeon in achieving his or her goal for the patient. Given its preference for absorption by water, it should be primarily used for precision cutting and ablating and not for haemostasis. It works best when it strikes tissue perpendicularly and hence will not work as effectively or at all if the angle of strike is acute. Charring and carbonisation do not allow the proper penetration of the laser into the tissues and should therefore be cleaned. Small bleeds can be managed (diameter 0.5 mm or less) with a defocussed beam, but bipolar cautery should be used for bigger vessels. Scanning technology if available provides the cleanest and most efficient way of cutting and ablating. Microspot usage is less efficient and causes more carbonisation. Power settings are computed by the laser to achieve the most efficient fluence for the tissue chosen in the system—it is best to leave these alone. The laser like any machinery can fail, and it is important to be able to troubleshoot problems when possible or seek an alternative option if it fails.

6.14 Conclusion

The CO_2 laser has revolutionised transoral laryngeal surgery. It is used for both benign and oncological purposes with exceptional results when the technology is mastered and applied appropriately. It has the ability to be used in free beam, magnified directly and passed through flexible fibres to handle the multitude of laryngeal pathologies that require a reliable, precise and effective surgical tool.

References

1. Patel CKN, Tien PK, McFee JH. CW high power CO_2 N_2-He laser. Appl Phys Lett. 1965;7:290–2.
2. Jako GJ. Laser surgery of the vocal cords: an excellent study with carbon dioxide laser on dogs. Laryngoscope. 1972;82:2204–15.

3. Strong MS. Laser management of premalignant lesions of the larynx. Can J Otolaryngol. 1974;3:560–3.
4. Strong MS. Laser excision of carcinoma of the larynx. Laryngoscope. 1975;85:1286–9.
5. Kleinsasser O. Microlaryngoscopy and endolaryngeal microsurgery. II. A review of 2500 cases. HNO. 1974;22:69–83.
6. Grossenbacher R. Initial experiences with endolaryngeal CO_2-laser surgery in circumscribed laryngeal cancer. Fortschr Med. 1983;101:1030–2.
7. Motta G, Esposito E, Cassiano B, Motta S. T1-T2-T3 glottic tumours: fifteen years' experience with CO_2 laser. Acta Otolaryngol Suppl. 1997;527:155–9.
8. Rudert H. Larynx and hypopharynx cancers – endoscopic surgery with laser: possibilities and limits. Arch Otorhinolaryngol Suppl. 1991;1:3–18.
9. Steiner W. Results of curative laser microsurgery of laryngeal carcinomas. Am J Otolaryngol. 1993;14:116–21.
10. Vaughan CW, Strong MS, Shapshay SM. Treatment of T1 and in situ glottic carcinoma: the transoral approach. Otolaryngol Clin N Am. 1980;13:509–13.
11. Davis RK. Endoscopic surgical management of glottic laryngeal cancer. Otolaryngol Clin N Am. 1997;30:79–86.
12. Ambrosch P. The role of laser microsurgery in the treatment of laryngeal cancer. Curr Opin Otolaryngol Head Neck Surg. 2007;15:82–8.
13. Trotti A, Bellm LA, Epstein JB, et al. Mucositis incidence, severity and associated outcomes in patients with head and neck cancer receiving radiotherapy with or without chemotherapy: a systematic literature review. Radiother Oncol. 1997;66(3):253–62.
14. Rosenthal DI, Lewin JS, Eisbruch A. Prevention and treatment of dysphagia and aspiration after chemoradiation for head and neck cancer. J Clin Oncol. 2006;24(17):2636–43.
15. Logemann JA, Pauloski BR, Rademaker AW, et al. Swallowing disorders in the first year after radiation and chemoradiation. Head Neck. 2008;30:148–58.
16. Langendijk JA, Doornaert P, Verdonck-de Leeuw IM, Leemans CR, Aaronson NK, Slotman BJ. Impact of late treatment-related toxicity on quality of life among patients with head and neck cancer treated with radiotherapy. J Clin Oncol. 2008;26(22):3770–6.
17. Pauloski BR, Rademaker AW, Logemann JA, et al. Relationship between swallow motility disorders on videofluorography and oral intake in patients treated for head and neck cancer with radiotherapy with or without chemotherapy. Head Neck. 2006;28(12):1069–76.
18. Einstein A. Zur quantentheorie der Strahlung. Physicalische Gesellschaft Zurich Miteilungen. 1916;18:46–62.
19. Anderson RR, Parrish JA. Selective photothermolysis: precise microsurgery by selective absorption of pulsed radiation. Science. 1983;220(4596):524–7. https://doi.org/10.1126/science.6836297.
20. Remacle M, Hassan F, Cohen D, Lawson G, Delos M. New computer-guided scanner for improving CO_2 laser-assisted microincision. Eur Arch Otorhinolaryngol. 2005;262(2):113–9.
21. Remacle M, Lawson G, Nollevaux MC, Delos M. Current state of scanning micromanipulator applications with the carbon dioxide laser. Ann Otol Rhinol Laryngol. 2008;117:239–44.
22. Rigual NR, Thankappan K, Cooper M, Sullivan MA, Doughty T, Popat SR, Loree TR, et al. Photodynamic therapy for head and neck dysplasia and cancer. Arch Otolaryngol Head Neck Surg. 2009;135:784–8.
23. Remacle M, Matar N, Delos M, Nollevaux MC, Jamart J, Lawson G. Is frozen section reliable in transoral CO(2) laser-assisted cordectomies? Eur Arch Otorhinolaryngol. 2010;267(3):397–400. https://doi.org/10.1007/s00405-009-1101-x. Epub 2009 Sep 27
24. Remacle M, Delos M, Lawson G, Jamart J. Accuracy of histological examination following endoscopic CO_2 laser-assisted laryngectomy. Oto-Rhino-Laryngologia Nova. 2002;12:16–20.
25. Remacle M, Ricci-Maccarini A, Matar N, Lawson G, Pieri F, Bachy V, Nollevaux MC. Reliability and efficacy of a new CO_2 laser hollow fiber: a prospective study of 39 patients. Eur Arch Otorhinolaryngol. 2012;269(3):917–21. https://doi.org/10.1007/s00405-011-1822-5. Epub 2011 Nov 6
26. Remacle M, Prasad VMN. Preliminary experience in transoral laryngeal surgery with a flexible robotic system for benign lesions of the vocal folds. Eur Arch Otorhinolaryngol. 2018;275(3):761–5. https://doi.org/10.1007/s00405-018-4900-0. Epub 2018 Feb 7
27. Sayin I, Fakhoury R, Prasad VM, Remacle M, Lawson G. Transoral robotic surgery for base of tongue neoplasms. B-ENT. 2015;Suppl 24:45–50.
28. Van der Vorst S, Prasad V, Remacle M, Bachy V, Lawson G. Functional outcomes after transoral robotic surgery for squamous cell carcinoma of the oropharynx. B-ENT. 2015;Suppl 24:15–9.
29. Fakhoury R, Prasad VM, Sayin I, Van der Vorst S, Remacle M, Lawson G. The da Vinci robotic system in head and neck surgery. B-ENT. 2015;Suppl 24:1–6.
30. Remacle M, M N Prasad V, Lawson G, Plisson L, Bachy V, Van der Vorst S. Transoral robotic surgery (TORS) with the Medrobotics Flex™ System: first surgical application on humans. Eur Arch Otorhinolaryngol. 2015;272(6):1451–5. https://doi.org/10.1007/s00405-015-3532-x. Epub 2015 Feb 8
31. Remacle M, Matar N, Lawson G, Bachy V, Delos M, Nollevaux MC. Combining a new CO_2 laser wave guide with transoral robotic surgery: a feasibility study on four patients with malignant tumors. Eur Arch Otorhinolaryngol. 2012;269(7):1833–7. https://doi.org/10.1007/s00405-011-1838-x. Epub 2011 Nov 20

Thyroplasty/Framework Surgery

7

G. R. R. Desuter and J. T. van Lith-Bijl

Key Points
- History and general consideration about thyroplasty.
- Type of materials and methods.
- The Montgomery thyroplasty.
- Surgical procedure.

In their 2001 landmark paper, the European Laryngological Society classified all laryngeal framework surgery [1].

They distinguished four different types of surgeries, improving voice by modifying the shape of larynx osteocartilaginous framework: (a) the approximation laryngoplasty aka *medialization thyroplasty* with or without arytenoid procedure; (b) the expansion laryngoplasty aka *lateralization thyroplasty*; (c) the relaxation laryngoplasty aka *shortening thyroplasty*; and (d) the tensioning laryngoplasty aka *elongation thyroplasty* or cricothyroid approximation.

The terms laryngoplasty and thyroplasties are interchangeable although some of these procedures involve other laryngeal structures than the thyroid cartilage. Clinical usage tends to favor the thyroplasty term. This is why the term "thyroplasty" will exclusively be used in this chapter.

7.1 The Medialization Thyroplasty (MT)

The medialization thyroplasty, also known as the Isshiki type 1 thyroplasty, represents as much as 95% of all types of thyroplasties realized in the world. This is due to the occurrence of its main indication, that is, the presence of a glottal gap or insufficiency.

Potentially all types of glottal insufficiencies (sulcus, scar, vocal fold immobility) can be treated by a MT, although the main indication of MT remains the vocal fold paralysis in abduction.

The basic principle of medialization thyroplasty consists in pushing the paralyzed vocal fold inwards true a fenestration performed within the lateral ala of the thyroid cartilage. The medialized vocal fold is maintained in a permanent position by the interposition of a material that is left in place at the end of surgery. By maintaining the paralyzed vocal fold in adduction, surgeons

G. R. R. Desuter (✉)
Voice and Swallowing Clinic, ENT Head and Neck Surgery Department, Cliniques Universitaires Saint-Luc, Brussels, Belgium

ENT Department, Universitair Ziekenhuis Antwerpen, Edegem, Belgium

Greenwood Clinic, Brussels, Belgium
e-mail: gauthier.desuter@uza.be, gauthier.desuter@outlook.be

J. T. van Lith-Bijl
Voice and Swallowing Clinic, ENT Head and Neck Surgery Department, Cliniques Universitaires Saint-Luc, Brussels, Belgium

M. Remacle, H. E. Eckel (eds.), *Textbook of Surgery of Larynx and Trachea*,
https://doi.org/10.1007/978-3-031-09621-1_7

Table 7.1 The different types of implants, their designer, and some reference papers [4–9]

Type of implant and technique	Designer (if applicable)	Reference article [4–9]
Medtronic Silastic Implant™	J. L. Netterville	Netterville JL, Stone RE, Luken ES, Civantos FJ, Ossoff RH (1993) Silastic medialization and arytenoid adduction: the Vanderbilt experience. A review of 116 phonosurgical procedures. Ann Otol Rhinol Laryngol 102:413–424
Hard silicone MTIS™	W. Montgomery	Montgomery WW, Blaugrund SM, Varvares MA (1993) Thyroplasty: a new approach. Ann Otol Rhinol Laryngol 102:571–579
Hydroxyapatite VoCom™ implant	C. W. Cummings	Cummings CW, Purcell LL, Flint PW (1993) Hydroxylapatite laryngeal implants for medialization. Preliminary report. Ann Otol Rhinol Laryngol 102:843–851
Titanium implant	G. Friedrich	Friedrich G (1999) Titanium vocal fold medialization implant: introducing a novel implant system for external vocal fold medialization. Ann Otol RhinolLaryngol 108:79–86
Gore-Tex™ (Polytetrafluoroethylene)	None/surgeon-specific technique	McCullogh TM, Hoffman HT (1998) Medialization laryngoplasty with expanded polytetrafluoroethylene. Ann Otol Rhinol Laryngol 107:427–432
Self-carved silastic block	None/surgeon-specific technique	Benninger MS, Manzoor N, Ruda M (2015) Short and long-term outcomes after silastic medialization laryngoplasty: are arytenoid procedures needed? J Voice 29N(2):236–40

restore a subglottic vault and a glottis closure during phonation that allows the creation of a subglottic pressure and a subsequent oscillation of the vocal fold mucosa, two conditions of a proper phonation.

Many materials have been proposed over the years since the first interposition of cartilage performed by Mr. Payr in 1915 [2].

Table 7.1 summarizes the different main materials that are used around the world. Some materials need bigger or smaller cartilage fenestration. Some are pre-molded and provided by the industry; others are self-carved per-operatively by the surgeon. Finally, some are self-anchored; others need stiches in order to be stabilized [3].

Some surgeons add to the medialization thyroplasty procedure, an arytenoid procedure whether an arytenoid adduction or an arytenoidopexy. These adjunctive procedures are aimed at addressing specifically the posterior part of the glottis.

Reports reveal good results for all of the materials described in Table 7.1, showing a rather low rate of reinterventions.

Unfortunately, the lack of standardized voice outcome indicators impedes proper comparison between materials and techniques so that, to our best knowledge, none of these can be declared as superior to others.

In 2018, the choice of the technique and material that will be used for a medialization thyroplasty is left to the discrepancy of surgeons. Their choice is usually based on their own experience and training.

The medialization thyroplasty technique known as the Montgomery Thyroplasty Implant System™ (MTIS) will be further detailed in this chapter.

The technique and type of implant are largely used and available over the world. It is growing in volume of use and reported a short learning curve and excellent postoperative voice outcomes [10, 11]. Although the MTIS provides not only a premolded hard silicone implant but also a step-by-step operative procedure, this procedure has been recently questioned in the literature [12, 13]. The procedure that will be explained in this book modifies the procedure according to this recent literature [14].

7.1.1 The Procedure

The procedure is performed under light sedation and local anesthesia. A particular attention will be offered to overweight and/or apneic patient for which sedation must be titrated in order to avoid any tongue ptosis causing apnea and desaturation. An anesthesiologist is present within the OR during the entire procedure. Oxygen and cardiopulmonary parameters are monitored continuously.

Patient is lying on his back with a neutral positioning of the head. Oxygen is administrated true a nasal probe fixed with tape.

In our experience, we do not proceed systematically under visual feedback of the larynx imposing trans-nasal simultaneous video-endoscopy. Patient's voice—the purpose of the procedure—will represent the sole feedback indicator. Video-endoscopic feedback will be reserved for difficult or doubtful cases.

All surgical steps correspond to the step-by-step surgical procedure described by Dr. Montgomery's initial paper and provided with the implants, sizers set, and surgical instrument set by Boston Medical Inc. [Montgomery® Thyroplasty Implant System: Instructions for Use. Boston Medical Products, Shrewsbury, MA, USA; MK-THYCAT-C; 05-2016]. These steps are filed at the federal Food and Drugs Administration (FDA) and were never modified since their initial filing.

Step 1 Prep and Drape

A local anesthesia is performed by subcutaneous and intramuscular infiltration of noradrenaline-lidocaine 2% at the level of the skin incision.

Skin is prep with a disinfectant substance from the sternum to the nose. Draping spares the mouth and nose to avoid any claustrophobic sensation that could be felt by the patient. Eyelids closure is secured by tape.

Light and sounds intensity is carefully reduced at its minimum within the OR.

Surgeon will regularly check the patient's vigilance by engaging conversation with him/her. Hypnotic conversation techniques can be used as wel.

Step 2 Incision

A 4–5 cm skin incision, crossing the midline, is performed at the level of the cricothyroid membrane. By doing a rather low incision, this will preserve the surgeon of a too superior cartilage fenestration which represents the biggest failure cause.

Step 3 Dissection and Exposure

Platysma is divided and dissected. An orthostatic retractor is placed to expose the field and maintain cutaneo-muscular platysma flaps.

Midline is dissected, and sternohyoid and omohyoid muscles are reclined with two retractors. In some occasions, an anterior jugular vein needs to be ligated to allow proper retraction of the strap muscles.

In female patient, usually presenting a rather flat shape of the thyroid cartilage, infrahyoid strap muscles don't need to be divided. In male patient, usually presenting a sharper thyroid cartilage shape, sternohyoid muscle needs to be partially divided to offer proper access to the lateral ala of the thyroid cartilage.

For both genders, the anterior lower part of the thyrohyoid muscle has to be divided to expose completely thyroid cartilage external perichondrium (Fig. 7.1).

Step 4 Location of "Key Point"

At this stage comes the time of the fenestration landmarks as described by Montgomery's instruction for use. The two first landmarks are on the midline. It consists of the upper thyroid notch superiorly and the lower midline edge of the thyroid cartilage inferiorly. The last and third midline's landmark consist of a point located at the exact mid distance of the two previous landmarks. This crucial point corresponds to the position of the anterior commissure of the vocal folds. The fenestration should never occur above this level.

The superior landmark -that will never be trespassed !- will be a line defined two points defined with the help of two-teeth calipers provided by the Montgomery Surgical Set (Fig. 7.2).

These calipers will be oriented perpendicular to the lower margin of the thyroid cartilage. One will mark a point before (point 1) the inferior thyroid tubercle marking the end of the oblique line and the second after (point 2) the same tubercle.

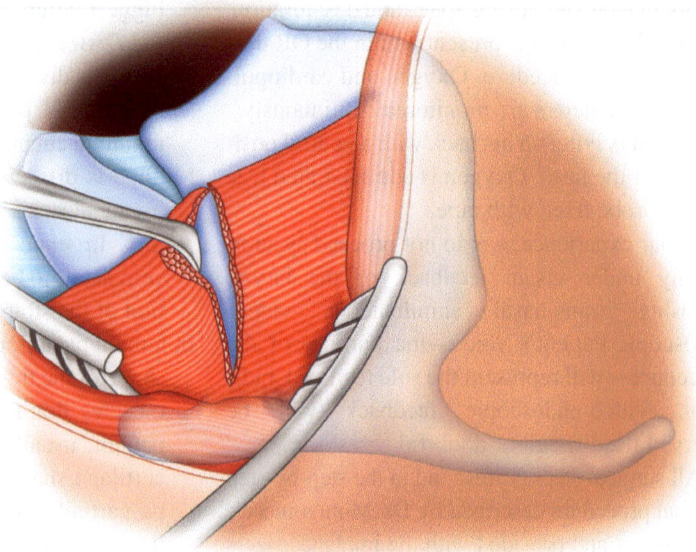

Fig. 7.1 Exposure of the lateral ala of the thyroid cartilage. Exposure of the lower border of the thyroid cartilage

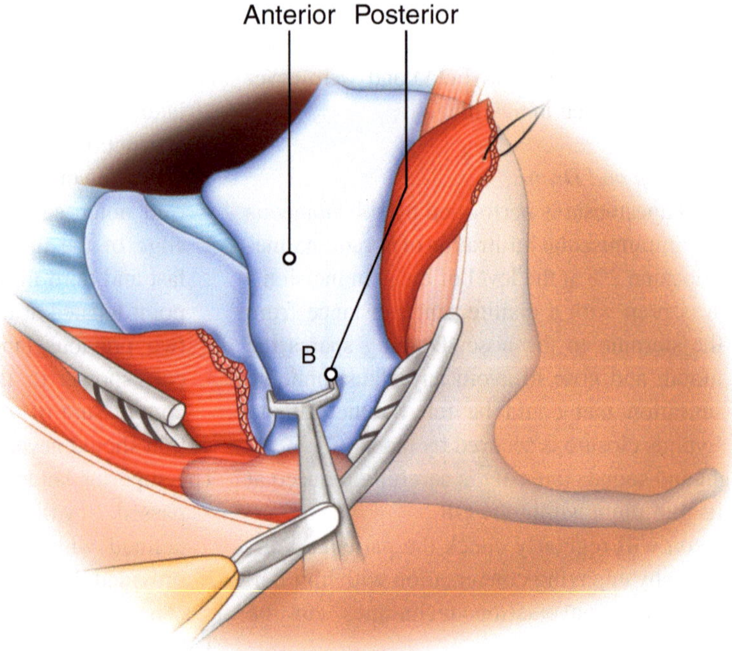

Fig. 7.2 Marking of two points (A and B) on both sides of the thyroid tuberculum using the Montgomery sizer corresponding to patient's gender. Make sure that the sizer is perpendicular to the lower edge of the thyroid cartilage. A cautery on the sizer can be used to mark. These two points will determine a line characterizing the superior border of the fenestration. Place the template approximately 5–6 mm from the midline

An imaginary line is drawn between points 1 and 2. This very same line represents the limit of the outline instrument, which is the upper limit of the implant. Measuring, with the caliper, from the anterior midline along the line connecting point 1 and 2, a cautery mark is made. This represents the "key point" described by Montgomery that corresponds with the anterior superior angle of the thyroplasty window.

The same line will also determine the orientation or angulation of the implant compared to the lower limit of the thyroid cartilage.

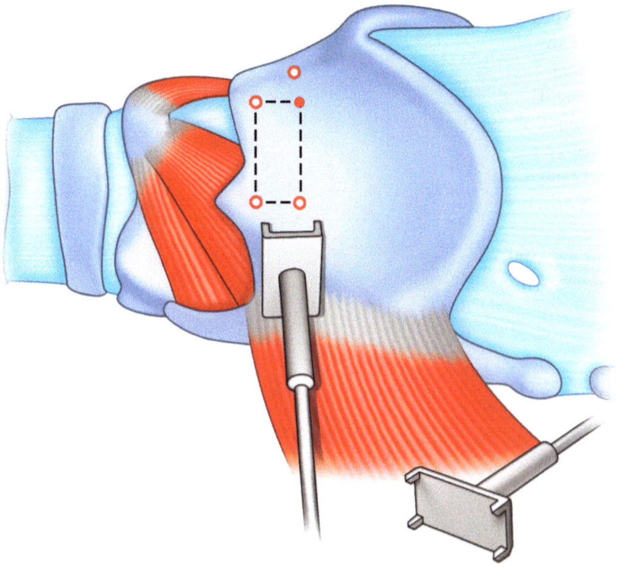

Fig. 7.3 The gender appropriate fenestration template instrument is guided along the line drawn between point A and B (see Fig. 7.2). The lower border of the template should be parallel to the lower border of the thyroid cartilage. The anterior border of the template should *not*, per se, be parallel to the midline

Step 5 Window Outline

An outline instrument, also provided by the Montgomery Surgical Set, will glide and make a translation below the imaginary line (Fig. 7.3). The window outline instruments measure 5 × 10 mm for females and 7 × 12 mm for males. The outline instrument is placed along the line so that its superior-anterior corner lies on the "key point" while its superior border follows the imaginary line. Cautery current is applied on the outline instrument making four marks designating the four corners of the window.

Step 6 Cutting the Window

Cutting is preferably achieved by using a three-teeth's saw to obtain sharp contours. A blur represents a valid alternative.

Step 7 Confirming the Window Size

The outline instrument is used as a template to check window's dimensions.

Step 8 Elevation the Inner Perichondrium

The inner perichondrium may be gently incised if elevation is not obtainable due to perichondrial calcification.

Step 9 Using of the Implant Measuring Devices (Sizers) to Determine the Implant Size

As sizer is engaged, patient is asked to phonate. Each sizer is applied—starting with the smaller size—until the ideal voice is obtained. The triangular portion of the sizer must point in the direction of the vocal process of the arytenoid (Fig. 7.4). The selected size is noted.

Step 10 Insertion of the Montgomery® Thyroplasty Implant

The implant is grasped with broad forceps, and the posterior tip of the triangular portion is inserted through the window in the direction of the vocal process of the arytenoid.

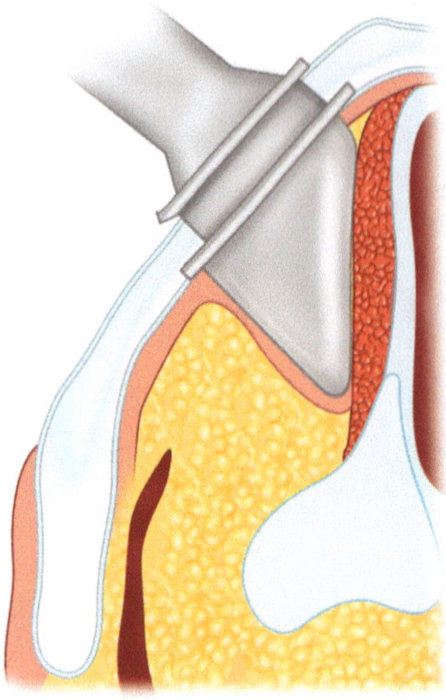

Fig. 7.4 Insert the dummy sizers and ask for voice feedback on a comfort pitch. Try to limit your assessments as it can cause a vocal fold edema that can mislead your vocal feedback. You might already have a sense of the initial size of your dummy by checking a preoperative CT scanner. If you have no CT scanner at your disposal, start with a middle size dummy

The middle plate of the implant's base is in the posterior rim of the window with the top and bottom of the base on either side of the thyroid ala.

The implant is held in position with the index (or thumb) of the non-dominant hand (Fig. 7.5). The implant inserter—also provided in the Montgomery thyroplasty surgical set—is located in the middle tier of the anterior base and is used to snap the implant in place.

A fiberoptic laryngoscopy is recommended at this particular time (Fig. 7.6).

Step 11 Repair

A suction drainage and a multilayer classical closure are advised (Fig. 7.7).

Step 12 Postoperative Care

A 24 hours drainage monitoring and a one-week oral antibiotics coverage is recommended.

Same-day surgery is not favored within the European healthcare environment because of the possibility of laryngeal edema or postoperative bleeding that could interfere with the laryngeal airway.

Postoperative voice therapy and regular voice assessment at 1, 6, and 12 months are advocated.

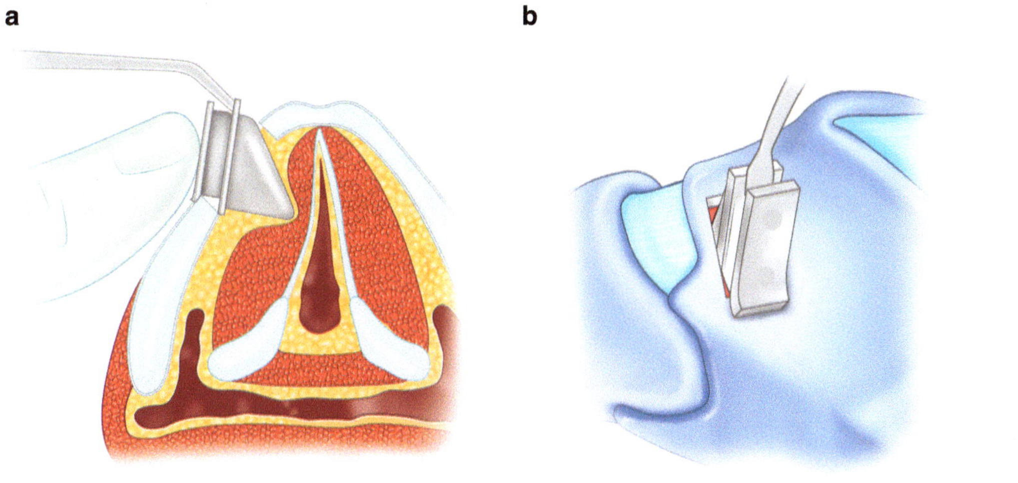

Fig. 7.5 (**a**, **b**) Insert the appropriate implant by stabilizing it posteriorly with your thumb and pressing the middle plate of the implant with the appropriate instrument provided by the Montgomery system. Patient maintains a Valsalva during the entire process

Fig. 7.6 Implant correctly inserted. Note its very anterior positioning

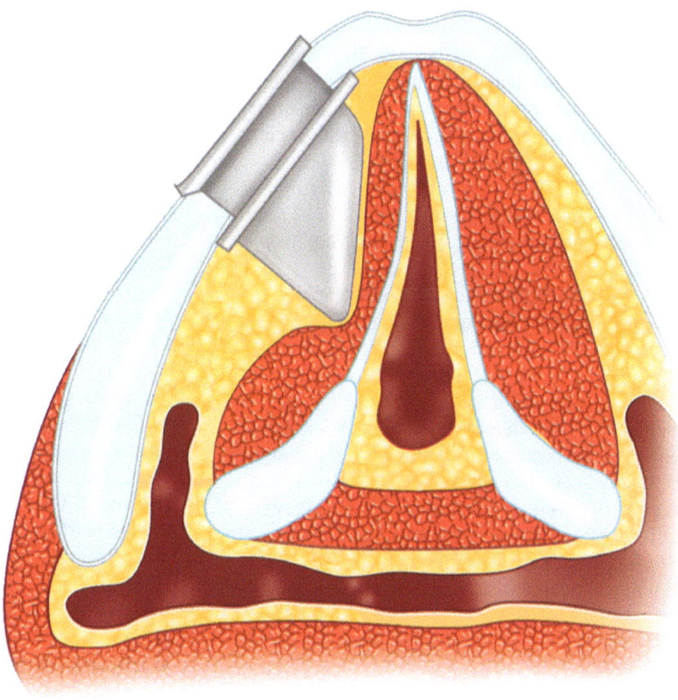

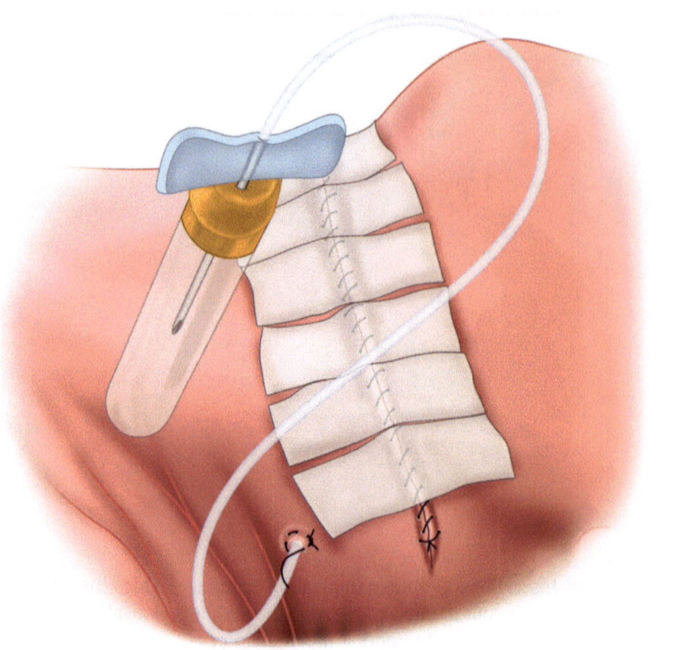

Fig. 7.7 Closing by a three planes suture (subglottic muscles, platysma, and skin). A 24h00 drainage suction drainage is advised

References

1. Friedrichs G, de Jong F, Mahieu H, Benninger M, Isshiki N. Laryngeal framework surgery: a proposal for classification and nomenclature by the phonosurgery committee of the European Laryngological Society. Eur Arch Otorhinolaryngol. 2001;258:389–96.
2. Desuter GRR. The Montgomery Thyroplasty Implant System: a 360° assessment. Doctoral Thesis, Universiteit Leiden, 21 Jan 2020. http://hdl.handle.net/1887/83254.
3. Payr E. Plastik am schildknorpel zur behebung der folgen einseitiger stimmbandlähmung. Dtsch Med Wochenschr. 1915;43:1265–70.
4. Netterville JL, Stone RE, Luken ES, Civantos FJ, Ossoff RH. Silastic medialization and arytenoid adduction: the Vanderbilt experience. A review of 116 phonosurgical procedures. Ann Otol Rhinol Laryngol. 1993;102:413–24.
5. Montgomery WW, Blaugrund SM, Varvares MA. Thyroplasty: a new approach. Ann Otol Rhinol Laryngol. 1993;102:571–9.
6. Cummings CW, Purcell LL, Flint PW. Hydroxylapatite laryngeal implants for medialization. Preliminary report. Ann Otol Rhinol Laryngol. 1993;102:843–51.
7. Friedrich G. Titanium vocal fold medialization implant: introducing a novel implant system for external vocal fold medialization. Ann Otol Rhinol Laryngol. 1999;108:79–86.
8. McCullogh TM, Hoffman HT. Medialization laryngoplasty with expanded polytetrafluoroethylene. Ann Otol Rhinol Laryngol. 1998;107:427–32.
9. Benninger MS, Manzoor N, Ruda M. Short and long-term outcomes after silastic medialization laryngoplasty: are arytenoid procedures needed? J Voice. 2015;29N(2):236–40.
10. Desuter G, Henrard S, Boucquey D, Van Boven M, Gardiner Q, Remacle M. Learning curve of medialization thyroplasty using a Montgomery™ implant. Eur Arch Otorhinolaryngol. 2015;272:385–90.
11. Desuter G, Zapater E, Van der Vorst S, et al. Very long-term voice handicap index voice outcomes after Montgomery thyroplasty: a cross-sectional study. Clin Otolaryngol. 2018; https://doi.org/10.1111/coa.13113.
12. Desuter G, Henrard S, Van Lith-Bijl JT, et al. Shape of thyroid cartilage influences outcome of Montgomery medialization thyroplasty: a gender issue. J Voice. 2017;31(2):245.e3–8.
13. Desuter G, Cartiaux O, Pierard J, et al. Accuracy of thyroid cartilage fenestration during Montgomery medialization thyroplasty. J Voice. 2010;34(4): 609–15.
14. Laccourreye O, Rubin F, van Lith-Bijl J, Desuter G. Keys to successful type-1 Thyroplasty with Montgomery® implant for unilateral laryngeal immobility in adults. Eur Ann Otorhinolaryngol Head Neck Dis. 2021;138(3):191–4. https://doi.org/10.1016/j.anorl.2020.10.001.

8 Surgical Management of Vocal Fold Scars

Antoine Giovanni and Alexia Mattei

Key Points

- Vocal fold microstructure is complex, particularly due to its foliated organization.
- Vocal fold scarring is a pathological entity characterized by reduced pliability of the vocal fold mucosa with a reduced mucosal wave and, occasionally, an incomplete glottic closure during phonation.
- A variety of treatment options have been developed in the last decades, but despite all efforts, it has not yet been possible to completely restore an unaltered VF structure and oscillation.
- Because surgical treatment is usually very difficult and the therapeutic outcome is to some extent unpredictable, conservative therapy should be the first line of treatment.

A. Giovanni · A. Mattei (✉)
Department of Oto-Rhino-Laryngology and Head and Neck Surgery, APHM, La Conception University Hospital, Marseille, France

Aix Marseille Univ, CNRS, LPL, Aix-en-Provence, France
e-mail: antoine.giovanni@ap-hm.fr; alexia.mattei@ap-hm.fr

8.1 Introduction

Vocal fold scarring is a pathological entity characterized by reduced pliability of the vocal fold mucosa with a reduced mucosal wave and, occasionally, an incomplete glottic closure during phonation. Regardless to the etiology, vibratory consequences will correspond to the degree of abnormality of the vocal fold structure. In the interest of simplification, it has been proposed different classifications for larynx diseases. These include the classification used to describe sulcus vocalis and the ELS classification used to describe endoscopic cordectomies [1–4]. A joint committee of members of the European Laryngological Society and the American Laryngological Association presented recently a simple and useful classification (Fig. 8.1):

- **Type I**: Atrophy of lamina propria with/without affected epithelium. This category includes conditions in which there is pliability of the vocal fold. These are characterized of incomplete glottic closure with bowing of the vocal fold on stroboscopic evaluation. These conditions are the various types of atrophy of the lamina propria, as these have been described by others [1, 2], and age-related vocal fold atrophy (presbylarynx). These include superficial sulcus, sulcus vergeture, sulcus vocalis, and mucosal bridge with/without sulcus.

M. Remacle, H. E. Eckel (eds.), *Textbook of Surgery of Larynx and Trachea*,
https://doi.org/10.1007/978-3-031-09621-1_8

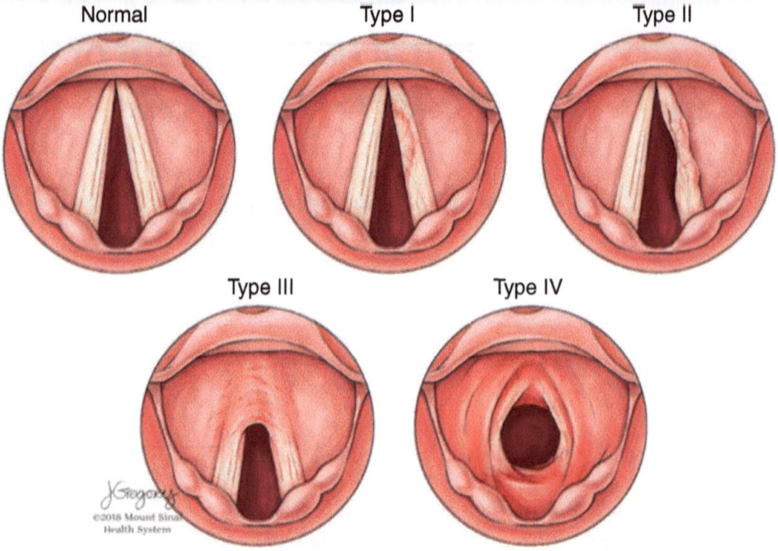

Fig. 8.1 ELS-ALA and ELS classification. (In Hantzakos 2019 [5])

- **Type II**: The epithelium, lamina propria, and muscle are affected. This category includes conditions that alter the pliability of the vocal folds. They result in stiffening of the mucosal wave, which may be secondary to phonotrauma, direct trauma, iatrogenic, postradiation, and chronic chemical irritation (smoking, reflux). These may vary from minimal changes noted on the epithelium and lamina propria with simple stiffening of the free vocal fold edge and minimal reduction of the mucosal wave, to partial or complete.
- **Type III**: Scar located on the anterior commissure, resulting in anterior glottal incompetence with or without affecting the mucosal wave on stroboscopy. It includes congenital or acquired laryngeal web and types Va and VI cordectomies and results in anterior involvement.
- **Type IV**: This category includes extended scar formation in both anteroposterior and rostro-caudal axis, with significant loss of vocal fold mass. It includes ELS type Vb–d cordotomies, as well as patients with voice deficiency after open vertical partial laryngectomy with extended vertical partial laryngectomy. This category also includes open subtotal partial laryngectomy with arytenoidectomy with contralateral cordectomy.

This classification is useful as it gives a simple framework in which almost all the clinical situations can be classified. If we focus mainly on type I and type II, we can summarize considering the deeper layer involved

Type I: Epithelium and lamina propria
Type II: Epithelium, lamina propria, and muscle

We can understand easily that biomechanical consequences will be different since type I is "characterized of incomplete glottic closure with bowing of the vocal fold on stroboscopic evaluation." But, in the paper presented, biomechanics characteristics remain unclear: "These may vary from minimal changes noted on the epithelium and lamina propria with simple stiffening of the free vocal fold edge and minimal reduction of the mucosal wave, to partial or complete." Coming back to what we know about the role of each layer of the vocal fold seems necessary.

8.2 Vocal Fold Healing

Vocal fold microstructure is complex [6, 7], particularly due to its foliated organization. According to Hirano's body-cover theory, the vocal folds comprise a superior layer ("cover") composed of the epithelium, basal membrane and the superior part of the lamina propria, and an inferior layer ("body") composed of the deep lamina propria and thyroarytenoid muscle, the two being separated by the intermediate layer of the lamina propria. This specific architecture allows the two functional units to vibrate independently and is found in the mid-part of the vocal folds. The anterior and posterior regions, which are the site of maculae flavae, show a different architecture which acts as a buffer. The proportions and organization of the extracellular matrix components largely determine the mechanical properties of the vocal folds. The superficial layer of the lamina propria is mainly composed of amorphous material poor in collagen fibers and elastin; the intermediate layer contains more elastic fibers and the deep layer more collagen fibers. Following laryngeal microsurgery, vocal fold scarring is sometimes observed, due to partial disappearance of the lamina propria, with the superficial and/or intermediate layer replaced by fibrous tissue, preventing mechanical uncoupling of the epithelium and muscle and thereby inducing vibration disorder (Fig. 8.2). Scar tissue may also be found without iatrogenic etiology: congenital or, more often, acquired, via a mechanism similar to that of cutaneous vergetures or as a result of trauma or chronic inflammatory phenomena.

Pathological scarring comprises three phases: inflammation, proliferation, and remodeling [8]. The first phase implicates inflammation factors such as interleukin 1β or TNFα, synthesized 4–8 h after injury. There is then increased expression of hyaluronan synthases 1 and 2, procollagens I and III, and cyclooxygenase 2, followed by massive recruitment of cells, mainly with fibroblastic characteristics, derived from the macula flava or remote tissue such as bone marrow. Density peaks at day 5–7 but may fail to fully restore the vocal fold. The fibroblasts then differentiate into myofibroblasts; the collagen and elastin bundles become disorganized, losing parallelism; the density of elastin, hyaluronic acid, fibromodulin, and decorin diminishes; fine type III collagen is replaced by type I; and fibronectin density increases. This is often accompanied by loss of volume and glottal defect. The vocal impact is disabling, especially for professional communicators, while current treatment possibilities are limited as the great complexity of vocal fold microstructure hinders the development of effective therapy.

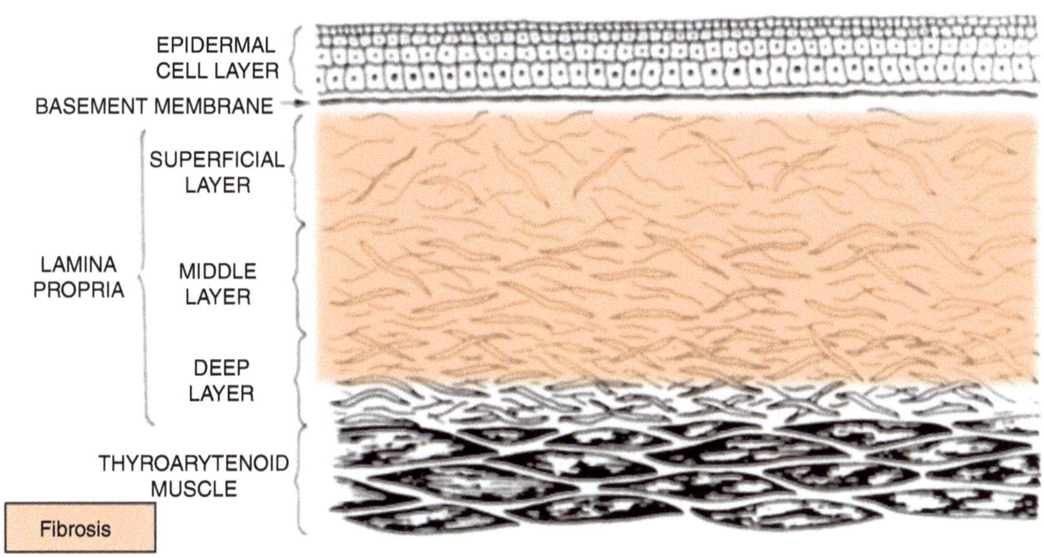

Fig. 8.2 Layered structure of the vocal folds and fibrosis localization. (From Friedrich G, Dikkers FG, Arens C, Remacle M, Hess M, Giovanni A et al. Vocal fold scars: current concepts and future directions. Consensus report of the phonosurgery committee of the European Laryngological Society. Eur Arch Otorhinolaryngol. 2013;270(9):2491–507 [6])

8.3 Biomechanical Consequences of Vocal Fold Scarring

In 1975, Hirano proposed his theory of voice production that is now known as the cover-body theory [7]. This has been the basis for understanding vocal fold mechanics and benign vocal fold pathology ever since. The location, extent, and depth of damage on each layer, therefore, alter the vocal fold vibration and determine the phonatory outcomes. Nevertheless, the exact role of each layer is not completely elucidated, and some further knowledge of the subtle interactions between layers are still to be completed.

Basically, it is widely admitted that there are two main mechanisms of vibration of the vocal fold (mechanism 1 and mechanism 2 according mainly to the contraction of the cricothyroid muscle). In mechanism 1 (chest register, i.e., in lower tones of the voice, near the fundamental frequency), despite the relative freedom of epithelium thanks to the superficial lamina propria, we can observe on stroboscopic evaluation or on high-speed video recordings that the epithelium vibrates at the same frequency and phase as the vocalis muscle. That actually means that the vibrating layer (cover layer to come back to the body-cover theory) is made of, from surface to depth, epithelium, lamina propria, and vocalis muscle. On the other hand, the non-vibrating layer (or support layer or "body layer") corresponds to the lateral chief of the thyroarytenoid muscle and the thyroid cartilage (Fig. 8.3). This mechanism is used for phonation around our usual fundamental frequency. The frequency of the produced voice (pitch) is determined by the progressive isometric contraction of the vocalis muscle.

At a certain pitch, according to the natural and acquired skills of the speaker, vocalis muscle cannot contract itself anymore, and the contraction of the cricothyroid muscle starts. Its action "pulls" forward the thyroid cartilage (and the vocalis as well), which causes a passive elongation of the vocalis and consequently a higher tension in the vibrating layer as a whole. It is not clearly demonstrated in the scientific literature, and large studies are missing, but it is "probable" that the vocalis muscle progressively disengages while cricothyroid muscle is contracting. This results in an apparent shift of the border between body and cover: in high tones, the vibrating layer is (at least apparently) made of epithelium, lamina propria, and a more or less thin medial part of the vocalis (Fig. 8.4). These points are of crucial importance regarding the biomechanical consequences of vocal fold scarring.

A scar can be modeled as a structural modification of the normal layered structure leading to a more rigid structure in one layer or connecting two different layers and disturbing their gradient of pliability. This rigid, fibrous part of the system may involve the epithelium only, the lamina propria in its different substructures, the vocal ligament, the vocalis muscle, and even the thyroarytenoid muscle. We can understand that biomechanical consequences will be significantly different as well as therapeutic opportunities. Consequently, it looks crucial to identify the considered layer and to more stratify the classifica-

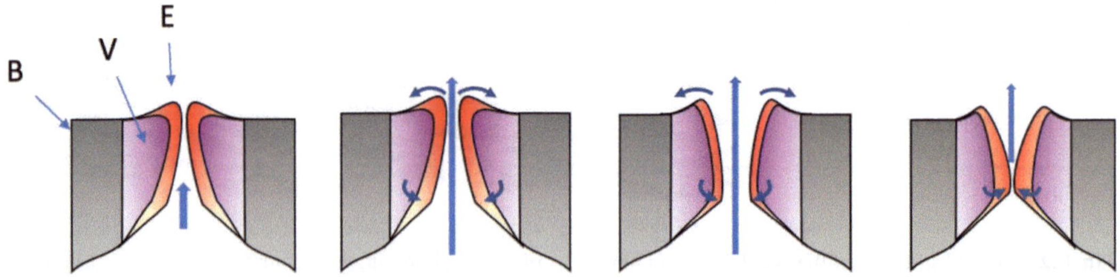

Fig. 8.3 Schematic view of the body-cover theory in vocal fold vibration. *B* body, *V* vocalis, *E* epithelium (V + E: cover)

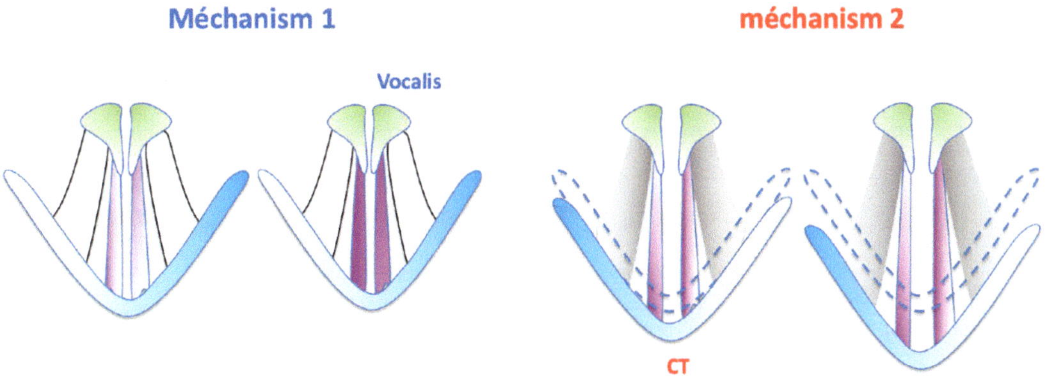

Fig. 8.4 Schematic view of the muscles involved in laryngeal mechanisms

tion proposed by the ELS and the ALA. To that end, we propose a more detailed classification allowing a better understanding of induced dysphonia and therapeutic options.

ELS-ALA type I involving epithelium and lamina propria may be split into:

- **Type I epithelium**: The scar involves only the epithelium of the vocal fold without significant alteration of the lamina propria. In stroboscopic examination, it is observed as a "rigid" zone looking stiffer compared to the mucosal undulation below.
- **Type I Reinke**: No more stroboscopic undulation ("stroboscopic silence") and a scar involving the entire width of the Reinke's space with loss of pliability gradient within the different layers. There is a glottal leakage due to the loss of vibration itself, but the global mass of the vocal fold is intact, i.e., contact between the vocal folds can be observed in cold light examination without significant gap. In some cases, the epithelium can be intact but without any degree of freedom that leads to the same stroboscopic silence.

ELS-ALA type II involving the epithelium, lamina propria, and muscle may be split into (Fig. 8.5 and Table 8.1):

- **Type II ligament**: The scar unites in a same rigid object the epithelium and the different layers of the lamina propria, including vocal ligament. Again, there is no more stroboscopic undulation. The differential diagnostic with the type I Reinke can be made thanks to the presence of the gap visible in cold light examination of the vocal folds. During a microsurgical exploration, palpation cannot manage to find a plane between the scar and the vocal ligament. For this type II ligament, therapeutics should include, in addition to a procedure on the scar itself, some kind of "volumation" of the vocal fold.
- **Type II muscle**: Here the vocal fold is made of a remaining part of the thyroarytenoid muscle covered with a more or less thin epithelium. Basically, this configuration is the one observed after a type III or type IV cordectomy. Paradoxically, this kind of "primitive" vibrator may be more efficient than the previous one, probably because the thyroarytenoid muscle is more pliable itself than a rigidified vocal ligament as in a type II cordectomy.

This classification is more complete that the ELS classification but seems, actually, more adapted to find out more or less homogeneous groups of patients with vocal fold scars. On the other hand, distinction between the different subtypes seems easy on the basis of the usual assessment of these lesions: cold light and stroboscopic examination and phonosurgical exploration.

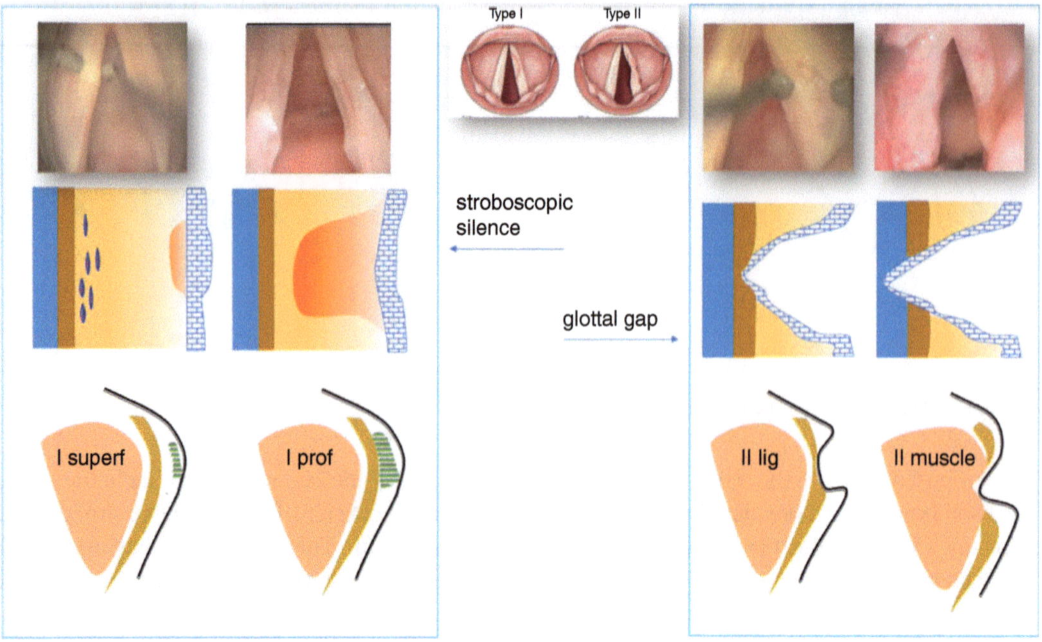

Fig. 8.5 Detailed classification of vocal fold scars

Table 8.1 Comparison of different classifications (Remacle and Arens [9], Hantzakos et al. [5] and ours)

	Remacle and Arens	ELS and ALA	Classification	Therapeutic options
Epithelium	I	I	I Epithelium	Scar dissection
Lamina propria			I Reinke	Scar dissection and/or medialization
Ligament	III	II	II Ligament	Medialization
Muscle			II Muscle	Medialization

8.4 Etiopathogenesis of Vocal Fold Scars

There is no general accepted classification of VF scars. Benninger et al. [10] distinguished the following causes of VF scarring: traumatic, neoplastic, iatrogenic, inflammatory, and miscellaneous. In its broader definition, vocal fold scarring may include vocal fold atrophy, congenital or acquired sulcus vocalis, iatrogenic or postsurgical scarring, and direct trauma, i.e., after prolonged intubation or as a result of radiation or chronic irritation on reflux disease. Even lesions caused by phonotrauma could be considered as a kind of scarring since they are linked to an altered healing after (or during) a trauma: although of different origin, the phonatory outcome is similar. This wide variety of pathologies under the same term may cause disturbance, and it is generally admitted that the term "scars" is reserved for sequelae following the healing after the initial trauma (surgery, direct trauma, pharyngo-laryngeal reflux). It is commonly admitted that exudative lesions and dysplastic or malignant lesions are excluded from the range of "vocal fold scars."

8.4.1 Iatrogenic Mechanisms

The most common cause for VF scars is sequelae after traumatic injuries by heterogenic mechanisms including external laryngeal trauma (fracture), internal laryngeal trauma (intubation), and phonotrauma as well as phonosurgery. In cancer surgery, extended resection of VF tissue with consecutive major scarring is mostly inevitable. Surgery for benign VF lesions has to avoid this by any means, carefully respecting phonosurgical principles since inadequate techniques and wrong indications can have disastrous consequences for the patient [11, 12]. Special care must be taken for the very trauma-sensitive superficial lamina propria. A study by Martinez-Arias et al. [13] described adherent epithelium to the deep VF tissue after laser-assisted surgery (CO_2 laser scanning technology) of benign lesions in 12 patients. Thermal trauma can damage the delicate lamina propria very easily. On the other hand, Benninger [14] and Remacle [15] showed that there are no differences in the functional outcomes between CO_2 laser and cold instrument surgery in benign VF lesions when proper settings and techniques are used. Other causes for acquired VF scars are chronic inflammatory processes due to laryngopharyngeal reflux, smoking, radiotherapy, toxic inhalants, etc. The aging process of the VFs does not necessarily lead to scars but very often to similar conditions by a combination of VF atrophy and an accumulation of traumas throughout life.

8.4.2 Congenital Theory of Epidermoid Cysts Evolution

Bouchayer and Cornut published in 1985 an elaborated concept of congenital VF lesions, suggesting epidermoid cysts as a common cause for different pathologic conditions [16]. They hypothesized that epidermoid cysts result from embryologic residuals of epithelial cells underneath the normal epithelium of the vocal fold. According to their theories, sulcus vocalis can be considered as an "open cyst," and what they refer to as vergeture results from an atrophic evolution of the cyst. If the ruptured VF cyst penetrates on both sides (superior and below the free margin of the VF), the mucosa between these two openings turns into a mucosal bridge [1, 16]. They underlined their theory with the typical early onset of this kind of dysphonia during childhood, some cases of familial occurrence, simultaneous findings of multiple lesions in both VFs, and association with other malformations, such as pathological vessels and micro-webs. This theory is summarized in Fig. 8.6.

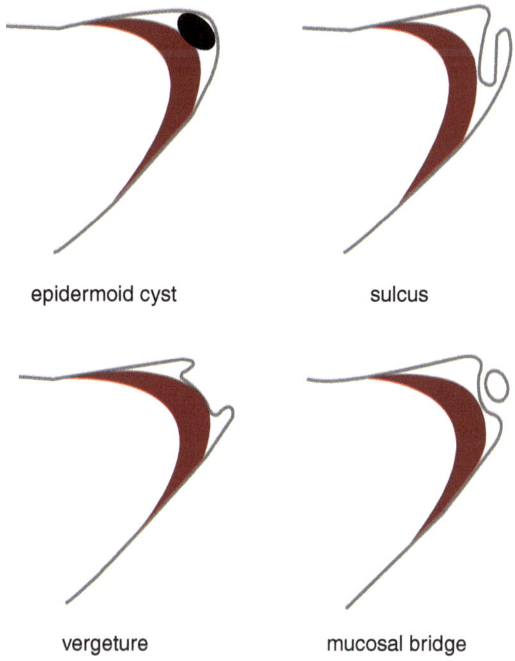

Fig. 8.6 Congenital lesions according to the concept of Bouchayer and Cornut [16]

8.4.3 Acquired Theory of Sulcus

Other authors have suggested that sulcus vocalis is acquired and results from local trauma and/or chronic inflammatory processes [17, 18]. Sato and Hirano [19] demonstrated that sulcus vocalis is associated with a degeneration of fibroblasts in the macula flava. Collagenous and elastic fibers, synthesized by fibroblasts in the maculae flavae, were decreased. They described the presence of many abnormal elastic fibers in the maculae flavae. This mechanism is similar to the age-related degeneration of the VFs. Giovanni [20] concluded that congenital and acquired lesions are complementary and that the decisive link is a specific weakness in the regulation mechanisms of fibrous tissue in the VF.

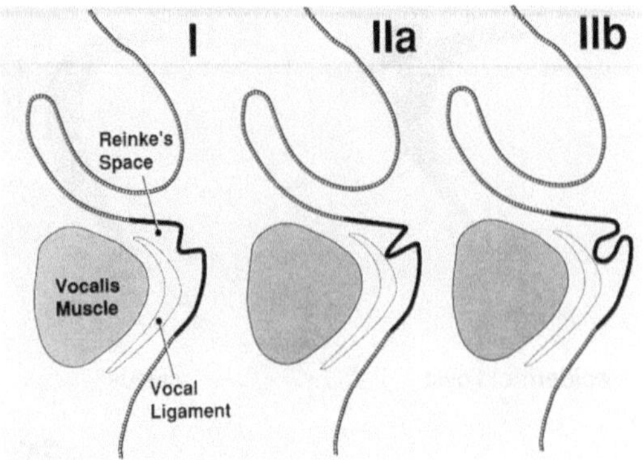

Fig. 8.7 Ford's classification [2]

Ford classified sulcus vocalis into three subtypes [2]: type I is a physiologic variant accentuated by atrophy but with intact lamina propria and an undisturbed mucosal wave. Type IIa (sulcus vergeture) is characterized by disappearance of a functional SLP. In most cases, the bottom of the vergeture is attached to the vocal ligament and leads to moderate dysphonia. Type IIb or true sulcus (pouch) extends more deeply into the vocal ligament and may even penetrate into the thyroarytenoid muscle. It disrupts the mucosal vibration and leads to severe dysphonia [20]. The incidence of sulcus vocalis could be considerably higher than commonly admitted: a recent study performed in 100 cadavers found sulcus vocalis in 39 cases with a pathological sulcus vocalis rate of 23 [21] (Fig. 8.7).

8.5 Therapeutic Options

8.5.1 General Principles

The major aim of all therapeutic procedures is primarily to increase loudness and vocal endurance, reduce air loss and vocal fatigue, and improve the voice aesthetics. The current therapeutic possibilities are reduced, the high complexity of the microstructure of the vocal cords contributing to the difficulty of finding an ideal treatment. From a functional view, the superficial lamina propria is the crucial structure of the VF, and the creation of a new gliding zone remains one of the major unsolved problems in phonosurgery. A variety of treatment options have been developed in the last decades. Despite all efforts, it has not yet been possible to completely restore an unaltered VF structure and oscillation. Because surgical treatment is usually very difficult and the therapeutic outcome is to some extent unpredictable, conservative therapy should be the first line of treatment. Voice therapy alone can be effective and satisfactory, but it might also be given as a supplementary postoperative treatment modality. It is usually based on the traditional holistic concepts primarily focusing on resonatory voice and breath supported voice coordination.

In any case, the first step in choosing a therapeutic option is the assessment of the patient's glottic and vocal situation. It is necessary to specify the vocal problem on the basis of the proposed classification, but it is also necessary to take into account the quality of the voice produced by the patient and especially what he feels about his/her vocal problem. It is generally prudent to perform a pre-therapeutic voice recording and ask the patient to complete a questionnaire such as Voice Handicap Index. Surgery should not be performed within 6 months after the scar formation, i.e., when the healing process is not yet complete. As the objective of surgery is to improve glottic closure and pliability of the VF, the treatment should be orientated towards the main clinical feature: either glottic gap or rigidity.

8.5.2 Treatment Options to Improve Pliability

When rigidity appears to be the major feature, the mucosal wave can be (at least theoretically) restored by lysing the scarred mucosa and creating a new layer between the epithelium and the vocal ligament to restore the body-cover relationship.

In the history of scars, first proposed technique has been the resection of the scar (micro-

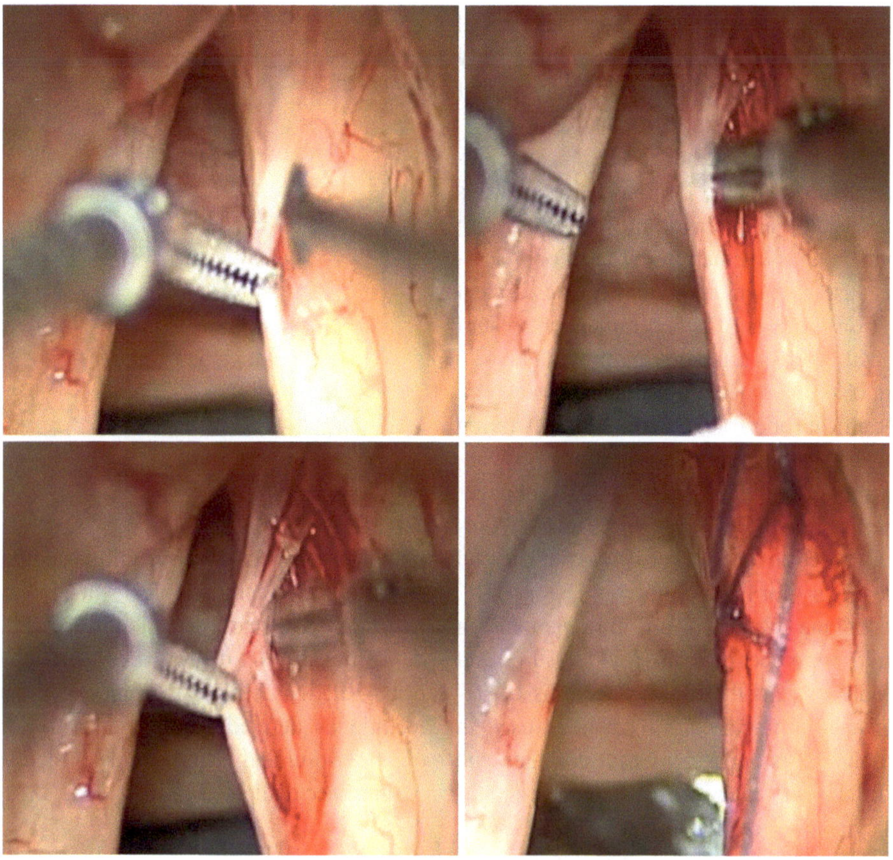

Fig. 8.8 Scar resection under microlaryngoscopy

flap technique). After careful dissection of the epithelium and resection of pathologic tissue, the flap is turned back and fixated with fibrin glue or a microstitch (Fig. 8.8). The major disadvantage of this technique is the unpredictable re-adhesion or even the creation of new scars as no filler or tissue is used for replacement of superficial lamina propria. This technique has recently be emphasized by Sulica [22]. Sataloff et al. developed a minimal invasive technique with the creation of subepithelial tunnels by elevating the scarred mucosa using blunt and sharp microinstruments [23]. The fat is inserted into these pockets with a forceps or a laryngeal syringe with a large diameter needle. The procedure itself resolves the scar by elevating the mucosa which restores the cover-body relationship thanks to the low-viscosity characteristics of fat. They found an improved wavelike vibration pattern with more regular periodicities at the free margins. Here again the problem consists in the resorbable nature of fat. Some other authors described mucosa grafting with an autogenous buccal mucosa graft. Reappearance of vibration takes several months but is not guaranteed in every case.

Another novel approach for the treatment of scars is the use of angiolytic lasers, i.e., PDL (pulsed dye laser) and PTP (potassium titanyl phosphate) [24–26]. A growing number of papers demonstrated a beneficial effect in treating cutaneous scars. Although the exact underlying mechanisms are not fully understood to date, experimental trials described the potential development of a sub-basement membrane cleavage plane, as well as the upregulation of proteins which may actively modulate mature fibrosis. However, this type of laser is currently not available routinely.

But, as every surgery, these techniques including manipulations of the lamina propria always bear the risk of an unfavorable outcome with even worsening the situation by additional scarring. Because of the unpredictability of a surgical intervention's results, it is recommended to start always with the less traumatizing procedure.

Corticosteroids injection in the scar itself can play an anti-fibrotic role. Steroid administration in microlaryngeal surgery for vocal scar prevention has a long history of use. In 1992, Bouchayer and Cornut already described the use of hydrocortisone injections in the vocal folds at the end of microsurgery for benign mucosal lesions [16]. This technique produced an improvement in vocal fold suppleness, vocal fold closure, and voice quality. In another field, injections of steroids such as triamcinolone have been used in hypertrophic scars and keloid with collagen and cell proliferation reduction mediated by alterations in cytokine secretion [27].

The development of in-office laryngology allows injections under local anesthesia and can be an elegant solution mainly in cases of relatively recent scarring (Fig. 8.9). After office steroids injection (methylprednisolone 40 mg/mL) in 12 patients with scarred vocal folds (under local anesthesia), Mortensen showed a significant improvement in voice grade, amplitude, and mucosal wave without any complications [28]. Another study from Young in 2016 evaluated 25 patients undergoing office-based dexamethasone (10 mg/mL) injection into the superficial lamina propria for mild/moderate vocal fold scar [29]. Most of the parameters including videostroboscopic parameters were improved after injection combined with voice therapy.

In some studies, autologous fat and low-grade cross-linked hyaluronic acid have been proposed for this purpose. Injections must be done superficially, into the scar tissue: the injectables should not act as fillers but create a new soft and pliable layer for restoration of the mucosal wave propagation. Some interesting results have been published but with a low replicability by other teams and relatively unpredictable results. Postoperative adhesion and scar formation were reduced by deposition of HA derivatives in the lamina propria [30]. It is precisely in these situations that techniques derived from regenerative medicine can be useful and have been described in the literature (see dedicated chapter) [31–33].

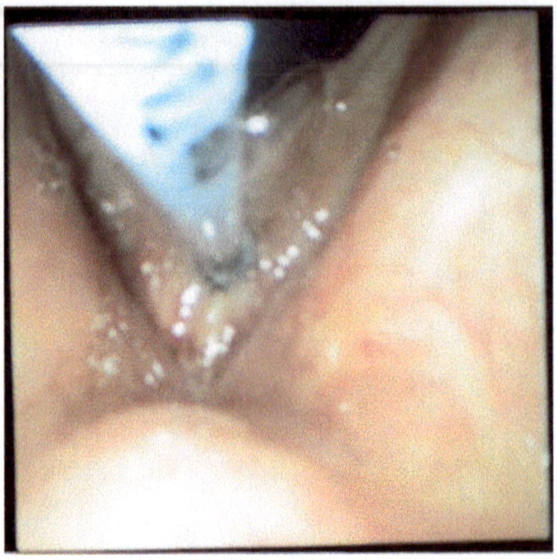

Fig. 8.9 In-office steroid injection

8.5.3 Treatment Options in Case of Glottic Leakage

In cases where an insufficient glottic closure is the predominant finding, medialization procedures proved to be very effective. These can either be performed with medialization thyroplasty or injection augmentation with some more or less absorbable material. Autologous materials have the big advantage of providing excellent biocompatibility. The most common autologous fillers used so far for treatment of VF scarring are autologous fat (with a strong preference on lateral fat injection compared to implantation near the vibratory margin) and fascia. Fat autografts are easy to harvest and show only minimal immunological reactivity. Glottic gap insufficiency diminishes after injection as the VF is placed medially and additional bulk is added to the VF (Fig. 8.10). It is possible as well to use hydroxyapatite or hyaluronic acid. In some cases, it is even necessary to propose a thyroplasty with, for instance, a Montgomery prosthesis.

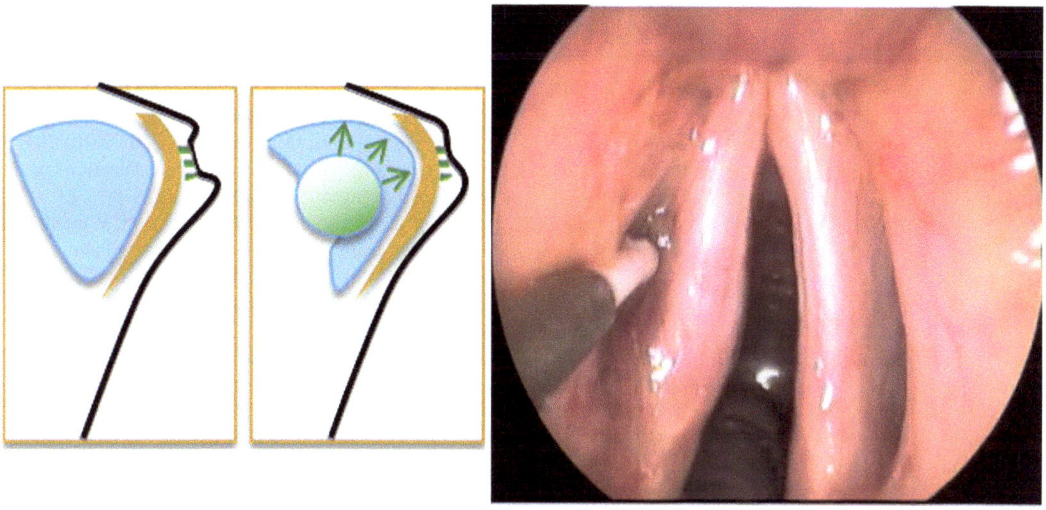

Fig. 8.10 Injection for medialization

References

1. Monday LA, Cornut G, Bouchayer M, Roch JB. Epidermoid cysts of the vocal cords. Ann Otol Rhinol Laryngol. 1983;92:124–7.
2. Ford CN, Inagi K, Khidr A, Bless DM, Gilchrist KW. Sulcus vocalis: a rational analytical approach to diagnosis and management. Ann Otol Rhinol Laryngol. 1996;105:189–200.
3. Remacle M, Eckel HE, Antonelli A, Brasnu D, Chevalier D, Friedrich G, Olofsson J, Rudert HH, Thumfart W, de Vincentiis M, Wustrow TP. Endoscopic cordectomy. A proposal for a classification by the Working Committee, European Laryngological Society. Eur Arch Otorhinolaryngol. 2000;257(4):227–31.
4. Remacle M, Van Haverbeke C, Eckel H, Bradley P, Chevalier D, Djukic V, De Vicentiis M, Friedrich G, Olofsson J, Peretti G, Quer M, Werner J. Proposal for revision of the European Laryngological Society classification of endoscopic cordectomies. Eur Arch Otorhinolaryngol. 2007;264:499–504. https://doi.org/10.1007/s00405-007-0279-z.
5. Hantzakos A, Dikkers FG, Giovanni A, Benninger MS, Remacle M, Sjögren EV, et al. Vocal fold scars: a common classification proposal by the American Laryngological Association and European Laryngological Society. Eur Arch Otorhinolaryngol. 2019;276(8):2289–92.
6. Friedrich G, Dikkers FG, Arens C, Remacle M, Hess M, Giovanni A, et al. Vocal fold scars: current concepts and future directions. Consensus report of the Phonosurgery Committee of the European Laryngological Society. Eur Arch Otorhinolaryngol. 2013;270(9):2491–507.
7. Hirano M. Phonosurgery: basic and clinical investigation. Otologia (Fukuoka). 1975;21:239–440.
8. Gugatschka M, Kojima T, Ohno S, Kanemaru S-i, Hirano S. Recruitment patterns of side population cells during wound healing in rat vocal folds. Laryngoscope. 2011;121(8):1662–7.
9. Arens C, Remacle M. Scarred larynx. In: Remacle M, Eckel H, editors. Surgery of the larynx and trachea. 1st ed. Berlin: Springer; 2010. p. 171–6.
10. Benninger MS, Alessi D, Archer S, et al. Vocal fold scarring: current concepts and management. Otolaryngol Head Neck Surg. 1996;115:474–82.
11. Friedrich G. Basic principles for indications in phonosurgery. Laryngorhinootologie. 1995;74:663–5.
12. Friedrich G, Remacle M, Birchall M, Marie JP, Arens C. Defining phonosurgery: a proposal for classification and nomenclature by the Phonosurgery Committee of the European Laryngological Society (ELS). Eur Arch Otorhinolaryngol. 2007;264:1191–200.
13. Martinez Arias A, Remacle M, Lawson G. Treatment of vocal fold scar by carbon dioxide laser and collagen injection: retrospective study on 12 patients. Eur Arch Otorhinolaryngol. 2010;267:1409–14.
14. Benninger MS. Microdissection or microspot CO_2 laser for limited vocal fold benign lesions: a prospective randomized trial. Laryngoscope. 2000; 110:1–17.
15. Remacle M, Arens C, Eldin MB, Campos G, Estomba CC, Dulguerov P, et al. Laser-assisted surgery of the upper aero-digestive tract: a clarification of nomenclature. A consensus statement of the European Laryngological Society. Eur Arch Otorhinolaryngol. 2017;274(10):3723–7.
16. Bouchayer M, Cornut G. Microsurgical treatment of benign vocal fold lesions: indications, technique, results. Folia Phoniatr (Basel). 1992;44:155–84.

17. Itoh T, Kawasaki H, Morikawa I, Hirano M. Vocal fold furrows. A 10-year review of 240 patients. Auris Nasus Larynx. 1983;10(Suppl):S17–26.
18. Nakayama M, Ford CN, Brandenburg JH, Bless DM. Sulcus vocalis in laryngeal cancer: a histopathologic study. Laryngoscope. 1994;104:16–24.
19. Sato K, Hirano M. Electron microscopic investigation of sulcus vocalis. Ann Otol Rhinol Laryngol. 1998;107:56–60.
20. Giovanni A, Chanteret C, Lagier A. Sulcus vocalis: a review. Eur Arch Otorhinolaryngol. 2007;264:337–44.
21. Sunter AV, Yigit O, Huq GE, Alkan Z, Kocak I, Buyuk Y. Histopathological characteristics of sulcus vocalis. Otolaryngol Head Neck Surg. 2011;145:264–9.
22. Andreadis K, Hoffman K, D'Angelo D, Sulica L. Sulcus vocalis: results of excision without reconstruction. Laryngoscope. 2020;130(9):2208–12.
23. Sataloff RT, Spiegel JR, Heuer RJ, et al. Laryngeal minimicroflap: a new technique and reassessment of the microflap saga. J Voice. 1995;9(2):198–204.
24. Prufer N, Woo P, Altman KW. Pulse dye and other laser treatments for vocal scar. Curr Opin Otolaryngol Head Neck Surg. 2010;18:492–7.
25. Zeitels SM, Burns JA. Office-based laryngeal laser surgery with the 532-nm pulsed-potassium-titanyl-phosphate laser. Curr Opin Otolaryngol Head Neck Surg. 2007;15:394–400.
26. Mortensen MM, Woo P, Ivey C, Thompson C, Carroll L, Altman K. The use of the pulse dye laser in the treatment of vocal fold scar: a preliminary study. Laryngoscope. 2008;118:1884–8.
27. Carroll LA, Hanasono MM, Mikulec AA, Kita M, Koch RJ. Triamcinolone stimulates bFGF production and inhibits TGF-[beta]1 production by human dermal fibroblasts. Dermatol Surg. 2002;28(8):704–9.
28. Mortensen M, Woo P. Office steroid injections of the larynx. Laryngoscope. 2006;116:1735–9.
29. Young W, Hoffman MR, Koszewski IJ, Whited CW, Ruel BN, Dailey SH. Voice outcomes following a single office-based steroid injection for vocal fold scar. Otolaryngol Head Neck Surg. 2016;155(5):820–8.
30. Hertegard S, Dahlqvist A, Goodyer E. Viscoelastic measurements after vocal fold scarring in rabbits—short-term results after hyaluronan injection. Acta Otolaryngol. 2006;126(7):758–63.
31. Mattei A, Magalon J, Bertrand B, Philandrianos C, Veran J, Giovanni A. Cell therapy and scarred vocal folds. Eur Ann Otorhinolaryngol Head Neck Dis. 2017;1879–296(17):30103–5.
32. Graupp M, Bachna-Rotter S, Gerstenberger C, Friedrich G, Fröhlich-Sorger E, Kiesler K, et al. The unsolved chapter of vocal fold scars and how tissue engineering could help us solve the problem. Eur Arch Otorhinolaryngol. 2016;273(9):2279–84.
33. Gugatschka M, Ohno S, Saxena A, Hirano S. Regenerative medicine of the larynx. Where are we Today? A review. J Voice. 2012;26(5):670.e7–670.e13.

Regenerative Procedures in Laryngology

9

Markus Gugatschka and David Hortobagyi

Key Points

- Regenerative medicine is a causal therapy approach that aims to restore organ integrity including function. As such this approach is rather rare, as most established therapies in the realm of laryngology are symptomatic only.
- Regenerative medicine bases on the following elements: cell therapy, material-based approaches, application of cytokines or growth factors, and, according to newer classifications, gene therapy.
- Tissue engineering can be seen as a subclass of regenerative medicine, combining the previously mentioned elements, with the purpose of replacing pathological tissue with an in vitro-fabricated fragment of healthy tissue.

9.1 What Is Regenerative Medicine? How Can It Be Useful in Laryngology?

Despite considerable progress in laryngological research, there remain several diseases and conditions that can only be treated symptomatically, among these are vocal fold (VF) scars, paresis, or sulcus to name a few. This relates to the fact that it is virtually impossible to study the human VF and its adjacent structures on a cellular or molecular level (see also Chap. 3 of this textbook). Likewise, most laryngeal examinations are still nowadays noninvasive and partly indirect such as laryngoscopy, stroboscopy, and voice analysis. It is evident though that before new treatment strategies can be established, we need to understand the microstructure and microphysiology of the VF during health and disease more in detail.

However, it is ethically not feasible to perform repeated biopsies in humans especially from the VF to study the consequences of therapeutic interventions. The difficult accessibility of the larynx also hampers further exploration. The consequences can be seen exemplarily in the case of laryngopharyngeal reflux: There are plenty of studies employing different diagnostic methods for often unspecific symptoms, leading to inconclusive results which lead to a highly unsatisfactory situation for the clinician.

Researchers started exploring laryngeal diseases at a cellular level and laryngeal tissue

M. Gugatschka (✉) · D. Hortobagyi
Division of Phoniatrics, ENT University Hospital Graz, Medical University Graz, Graz, Austria
e-mail: markus.gugatschka@medunigraz.at

M. Remacle, H. E. Eckel (eds.), *Textbook of Surgery of Larynx and Trachea*,
https://doi.org/10.1007/978-3-031-09621-1_9

engineering in the early 2000s, resulting in a considerable number of publications [1, 2]. In general, methods of *tissue engineering* and *regenerative medicine* (often referred to as TERM) are defined as methods to "repair, replace, or regenerate cells, tissues, or organs to restore impaired function" [3]. This can be done by both in vivo and ex vivo reactivation of developmental processes. Usually regenerative medicine is categorized into three elements [4], which are as follows:

- *Cell therapy*
- *Material-based approaches (scaffolds, gels, polymers)*
- *Use of cytokines and growth factors*
- *(Gene [modulation] therapies)*

Due to recent developments, a newer classification might also include *gene (modulation) therapies* as a separate point. In reality these approaches are used mutually with considerable overlap between them.

9.2 Which Laryngeal Diseases Should Be Addressed?

There are a number of diseases which might be a potential target for TERM. For didactical reasons, we decided to discuss in the following several clinically relevant laryngeal diseases and point out possible implications of TERM. As current treatment strategies are described in other chapters of this textbook, we will solely focus on experimental and possibly upcoming developments.

9.2.1 Vocal Fold Scar

Scar tissue formation can be, depending on its expansion, accompanied by significant deterioration of oscillatory functions of the VF and consequently cause dysphonia. The physiological vibratory functions of the affected VF are diminished or even suspended; the affected VF appears laryngoscopically stiffened with an altered surface.

At a cellular level, VF scarring is associated with a differentiation of the vocal fold fibroblasts (VFF) into fibrotic VF fibroblasts, or "myofibroblasts." This has a significant impact on the extracellular matrix metabolism as fibrotic VFF alter their expression profile. As a consequence, lower concentrations of hyaluronic acid (HA), decorin, and elastin were described in scar tissue [5]. On the other hand, scar tissue contains a higher amount of collagen fibers. In a healthy *lamina propria*, these fibers are aligned in parallel to the VF edge, whereas histological examinations have shown that collagen fibers follow a disordered pattern in scar tissue. This results in an impairment of viscoelastic properties, leading to irregular oscillation and a dysphonic voice.

There are many factors influencing wound healing or scar formation, among them is age. According to in vitro studies, myofibroblasts of younger rodents produced significantly higher amounts of (scar protective) HA when compared to an aged group [6]. In addition, myofibroblasts of younger rats showed a superior response to the anti-fibrotic cytokine hepatocyte growth factor (HGF) [7].

9.2.1.1 Cell Therapy

The concept underlying cell therapy is that scarred VF will regenerate and rebuild the layers of the *lamina propria* given the right trigger. However, it is important to have in mind that after a severe injury, the VF will rather be re-epithelialized than regenerate the *lamina propria* layers. Based on clinical knowledge, one can assume that in mature VF scar, the typical architecture of the *lamina propria* is no longer existent.

Cell therapy was used as early as 2004 to improve VF pliability. Chetri et al. treated injured/scarred VF in an animal model with three weekly injections of buccal mucosal fibroblasts [8]. Results showed improved VF pliability and near-normal mucosal wave propagation. The same group published in 2011 the use of autologous cultured fibroblasts from the oral mucosa in an uncontrolled trial including five patients and reported improved mucosal wave and VHI scores [9].

Later on, as different kinds of stem cells became more easily available, various studies were undertaken, again starting in animal models [4]. It also needs to be mentioned that many of these studies were done in acute injury settings rather than in chronic VF scar which has important implications on the findings of these publications. However, most studies reported positive effects in a variety of histological, molecular, and biomechanical parameters [10–13].

More recent studies transferred the use of stem cells for VF scar restoration into the human setting [14, 15]. The groups included were usually small (<17 patients) with a broad range of diseases. No control groups were included. Both studies reported no severe side effects following the procedures. However, based on the study settings, no conclusions about the efficacy of the treatment can be drawn. Improvements were mainly found in subjective scores such as the Voice Handicap Index (VHI). Standardized study protocols and procedures would be strongly needed, which could presumably be only reached in a multicenter approach.

9.2.1.2 Material-Based Approaches (Scaffolds, Gels, and Polymers)

The advances in biotechnologies led to the development of a newer generation of biocompatible materials. Suitable compounds could enlarge the therapeutic amatory considerably. An ideal candidate would promote wound healing and induce VF tissue regeneration by delivering (stem) cells or bioactive factors to the site of pathology. It would furthermore navigate the controlled release of these factors and guarantee that cells stay longer at the site of injection. Injectable bioactive and biodegradable polymers and hydrogels have significant advantages over traditional implantation materials. By minimizing the invasiveness and potential trauma to the VF, they limit the risk of secondary scarring and infection with providing easy practice and patient accessibility at the same time [16].

Injectable hydrogels in the realm of VF tissue regeneration were mainly focused on hyaluronic acid (HA) and its derivatives due to their important role in VF biology. The osmotic, viscoelastic, and space filling properties of HA are critical during phonation as they determine thickness, shape, and viscosity of the VF [17, 18]. Whereas many HA-based products were mainly used as fillers, they provide a broader therapeutical spectrum when used as a carrier for bioactive factors or cells.

Modifications of the carboxylic acids on the HA backbone lead to a new derivative, Carbylan-S. Acute injury models in rabbit models showed less fibrosis formation when Carbylan-SX hydrogel (Carbylan-S cross-linked with PEGDA) was applied directly after injury when compared to control substances [19]. Further work was done on another derivative, Carbylan-GSX. Experiments under 2D and 3D conditions explored biological behavior of encapsulated human VFF, reporting that Carbylan-GSX did not induce toxicity or inflammation. Carbylan-GSX-treated rabbit VF exhibited significantly better viscoelastic properties after 6 months, probably due to an enhanced healing process following prophylactic application at the time of surgery [20].

9.2.1.3 Use of Cytokines and Growth Factors

Cytokines and growth factors have been studied extensively in vitro and in vivo throughout the past 20 years, mostly in the field of VF scar research and to a minor degree in age-related VF atrophy. Once established, possible candidates might be used in an outpatient clinical setting. Hepatocyte growth factor (HGF) [21, 22] and basic fibroblast growth factor (bFGF) [23, 24] are to date the most extensively studied substances. HGF is a multifunctional polypeptide involved in embryogenesis, angiogenesis, organ regeneration, and wound healing. It has proved its antifibrotic efficacy in prevention or resolution of fibrosis of the liver, kidney, and lungs in animal models. In terms of VF fibrosis, HGF showed increased HA production and decreased collagen production in VF fibroblasts (canine in vitro trial) [22]. Due to insufficient retention times of HGF at the site of injection, drug delivery systems in form of hydrogels were developed [25]. In a canine model, beneficial effects in terms of histologic evaluation and vibration were observed injecting HGF 1 month after injury. Another study explored local tissue response as well as blood transmission of topically administered HGF. The study showed that HGF administered to the rat VF disappeared after 7 days with only minimal transmission to the blood [26]. It was Shigeru Hirano who published in 2017 the first prospective clinical trial including 18 patients (VF scar and sulcus). During the follow-up time of 6 months, no major local or systemic safety concerns were detected, and several outcome parameters (VHI-10, GRBAS scale) were improved [27].

Similar to HGF, bFGF exerts its effects via VF fibroblasts and HA production [28]. Several studies showed positive effects to reduce scar formation after injury (porcine model) [29], as well as in the chronic VF scar setting [28]. Several clinical studies reported positive effects up to 1 year after treatment [30, 31]. However, to date, human recombinant HGF is sold only in Japan, where it is approved for treatment of skin ulcers and burn injuries.

As indicated above, clinical trials performed so far showed promising results when using HGF and bFGF. There remains however uncertainties which need to be worked out by increasing sample sizes. A known disadvantage of these cytokines is their short half-life caused by their rapid resorption in vivo, which makes repeated injections mandatory [32]. Other issues which need to be resolved are optimal dosage and delivery methods (saline solution, carrier gel, etc.).

9.2.1.4 Gene (Modulation) Therapy

At the foremost edge of technology today is genome editing. This technique bases on a precise manipulation of targeted genes with the aid of molecules, which can be seen as a kind of "genetic scissor." In an animal experiment, a (small interfering) siRNA-liposome complex was injected locally into previously induced scar tissue, with the aim to suppress SERPINH-1. This molecule is responsible for the correct folding of collagen. Via gene silencing, a reduced collagen accumulation and therefore an improved wound healing were shown [33].

9.2.2 Vocal Fold Paresis

Current surgical-based therapies for VF paresis intend to place the VF in an appropriate position to minimize symptoms in case of unilateral VC paresis or to ablate them partially in case of bilateral VF paresis. Synkinetic reinnervation, i.e., mislead reinnervation, is one cause of poor functional recovery after RLN injury.

9.2.2.1 Cell Therapy

Regenerative medicine aims to restore muscle mass and neuromuscular function with unpaired mobility. Muscle progenitor cells were regarded as suitable cell type. Several groups injected autologous muscle progenitor cells into laryngeal muscles and found that they survived in their new muscle, attenuated atrophy, fused with the native myofibers, and enhanced reinnervation (rat studies) [34, 35]. These positive findings were recently corroborated in larger animal studies (canines) [36].

9.2.2.2 Use of Cytokines and Growth Factors

Another way towards nerval rehabilitation is the application of nerve growth factors. Naturally, following laryngeal nerve injury, differences in gene expression of several neurotrophic factors in laryngeal muscles were reported [37]. In a therapeutic manner, these neurotrophic factors can be targeted to prevent misdirected reinnervation. It is known that glial-derived neurotrophic factor (GDNF) is elevated in rat laryngeal muscles during RLN reinnervation. Hernandez-Morato and coworkers injected anti-GDNF antibody to the PCA 3 days after RLN transection and anastomosis [38]. They found that early arriving axons bypassed the PCA and entered the LTA leading to less synkinetic innervation.

The local administration bears the advantage that systematic side effects are rare. The adverse side, however, is the need for repeated injections since the factors are quickly absorbed. Gene therapy aims to circumvent this problem by altering the behavior of local cells so that they secrete the growth factors by themselves. Studies suggest that this method might increase the delivery of the specific growth factor to the site of the lesion and therefore improve neuronal recovery [39].

Furthermore, the oral intake of nimodipine showed interesting results. It is a calcium channel antagonist which was originally used to treat arterial hypertension. Its precise mechanism in recurrent laryngeal nerve injury is, to date, still not fully understood. The alteration of Ca^{2+} channels is presumed to improve the axonal growth at the nodes of Ranvier. A meta-analysis suggested that nimodipine has a positive impact on VF reinnervation. It also emphasized the need for further randomized clinical studies to draw further conclusions [40].

9.2.3 Laryngeal Transplantation/ Carcinoma

Curative approaches in malignant diseases aim to eliminate all tumor cells. This is particularly difficult to achieve in advanced stages of laryngeal cancer as surgery comes often along with substantial tissue defects resulting in difficulties in swallowing, breathing, or phonation. Laryngeal transplantation may open new therapeutic opportunities to preserve complete laryngeal functionality after laryngectomy (including non-malignant cases such as severe laryngeal trauma and stenosis). There remain however substantial obstacles to be overcome before transplantation will find broader acceptance. These are in detail the modulation of the recipients' immune system to allow tolerance while maintaining immunosurveillance, as well as attempts to restore glottic function by, e.g., selective innervation or electrical pacing.

To date only two secured cases of successful laryngotracheal allotransplantations were published in the literature [41]. Even if both patients reported improved quality of life, they have remained dependent on tracheostomy due to incomplete VF movement. Besides ethical considerations, there are also other difficulties, such as shortage of organ donors impeding advances in this field. Some of these issues might be circumvented by the transplantation of tissue-engineered larynges [42].

A tissue-engineered, artificial larynx needs to have the same anatomical features as a "natural" larynx to fulfill all requirements. These are plentiful and comprise the engineering of an adequate housing/framing, functionally intact VF mucosa, agonistic and antagonistic muscles, and, maybe most importantly, a selective innervation.

Creating an adequate framework is maybe the easiest task. Autologous cartilage can be used and has the advantage of not only being biocompatible but can also provide stability to withstand mechanical stress. Synthetically manufactured scaffolds provide a viable alternative in order to overcome this difficulty [42]. Developments were made recently when it comes to tissue-engineered laryngeal mucosa: Ling et al. isolated human VF fibroblasts and epithelial cells and co-cultivated them in vitro. This way, a VF mucosa, which was able to restore viscoelastic properties, could be bioengineered [43]. Presumably, proper vascularization might be the next goal when it comes to bioengineered mucosa.

For a successful laryngeal transplantation, the retrieval of the laryngeal function needs to be accomplished. Even though efforts considering reinnervation of limb muscles have been described in the literature, a complete regeneration has not yet been succeeded [44]. Since phonation, respiration, and swallowing are complex processes which need exact temporospatial coordination, a laryngeal transplant reinnervation might be even more challenging and is currently inconceivable. Tissue-engineered muscles and their reinnervation are possible solutions to this problem.

9.3 Outlook

During the last 20 years, we gained significant insight into microphysiology and pathophysiology of the larynx. Preclinical experiments using animal and cell culture models led to first clinical applications. We want to emphasize again the importance of gaining a deeper knowledge of VF biology before going into clinical trials using, e.g., different cytokines and/or (stem) cells. Recent developments in VF fibrosis models [45] or phonomimetic bioreactors [46, 47] pave the way towards this goal. Organotypic models of the laryngeal mucosa are another powerful tool to better understand VF biology and to test drugs before going into clinical trials [43, 48].

Non-standardized study protocols, different surgical techniques, and non-homogenous cohorts will lead ultimately to poor data which makes it difficult to estimate the therapeutical success. The complexity of the field makes it mandatory to establish collaborations between clinicians, biologists, and engineers, as no profession can manage the challenges alone. Interdisciplinary teams need to work on scaffolds, gels, and matrices that are biocompatible with the unique microenvironment of the human larynx and are suitable for the delivery of cytokines, growth factors, and cells.

References

1. Hirano S, Bless DM, Rousseau B, Welham N, Scheidt T, Ford CN. Fibronectin and adhesion molecules on canine scarred vocal folds. Laryngoscope. 2003;113(6):966–72.
2. Hirano S, Bless DM, Rousseau B, Welham N, Montequin D, Chan RW, et al. Prevention of vocal fold scarring by topical injection of hepatocyte growth factor in a rabbit model. Laryngoscope. 2004;114(3):548–56.
3. Mason C, Dunnill P. A brief definition of regenerative medicine. Regen Med. 2008;3(1):1–5.
4. Fishman JM, Long J, Gugatschka M, De Coppi P, Hirano S, Hertegard S, et al. Stem cell approaches for vocal fold regeneration. Laryngoscope. 2016;126(8):1865–70.
5. Chen H, Erndt-Marino J, Diaz-Rodriguez P, Kulwatno J, Jimenez-Vergara AC, Thibeault SL, et al. In vitro evaluation of anti-fibrotic effects of select cytokines for vocal fold scar treatment. J Biomed Mater Res B Appl Biomater. 2019;107(4):1056–67.
6. Gugatschka M, Ainodhofer H, Gruber HJ, Graupp M, Kieslinger P, Kiesler K, et al. Age effects on extracellular matrix production of vocal fold scar fibroblasts in rats. Eur Arch Otorhinolaryngol. 2014;271(5):1107–12.
7. Graupp M, Kiesler K, Friedrich G, Ainodhofer H, Gruber HJ, Kieslinger P, et al. Vocal fold fibroblast response to growth factor treatment is age dependent: results from an in vitro study. J Voice. 2014;28(4):420–3.
8. Chhetri DK, Head C, Revazova E, Hart S, Bhuta S, Berke GS. Lamina propria replacement therapy with cultured autologous fibroblasts for vocal fold scars. Otolaryngol Head Neck Surg. 2004;131(6):864–70.
9. Chhetri DK, Berke GS. Injection of cultured autologous fibroblasts for human vocal fold scars. Laryngoscope. 2011;121(4):785–92.
10. Bartlett RS, Guille JT, Chen X, Christensen MB, Wang SF, Thibeault SL. Mesenchymal stromal cell injection promotes vocal fold scar repair without long-term engraftment. Cytotherapy. 2016;18(10):1284–96.
11. Kanemaru S, Nakamura T, Omori K, Kojima H, Magrufov A, Hiratsuka Y, et al. Regeneration of the vocal fold using autologous mesenchymal stem cells. Ann Otol Rhinol Laryngol. 2003;112(11):915–20.
12. Gaston J, Quinchia Rios B, Bartlett R, Berchtold C, Thibeault SL. The response of vocal fold fibroblasts and mesenchymal stromal cells to vibration. PLoS One. 2012;7(2):e30965.
13. Hertegard S, Cedervall J, Svensson B, Forsberg K, Maurer FH, Vidovska D, et al. Viscoelastic and histologic properties in scarred rabbit vocal folds after mesenchymal stem cell injection. Laryngoscope. 2006;116(7):1248–54.
14. Hertegard S, Nagubothu SR, Malmstrom E, LeBlanc K. Treatment of vocal fold scarring with autologous bone marrow-derived human mesenchymal stromal cells-first phase I/II human clinical study. Stem Cell Res Ther. 2020;11(1):128.
15. Mattei A, Bertrand B, Jouve E, Blaise T, Philandrianos C, Grimaud F, et al. Feasibility of first injection of autologous adipose tissue-derived stromal vascular fraction in human scarred vocal folds: a nonrandomized controlled trial. JAMA Otolaryngol Head Neck Surg. 2020;146(4):355–63.
16. Li L, Stiadle JM, Lau HK, Zerdoum AB, Jia X, Thibeault SL, et al. Tissue engineering-based therapeutic strategies for vocal fold repair and regeneration. Biomaterials. 2016;108:91–110.
17. Chan RW, Gray SD, Titze IR. The importance of hyaluronic acid in vocal fold biomechanics. Otolaryngol Head Neck Surg. 2001;124(6):607–14.
18. Gray SD, Titze IR, Chan R, Hammond TH. Vocal fold proteoglycans and their influence on biomechanics. Laryngoscope. 1999;109(6):845–54.
19. Hansen JK, Thibeault SL, Walsh JF, Shu XZ, Prestwich GD. In vivo engineering of the vocal fold extracellular matrix with injectable hyaluronic acid hydrogels: early effects on tissue repair and biomechanics in a rabbit model. Ann Otol Rhinol Laryngol. 2005;114(9):662–70.
20. Thibeault SL, Klemuk SA, Chen X, Quinchia Johnson BH. In vivo engineering of the vocal fold ECM with injectable HA hydrogels-late effects on tissue repair and biomechanics in a rabbit model. J Voice. 2011;25(2):249–53.
21. Kishimoto Y, Hirano S, Kitani Y, Suehiro A, Umeda H, Tateya I, et al. Chronic vocal fold scar restoration with hepatocyte growth factor hydrogel. Laryngoscope. 2010;120(1):108–13.
22. Hirano S, Bless DM, Heisey D, Ford CN. Effect of growth factors on hyaluronan production by canine

vocal fold fibroblasts. Ann Otol Rhinol Laryngol. 2003;112(7):617–24.
23. Hirano S, Tateya I, Kishimoto Y, Kanemaru S, Ito J. Clinical trial of regeneration of aged vocal folds with growth factor therapy. Laryngoscope. 2012;122(2):327–31.
24. Hirano S, Kishimoto Y, Suehiro A, Kanemaru S, Ito J. Regeneration of aged vocal fold: first human case treated with fibroblast growth factor. Laryngoscope. 2008;118(12):2254–9.
25. Ohno T, Hirano S, Kanemaru S, Yamashita M, Umeda H, Suehiro A, et al. Drug delivery system of hepatocyte growth factor for the treatment of vocal fold scarring in a canine model. Ann Otol Rhinol Laryngol. 2007;116(10):762–9.
26. Mizuta M, Hirano S, Kishimoto Y, Hiwatashi N, Tateya I, Kanemaru S, et al. Pharmacokinetics and safety of human recombinant hepatocyte growth factor administered to vocal folds. Laryngoscope. 2014;124(9):2131–5.
27. Hirano S, Kawamoto A, Tateya I, Mizuta M, Kishimoto Y, Hiwatashi N, et al. A phase I/II exploratory clinical trial for intracordal injection of recombinant hepatocyte growth factor for vocal fold scar and sulcus. J Tissue Eng Regen Med. 2018;12(4):1031–8.
28. Suehiro A, Hirano S, Kishimoto Y, Tateya I, Rousseau B, Ito J. Effects of basic fibroblast growth factor on rat vocal fold fibroblasts. Ann Otol Rhinol Laryngol. 2010;119(10):690–6.
29. Erndt-Marino JD, Jimenez-Vergara AC, Diaz-Rodriguez P, Kulwatno J, Diaz-Quiroz JF, Thibeault S, et al. In vitro evaluation of a basic fibroblast growth factor-containing hydrogel toward vocal fold lamina propria scar treatment. J Biomed Mater Res B Appl Biomater. 2018;106(3):1258–67.
30. Kanazawa T, Komazawa D, Indo K, Akagi Y, Lee Y, Nakamura K, et al. Single injection of basic fibroblast growth factor to treat severe vocal fold lesions and vocal fold paralysis. Laryngoscope. 2015;125(10):E338–44.
31. Ban MJ, Park JH, Kim JW, Park KN, Lee JY, Kim HK, et al. The efficacy of fibroblast growth factor for the treatment of chronic vocal fold scarring: from animal model to clinical application. Clin Exp Otorhinolaryngol. 2017;10(4):349–56.
32. Xu H, Fan GK. The role of cytokines in modulating vocal fold fibrosis: a contemporary review. Laryngoscope. 2021;131(1):139–45.
33. Kishimoto Y, Yamashita M, Wei A, Toya Y, Ye S, Kendziorski C, et al. Reversal of vocal fold mucosal fibrosis using siRNA against the collagen-specific chaperone Serpinh1. Mol Ther Nucleic Acids. 2019;16:616–25.
34. Halum SL, Naidu M, Delo DM, Atala A, Hingtgen CM. Injection of autologous muscle stem cells (myoblasts) for the treatment of vocal fold paralysis: a pilot study. Laryngoscope. 2007;117(5):917–22.
35. Halum SL, Hiatt KK, Naidu M, Sufyan AS, Clapp DW. Optimization of autologous muscle stem cell survival in the denervated hemilarynx. Laryngoscope. 2008;118(7):1308–12.
36. Paniello RC, Brookes S, Bhatt NK, Bijangi-Vishehsaraei K, Zhang H, Halum S. Improved adductor function after canine recurrent laryngeal nerve injury and repair using muscle progenitor cells. Laryngoscope. 2018;128(7):E241–6.
37. Vega-Cordova X, Cosenza NM, Helfert RH, Woodson GE. Neurotrophin expression of laryngeal muscles in response to recurrent laryngeal nerve transection. Laryngoscope. 2010;120(8):1591–6.
38. Hernandez-Morato I, Tewari I, Sharma S, Pitman MJ. Blockade of glial-derived neurotrophic factor in laryngeal muscles promotes appropriate reinnervation. Laryngoscope. 2016;126(10):E337–42.
39. Araki K, Suzuki H, Uno K, Tomifuji M, Shiotani A. Gene therapy for recurrent laryngeal nerve injury. Genes (Basel). 2018;9(7):316. https://doi.org/10.3390/genes9070316.
40. Rosen CA, Smith L, Young V, Krishna P, Muldoon MF, Munin MC. Prospective investigation of nimodipine for acute vocal fold paralysis. Muscle Nerve. 2014;50(1):114–8.
41. Krishnan G, Du C, Fishman JM, Foreman A, Lott DG, Farwell G, et al. The current status of human laryngeal transplantation in 2017: a state of the field review. Laryngoscope. 2017;127(8):1861–8.
42. Hamilton NJI, Birchall MA. Tissue-engineered larynx: future applications in laryngeal cancer. Curr Otorhinolaryngol Rep. 2017;5(1):42–8.
43. Ling C, Li Q, Brown ME, Kishimoto Y, Toya Y, Devine EE, et al. Bioengineered vocal fold mucosa for voice restoration. Sci Transl Med. 2015;7(314):314ra187.
44. Zuo KJ, Willand MP, Ho ES, Ramdial S, Borschel GH. Targeted muscle reinnervation: considerations for future implementation in adolescents and younger children. Plast Reconstr Surg. 2018;141(6):1447–58.
45. Graupp M, Gruber H, Weiss G, Kiesler K, Bachna-Rotter S, Friedrich G, et al. Establishing principles of macromolecular crowding for in vitro fibrosis research of the vocal fold lamina propria. Laryngoscope. 2015;125(6):E203–9.
46. Kirsch A, Hortobagyi D, Stachl T, Karbiener M, Grossmann T, Gerstenberger C, et al. Development and validation of a novel phonomimetic bioreactor. PLoS One. 2019;14(3):e0213788.
47. Zerdoum AB, Tong Z, Bachman B, Jia X. Construction and characterization of a novel vocal fold bioreactor. J Vis Exp. 2014;(90):e51594.
48. Lungova V, Chen X, Wang Z, Kendziorski C, Thibeault SL. Human induced pluripotent stem cell-derived vocal fold mucosa mimics development and responses to smoke exposure. Nat Commun. 2019;10(1):4161.

Voice Feminization and Masculinization

10

Raja Fakhoury, Vyas M. N. Prasad, Marc Remacle, and James P. Thomas

Key Points

- Voice therapy is an essential part of the management of patients who have committed to and undergone treatment to fully alter their gender.
- The mainstay of treatment for masculinization is indeed hormonal. Masculinization surgery therefore is rarer compared to feminization and is usually performed in cases of mutational voice disorders and puberphonia.
- Isshiki's type IV thyroplasty raises the fundamental frequency, but medium- to long-term follow-up shows declination of pitch.
- The glottoplasty described by Wendler aims to de-epithelialize the anterior half of the true vocal folds either using cold steel or laser (CO_2) and thereafter utilizing sutures to approximate the folds creating an anterior glottic web. The procedure is based on the principle of reducing the effective mass of the vibrating folds thereby raising the pitch.
- The complexities involved in achieving this success require a careful understanding of the role of the multidisciplinary team that is patient-centric and places its emphasis on not purely pitch surgery but a holistic treatment pathway.
- The feminization laryngoplasty consists in reducing the size of the larynx to a more female size in its cross-sectional dimension and shortening the length of the vibratory vocal fold.
- Isshiki's type III thyroplasty, pushing back the anterior commissure and relaxing the vocal folds, is the mainstay for pitch lowering surgery and voice masculinization.

R. Fakhoury
Department of Clinical Otorhinolaryngology Head & Neck Surgery, Saint George Hospital University Medical Center, Beirut, Lebanon
e-mail: Rafakhoury@stgeorgehospital.org

V. M. N. Prasad
Department of Otorhinolaryngology Head & Neck Surgery, Singapore Medical Center, Singapore, Singapore

M. Remacle (✉)
Department of Otorhinolaryngology Head & Neck Surgery, Centre Hospitalier de Luxembourg, Luxembourg, Luxembourg

J. P. Thomas
Voicedoctor, Portland, OR, USA
e-mail: thomas@voicedoctor.net

M. Remacle, H. E. Eckel (eds.), *Textbook of Surgery of Larynx and Trachea*,
https://doi.org/10.1007/978-3-031-09621-1_10

10.1 Voice Feminization and Masculinization

Vyas M. N. Prasad, Marc Remacle
and Raja Fakhoury

10.1.1 Introduction

Voice is a critical feature in the identification, perception and recognition of an individual's gender. It is an essential factor in contributing to a holistic image of the person subjectively and objectively. Its impact physically, emotionally and socially cannot be overstated and, in this regard, is seen as the completion of the long and often challenging journey of the transgender patient [1, 2].

This chapter aims to provide the readership with the basis of voice feminization and masculinization, a brief history and background of therapy with a focus on the authors experience in both therapies, pitfalls and pearls from surgery and a discussion on future improvements [3].

10.1.1.1 Background

Transsexualism, attitudes to the former and definitions have undergone changes in keeping with our better understanding of this group of gender dysphorias. The Diagnostic and Statistical Manual of Mental Disorders Version IV (DSM-IV) has replaced the term transsexualism to gender identity disorder in adolescents and adults. Prior terminology including primary and secondary transsexualism has been abandoned for more modern, applicable and appropriate terminology [4, 5]. Transgender or sex reassignment surgery has been performed for over a century with mixed results initially but, over time and with advancements in surgical technique and hormonal therapies, has developed into a well-established multi-specialty process with excellent results. Voice alteration is one of the many changes that the transgender patient undergoes. In the past, the focus was to suppress the natural hormonal release and replace it with the opposing sex hormone. Included in this process was the surgical removal of the gonads and administration of inhibitors and analogues accordingly. A lengthy patient journey awaited these patients with multiple operations to alter their physical state to essentially transform them into the desired gender. In the case of male-to-female (MtF/trans woman) transgender patients, this would include orchidectomy, penectomy, feminizing genitoplasty, breast augmentation, facial feminization and so on. Conversely, the female-to-male (FtM/trans man) subject would undergo a series of procedures which involved the development of male physical features with the consequent loss of female feature such as a mastectomy, salpingo-oopherectomy and phalloplasty [6, 7].

Hormone replacement therapy in FtM patients has historically been the primary treatment. Androgen therapy alters the secondary sexual characteristics with alteration in hair pattern, fat and muscle distribution and voice. The alteration to voice is irreversible, and without androgen therapy, many trans men patients find themselves still being perceived as female despite all other attributes being masculine [8].

The same however cannot be said of the MtF patient. Hormone therapy has little to no impact structurally in the alteration of the trans female voice as the effects of testosterone exposure during puberty are irreversible to the larynx. Hormone therapy may however alter self-perception of MtF patients with the development of female sexual characteristics such as breast development and living as a woman. Hence, despite the lack of physical alteration to the larynx, voice intervention is delayed to optimize the patient mentally [9].

10.1.1.2 The Physics of Transgender Voice Alteration

The true vocal folds comprise a pair of multilayered structures that are part gelatinous, ligamentous and muscular. They have a viscosity within the superficial layer that allows for vibratory activity and can be stretched, shortened, thickened and thinned according to the needs of use. Like the strings on a musical instrument, they follow the laws of physics and, in so doing, produce pitch which can be altered over a range of frequencies. The length of the vocal folds is altered by relaxing or tensing the folds and pitch rises with reduced length and drops with a longer fold. The constant feature of this system is the underlying mass of the vocal folds or at least the mass of the vibratory segment. The tension of the folds is altered by the cricothyroid muscle (the only intrinsic muscle of the larynx found outside it) [10]. Lesser effects on vocal fold tension are seen with the contraction of the vocalis and thyroarytenoid muscles with mild pitch increment. In this regard, the principles of surgery are primarily to alter the mass of the vibrating fold and relax or stretch the folds with concomitant changes in length.

The vocal tract beyond childhood is also influenced and altered by the release of the sex hormones during puberty with descent of the larynx in the male, elongating the pharynx and reducing the fundamental frequency. The female vocal tract does not descend as much, and there is little change structurally to that of the infant. Raising or lowering the larynx with respect to the hyoid bone can alter the fundamental frequency in this regard [11].

10.1.2 Voice Therapy

Voice therapy is an essential part of the management of patients who have committed to and undergone treatment to fully alter their gender. It aims not only to instruct the patient on how to manage their altered voices in various conversational settings but also to master vocal cues, control of breathing, flow phonation, 'feminine' and masculine cues and vocabulary and emotional aspects that are so intrinsically linked to perceptions of gender through voice [12]. Paralaryngeal muscle exercises also help with pitch alteration in raising the larynx in the MtF subject, shortening the vocal tract and narrowing the pharynx. Voice therapy and counselling is initiated prior to any surgical procedure and continued thereafter until the desired result is achieved with careful consideration of other co-factors that may preclude a good outcome including the ingestion of alcohol and smoking.

10.1.2.1 Pitch Perception and Gender Recognition

The fundamental frequency in males range from 80 to 165 Hz, while that of females is about 145–275 Hz. Culture, language and size of the individual (xrf. directly proportional to size of the vocal tract and inversely related to fundamental frequency) account for the variation in fundamental frequency. Pitch perception and gender recognition do not always correspond with some trans females who, despite having deeper voices (e.g. smokers), are perceived as female and feminine. There is also a range where fundamental frequency is shared between males and females, i.e. 145–165 Hz [13]. The 'telephone test' is often cited as a useful measure in assessing if the transgender patient has the vocal characteristics ascribed to the particular gender. It is a non-visual test and has been used to assess the success of voice surgery and therapy.

10.1.3 Surgery

The surgical treatment of transgender patients for voice alteration is often performed after they have undergone the comprehensive array of procedures and hormonal therapies which make up the complex transformation that this patient group warrants. As mentioned before, the mainstay of treatment for masculinization is indeed hormonal. Masculinization surgery therefore is rarer compared to feminization and is usually performed in cases of mutational voice disorders and puberphonia when the patient has a feminine voice despite normal androgen levels (innately or therapeutically) or when response to androgens in FtM patients is suboptimal.

Isshiki described in his seminal work the principles of thyroplasty surgery and the operations that altered pitch, namely, the types III and IV—relaxation and tensing procedures. These principles continue to hold true in keeping with the physics and physiology behind voice but have been modified by various other laryngologists over time [14, 15].

10.1.3.1 Preoperative Assessment

A thorough history and examination of the patient undergoing voice surgery are mandatory with input by an endocrinologist and psychologist where necessary. Prior videolaryngostroboscopic (VLS) examination of the patient with recording facilities for comprehensive documentation is very useful. Voice assessment is evaluated, and while several protocols—local, national or international—exist, we utilize the European Laryngological Society's Committee on Phoniatrics [16]. This is a multidimensional set of minimal basic measurements suitable for 'common' dysphonias. It consists of five different categories: perception (grade, roughness, breathiness); videostroboscopy (closure, regularity, mucosal wave and symmetry); acoustics (jitter, shimmer, F0 range and softest intensity); aerodynamics (phonation quotient); and subjective rating (Voice Handicap Index (VHI), Visual Analogue Scale (VAS)).

The lowering of pitch when pressure is applied to the anterior thyroid cartilage backward during phonation (manual or Gutzman's test) should lower the pitch and may predict success from relaxation thyroplasty [17].

Laryngeal shave or chondrolaryngoplasty, although not a pitch-altering procedure, is often performed at the same sitting as feminization surgery to reduce the laryngeal prominence. Some procedures combine pitch raising and prominence reduction as part of the single operation [18].

10.1.3.2 Voice Questionnaires

Several voice questionnaires have been used in transgender patients including gender nonspecific ones such as the Voice Handicap Index and Voice-Related Quality of Life (VRQOL) [19, 20]. The Transgender Self-Evaluation Questionnaire (TSEQ) was the progenitor of transgender self-administered questionnaires adapted from the well-established VHI. Thereafter, the Transsexual Voice Questionnaire (TVQ^{MtF}) was developed from the TSEQ and is a validated patient-reported outcome measurement tool consisting of three categories: anxiety and avoidance, gender identity and voice quality. A lower total score reflects a better outcome [21, 22]. The TVQ^{MtF} is an MtF questionnaire however. There is a significant paucity in the literature of FtM questionnaire-based studies despite the fact that androgen therapy is not always successful, and this group of patients does indeed benefit from voice therapy and surgery when indicated. It is postulated that the VHI and VR-QOL are used in this group.

10.1.3.3 Informed Consent

The management of patients is multidisciplinary, and all available options (medical, surgical and behavioural) should be explored and where possible offered. Some MtF patients respond well to voice and behavioural therapy and can function albeit with some difficulty in falsetto. Similarly, psychotherapy at a younger age has been shown to reduce the need for surgery in puberphonia. Botox injections have been explored to paralyse the cricothyroid muscle and lower the pitch as has injection laryngoplasty [23–25]. The aims of surgery, risks versus benefits, are clearly explained, and it is worthwhile in selected cases for the patient to meet previously treated subjects.

10.1.4 Voice Feminization

Initially, surgery for voice feminization was primarily aimed at altering the length and tension of the vocal fold through open procedures. These procedures were often combined with the laryngeal shave. The concept of tightening the vocal fold by stretching it and creating a response that was an exaggeration of the cricothyroid was the basis of Isshiki's type IV thyroplasty [14]. The initial results of this procedure did indeed raise the fundamental frequency, but medium- to long-term follow-up showed declination of pitch potentially related to cricoarytenoid joint being a mobile entity, the stretch/tensing of the vocal fold regressing naturally over time and the added effect of fold lengthening which in turn lowers pitch. Reduction of the vibrating mass of the vocal fold provided an alternative to raising tension, and several procedures, both open and endoscopic, have been used with varying success. Several procedures have been described with varying short- and long-term success. They include tension-increasing procedures (cricothyroid approximation, laser tightening and anterior commissure advancement); mass reduction procedures; laser debulking and vocal webbing and the feminization laryngoplasty which is a reduction of the anterior part of the larynx including the thyroid cartilage, the vocal folds and the ventricular folds [26].

10.1.4.1 Voice Feminization: The Different Procedures

Cricothyroid Approximation (CTA)

This open procedure was popularized almost 50 years ago and was based on the principle of stretching the vocal folds, raising their tension (despite the consequent increase in length with a physical effect of lowering pitch) and consequently raising the pitch. Variations on Isshiki's type IVa procedure abound with subtle differences, but the concept remains the same—the cricothyroid muscle being made redundant and the gap between the thyroid and cricoid effaced.

Procedure

A horizontal anterior neck skin crease incision is performed at the level of the cricothyroid membrane. The dissection is performed to allow for a clear appreciation of the anterior aspect of the thyroid cartilage including the thyroid prominence and the cricoid ring. This anatomical region is relatively safe. The operation involves closing the gap between the thyroid and cricoid using a variety of sutures (non-absorbable, metal wires), titanium plates, silicone buttresses and so on. The principle is to stretch the vocal folds increasing their tension primarily. A tracheal shave can be incorporated using the same incision as rotation of the thyroid cartilage increases the laryngeal prominence. The CTA has been shown to increase pitch but has been associated with a monotonous pitch often described as falsetto and, initially, often described 'unfeminine female' with a reduced range and consequent irreversible loss of function of the cricothyroid muscle. In patients where pitch has started to drop after CTA, revision vocal feminization using other treatment modalities can be difficult if they involve other types of laryngeal framework surgery (FemLar/anterior partial laryngectomy) as fusion of the cricoid to the thyroid can require powered instrumentation (e.g. drills and saws) to separate the two.

Cricothyroid Subluxation

Cricothyroid subluxation described by Zeitels et al. was initially used an adjunctive treatment for the paralysed vocal fold increasing the length and tension of the fold after medialization thyroplasty [27]. Conceptually, it was meant to replicate the action of the cricothyroid muscle producing counter tension on the thyroarytenoid muscle. As a result, it raised the fundamental frequency of the patient and improved the dysphonia often seen in medialization thyroplasty. It is rarely performed for voice feminization surgery alone.

Anterior Commissure Advancement

The procedure had been designed to close the glottic chink seen in vocal fold bowing amongst the elderly but was adapted to raise pitch. It was first described by Le Jeune and modified by Tucker [28, 29]. The procedure is rarely if at all used currently. It was based on a medial 'springboard' flap of thyroid cartilage, initially inferiorly based but thereafter modified as an anterior based flap by Tucker, held in place by a silastic shim. The flap could be brought forward to stretch the anterior commissure to raise the pitch and approximate the vocal folds or pushed inward for relaxation of the vocal folds and pitch lowering. Anterior commissure advancement did help raise the comfortable speaking pitch but inevitably caused protrusion of the laryngeal prominence.

Webbing Procedure (Wendler's Glottoplasty)

This procedure, first described by Wendler, aims to de-epithelialize the anterior half of the true vocal folds either using cold steel or laser (CO_2) or thereafter utilizing sutures to approximate the folds creating an iatrogenic anterior glottic web [30]. The procedure is based on the principle of reducing the effective mass of the vibrating folds thereby raising the pitch. Variations and modifications of Wendler's procedure have been described including de-epithelialization with injection laryngoplasty to bring the two folds into contact and thus obviating the need for sutures and the adjunctive use of Botox to limit voice use postoperatively [31–35]. This procedure, done under general anaesthesia, endoscopically requires some experience in transoral laryngeal suturing techniques. The laryngeal laryngoplasty (26) and the laryngeal voice adjustment technique (LAVA) [36, 37] which is complementary to these techniques are repeated after this subchapter

The authors have considerable experience in this procedure and have adopted it over the CTA as their procedure of choice in MtF patients. The procedure is performed under general anaesthesia with jet ventilation as a day-case procedure where possible. We place the patient in suspension with rigid laryngoscope and thereafter de-epithelialize the anterior third to half of the membranous true vocal fold on its superior, inferior and medial (i.e. free edge) surfaces bilaterally. We prefer the CO2 laser (Lumenis AcuBlade™, Santa Clara, CA, USA) in scanning continuous mode with a 2 mm beam. Care is taken not to damage the vocal ligament. Thereafter, the corresponding tissue of the vocal folds is firmly sutured to obtain a 'V'-shaped anterior commissure. A pair of laparoscopic forceps is used as a needle holder, and a knot pusher designed for endolaryngeal surgery (Ethicon, NJ, USA) is inserted to drive the knots into place securing the sutures in place. Four 3.0 resorbable sutures (two on either side) are needed. One thread is passed through the vocal ligament at the junction of the anterior and middle third. The second is passed more anteriorly to the first. These steps are repeated on the contralateral side. The anterior thread is then ligated through one knot, inferior to the glottic plane and one superiorly. This is similarly repeated for the posterior two threads. We use fibrin sealant to strengthen the suture (Figs. 10.1.1, 10.1.2, 10.1.3, 10.1.4, 10.1.5, 10.1.6, and 10.1.7).

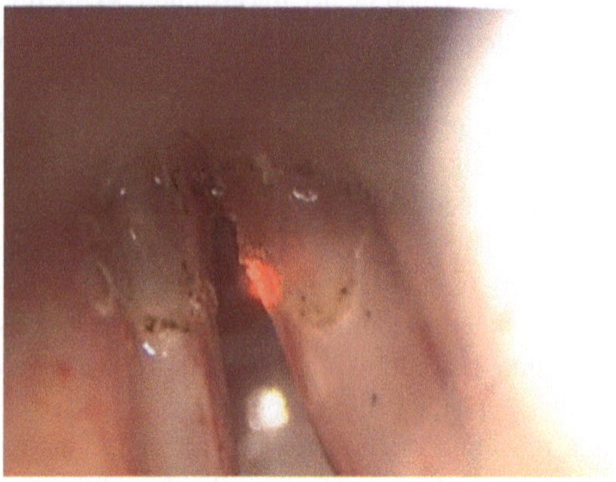

Fig. 10.1.1 Laser de-epithelialization of medial and superior vocal fold

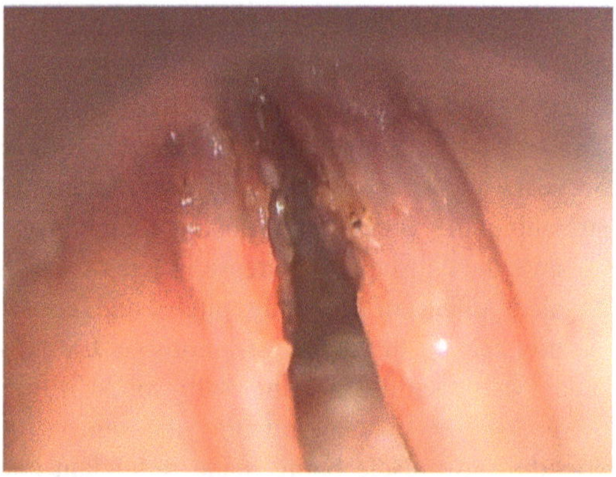

Fig. 10.1.2 Completion of laser de-epithelialization

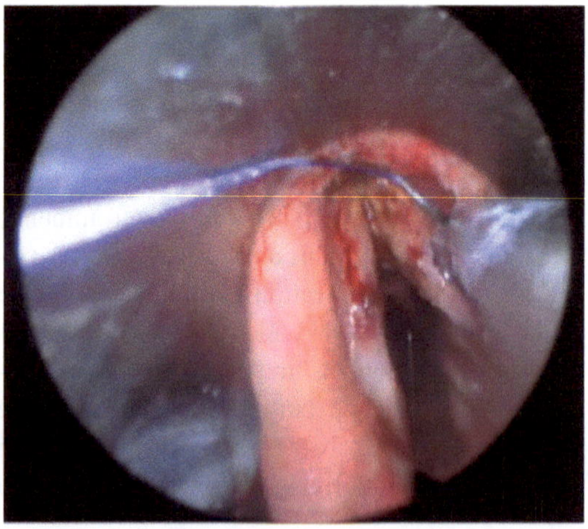

Fig. 10.1.3 Suturing of posterior web

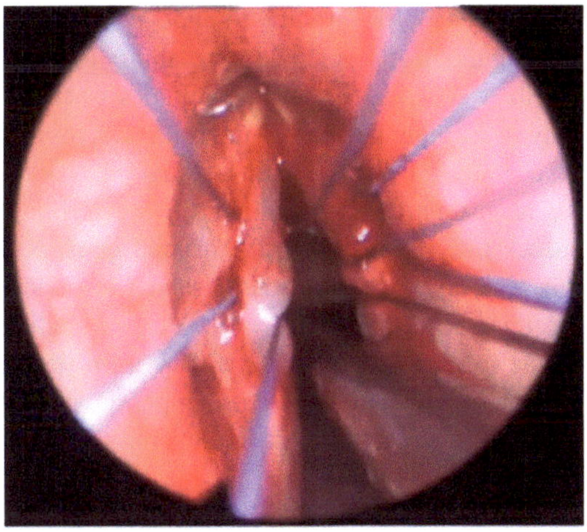

Fig. 10.1.4 All four pairs of sutures in place

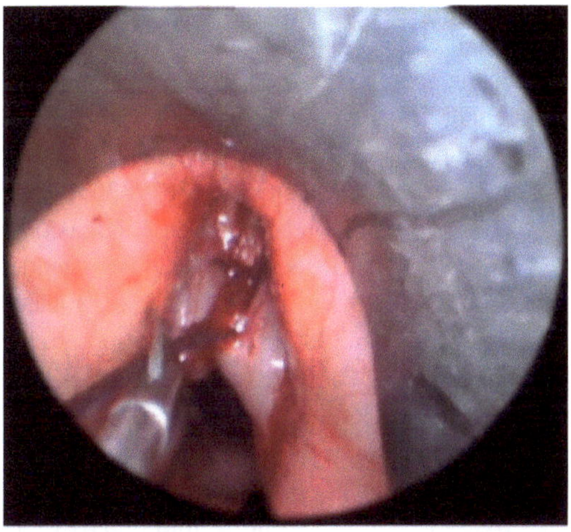

Fig. 10.1.5 Knotting of sutures

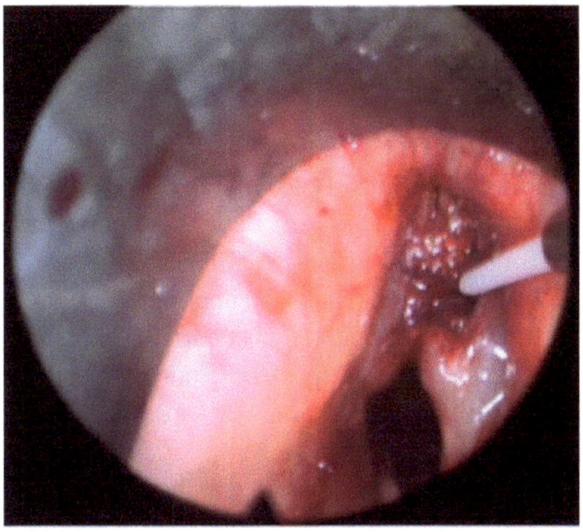

Fig. 10.1.6 Application of fibrin glue

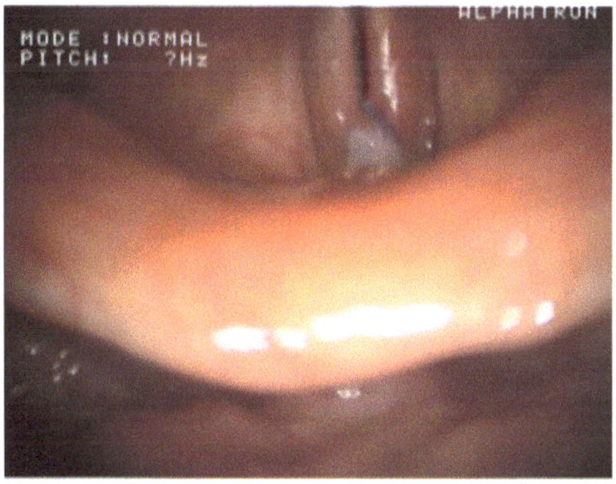

Fig. 10.1.7 Postoperative view after 1 week

The patients are advised to strictly adhere to a 10-day voice rest. Although the duration is empirical, we have found it useful to avoid the possibility of dehiscence of the suture points. Postoperative broad-spectrum antibiotics for a week (e.g. co-amoxiclav 1 g tds) are also prescribed as well as twice daily proton pump inhibitors (6 weeks) and inhaled steroids (1 week).

Voice assessment was based on acoustic and aerodynamic analysis with patient self-administered VHI and Hirano's GRBAS scale by our speech pathologists. We found that our patients did not have a significant change on their VHI possibly because this validated questionnaire was not designed with the transgender patient in mind. This was despite the fact that they had a significant improvement in their F0 (median F0 increased from 139 to 191 Hz). Three of our patients in our series between 2006 and 2008 encountered degradation of F0. They were all older (age > 45 years), and two of them continued to smoke. In our follow-up study between 2009 and 2012, we demonstrated effective pitch increase in our two groups of patients but a greater increase in a younger group (means 28.6 years vs. 51.9 years) after an average follow-up of 9.2 months supporting the fact that transgender voice feminization surgery may be better at a younger age. We did not encounter any significant complications in this study, but three patients did undergo revision glottoplasty, two because of early breakdown of the suture line and the third for insufficient pitch elevation.

A further review of 31 patients who underwent this procedure between 2015 and 2018 was performed. Fourteen patients completed the study where the aim was to assess their satisfaction with the procedure at least 6 months after using the TSEQ. The study showed a high rate of satisfaction after surgery with a mean TSEQ score of 51.3 ± 21.37 (range 33–113). The majority of the patients rated their voice as female (28.6% very female and 35.7% somewhat female), while 28.6% felt they were gender neutral and 7.1% somewhat male. Patient's satisfaction post-surgery was not affected by age groups, time to evaluation, smoking status and hormonal therapy [unpublished date—presented at the AAO-HNSF as a Free Paper 2020].

10.1.5 Post-treatment Follow-Up

Patients who undergo any treatment for transgender voice are usually followed up in the multidisciplinary setting. Our experience is that most patients are better at gauging the success of their respective therapies, and in that regard, subjective questionnaires prove to be better yardsticks of therapeutic benefit as opposed to other non-patient-based assessments including acoustic and aerodynamic studies. The mere focus on their pitch range and fundamental frequency without taking into consideration formant frequencies, breathiness, prosody and their own overall subjective rating and satisfaction has been shown in several studies to be a poor yardstick for success. However, tests such as the 'telephone test' do have their place where gender identification is made on non-visual cues [39].

10.1.6 Conclusion

Voice can be viewed as the final piece in the complex mosaic that makes up the transgender puzzle. It defines the gender in a non-visual way and in this regard is difficult to hide or disguise. Getting the 'right' voice with the ability to transmit the right gender cues and attitudes when not only conversing but expressing sounds, sighs and other vocalizations (yawning, coughing, sneezing and laughing) is paramount in being able to successfully transition to the desired gender. In this regard, the complexities involved in achieving this success require a careful understanding of the role of the multidisciplinary team that is patient-centric and places its emphasis on not purely pitch surgery but a holistic treatment pathway.

10.1.7 References

1. Dacakis G, Oates J, Douglas J. Beyond voice: perceptions of gender in male-to-female transsexuals. Curr Opin Otolaryngol Head Neck Surg. 2012;20(3):165–70. https://doi.org/10.1097/MOO.0b013e3283530f85.
2. Winter S, Diamond M, Green J, Karasic D, Reed T, Whittle S, Wylie K. Transgender people: health at the margins of society. Lancet. 2016;388(10042):390–400. https://doi.org/10.1016/S0140-6736(16)00683-8.
3. Davies S, Goldberg J. Clinical aspects of transgender speech feminization and masculinization. Int J Transgenderism. 2006:9:3–4, 167–96. https://doi.org/10.1300/J485v09n0308.
4. Kraus C. Classifying Intersex in DSM-5: critical reflections on gender dysphoria. Arch Sex Behav. 2015;44(5):1147–63. https://doi.org/10.1007/s10508-015-0550-0.
5. Davy Z. The DSM-5 and the politics of diagnosing transpeople. Arch Sex Behav. 2015;44(5):1165–76. https://doi.org/10.1007/s10508-015-0573-6.
6. Prince JCJ, Safer JD. Endocrine treatment of transgender individuals: current guidelines and strategies. Expert Rev Endocrinol Metab. 2020:1–9. https://doi.org/10.1080/17446651.2020.1825075.

7. Pan S, Honig SC. Gender-affirming surgery: current concepts. Curr Urol Rep. 2018;19(8):62. https://doi.org/10.1007/s11934-018-0809-9.
8. Defreyne J, T'Sjoen G. Transmasculine hormone therapy. Endocrinol Metab Clin North Am. 2019;48(2):357–75. https://doi.org/10.1016/j.ecl.2019.01.004.
9. Hamidi O, Davidge-Pitts CJ. Transfeminine hormone therapy. Endocrinol Metab Clin North Am. 2019;48(2):341–55. https://doi.org/10.1016/j.ecl.2019.02.001.
10. Kitajima K, Tanabe M, Isshiki N. Cricothyroid distance and vocal pitch. Experimental surgical study to elevate the vocal pitch. Ann Otol Rhinol Laryngol. 1979;88(1 Pt 1):52–5. https://doi.org/10.1177/000348947908800109.
11. Isshiki N, Taira T, Tanabe M. Surgical alteration of the vocal pitch. J Otolaryngol. 1983;12(5):335–40.
12. Hancock AB, Garabedian LM. Transgender voice and communication treatment: a retrospective chart review of 25 cases. Int J Lang Commun Disord. 2013;48(1):54–65. https://doi.org/10.1111/j.1460-6984.2012.00185.x.
13. Thomas J. Feminizing laryngoplasty, Chapter 22. In: Nerurkar N, Roychoudhury A, editors. Textbook of laryngology, 1st ed. Jaypee; 2017. p. 222–9.
14. Isshiki N, Morita H, Okamura H, Hiramoto M. Thyroplasty as a new phonosurgical technique. Acta Otolaryngol. 1974;78(5–6):451–7. https://doi.org/10.3109/00016487409126379.
15. Isshiki N, Tanabe M, Ohkawa M, Kita M. Laryngeal framework surgery for voice disorders. Auris Nasus Larynx. 1985;12 Suppl 2:S217–20. https://doi.org/10.1016/s0385-8146(85)80062-6.
16. DeJonckere PH, Crevier-Buchman L, Marie JP, Moerman M, Remacle M, Woisard V; European Research Group on the Larynx. Implementation of the European Laryngological Society (ELS) basic protocol for assessing voice treatment effect. Rev Laryngol Otol Rhinol (Bord). 2003;124(5):279–83.
17. Isshiki N. Phonosurgery – theory and practice. Tokyo: Springer; 1989.
18. Kunachak S, Prakunhungsit S, Sujjalak K. Thyroid cartilage and vocal fold reduction: a new phonosurgical method for male-to-female transsexuals. Ann Otol Rhinol Laryngol. 2000;109(11):1082–6. https://doi.org/10.1177/000348940010901116.
19. Jacobson BH, Johnson A, Grywalsky C, et al. The voice handicap index (VHI): development and validation. Am J Speech Lang Pathol. 1997;6:66–70.
20. Hogikyan ND, Sethuraman G. Validation of an instrument to measure voice-related quality of life (V-RQOL). J Voice. 1999;13(4):557–69. https://doi.org/10.1016/s0892-1997(99)80010-1.
21. Dacakis G, Davies S, Oates JM, Douglas JM, Johnston JR. Development and preliminary evaluation of the transsexual voice questionnaire for male-to-female transsexuals. J Voice. 2013;27(3):312–20. https://doi.org/10.1016/j.jvoice.2012.11.005.
22. Dacakis G, Oates JM, Douglas JM. Further evidence of the construct validity of the Transsexual Voice Questionnaire (TVQ^{MtF}) using principal components analysis. J Voice. 2017;31(2):142–8. https://doi.org/10.1016/j.jvoice.2016.07.001.
23. Pau H, Murty GE. First case of surgically corrected puberphonia. J Laryngol Otol. 2001;115(1):60–1. https://doi.org/10.1258/0022215011906821.
24. van den Broek EM, Vokes DE, Dorman EB. Bilateral in-office injection laryngoplasty as an adjunctive treatment for recalcitrant puberphonia: a case report and review of the literature. J Voice. 2016;30(2):221–3. https://doi.org/10.1016/j.jvoice.2015.03.019.
25. Hamdan AL, Khalifee E, Ghanem A, Jaffal H. Injection laryngoplasty in patients with puberphonia. J Voice. 2019;33(4):564–6. https://doi.org/10.1016/j.jvoice.2018.02.017.

26. Thomas JP, Macmillan C. Feminization laryngoplasty: assessment of surgical pitch elevation. Eur Arch Otorhinolaryngol. 2013;270(10):2695–700. https://doi.org/10.1007/s00405-013-2511-3.
27. Zeitels SM, Hillman RE, Desloge RB, Bunting GA. Cricothyroid subluxation: a new innovation for enhancing the voice with laryngoplastic phonosurgery. Ann Otol Rhinol Laryngol. 1999;108(12):1126–31. https://doi.org/10.1177/000348949910801206.
28. LeJeune FE, Guice CE, Samuels PM. Early experiences with vocal ligament tightening. Ann Otol Rhinol Laryngol. 1983;92(5 Pt 1):475–7. https://doi.org/10.1177/000348948309200513.
29. Tucker HM. Anterior commissure laryngoplasty for adjustment of vocal fold tension. Ann Otol Rhinol Laryngol. 1985;94(6 Pt 1):547–9. https://doi.org/10.1177/000348948509400604.
30. Wendler J. Vocal pitch elevation after transsexualism male to female. In: Proceedings of the European Phoniatricians; Salsomaggiore, Italy, 1990.
31. Remacle M, Matar N, Morsomme D, Veduyckt I, Lawson G. Glottoplasty for male-to-female transsexualism: voice results. J Voice. 2011;25(1):120–3. https://doi.org/10.1016/j.jvoice.2009.07.004.
32. Mastronikolis NS, Remacle M, Biagini M, Kiagiadaki D, Lawson G. Wendler glottoplasty: an effective pitch raising surgery in male-to-female transsexuals. J Voice. 2013;27(4):516–22. https://doi.org/10.1016/j.jvoice.2013.04.004.
33. Anderson J. Endoscopic laryngeal web formation for pitch elevation. J Otolaryngol. 2007;36(1):6–12. https://doi.org/10.2310/7070.2006.0153.
34. Anderson JA. Pitch elevation in trangendered patients: anterior glottic web formation assisted by temporary injection augmentation. J Voice. 2014;28(6):816–21. https://doi.org/10.1016/j.jvoice.2014.05.002.
35. Meister J, Hagen R, Shehata-Dieler W, Kühn H, Kraus F, Kleinsasser N. Pitch elevation in male-to-female transgender persons-the Würzburg approach. J Voice. 2017;31(2):244.e7–244.e15. https://doi.org/10.1016/j.jvoice.2016.07.018.
36. Orloff LA, Mann AP, Damrose JF, Goldman SN. Laser-assisted voice adjustment (LAVA) in transsexuals. Laryngoscope. 2006;116(4):655–60. https://doi.org/10.1097/01.mlg.0000205198.65797.59.
37. Koçak I, Akpınar ME, Cakır ZA, Doğan M, Bengisu S, Celikoyar MM. Laser reduction glottoplasty for managing androphonia after failed cricothyroid approximation surgery. J Voice. 2010;24(6):758–64. https://doi.org/10.1016/j.jvoice.2009.06.004.
38. Friedrich G, de Jong FI, Mahieu HF, Benninger MS, Isshiki N. Laryngeal framework surgery: a proposal for classification and nomenclature by the Phonosurgery Committee of the European Laryngological Society. Eur Arch Otorhinolaryngol. 2001;258(8):389–96. https://doi.org/10.1007/s004050100375.
39. Meister J, Kühn H, Shehata-Dieler W, Hagen R, Kleinsasser N. Perceptual analysis of the male-to-female transgender voice after glottoplasty-the telephone test. Laryngoscope. 2017;127(4):875–81. https://doi.org/10.1002/lary.26110.

10.2 The Rationale for Feminization Laryngoplasty

James P. Thomas

Once exposed to testosterone, typically during puberty, the thyroid cartilage enlarges, both increasing the internal luminal size of the larynx and altering the neck profile by visible protrusion of the Adam's apple. The vocal cords elongate and thicken, lowering the comfortable speaking pitch and lowest vocal pitch. There is usually a reduction of the upper vocal range or at least a change in the quality of the upper vocal range since thicker vocal cords must be stretched tighter to produce the same pitch. The relaxed laryngeal position drops lower in the neck increasing the internal length of the pharyngeal chamber, a longer chamber selectively amplifying the lower notes.

In individuals identifying as female gender (whether genetically male, intersex or female), speech therapy or self-practice may result in learning to produce a desirable speaking vocal pitch and resonance, masking these changes induced by testosterone. These techniques utilize active compensatory muscle contraction of intrinsic and cervical muscles and require ongoing effort. Some individuals are successful in developing a habitual contraction, to the point of requiring conscious effort to lower their larynx and speak with their 'male voice' while perhaps most others develop ongoing fatigue from these attempts at maintaining female pitch and resonance through tonic muscle contraction. Some individuals are rather unable to accomplish this task. Even when successful, some individuals remain fearful of letting their guard up for even a moment in a sensitive situation where a masculine voice would be inappropriate. As an ideal, after transition, comfortable speech would occur at a feminine pitch and with a feminine quality without having to think about contracting several muscles before every phonation.

The fundamental frequency of speech is one distinctive parameter in determination of a male versus female voice [1, 2]. A number of pitch-altering surgeries have been pursued to address this frustration including cricothyroid approximation (CTA) [1–8], anterior commissure advancement [9] and vocal cord webbing [10–12].

CTA is one of the most common surgeries currently used to change the relaxed pitch of the voice. The normal action of the cricothyroid muscle is to lengthen the vocal cord [13]. The vocal quality produced by this increase in tension of the vocal cord is called falsetto. Bringing the thyroid cartilage and cricoid cartilage into approximation in the anterior midline, CTA surgery effectively sutures the cricothyroid muscle into a permanent position of contraction, although the degree is variable.

Some of the positive attributes of CTA surgery include the following. It is relatively easy to perform the surgery with the anatomy located very close beneath the skin. Surgeons inexperienced with the procedure can perform it relatively well.

There is minimal discomfort with the procedure, and it may be performed under local anaesthesia. The patient may speak during the procedure if the surgeon has a desire to attempt to 'tune' the pitch during the procedure, although for many 'CTA surgery is typically performed with intentional hyper-elevation of pitch in anticipation of gradual relaxation of the induced vocal fold tension over time' [14]. Because it is relatively easy to perform, is relatively safe from surgical complications and can be performed in a relatively short time, surgical costs associated with the procedure are low.

I began performing CTA surgery in 2001 for male-to-female transgender patients wishing to speak comfortably at a higher pitch in day-to-day conversation. I reviewed results on 23 patients in 2003 for a presentation (Thomas, J.P. Cricothyroid approximation & other phonosurgical procedures to alter the transgender voice. Biennial meeting of the Harry Benjamin International Gender Dysphoria Association, Inc. (HBIGDA), September 12, 2003, Ghent, Belgium). I noted that in aggregate, there was elevation of the comfortable speaking pitch by 7 semitones, although this ranged from a lowering of the speaking pitch by 2 semitones in one patient to an elevation of pitch by 18 semitones in one patient. The range was wide and seemingly unpredictable. To most patient's relief, individuals also lost an average of nine semitones from the bottom of their speaking range, providing a speaking pitch not at risk for a sudden drop in pitch.

Significant issues were noted with the CTA procedure. Some patients experience an initial pitch elevation that fades back to a baseline pitch over a few months, ultimately experiencing no permanent change in their voice at all. This occurred in about one third of patients despite vocal cords that remained visibly stretched on endoscopy. Neumann et al. also noted about one third of patients had a neutral pitch and about one third failed to gain in pitch [15]. They appeared to have lost pitch elevation by losing internal tension. I noted that the cricothyroid suture was not the cause of failure to raise pitch based on observations of patients of my own and others that I attempted to surgically revise. During attempted surgical revisions on my own and other surgeon's patients with this complaint, the cricothyroid space remained ablated, typically with the cricoid and thyroid cartilage fused in the anterior midline. Even with various suturing techniques including metal sutures, bolstered sutures and single or multiple sutures, none of the sutures had pulled out.

Another problematic issue was that many patients with successful pitch elevation spoke with an unnatural, hyper-elevated pitch ranging from an extreme falsetto to a mild falsetto quality of their voice. For some surgeons, 'CTA surgery is typically performed with intentional hyper-elevation of pitch in anticipation of gradual relaxation of the induced vocal fold tension over time' [14].

Some of my patients describe it as a 'gay male' sound.

An uncommon problem was observed related to the cricothyroid joint. The joint appears to become so fixed, perhaps subluxed, such that an individual may almost completely lose the ability to change pitch and volume at all, leaving them with a monotonal voice (primary author's observation).

At best, I reasoned that the post CTA patient forfeits the use of her cricothyroid muscle so all pitch changes must now be produced by tensioning the thyroarytenoid muscle. Because I felt these issues were significant vocal compromises for the patients, I looked for an alternative approach that would raise the comfortable speaking pitch.

There are various types of lasers and various modalities for using lasers on the vocal cords. One type of laser treatment, LAVA, attempts to increase vocal pitch through a thinning and tightening of the vocal cords. Increases in fundamental frequency with this technique tend not to be as large as with other surgical methods [14]. One advantage is that no external incision is required. In one of my patients whose pitch spontaneously returned to the masculine range after CTA, the addition of the LAVA procedure brought her comfortable speaking pitch back up toward the female range again temporarily. So it is possible that some combination of procedures might be beneficial. See also [16].

A proposed fundamental frequency range for adult females is 145–275 Hz (D3-C#4) and for males 80–165 Hz (D#2-E3) [16]. This leaves an area of overlap from 145 to 165 Hz (D3-E3) where fundamental frequency alone might not be sufficient to determine the sex of a patient. This is important as transgender patients with F0 as high as 181 Hz have been perceived as male. 'It appears that it is the interaction between F0, F0 range, intonation and resonance that ultimately determines the perception of the speaker as female' [17]. Addressing these components as complements to each other would represent a more desirable approach to voice modification compared to fundamental pitch change alone.

Resonant frequency also affects the gender perception of voice. This is especially true in the grey area where normal male and female speaking pitches overlap [18]. The resonant frequency is inversely related to the length of the resonant tube, the pharynx [19]. Speech therapy techniques have been used to modify the mouth opening and tongue placement [17]. Gunzburger noted that when comparing transexuals' male vs. female voice, the resonance patterns change [20]. He hypothesized that this was accomplished by practiced manipulation of oropharyngeal shape and the elevation of the larynx [2, 20]. Elevation of the larynx enables higher resonant frequency of the pharynx, as the length of the resonant tube is decreased [21].

In transgender patients particularly adept at creating a female voice quality, I noted an ability to maintain with muscle tension two pharyngeal parameters: elevation of the larynx and narrowing of the pharynx. Based on a personal communication with Robert Bastian discussing this idea, I began to suspend the larynx higher in the neck (thyrohyoid elevation component). This might address one of the parameters, length of the pharyngeal chamber, leaving to the patient to address the diameter of the chamber with muscle contraction if possible.

I have tried to reduce the diameter of the pharyngeal chamber in one patient, but I have not worked out a reliable technique to accomplish narrowing. Perhaps I removed an insufficient amount of tissue.

Somyos Kunachak in Thyroid Cartilage and Vocal Fold Reduction [22] proposed an open laryngoplasty to alter pitch. This procedure reduced the size of the larynx to a more female size in its cross-sectional dimension and shortened the length of the vibratory vocal fold. It possibly tensioned the vocal fold. It preserved the use of the cricothyroid muscle. Perhaps it thinned the vocal folds. Based primarily on this article, I began to perform what developed into a procedure termed feminization laryngoplasty or, as my first patient called it, 'FemLar'.

10.3 Feminization Laryngoplasty: Technique [23]

James P. Thomas

10.3.1 Preoperative

After an appropriate history, the patient's voice is recorded reading a standardized passage (Man's First Boat). Comfortable speaking pitch, attempted best female voice, vocal pitch range, maximum and minimum volumes, maximum phonation time and vegetative sounds are recorded. The vocal cords are then visualized and video recorded with flexible laryngoscopy including stroboscopy at a variety of pitches and volumes. Alternatives to surgery and the possible risks are discussed. Patients attend a 1-h voice education discussion with a speech therapist prior to surgery.

10.3.2 Surgery

Location All surgeries have been performed in a Medicare-certified, outpatient surgical centre. The procedure is typically 2 h long.

Anaesthesia The procedure is performed under general endotracheal anaesthesia using a 6-0 endotracheal tube.

Antibiotics All patients are given gentamicin and clindamycin at the beginning of the case if there are no drug allergies to either medication. 600 mg of clindamycin is administered IV over 10 min, and 80 mg of gentamicin is placed in the first litre of IV fluids. (Since this cohort of patients, I have changed to clindamycin and Claforan at the time of surgery with 7 days of postoperative oral therapy with either cefuroxime or levofloxacin.) Typically, the litre of fluid had been administered around the time of entry into the airway. The wound is irrigated with normal saline containing 100,000 units per litre of bacitracin prior to closure.

Steroids 10 mg of dexamethasone are given intravenously at the beginning of surgery. Oral prednisone or methylprednisolone is given in selected cases if significant swelling develops postoperatively.

Technique (All photos are taken from the perspective of the anaesthetist at the head of the table.)

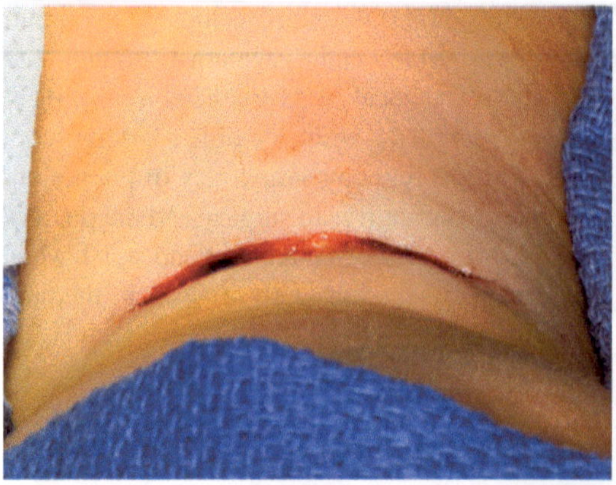

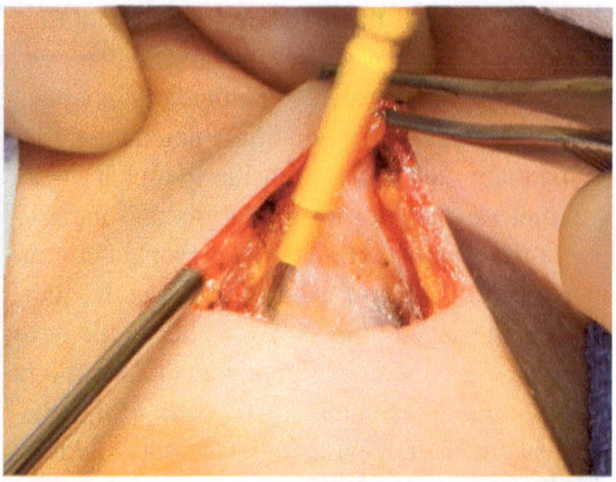

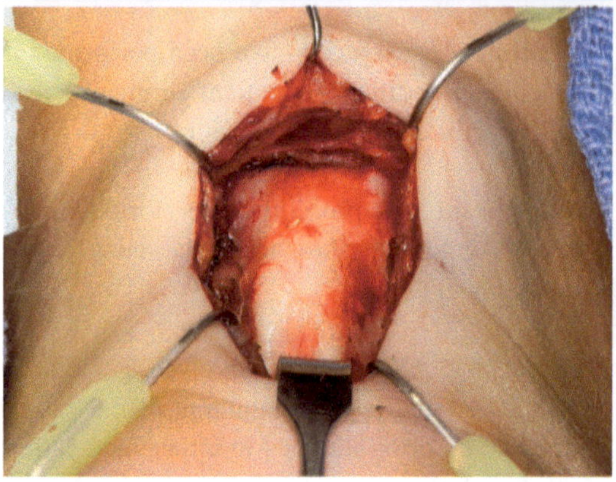

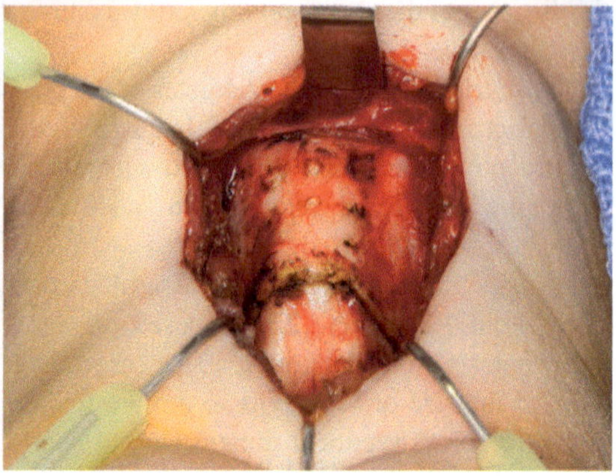

An approximately 5 cm incision is placed in or parallel to a skin crease directly in the midline and flaps developed at a level beneath the platysma. Strap muscles are separated in the midline exposing anatomy from the hyoid bone to the upper cricothyroid membrane. The midline is marked with a Bovie cautery, and secondary marks are placed 5–7 mm lateral to the midline on each side. I have also marked the upper incision to remove the upper alae of the thyroid cartilage.

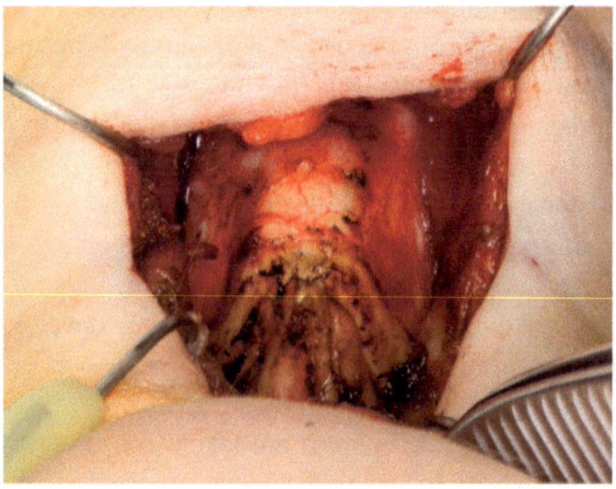

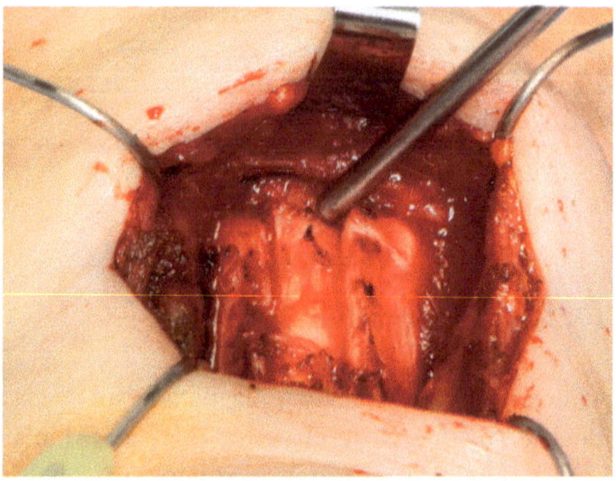

If a thyrohyoid elevation is planned, the upper portions of the thyroid cartilage may be removed at this point (or later after division of the thyroid cartilage in the midline). The thyroid cartilage is divided vertically with an oscillating saw about 5–7 mm on either side of the midline with the saw kerf removing about 1 additional millimetre of cartilage. The goal is to narrow the internal aperture of the laryngeal glottis by collapsing the thyroid alae medially.

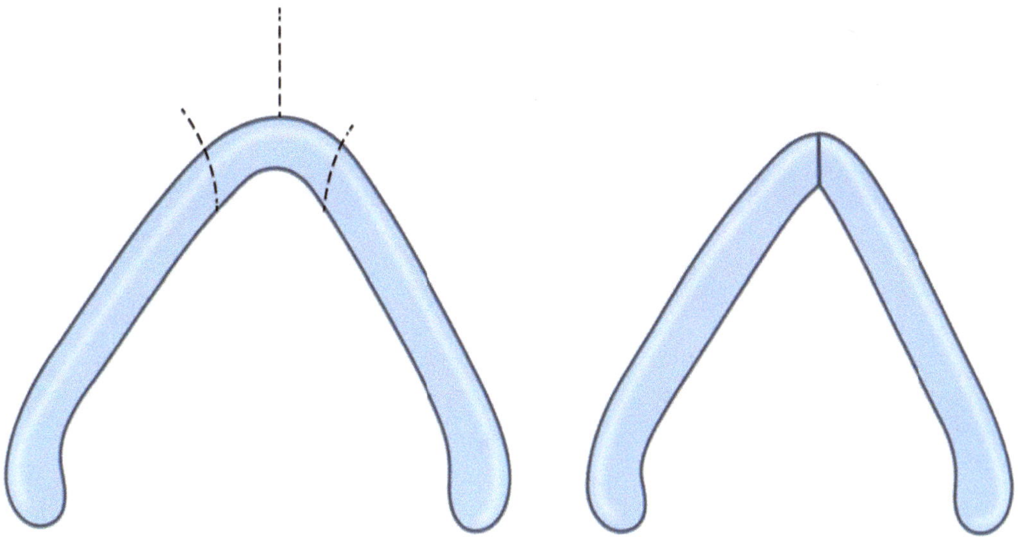

Beveling the cuts Cuts placed at a 90° angle to the cartilage allow only the inner thyroid lamina to approximate. The inner lamina is more contoured than the outer lamina with an internal bulge inferior to the vocal cords. A 90° cut thus prevents an airtight closure unless these contours are then removed with a cutting burr. By comparison, direct sagittal cuts allow only the outer lamina to approximate when the alae are collapsed back into the midline. Consequently, I attempt to bevel the cuts between these two planes to allow complete, airtight closure of the new anterior larynx in the midline.

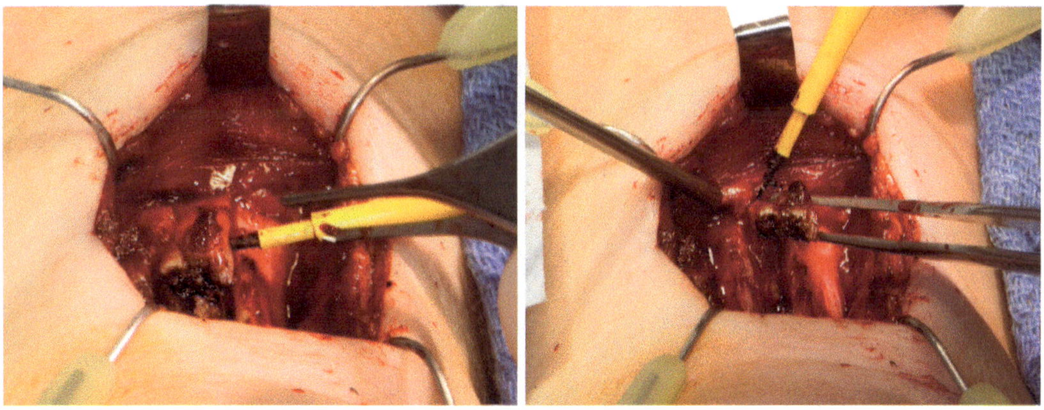

With electrocautery, the strip of anterior thyroid cartilage is elevated away from the soft tissue and removed. This removal of the vertical anterior thyroid cartilage segment will both narrow the internal laryngeal aperture and very effectively remove the Adam's apple contour (more completely than a 'tracheal shave'). The airway is not typically entered; though if it is, penetration usually occurs in the thinnest area, which is just superior to the anterior commissure.

The thyroid alae may be retracted laterally for a better view of the internal glottis. The vocal cord anterior ligaments are identified.

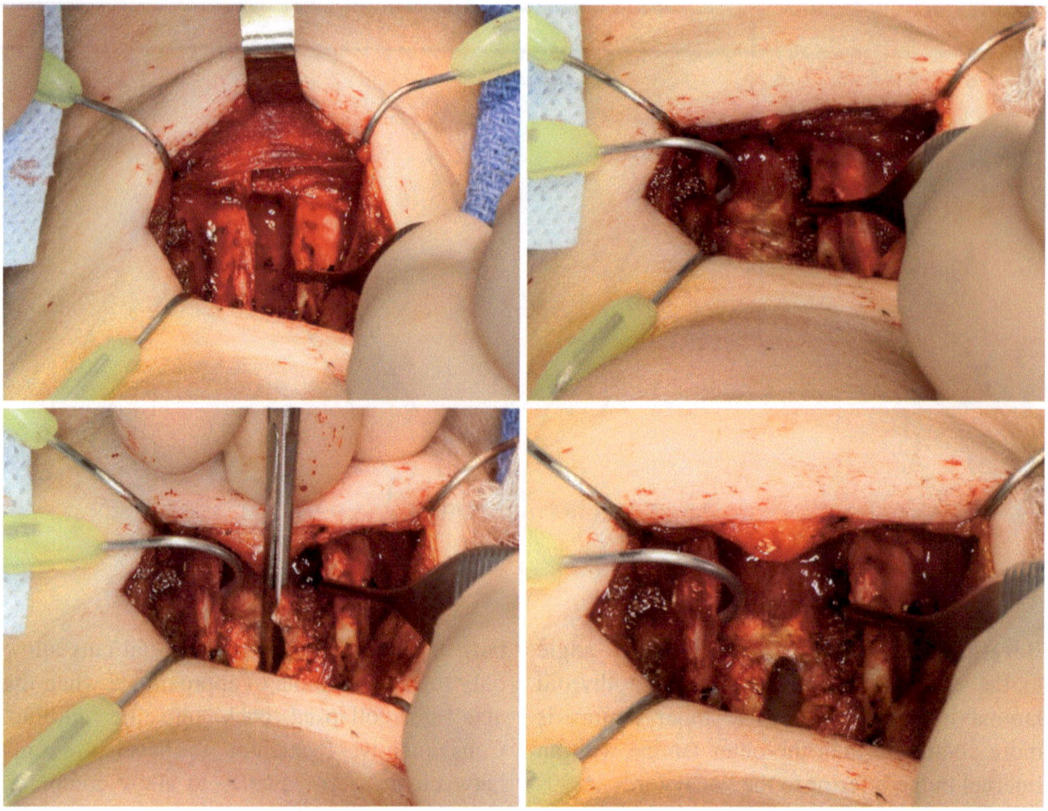

The airway is incised just superior to the anterior commissure. I extend this midline incision superiorly through the anterior commissure of the false vocal cords for a view of the endotracheal tube and the true vocal cords from above.

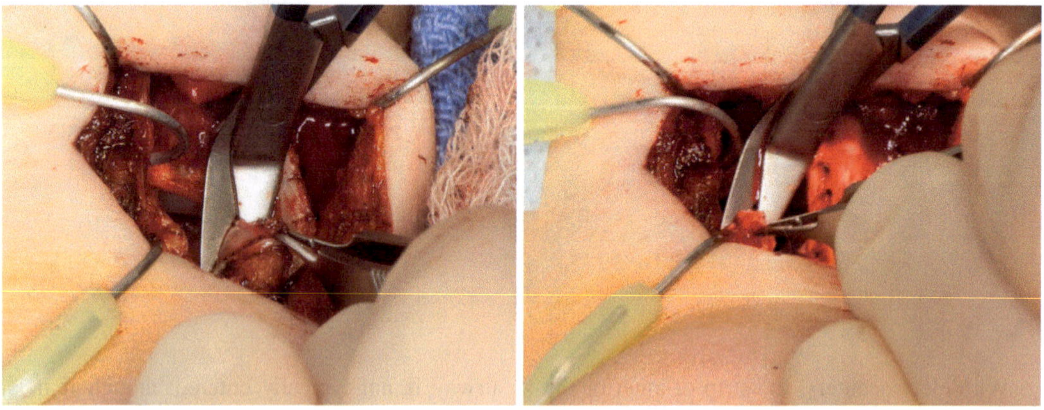

I remove approximately the anterior 1/3 of each false vocal cord, likely including the saccule. This reduces the diameter of the supraglottis after surgery. During surgery, this also provides an improved view of the true vocal cords and more space to manipulate needles within the larynx.

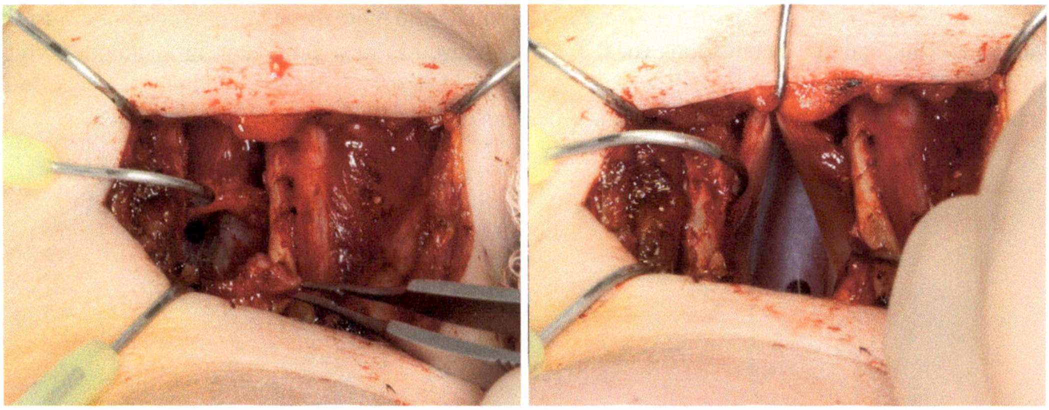

I prefer to maintain the anterior glottic ligament intact so that I can pull symmetrically on the vocal cords with a hook. I assess how much of the anterior vocal cord needs to be removed in order to collapse the thyroid alae back into the midline while maintaining tension on the vocal cords.

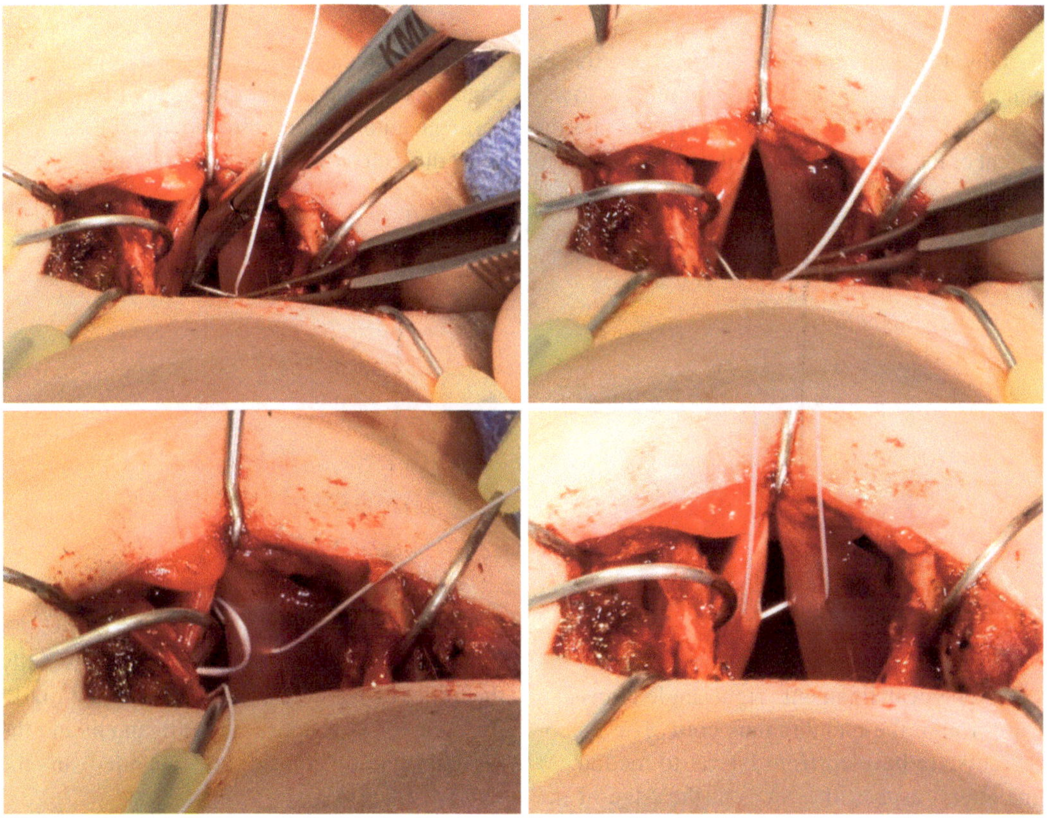

As I stretch them, I use one half of a double-ended 4-0 polytetrafluoroethylene (Gore-Tex) suture to mark the perceived 50–60% location along the membranous vocal cords as measured from the anterior commissure. I try to include the vocal ligament in this suture not only to maintain a symmetric length to the neo-vocal cords but also to maintain the vibratory margins vertical symmetry. My anticipated goal is to remove about 40–50% of the anterior membranous vocal cord. With removal of the anterior thyroid cartilage, the anterior-posterior dimension of the larynx will be smaller, so more membranous vocal cord must be removed to raise pitch than in a straight thyrotomy where only a small amount of vocal cord resection will raise pitch to some degree.

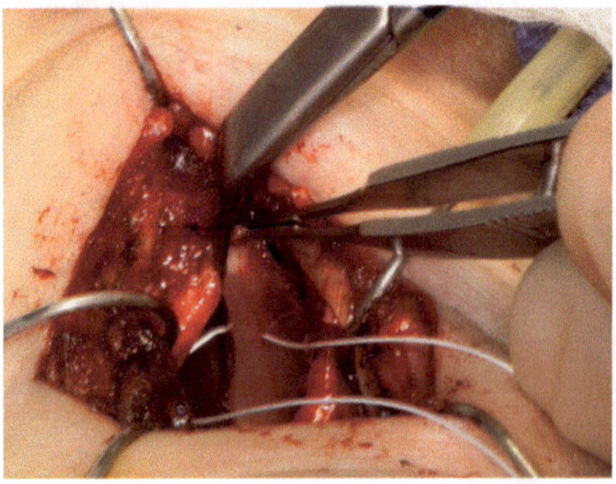

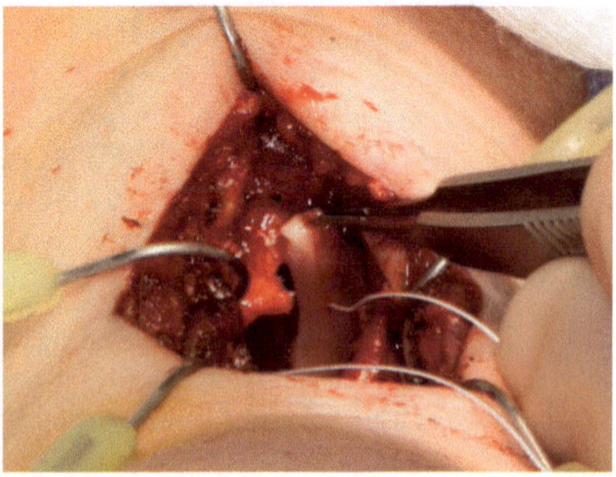

I divide the anterior commissure, attempting to minimize the length of the incision inferior to the vocal ligaments. My goal is to keep the inferior extent of the excision beneath the lower boundary of the thyroid cartilage. If the subglottic incision continues beyond the inferior edge of the thyroid cartilage into the cricothyroid membrane, it is more difficult to obtain an airtight closure.

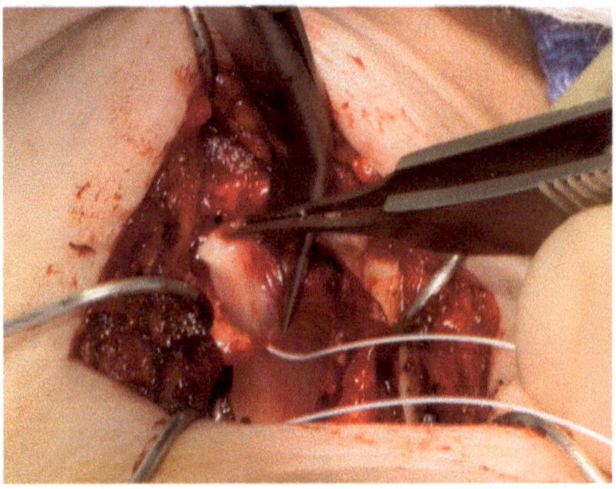

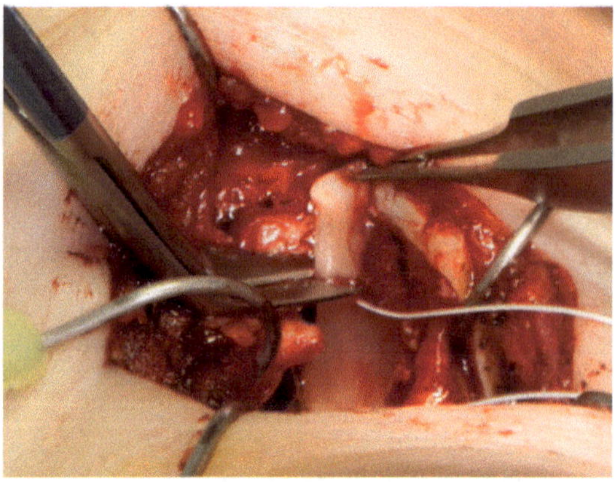

While tensioning each cord by grasping the anterior vocal ligament, right-angled scissors cut through the membranous cord. The mucosal cuts are beveled from lateral to medial. At the lateral aspect, the cut is at the edge of the inner lamina of the thyroid cartilage. Medially the cut exits the cord just anterior to the marking suture. The mucosa, vocal ligament and the thyroarytenoid muscle are included in the removal.

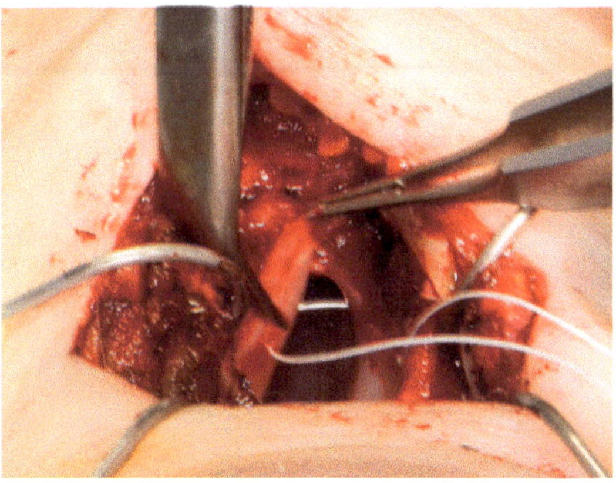

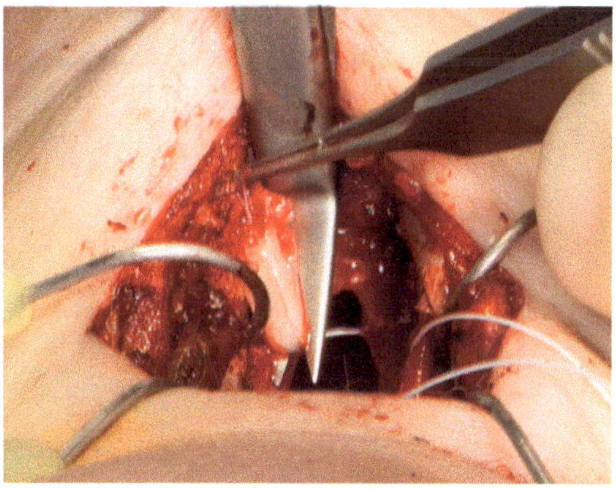

An identical amount is removed from the opposite vocal cord.

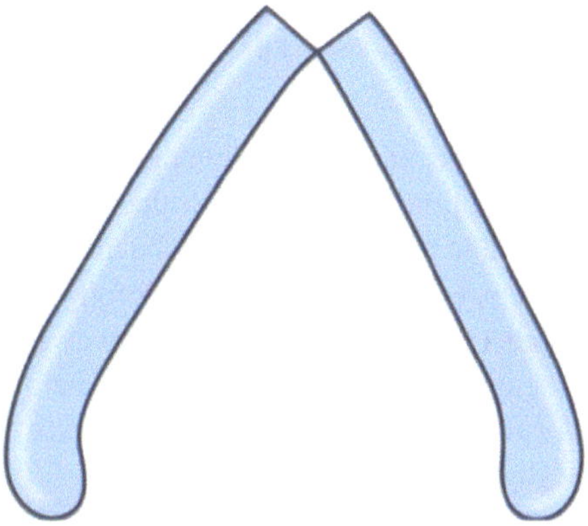

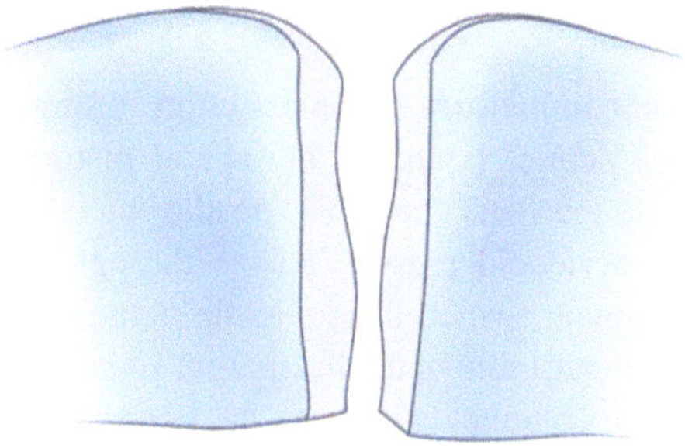

The cut edges of the thyroid cartilage are laid back together into their future position to check first for accurate coaptation. The cartilage is typically thicker just inferior to the attachment of the vocal cords. If tight closure is precluded by an inappropriate saw angle or because of any variation of thickness in the cartilage, these are removed or adjusted with a burr at this time.

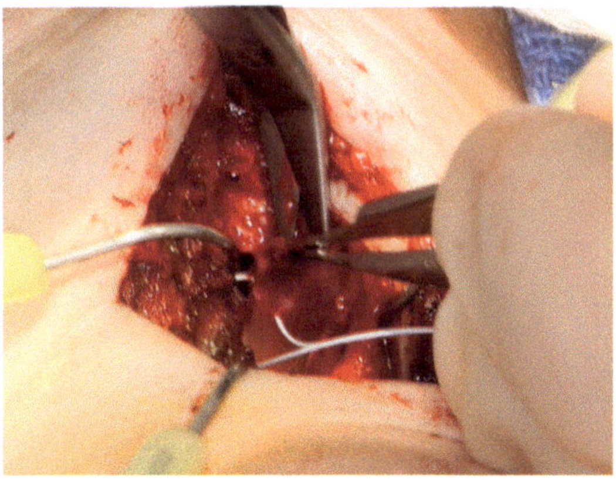

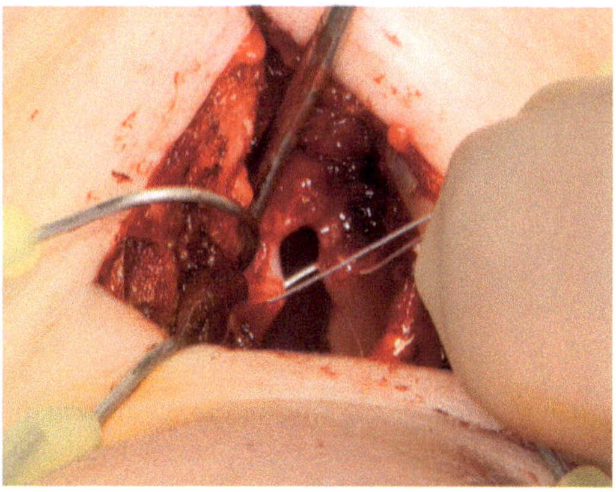

Secondly, the vocal cords are stretched as the thyroid lamina are brought back together to verify they are not too long to be placed under tension when secured against the inner thyroid lamina.

If they will not be under adequate tension, then more vocal cord can be removed. At times, the issue seems to be too much tissue bulk. I then grasp the central thyroarytenoid muscle, place it on a stretch and remove or debulk some additional muscle, typically nearly the anterior half of the thyroarytenoid muscle.

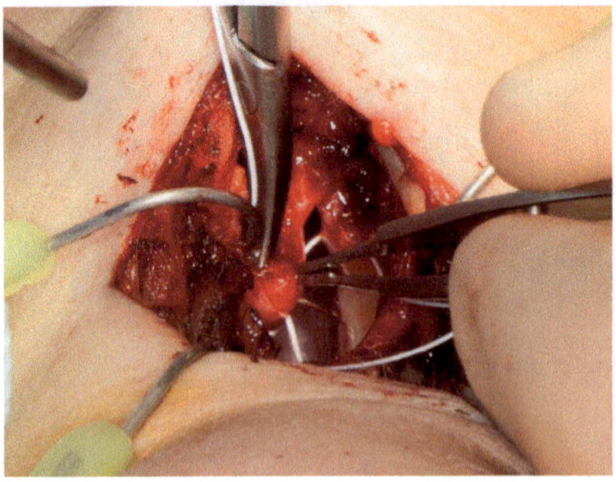

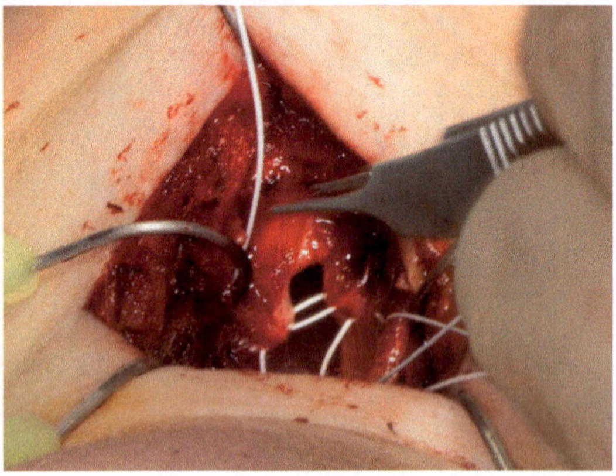

Anterior commissure reconstruction Using a Gore-Tex suture, I place a horizontal mattress suture into the vocal cords. The needle enters the left thyroarytenoid muscle, passes through the vocal ligament (which feels slightly dense) and includes about 1 mm of medial margin vocal cord epithelium. I attempt to exit at what I perceive to be the upper vibratory lip of the membranous vocal cord. This passes into the opposite cord in a similar location beginning with the vocal cord epithelium and passes out through the thyroarytenoid muscle. I repass the needle back following a path about 1 mm inferior at what I perceive will be the new inferior vibratory lip of the membranous vocal cord. Both ends of this first suture exit the left thyroarytenoid muscle.

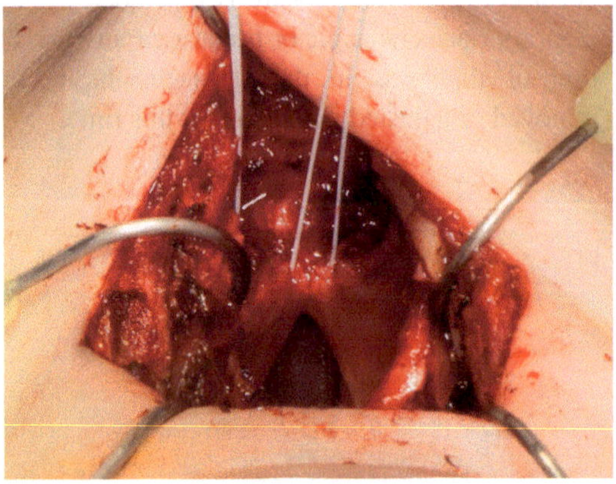

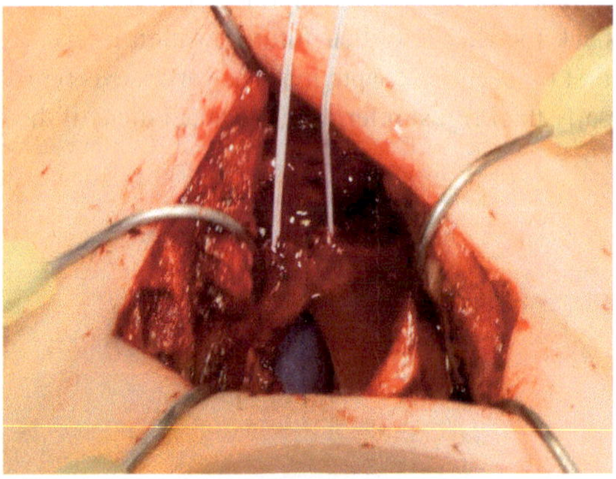

If I pull on the marking suture, I can visualize the neo-vocal cords (left photo). I remove the Gore-Tex marking suture, reusing it and passing it in opposition using a similar pathway beginning with the right thyroarytenoid muscle. At the conclusion, both ends of one suture exit the left vocal cord, and both ends of the other suture exit the right vocal cord. Pulling on these brings the new anterior commissure together.

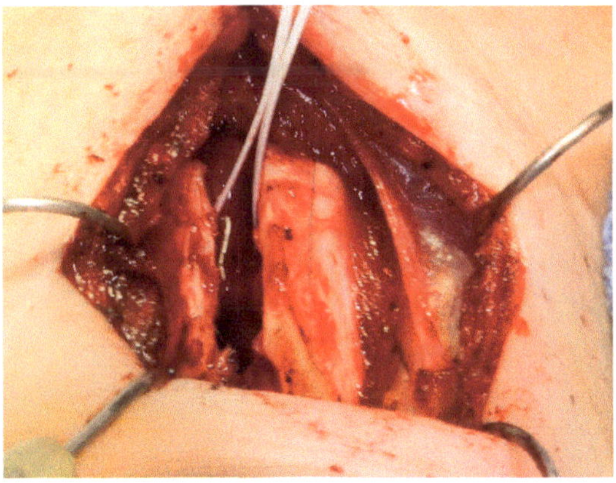

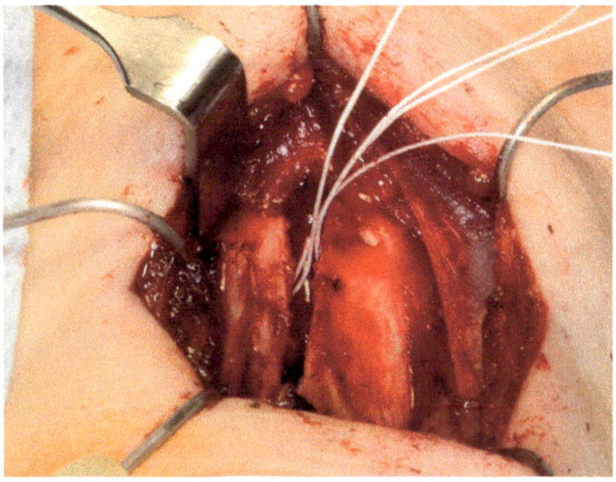

One reason that I use Gore-Tex is that when the thyroid alae are brought back together, the slipperiness of the Gore-Tex allows it to slide between the cartilages.

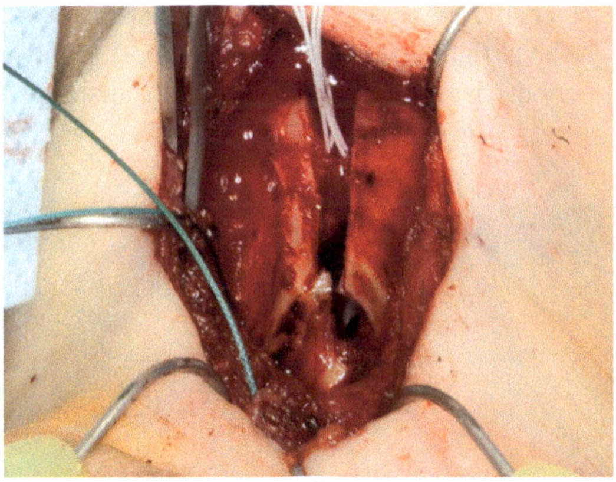

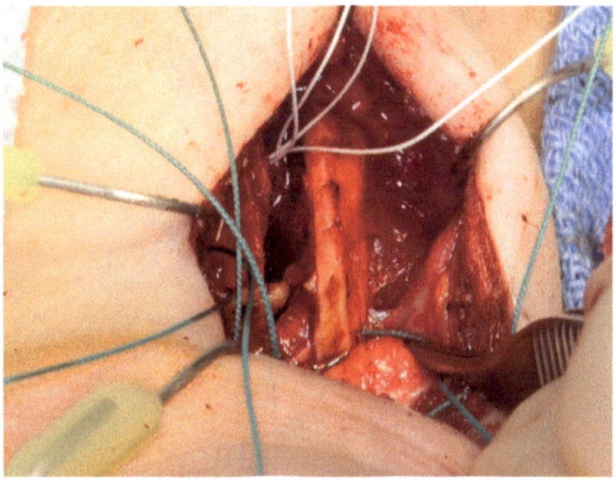

Thyrohyoid elevation: Muscles are elevated from the anterior inferior half of the hyoid bone with electrocautery. Strap muscles are divided at their insertion along the inferior edge of the hyoid bone for 15 mm either side of midline.

Closure: For closure of the thyroid cartilage, two 1-mm holes are drilled in the new anterior edge of each thyroid cartilage: one inferior at the level of the subglottis and one superior at the level of the false vocal cords. Each hole is angled toward the midline internally. To create the thyrohyoid elevation, two additional holes are placed along each superior border of the thyroid cartilage where the upper wings were removed. The softer the cartilage, the further from the upper cut edge of thyroid cartilage I place these holes to avoid tear-out later when tightening. Four holes are drilled into the hyoid bone, two on either side of the midline. These are angled slightly inferiorly to allow passage of the large needle on 0-Ethibond sutures.

Four braided, 0-Ethibond sutures are individually passed through each hole in the superior edge of the thyroid cartilage and passed through a corresponding hole in the hyoid bone. No sutures are tied yet.

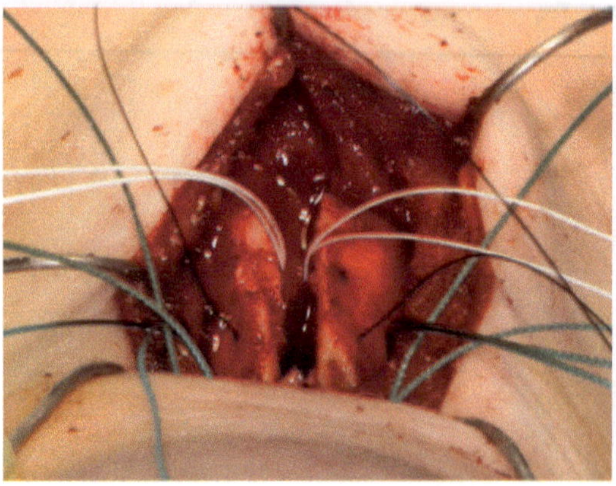

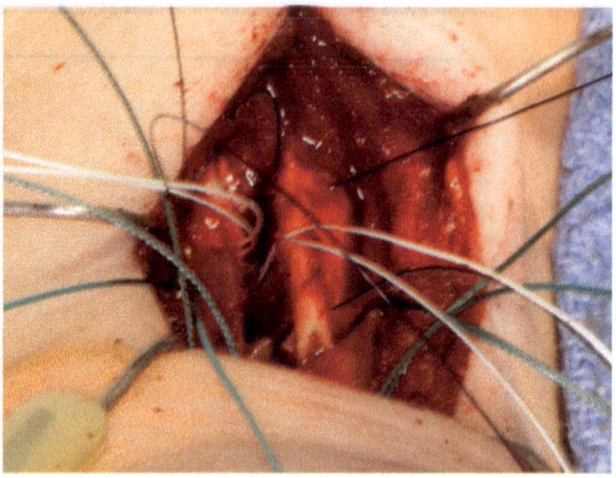

A 4-0 nylon or monofilament polyglyconate suture is placed through the upper holes in the superior thyroid cartilage and internally includes the cut edges of the false vocal cords with the intent of pulling this up against the inner thyroid lamina during closure. Another 4-0 nylon suture is passed through the inferior holes and includes the cut edge of the subglottic mucosa, again with the intent that the mucosa will reattach to the inner thyroid perichondrium and that there will be an airtight seal in the immediate postoperative period. I leave this needle attached temporarily.

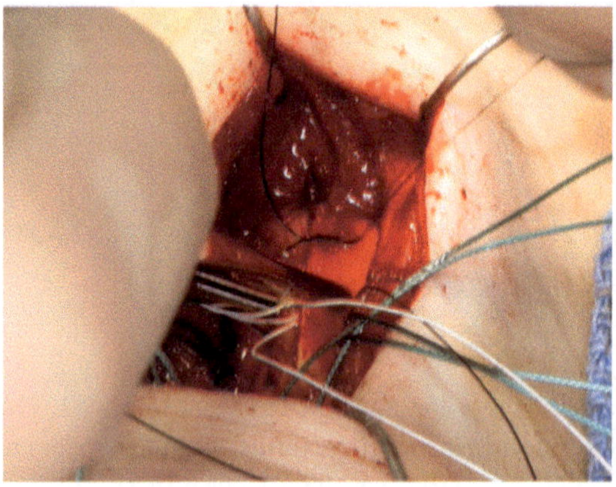

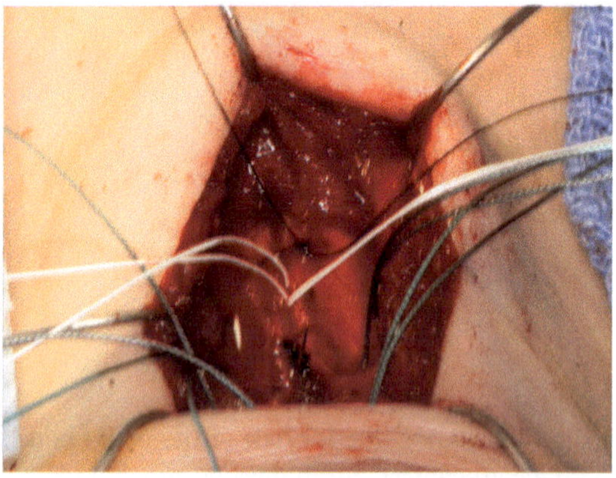

With all sutures in place, closure commences by bringing the cut edges of the thyroid cartilage together. The lower nylon suture is tied while an assistant squeezes the thyroid cartilage alae together with a forceps (above left photo). The upper suture is then tied securing the thyroid cartilage. With the needle still on this upper suture, I pass the needle through the tissue near the base of the epiglottis at the superior edge of the thyroid cartilage and secure it to the thyroid cartilage.

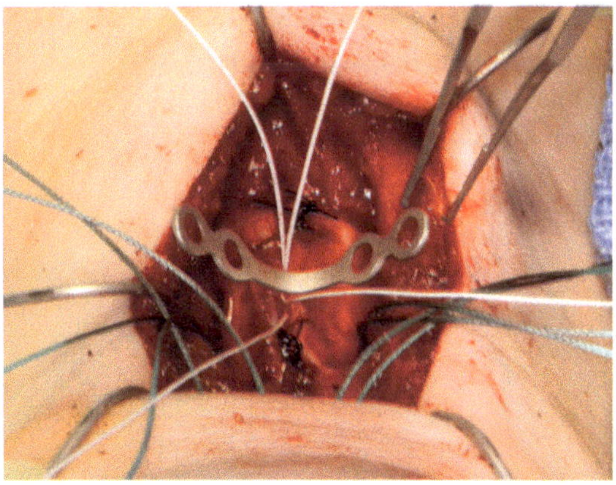

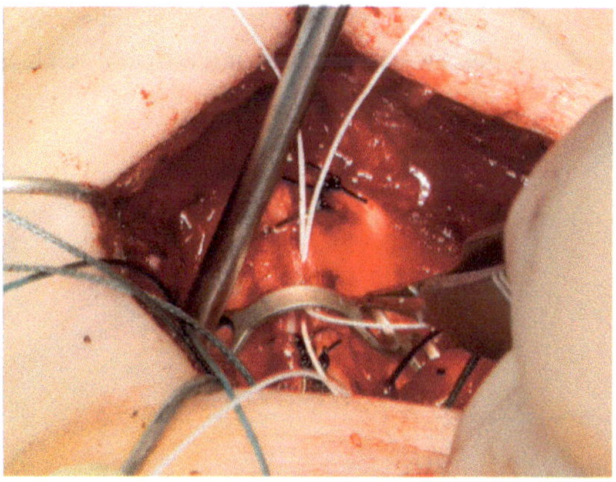

A four-hole, dog bone-shaped plate is bent to the shape of the newly angled anterior thyroid cartilage. It is placed preferably at the same level as the original attachment of the anterior commissure. I prefer self-tapping screws, which are placed bilaterally.

At this point, the slipperiness of the Gore-Tex suture presents its advantage, the ability to slide between the coapted edges of the thyroid cartilage. The Gore-Tex sutures are tightened and tied around the plate to pull the anterior commissure against the inner thyroid perichondrium. I have tried unsuccessfully to monitor the tensioning during this portion of the procedure with a flexible endoscope, but with the patient paralyzed, the soft tissues of the pharynx and larynx collapse onto the end of the endoscope precluded an adequate view of the glottis during the tightening.

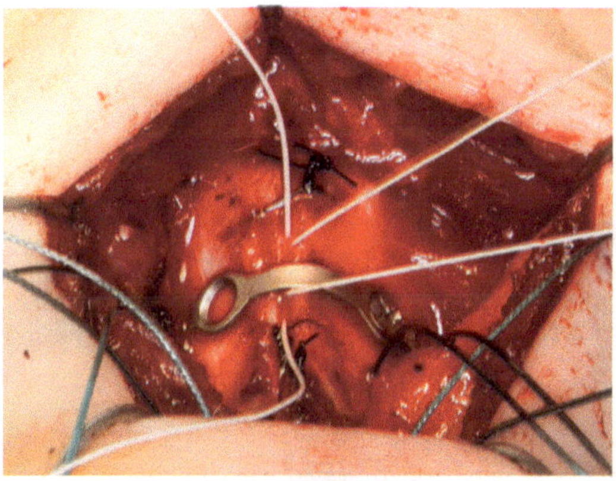

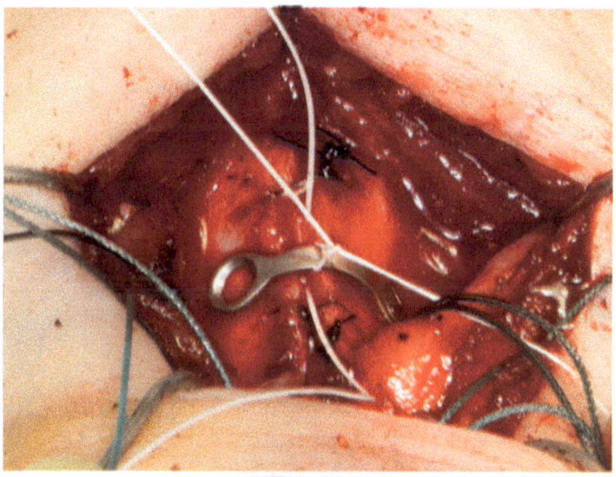

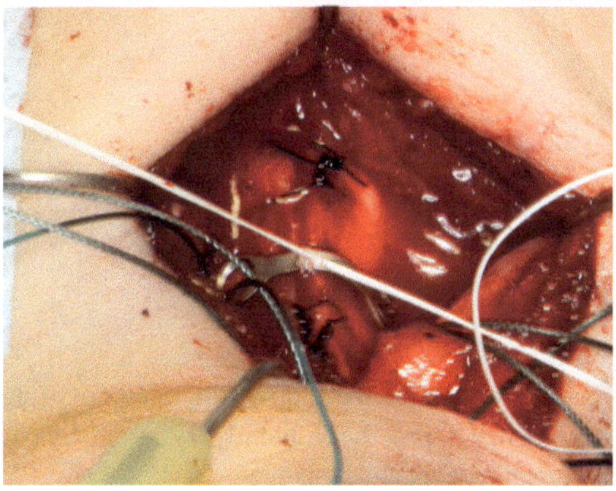

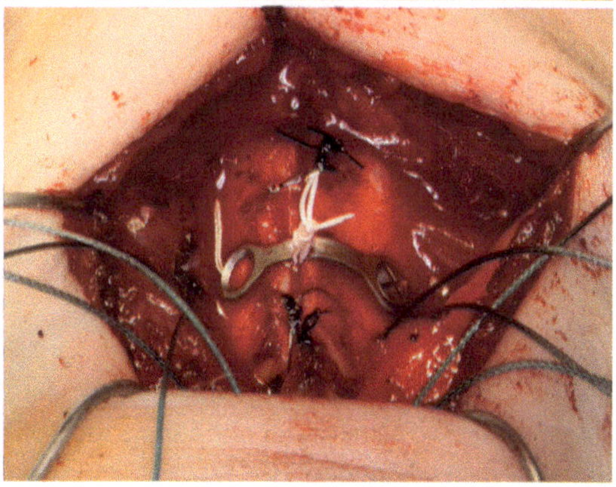

The 0-Ethibond sutures are then tightened and tied, pulling the larynx superiorly in the neck. Typically the thyroid cartilage does not quite reach the hyoid bone.

The wound is irrigated with saline solution containing bacitracin. The strap muscles are re-approximated and can be slightly plicated, pulled superiorly and reattached to the hyoid bone under some tension. Subcutaneous tissues are closed with 4-0 Monocryl.

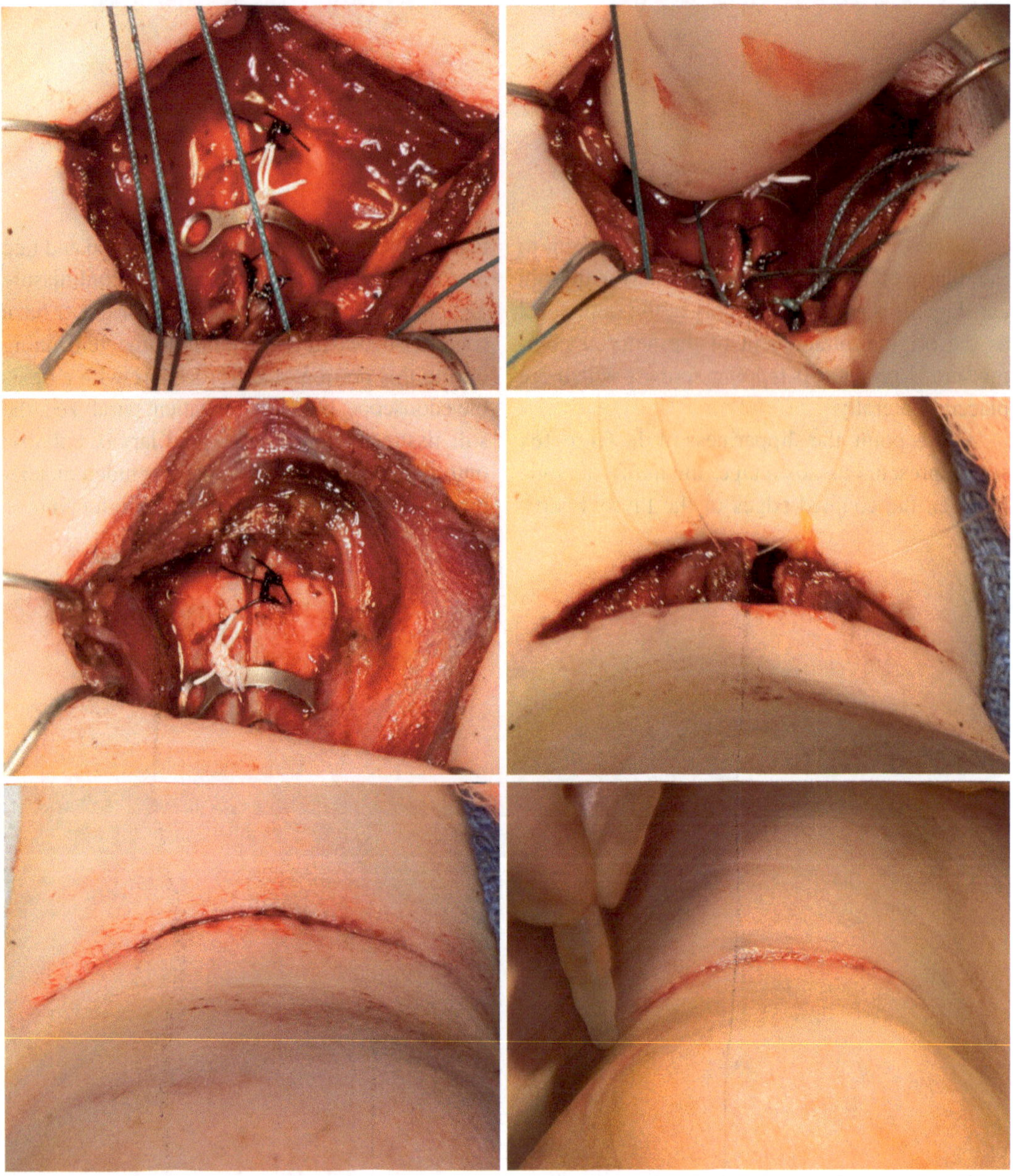

The skin is closed with a running subcuticular suture, either 4-0 Monocryl. I place some form of cyanoacrylate on the skin.

A nasogastric tube is passed momentarily into the stomach and the contents aspirated. She is extubated deep and awakened.

10.3.3 Postoperative

Surgery is performed as an outpatient. Each patient is discharged after approximately 1 h into the care of a friend, family or a professional caregiver. Because of the general anaesthetic, she must remain with someone for the first 24 h postoperatively. Most stay in a nearby hotel of their choosing. Postoperatively each patient is examined with flexible laryngoscopy every day for 3 days. I see them again 6 days postoperatively, and then she is free to return home if there are no complications.

Two weeks of complete voice rest are suggested. Pain is typically fairly minimal (though individually variable). A narcotic is prescribed for use as either pain or cough suppression. My postoperative instructions include instructions to avoid coughing. Nothing heavier than 10 pounds is to be lifted for 1 month. Other forms of straining, such as Valsalva manoeuvre, are strongly discouraged. I ask that she not be electively intubated for a period of 3 months. If intubated for general anaesthesia, she should request a number 6 endotracheal tube be used.

Acoustic data is taken from patients who subsequently return for scheduled follow-ups beyond the 2-week window. Voice samples are also accepted from patients who complete a recording by reading a voice analysis script. Recordings have been accepted on a wide range of media including computer files, video Hi8 tapes, cassettes, microcassettes, CDs and DVDs. Quality and background noise are variable. I have utilized software with Skype if the patient does not have recording capabilities, although cell phones and Skype seem to have automatic volume dampening that hampers assessment of some of the vocal parameters.

10.3.4 Caveats and Thoughts

Anaesthesia My initial FemLar procedure was performed under local anaesthesia. Although this is a feasible approach in terms of minimal pain during and after the surgery, the seeming risk of tearing the vocal cords while suturing them, if the patient tries to speak at an inappropriate moment, seems to outweigh the benefits of this approach. After the first patient, general endotracheal anaesthesia was used largely to prevent vocal cord movement at an inappropriate time.

Dividing the cartilage The thyroid cartilage is not calcified in some young patients, and a knife may be used. Over a number of patients, I placed the cuts further and further laterally trying to further narrow the larynx, until in one patient, after removing 10 mm either side of midline, I could not approximate the inferior cut edge of the thyroid cartilage. The upper edge of the cricoid cartilage lies internal to the lower thyroid cartilage, and the external diameter of the cricoid cartilage precluded complete closure.

Currently, the vertical incisions in the thyroid cartilage are generally placed about 5–6 mm either side of the midline. The amount removed varies with the perceived size of the thyroid cartilage. In very large thyroid cartilages and in cartilages with a very acute anterior angle, the vertical thyroid cartilage incision tends toward 7 or 8 mm from the midline. In small or very flat thyroid cartilages, perhaps only 5 or 6 mm are removed. At the typical beveled angle, in the average person, this removed piece of cartilage measures about 10 mm in width across the outer table of the thyroid cartilage and about 5 mm in width on the inner table. The width or kerf of the saw blade itself is about 1 mm.

Revisions Revisions are possible. In my first patient, I conservatively removed additional vocal cord over three surgeries until we reached the pitch that she desired. I presently consider about 50% of membranous cord to be the appropriate amount to remove.

Prior CTA surgery If a patient has had a prior CTA surgery, the cricoid and thyroid cartilage are typically fused. Even if they can be pried apart or even if they are sawed apart, in my experience, the cricothyroid joint has typically been immobilized long enough that the joint is non-functional. The cricothyroid muscle can no longer modify the vocal cord length. Dissecting apart this fusion sometimes lowers the pitch back into a male speaking range: certainly not desirable in most cases. Consequently, if there has been a prior cricothyroid approximation, I now leave the approximation intact. I utilize a midline thyrotomy division and do not remove any additional thyroid cartilage. The cricothyroid fusion limits opening of the thyroid cartilage and surgical exposure. I try to gain additional pitch elevation solely through removal of anterior membranous vocal cord and typically remove about 20% of the length.

Taking apart a cricothyroid fusion from a prior CTA, however, may not be a reliable way to lower the pitch, again because of cricothyroid joint fixation. There is an uncommon patient wishing to return to a lower or male speaking pitch. If after taking apart a cricothyroid fusion under local anaesthesia there is no or insufficient pitch drop, I place two vertical thyrotomy incisions and remove 1–3 mm of cartilage from one or both sides which drops the tension in the vocal cords.

This issue of cricothyroid joint fusion is also the reason I discourage 'trying the CTA surgery first'. The CTA procedure causes loss of use of one of the most important muscles for changing pitch. The postoperative CTA patient has only the thyroarytenoid muscle remaining to change pitch. The postoperative FemLar patient has both a shortened thyroarytenoid muscle available and a cricothyroid muscle available to alter pitch.

Dividing the vocal cords In early cases, I divided the anterior commissure early in the procedure so that I could widely open the larynx for a view. The very first time I cut the membranous vocal cords, the mucosa contracted all the way back to the vocal process, an unsettling manoeuvre that makes the vocal cord seem to disappear. It is possible to re-grasp the mucosa and the vocal ligament. However, resecting the anterior vocal cord one at a time seemed also to be a possible contribution to the likelihood of postoperative asymmetry between the vocal cords. Thus, I now place the marking suture in the mid-portion of the vocal cords in everyone before removing the anterior vocal cords. It acts as a marker for where I intend to place a cut as well as the suture to maintain symmetry. This also defines for me the area of the vocal ligament. When the vocal cord is cut, it not only contracts posteriorly toward the vocal ligament, it also flattens out against the lateral aspect of the thyroid cartilage. It can be difficult to locate the vertical level of the vocal ligament after releasing it.

Suturing the new anterior commissure In early cases I placed an additional suture into each vocal cord in order to tension the thyroarytenoid muscle separately from the new anterior commissure. Before placing the opposing horizontal mattress sutures which create the new anterior commissure, I drilled two additional holes into the thyroid cartilage at the level of the anterior commissure. I passed a nylon suture through the cut anterior end of the thyroarytenoid muscle. This was brought out of the glottis and passed into the thyroid cartilage from externally to internally and then back out of the thyroid cartilage via the other hole. As this suture was tightened, the central portion of the thyroarytenoid muscle was pulled up to the cut edge of the inner thyroid lamina. If there was too much thyroarytenoid muscle, such that it could be pulled out along the cut edge of the thyroid cartilage, then the suture was cut and more thyroarytenoid muscle resected. This type of suturing made further work internally more difficult since if the thyroid alae were pulled laterally for exposure after suturing the thyroarytenoid muscle, this suture would tear out of the muscle. I remain unconvinced that it added any pitch gain and it added time and technical difficulty to the procedure.

Voice rest With the initial patients, I did not suggest any voice rest. Many patients when they initially speak have a deeper comfortable speaking pitch, presumably because of the easily visualized swelling of the transected vocal cords.

Some patients seem to have tight enough vocal cords with minimal swelling and have a higher pitch even the first week after surgery. One patient, with an initial great result, began singing 1 week after surgery. She felt a pop and noted that her comfortable speaking pitch dropped. Since that time, I have requested 2 weeks of voice rest, and a number of patients have voluntarily undergone 3 weeks of voice rest if their occupational lowed.

Subcutaneous emphysema This might result from lack of an airtight closure or from an aggressive cough. Some patients will feel a need to cough from a tickle, or to clear secretions, or to clear a blood clot from the internal incision or even from a sensory illusion, the result of the swelling that places the anterior cords in apposition to each other. Isolated or infrequent coughing does not necessarily cause a problem. However, heavy or ongoing coughing may lead to subcutaneous emphysema. I have managed this with expectant waiting or on an occasion with placement of a drain. If air is leaking from internally, there also seems to be a higher associated rate of infection.

Postoperative airway compromise All of the iatrogenic airway compromise I have seen has been from supraglottic oedema and principally from oedema on the posterior aspect of the arytenoids. I believe there are two probable aetiologies for this oedema. One is infectious. The other seems to be from extension of the resection along the superior edge of the thyroid cartilage toward the superior thyroid cornu. After realizing that some supraglottic oedema is a result of surgical dissection posteriorly along the superior border of the thyroid cartilage, I began to remove only the anterior two thirds of the upper thyroid ala. I feel that I can still elevate and suspend the larynx from the hyoid bone without removing thyroid cartilage all the way to the superior cornu.

Oedema seems to peak on postoperative day number 3. Infections seem to be identifiable by day 3 or else an infection tends not to occur. I have not seen any airway compromise from oedema at the level of the glottis either early or late.

After one infection, where I inadequately drained a subcutaneous collection of purulence, the following day I placed a temporary tracheostomy and drained a deeper collection of purulence beneath the strap muscles. For a number of patients after this, I then placed a drain at the time of skin closure. This drain seemed to make no positive difference in the rate of infection and perhaps increased the rate of infection, so I have not been placing drains since. After switching preoperative antibiotics to a combination of clindamycin and a third-generation cephalosporin, combined with 7 days of postoperative cefuroxime or levofloxacin, I have encountered no severe infections.

I very aggressively try to ensure an airtight closure of the incision into the larynx. My present management approach is that if on endoscopic examination on postoperative day number 2 or number 3 there is any suggestion of infection including either supraglottic oedema, supraglottic erythema, increasing pain, subcutaneous fullness or subcutaneous fluid collection, then I will treat aggressively for presumed infection. This includes needle aspiration of any potential subcutaneous fluid collection and culture, and I start oral antibiotics.

In all cases of infection persisting beyond 10 days, I have ultimately returned the patient to surgery and removed the hardware or suture that was associated with the ongoing infection. The plate and Gore-Tex sutures, if removed after 1 month, are no longer needed, and the anterior commissure remains well attached.

One patient felt moderately short of breath yet had only typical mild supraglottic swelling, not enough to cause symptoms of an airway restriction. After a strong cough expectorated a clot, which must have been present in one of the bronchi, her sense of dyspnoea resolved.

Asymmetry I noticed varying degrees of asymmetry of the vocal cords on stroboscopy of patients from my very first procedure. While sometimes asymptomatic, there can be some pitch where asymmetric cords cause dysphonia, specifically diplophonia. If this is at the comfortable speaking pitch, the patient may learn to elevate or lower the pitch slightly to avoid the rough spot. Initially, when severe enough, I tried to correct the asymmetric tension with a revision surgery. Fifteen of the first 69 patients received a revision surgery. This correction of asymmetry was difficult to accomplish with scar tissue from the initial surgery being present, and it was difficult to judge the exact amount to remove.

On one patient with particularly severe dysphonia after an infection, I utilized an office laser to create a burn on the superior surface of the looser vocal cord, which tightened, correcting the dysphonia. It also raised the pitch slightly.

Since then, I have used the pulsed dye laser but more recently have preferred a KTP laser for vocal cord tightening. Using a flexible laser fibre passed through a flexible laryngoscope has proven to be a very cost-effective means of correcting surgical asymmetries.

The laser can also be applied bilaterally to raise the pitch. If I tighten both sides, I frequently can obtain an additional semitone of pitch elevation. This office laser procedure may be repeated after 2–3 months. I don't know the limit of how much pitch elevation may be obtained with additional treatment(s).

Elevation of the larynx On the first patient which I tried a thyrohyoid elevation, I was able to elevate the larynx just by passing sutures through the upper thyroid cartilage and the hyoid bone, but in my second patient and in many patients since, the upper edge of the thyroid cartilage abuts the hyoid bone precluding additional elevation. I presently consistently remove one vertical centimetre of upper thyroid cartilage, which gives additional room to raise the larynx in the neck. It also gives the appearance during surgery of a more typical female sized thyroid cartilage.

Elevation of the larynx changes only one of several anatomical features that contribute to resonant frequency. Other anatomical differences that affect resonance (i.e. the sinuses) cannot easily be surgically manipulated to produce a more feminine resonance. However, one anatomic area that might also be surgically manipulated is the diameter of the pharynx. There may be a way to plicate the pharyngeal walls and narrow the circumferential dimension of the pharynx, improving resonance of higher pitches. Or perhaps one might devise a subcutaneous augmentation to narrow the pharyngeal diameter in a way analogous to an obese person's narrowed pharynx.

Most patients note a loss of volume, both in everyday speech and for a yell. In most cases she cannot replicate the volume of her previous voice. Subjectively, some patients are pleased with the softness of their new voice or may consider it a reasonable trade-off.

Numerous patients did not initially perceive a change in their voice after surgery. I suspect we are used to hearing our voices via internal bone conduction. Additionally, FemLar does not change the accent or character of the voice after surgery. While documentation is important in many respects (for the surgeon to learn what works, legal documentation, etc.), it is invaluable to the patient as well to hear the difference in pitch on a recording. After hearing the pre- and postoperative recordings, many patients gain confidence in her new voice.

10.3.5 Conclusion

Feminization laryngoplasty, including a thyrohyoid elevation component and possibly a later postoperative laser tuning, is a surgical technique designed for individuals wishing to transition from a male to female voice by increasing the fundamental and resonant frequencies of her voice.

10.3.6 Online Media References

Voice samples are available at http://www.voicedoctor.net/Surgery/Pitch/Feminization-Laryngoplasty.

10.3.7 References

1. Wagner I, Fugain C, Monneron-Girard L, Cordier B, Chabolle F. Pitch-raising surgery in fourteen male-to-female transsexuals. Laryngoscope. 2003;113:1157–165. https://doi.org/10.1097/00005537-200307000-00011.
2. Brown M, Perry A, Cheesman AD, Pring T. Pitch change in male-to-female transsexuals: has phonosurgery a role to play? Int J Lang Comm Dis. 2000;35(1):129–36. https://doi.org/10.1080/136828200247296.
3. Isshiki N, Morita H, Okamura H, Hiramoto M. Thyroplasty as a new phonosurgical technique. Acta Otolaryng. 1974;78(1):451–7. https://doi.org/10.3109/00016487409126379.
4. Isshiki N, Taira T, Tanabe M. Surgical alteration of the vocal pitch. Otolaryngol Head Neck Surg. 1983;5(3):35–40.
5. Isshiki N. Mechanical and dynamic aspects of voice production as related to voice therapy and phonosurgery. J Voice. 1998;12(2): 125–37.
6. Neumann K, Welzel C, Berghaus A. Operative voice pitch raising in male-to-female transsexuals. A survey of our technique and results. HNO. 2003;51(1):30–7.
7. Matai V, Cheesman AD, Clarke PM. Cricothyroid approximation and thyroid chondroplasty: a patient survey. Otolaryngol Head Neck Surg. 2003;128(6):841–7.
8. Yang CY, Palmer AD, Murray KD, Meltzer TR, Cohen JI. Cricothyroid approximation (CTA) to elevate vocal pitch in male-to-female transsexuals: results of surgery. Ann Otol Rhinol Laryngol. 2002;111(6):477–85.
9. Tucker HM. Anterior commissure laryngoplasty for adjustment of vocal fold tension. Ann Otol Rhinol Laryngol. 1985;94:547–9.
10. Donald PJ. Voice change surgery in the transsexual. Head Neck Surg. 1982;4(5):433–7.
11. Gross M. Pitch-raising surgery in male-to-female transsexuals. J Voice. 1999;13(2): 246–50.
12. Remacle M, Matar N, Morsomme D, Verduyckt I, Lawson G. Glottoplasty for male-to-female transsexualism: voice results. J Voice. 2011;25(1):120–3.
13. Hong KH, Ye M, Kim YM, Kevorkian KF, Kreiman J, Berke GS. Functional differences between the two bellies of the cricothyroid muscle. Otolaryngol Head Neck Surg. 1998;118(5):714–22.
14. Orloff L, Mann A, Damrose J, Goldman S. Laser-aided voice adjustment (LAVA) in transsexuals. Laryngoscope. 2006; 116: 655–60. https://doi.org/10.1097/01.mlg.0000205198.65797.59.
15. Neumann K, Welzel C. The importance of the voice in male-to-female transsexualism. J Voice. 2004;18(1):153–67.
16. Koçak I, Akpınar ME, Cakır ZA, Doğan M, Bengisu S, Celikoyar MM. Laser reduction glottoplasty for managing androphonia after failed cricothyroid approximation surgery. J Voice. 2010;24(6):758–64.
17. Dacakis G. Long-term maintenance of fundamental frequency increases in male-to-female transsexuals. Voice. 2000;4:549–56.
18. Wolfe VI, Ratusnik DL, Smith FH, Northrop G. Intonation and fundamental frequency in male-to-female transsexuals. J Speech Hear Disord. 1990;55(1):43–50.
19. Lawrence A. 2004. http://www.annelawrence.com/twr/voicesurgery.html.
20. Günzburger D. Voice adaptation by transsexuals. Clin Linguist Phon. 3(2):163–72.
21. Carew L, Dacakis G, Oates J. The effectiveness of oral resonance therapy on the perception of femininity of voice in male-to-female transsexuals. J Voice. 2007;21(5):591–603.
22. Kunachak S, Prakunhungsit S, Sujjalak K. Thyroid cartilage and vocal fold reduction: a new phonosurgical method for male-to-female transsexuals. Ann Otol Rhinol Laryngol. 2000;109(11):1082–6.
23. Thomas JP. 21 feminization laryngoplasty – technique. voicedoctor.net.

10.4 Laser-Assisted Voice Adjustment (LAVA)

Marc Remacle and Vyas M. N. Prasad

Orloff et al. [1] described the use of the CO_2 laser in ablating the superior vocal fold mucosa extending up to the ventricle. Some reduction of the thyroarytenoid muscle inevitably occurs resulting in tightening of the vocal fold and reduction of the vocal fold mass—raising pitch. Performed entirely endoscopically, the procedure obviates the need for a neck incision, but it is a procedure where pitch increase may not be sufficient nor long lasting (Figs. 10.4.1 and 10.4.2). Several authors have however mentioned that this procedure, effectively a laser reduction glottoplasty, can be used as an adjunct to a CTA and, when more aggressively performed involving thyroarytenoid obliteration, provides sustained pitch elevation.

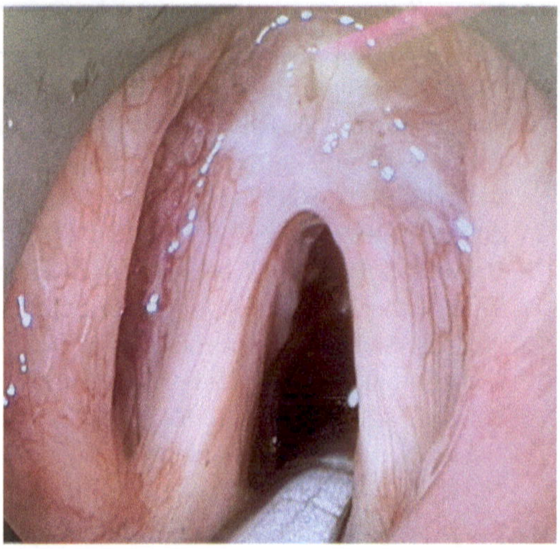

Fig. 10.4.1 Aspect before LAVA with previous glottoplasty

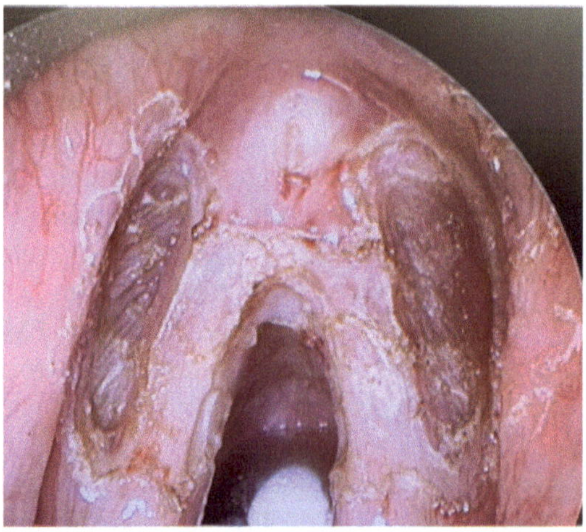

Fig. 10.4.2 Immediate aspect after LAVA procedure

10.4.1 Reference

1. Orloff LA, Mann AP, Damrose JF, Goldman SN. Laser-assisted voice adjustment (LAVA) in transsexuals. Laryngoscope. 2006;116: 655–60.

10.4.2 Summary: Voice Feminization

The above procedures have been either used or abandoned or continue to be used based on the expertise, experience and results of the laryngologists who perform them. Vocal fold feminization is however not a purely surgical process and should be viewed as a process that may require surgery depending on the patient's needs. As mentioned above, these procedures vary in their skill level, their ability to raise pitch adequately and maintain an acceptable vocal range and their appropriate resonance and have long-term stability of voice.

10.5 Voice Masculinization

Marc Remacle, Raja Fakhoury
and Vyas N. M. Prasad

10.5.1 Voice Masculinization

Masculinization of the voice is reflected by the lowering of the fundamental frequency and is primarily caused by exposure to androgens—namely, testosterone. Surgery is rarely required but is nevertheless an important treatment consideration in trans males who have not responded adequately to androgen treatment. Voice and behavioural therapy are equally important as are exercises to help depress the larynx, elongating the vocal tract and lowering the resonance of the vocal tract. Relaxation thyroplasty was attempted by Tucker [1], where a superiorly based 'diving board'-shaped flap was made in the midline of the thyroid cartilage and pushed into the larynx. Isshiki's type III thyroplasty, based on the same principle of pushing back the anterior commissure and relaxing the vocal folds, became the mainstay for pitch lowering surgery [2, 3, 4]. The author's experiences of relaxation thyroplasty (mainly in post-pubertal males with puberphonia/mutational falsetto) have been good with most patients registering an acceptable drop in fundamental frequency that is sustained over time [5, 6].

10.5.1.1 Relaxation Thyroplasty

This procedure is essentially a modified type III (i.e. IIIB thyroplasty based on the European Laryngological Society classification system [6]) (Fig. 10.5.1). We prefer to perform the procedure under general anaesthesia using a laryngeal mask airway to allow for inspection of the larynx intraoperatively with a digital distal chip on tip flexible nasendoscope with video recording capability.

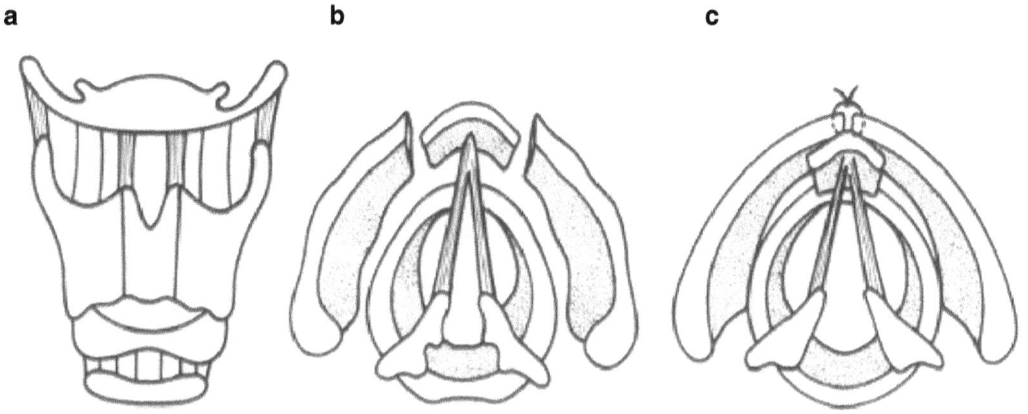

Fig. 10.5.1 (**a**) Paramedian incisions alonf the anterior commissure. (**b**) Relaxation of the anterior commissure into the larynx. (**c**) The relaxation is secured by approximation of the thyroid cartilages alae

Other surgeons however prefer the biofeedback of having the patient phonate while operating under sedation and local anaesthesia.

The salient steps of this procedure as with most anterior neck procedures are to incise the skin in a horizontal neck crease where possible, equidistant from the midline and at the lower border of the thyroid cartilage over the cricothyroid membrane. Skin flaps are raised and exposure of the larynx up to the superior margin of the thyroid cartilage without the need to cut the strap muscles but merely separating them. The thyroid cartilage is cut vertically, 5 mm either side of the midline along the entire length. Important landmarks are the thyroid notch and the inferior rim of the thyroid cartilage. Calcified cartilage may require a fine side-end burr or a sagittal saw. The cuts extend through the outer perichondrium but do not transgress the inner perichondrium. Thereafter, the anterior 1 cm of inner perichondrium is carefully elevated from the posterior cartilage segment with attached Broyle's ligament. This is retrodisplaced into the larynx, and the posterior segments are allowed to override it on either side laterally (Fig. 10.5.2). Endoscopic evaluation of the larynx using the aforementioned video endoscope is performed through an aperture in the LMA's connecting tubes (Fig. 10.5.3). The degree of retrusion is noted, and thereafter, the segments of thyroid cartilage lateral to the anterior segment are secured in position over the middle segment

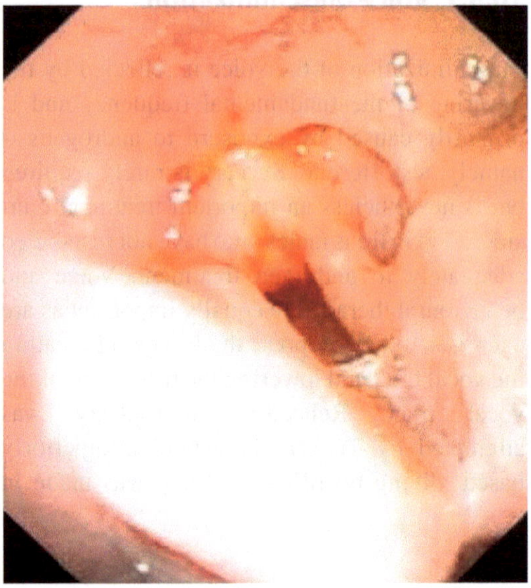

Fig. 10.5.3 Videoscope transoral viewing of the vocal folds after relaxation thyroplasty

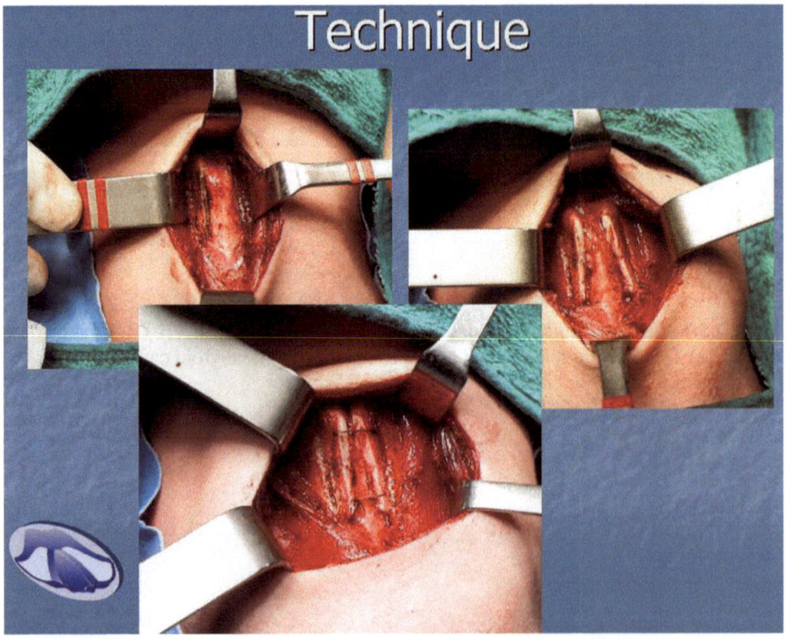

Fig. 10.5.2 Surgical view of relaxation thyroplasty, type III

with a non-absorbable monofilament suture (Nylon 3-0). We do insert a small suction drain and have found the application of fibrin glue over the retrusion helpful in reducing any bleeding/haematoma formation.

Patients are advised a week of low-intensity voicing after discharge and placed on a 5-day course of oral broad-spectrum antibiotics, steroid inhalers and proton-pump inhibitors empirically. Thereafter, patients undergo voice therapy after surgery to optimize the functional results with the new glottic configuration.

We reported a series from 2001 to 2008 on seven male patients who underwent the above-mentioned procedure with a mean age of 21 years after failure of behavioural management. Outcome was assessed based on the change to fundamental frequency, F0 and the VHI. The mean fundamental frequency was lowered from 187 to 104 Hz ($p < 0.001$) while the mean VHI improved from 70 to 21 [7].

10.5.1.2 Other Procedures

A variation of the Tucker procedure by Kocak et al. [8] describes a more stable 'rhomboid'-shaped cartilage window centred around the anterior commissure—the window anterior commissure relaxation laryngoplasty. Injection of hyaluronic acid into the vocal folds to increase their mass has also shown pitch reduction, but long-term results are yet to be published [9].

10.5.1.3 Summary: Voice Masculinization

Voice masculinization is usually performed as an open procedure with the type III thyroplasty being the most popular operation. It is advocated in recalcitrant cases of puberphonia unresponsive to voice and psychological therapy or in inadequately androgen-responsive FtM transgender patients.

10.5.2 References

1. Tucker HM. Anterior commissure laryngoplasty for adjustment of vocal fold tension. Ann Otol Rhinol Laryngol. 1985;94:547–9.
2. Isshiki N. Phonosurgery. Theory and practice. Tokyo, Japan: Springer; 1989.
3. Isshiki N, Taira T, Tanabe M. Surgical treatment for vocal pitch disorders. In: Fujimura O, editors. Vocal physiology: voice productions, mechanisms and functions. New York, NY: Raven Press; 1988. p. 449–58.
4. Remacle M, Matar N, Morsomme D, Veduyckt I, Lawson G. Glottoplasty for male-to-female transsexualism: voice results. J Voice. 2011;25(1):120–3.
5. Mastronikolis NS, Remacle M, Biagini M, Kiagiadaki D, Lawson G. Wendler glottoplasty: an effective pitch raising surgery in male-to-female transsexuals. J Voice. 2013;27(4):516–22.
6. Friedrich G, de Jong FI, Mahieu HF, Benninger MS, Isshiki N. Laryngeal framework surgery: a proposal for classification and nomenclature by the Phonosurgery Committee of the European Laryngological Society. Eur Arch Otorhinolaryngol. 2001;258:389–96.
7. Remacle M, Matar N, Verduyckt I, Lawson G. Relaxation thyroplasty for mutational falsetto treatment. Ann Otol Rhinol Laryngol. 2010;119:105–9.
8. Kocak I, Dogan M, Tadihan E, Alkan Cakir Z, Bengisu S, Akpinar M. Window anterior commissure relaxation laryngoplasty in the management of high-pitched voice disorders. Arch Otolaryngol Head Neck Surg. 2008;134:1263–9.
9. van den Broek EM, Vokes DE, Dorman EB. Bilateral in-office injection laryngoplasty as an adjunctive treatment for recalcitrant puberphonia: a case report and review of the literature. J Voice. 2016;30(2):221–3.

11 Exercise-Induced Laryngeal Obstruction

John-Helge Heimdal, Robert Maat, Magnus Hilland, and Leif Nordang

Key Points

- The larynx normally adapts to increased airflow during activity by abduction of the aryepiglottic and vocal folds.
- Breathing problems may be due to malfunction of this adaptive mechanism in a larynx that is otherwise normal.
- The term exercise-induced laryngeal obstruction is an umbrella term commonly used for this condition (see definition).
- The continuous laryngoscopy exercise (CLE) test is the gold standard for diagnostic measures.
- Reports indicate that EILO is a relatively prevalent entity, affecting adolescents or young adults in all activity levels.
- Different treatments have been described including breathing technique training by speech therapists and individual training programs with use of inspiratory muscle strength training devices.
- Selected cases with severe supraglottic EILO may be treated successfully with supraglottoplasty.
- There still is a need for further evidence regarding selection criteria and effects of different treatment modalities.

J.-H. Heimdal (✉)
Department of Surgery, Haukeland University Hospital, Bergen University, Bergen, Norway

Department of Otorhinolaryngology Head and Neck Surgery, Haukeland University Hospital, Bergen University, Bergen, Norway
e-mail: john.heimdal@helse-bergen.no

R. Maat
Department of Otolaryngology, Saxenburgh Medical Center, Hardenberg, The Netherlands

M. Hilland
Department of Otolaryngology, Haukeland University Hospital, Bergen, Norway

L. Nordang
Department of Surgical Sciences, Otorhinolaryngology and Head & Neck Surgery, Uppsala University, Uppsala, Sweden
e-mail: leif.nordang@akademiska.se

M. Remacle, H. E. Eckel (eds.), *Textbook of Surgery of Larynx and Trachea*,
https://doi.org/10.1007/978-3-031-09621-1_11

11.1 Background

Inducible laryngeal obstruction is a complex condition triggered by a variety of disorders and described with different terms [1]. The terminology used in historical reports on respiratory distress indicates causality by psychogenic factors. Reviews often include reference to Dunglison who in 1844 in a textbook described a disorder as "hysteric croup" [2] and Patterson and co-workers who illustrated attacks with inspiratory wheeze, worsened by infection or emotional distress in a case report entitled "Munchausen stridor" [3].

Often used terms are vocal cord dysfunction (VCD) [4] and paradoxical vocal cord motion (PVCM) [5]. These terms indicate obstruction at the glottic level. An International Task Force presented in 2013, the International Consensus Conference Nomenclature [6], providing definitions and recommendations concerning the term inducible laryngeal obstruction (Ilo). The report introduces exercise as a potential inducer for laryngeal obstruction, hence the term exercise-induced laryngeal obstruction (EILO). This chapter will focus mainly on this type of laryngeal obstruction.

11.1.1 Exercise (E) as Inducer (I) for Laryngeal (L) Obstruction (O) (EILO)

Ventilation increases during exercise, and the larynx quickly adapts to the request for increased airflow (hyperpnea) [7]. The epiglottis tilts forward, and the aryepiglottic folds are elongated and thinned [8]. The area of the glottis enlarges and forms a rhomboid appearance due to the elongation and abduction of the vocal folds. Intrinsic muscles, particularly the posterior crico-arytenoid (PCA) muscles, are involved. Dysfunction of this adaptive process may cause obstruction of the larynx, a phenomenon now recognized as EILO [9]. Obstruction can be demonstrated at the glottic as well as at the supraglottic level and simultaneously at both levels [10].

11.1.2 Symptoms

Dyspnea is the most frequent symptom, and stridor occurs in more than one half of EILO cases. Symptoms normalize quickly after cessation of exercise [11, 12]. This is in contrast to breathlessness due to central airway obstruction, e.g., exercise-induced asthma (EIA). This condition causes elongated and noisy expirium and often peaks at several minutes after the exercise has ceased [13]. EILO is unfortunately often unnoticed and misdiagnosed as EIA. Knowing the clinical features of EILO versus EIA is important in order to differentiate these two conditions. EILO patients typically develop symptoms during intense exercise. Griffin and co-workers have described typical clinical EILO features as follows: difficulties related to "breathing in or filling the lungs," upper chest discomfort, throat tickle or constriction, inspiratory wheeze or stridor, dry cough, and lack of relief with standard asthma therapy [14].

11.1.3 Differential Diagnosis

The most frequent misdiagnosis of EILO is EIA. It is important to note that the two conditions may co-exist [15]. Intra-thoracic pathology is also an important differential diagnosis to laryngeal obstruction if there are normal findings on laryngoscopy during exercise in patients experiencing respiratory distress [10, 16].

11.1.4 Evaluation

Sophisticated methods of video laryngoscopy allow examiners to visualize the larynx in situations where it previously was unreachable for examination [17, 18]. Visualization of laryngeal structures during ongoing exercise is the "gold standard" for diagnosing EILO. Direct observation of the larynx as symptoms develop can clarify causal mechanisms and help develop evidence-based approaches to therapy [19, 20]. Exercise-induced airflow constraint in an otherwise healthy larynx may become visible only at high airflow levels. Since airflow and symptoms decrease rapidly after exercise [21], both pre- and post-exercise laryngeal examinations may not reveal pathology as to laryngeal function during exercise. There is therefore a risk of false negative results from pre- and post-exercise laryngoscopies.

11.1.5 The Continuous Laryngoscopy Exercise (CLE) Test

This test is an integrated set-up combining equipment for laryngoscopy, video, and sound recording (in some laboratories also including an ergospirometry unit) [18] (Fig. 11.1a). A headset or helmet and a facemask can serve to secure the laryngoscope to the head of the test subject to prevent movements of the endoscope and camera while the test subject is performing exercise.

An adrenergic agonist is applied in the nostrils before the test, and the nasal cavity is anaesthetized with lidocaine. An open silicon plug in the facemask enables the physician to advance the endoscope through the nasal cavity and further into the oropharynx. The laryngoscope is placed and fixed in an ideal position just above the larynx. The test is considered successful if the patient can reproduce his or her respiratory complaints. If combined with ergospirometry, the test result should indicate exhaustion, preferably supported by a plateau in oxygen consumption and/or the heart rate response.

The type of exercise used in the laboratory should ideally be comparable to the symptom-triggering activity [17]. This is not always possible due to limitations of the equipment or laboratory facilities. The easiest valid set-up is probably the stationary bicycle as the upper body and head of the test person are relatively motionless during this activity. A treadmill and a headgear for fixation of the endoscope with a camera may be sufficient as well (Fig. 11.1b). Sophisticated cameras and recording features developed during recent years have enabled investigators to perform laryngoscopy in different exercise situations, including swimming and rowing [22, 23].

11.1.6 CLE Test Evaluation

Several methods are available for evaluation for the CLE test, e.g., the EILO grading scale

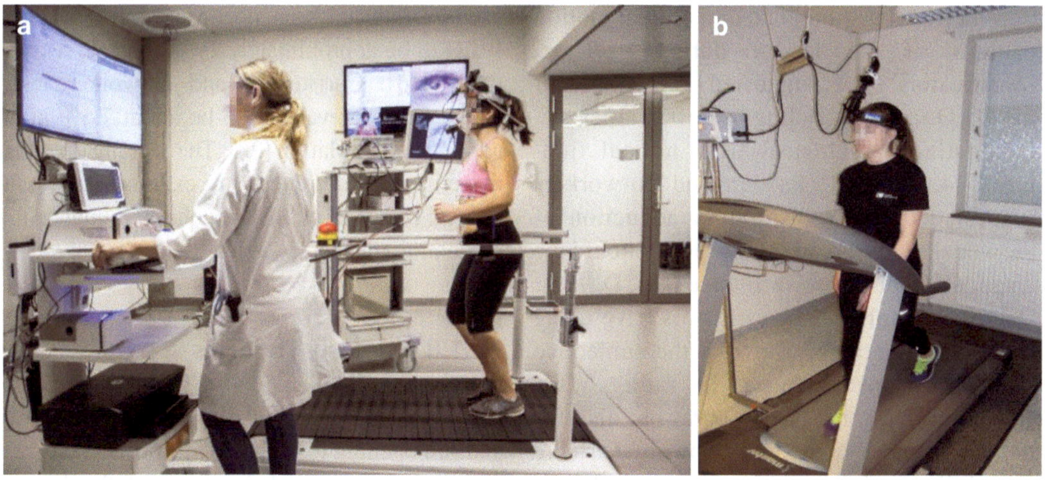

Fig. 11.1 CLE test. (**a**) A flexible laryngoscope fixed in an ideal position to a headgear as shown. A connection to a video camera or use of a video-in-tip endoscope (as shown) makes it possible for the observer to follow the laryngeal motions during the exercise test. In this example, a flow sensor is connected to the facemask in order to perform an ergospirometry (exercise test). (**b**) A more basic equipment sufficient for performing the CLE test on a treadmill

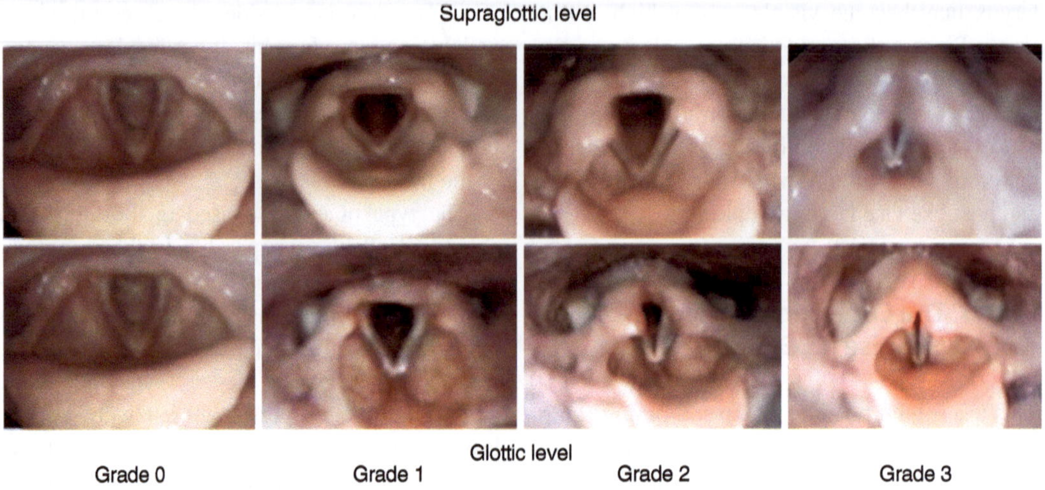

Fig. 11.2 Evaluation of laryngeal obstruction. The evaluation as suggested by Maat and colleagues, estimating the obstruction separately at supraglottic level (motion of the aryepiglottic folds) and glottic level (motion of vocal folds). Grading as shown from 0 to 3 at each level can be performed twice during test and all four scores summed to total score [24]

established by Maat and co-workers [24] and EILOMEA established by Christensen and co-workers [25]. Regardless of the method used, it is helpful for the observers to use predefined scores or schemes when observing the larynx motions during the test (Fig. 11.2). Unfortunately, there is no consensus in literature regarding classification or differentiations between pathological and normal motion patterns of the larynx during exercise. Investigators have suggested guidelines for the EILO scores including "cutoff" values differentiating pathological from normal findings [24, 26]. MC Fadden and co-workers suggested that any inspiratory adduction of the vocal folds greater than 50% should be diagnostic for exercise-induced VCD [16]. One of the problems investigators have using the scales mentioned above is the subjective score decisions included in rating. This applies not only for the observer but also for the test subject or patient showing variable tolerability for laryngeal obstruction [24, 26]. Objective measures of resistance over the larynx during exercise may help sort out questions concerning pathological versus normal motions of the larynx during exercise [27].

11.1.7 Epidemiology

Exercise-induced dyspnea is a problem among the general adolescent population as well as athletes. Both EIA and EILO are causes of exertional dyspnea in these cases. Johansson and co-workers performed a cross-sectional study among adolescents and estimated prevalence of exercise-induced bronchoconstriction (EIB) and EILO to be approximately 19% and 6%, respectively [15]. Christensen and co-workers estimated EILO prevalence to be about 7.5% in an adolescent population [28]. The varying diagnostic criteria, differences in examinations, and referral biases in published cohorts influence the epidemiological data [29].

11.1.8 Etiology Theories

Laryngeal closure for the protection of the airway and full opening to optimize airflow and exercise performance are vital functions of the larynx. These mechanisms are complex, and it is therefore likely that many factors play a role in the different manifestations of EILO. It is possible that etiological factors relate to a diversity of anatomical, aerodynamic, neurological, and psychological mechanisms [29]. Clinical observations of EILO compared with proven medicinal facts and clinical experience with analogous conditions may give an indication as to etiology. For overview purposes, supraglottic and glottic level types are discussed separately in the following although they are anatomically connected and often observed simultaneously.

11.1.8.1 EILO at the Supraglottic Level

The Venturi effect of the Bernoulli principle describes in a simplified model the forces acting upon walls of the larynx. The action of intrinsic muscles, stability of ligaments, and rigidity of cartilage will normally maintain patency of the larynx during the respiratory cycle. Disturbances in the neural control of the aryepiglottic folds have been suggested as a cause for supraglottic prolapse into the laryngeal inlet [30, 31]. Reidenbach suggested that insufficient anchorage could lead to pathological instability of the aryepiglottic folds [32]. Smith and co-workers observed the similarity between supraglottic laryngeal collapse during exercise and laryngomalacia (LM) and termed the condition exercise-induced laryngomalacia (EIL) [33]. The authors discussed in a follow-up study etiological mechanisms for EIL concluding that this may be a subtype of LM involving physiological changes in supraglottic dynamics. They suggested prerequisite conditions as a combination of high airflow, anatomical variants, and/or decreased supraglottic neuromuscular tonus [19]. This implies that athletes during exercise could generate enough inspiratory force to pull the posterior part of the aryepiglottic folds into the larynx [19]. Indeed, reminiscences of LM were found in adolescents who had CLM in childhood, indicating that there is a connection between supraglottic EILO and CLM [34]. Others have suggested that edematous/swollen mucosa of the arytenoids may initiate prolapse of the aryepiglottic folds and/or epiglottic posterior displacement [30, 35, 36].

11.1.8.2 EILO at the Glottic Level

The adaption of the larynx to exercise includes maximal abduction of the vocal folds forming a rhomboid area at the rima glottidis. An inappropriate narrowing, partial, or even total (spastic) closure of the rima glottidis ultimately causes respiratory distress [37, 38]. Observations from CLE tests have revealed that the normal laryngeal adaption to exercise, i.e., abduction of the vocal folds, fails and/or inappropriate adduction of the vocal folds appears in some individuals.

Central nervous system reflexes may play a role; they are important for laryngeal function concerning respiration, swallowing, and the protection of the lower airway. The closure of the glottis is part of the protective laryngeal adductor reflex [39]. Stimulation of sensory nerve endings in the upper or lower respiratory tract may stimulate local reflexes, leading to laryngeal closure [40–43]. A hyper-functional reflex has been suggested as a potential cause for EILO because different triggers like odors, perfumes, gastroesophageal reflux and infections, and exercise-induced stress can initiate this phenomenon [44–47]. Alternatively, alteration of the laryngeal adductor reflex may play a role [37, 48].

Breathing cold air may be an etiological factor. Subjects involved in winter sports such as cross-country skiing, biathlon, and alpine skiing seem to be over-represented. These findings correspond partly to the descriptions given by Rundell and co-workers, reporting that inspiratory stridor was more prevalent in outdoor athletes than in indoor athletes [49].

Psychological conditions or functional disorders as well as neurological diseases can cause paradoxical vocal fold motion. Maschka and co-workers proposed a classification scheme, later modified by Koufman and Block [50, 51]. The scheme separates paradoxical vocal fold motion based on possible etiology, both organic and nonorganic.

Vocal folds are under both autonomic and voluntary control, and therefore suggestion of a functional component is reasonable [52]. Elite athletes may subconsciously convert performance anxiety into laryngeal closure, providing a physiological mechanism for "choking" during sport [16].

Fatigue of abducting muscles of the larynx is also a reasonable explanation when taking into account the forces acting at the abducted vocal folds. The active process of laryngeal unfolding in the inspiratory phase of the respiratory cycle starts from an equilibrium in passive forces at the end of each expiration [53]. Observations from a large number of CLE tests indicate that there are inward directed forces (observed as medial traction) acting especially at the anterior third of the vocal folds. Bent and co-workers hypothesized that well-trained athletes, who could generate high airflow through the larynx for a longer period, were more likely to get EILO [19]. Beaty et al. argued that EILO was related to high inspiratory airflow and that physically active people therefore are more likely to be affected [54]. Breathing patterns that induce high airflow through the larynx correspond well to EILO [55].

11.2 Treatments

There are no published randomized controlled treatment trials on EILO. Many reports are anecdotal and retrospective reviews often based on small sample-sized studies with subjective reported outcome measures [9, 56]. Sparsely defined etiological factors lead to treatment modalities that differ widely. The heterogeneity of findings when investigating EILO patients indicates that phenotypic classification is important in order to provide personalized treatment and increase the success rates [6]. Use of a multidisciplinary team (MDT) approach for treating EILO has been suggested [57]. The management flowchart illustrates that decision-making may be complicated (Fig. 11.3).

The common goal for treatment is to relieve the experience of exercise-induced respiratory symptoms. The CLE test not only provides a diagnostic tool but also represents a therapeutic device. Looking at the video recording after the test and having the mechanisms of laryngeal obstruction explained are helpful and reassuring for many EILO patients with a mild or moderate

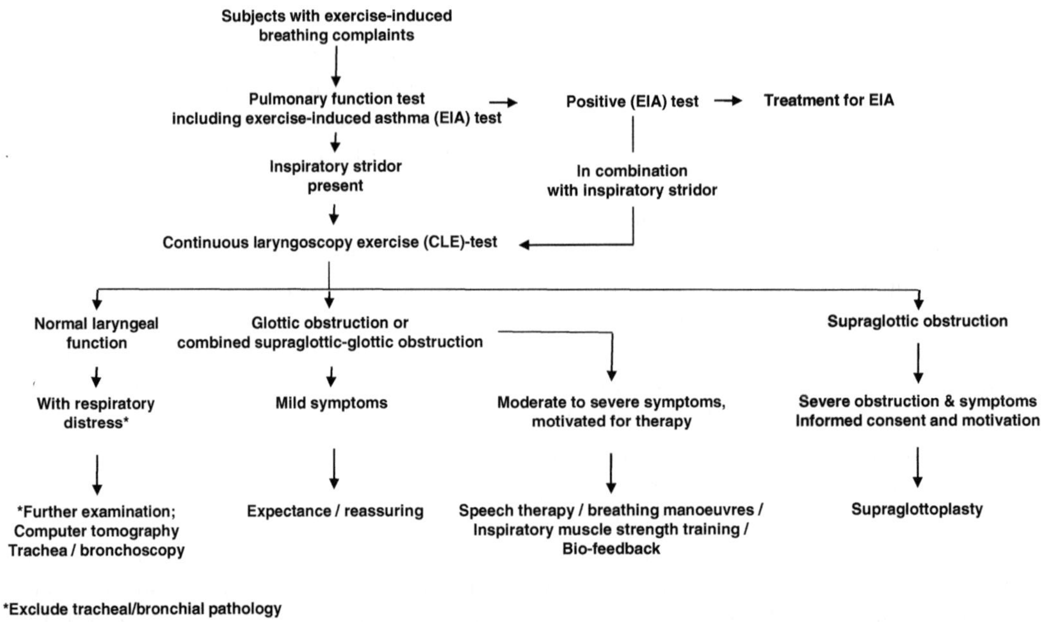

Fig. 11.3 Process of evaluation. The flowchart shows a suggested process of evaluation, decision-making, and treatment for EILO patients

condition [58]. Biofeedback techniques may be useful in this aspect [59]. It is also important to identify the problem as EILO and not asthma in patients who otherwise are treated inappropriately with anti-asthmatic drugs [55].

Treatment for gastroesophageal reflux has been reported to be efficacious by some authors [60] but not by others [61].

Psychological mechanisms may have an etiological role in EILO. Psychotherapy certainly plays a role in the management of the condition, although further investigations are advocated [62].

Speech language intervention for EILO can be a course of guided therapy tailored to the patient, including specific breathing techniques that optimize laryngeal relaxation and efficient breathing [63].

Inspiratory muscle strength training (IMST) may be an efficient treatment for EILO patients. This assumption depends on the theory that laryngeal muscles are strengthened and the laryngeal aperture is increased during inspiratory phase by using IMST. Sandnes and co-workers reported an effect in 22 of 28 athletes in a recent study. The effect was especially evident in the glottic subtype of EILO [64]. The authors advocated that further controlled studies are required in order to establish IMST as an effective treatment for glottic EILO.

11.2.1 Surgical Treatment

Smith and co-workers published a paper in 1995 describing supraglottoplasty as a treatment for patients with EIL. Removal of the corniculate cartilages by laser resulted in improvement in aerobic endurance as measured by physical fitness testing [33]. Bent and co-workers in their paper in 1996 reported beneficial effects of supraglottoplasty in two patients. The procedures are comparable to those used in children with CLM. Maat and co-workers later established this treatment for patients with severe supraglottic EILO who were strongly motivated for surgery [65]. The surgical method used by Maat and co-workers includes an incision in the aryepiglottic folds bilaterally close to the rim of the epiglottis and a circle-shaped mucosal incision at the top of the cuneiform tubercle, thereby removing redundant mucosa (see detailed procedure description) (Fig. 11.4).

The aim of the surgical procedures for EILO is to reduce the risk of supraglottic collapse and to improve the air passage through the larynx. The principles are to increase the diameter of the laryngeal inlet and reduce the adduction ability of the aryepiglottic folds, furthermore to make the edges of the plicas less flexible or flaccid, and if required to reduce the length of the epiglottis and rotate it anteriorly toward the tongue base.

Results from the early studies on supraglottoplasty for EILO were encouraging, and surgical treatment for supraglottic EILO was therefore established. Follow-up studies have later shown that the treatment has a long-lasting effect [58, 64]. In recent years, more ENT surgeons and research groups have gained experience with surgical treatment for EILO [66–70].

A pre-operative CLE test is mandatory before each surgical procedure to reveal the supraglottic collapse. It also enables the surgeon to adjust the procedure exclusively for each patient.

The supraglottoplasty is performed under general anesthesia by suspension laryngoscopy [65]. The laryngoscope is introduced and suspended in a position that exposes the aryepiglottic folds or epiglottis. The operating microscope enhances the operating field and enables the surgeon to perform an accurate procedure. Technically, the operation can be performed by using either scissors or laser (for more details, see below).

11.2.2 Detailed Description of the Procedure

See Fig. 11.4:

1. Introduce a Lindholm/Benjamin laryngoscope into the vallecula and lift anteriorly making sure you are exposing both aryepiglottic folds and the epiglottis. It may be easier to visualize one side at the time. Start laser/micro spot and adjust to required energy (normally, 2–4 W). Care is taken to avoid scarring. It is recommended to protect the posterior

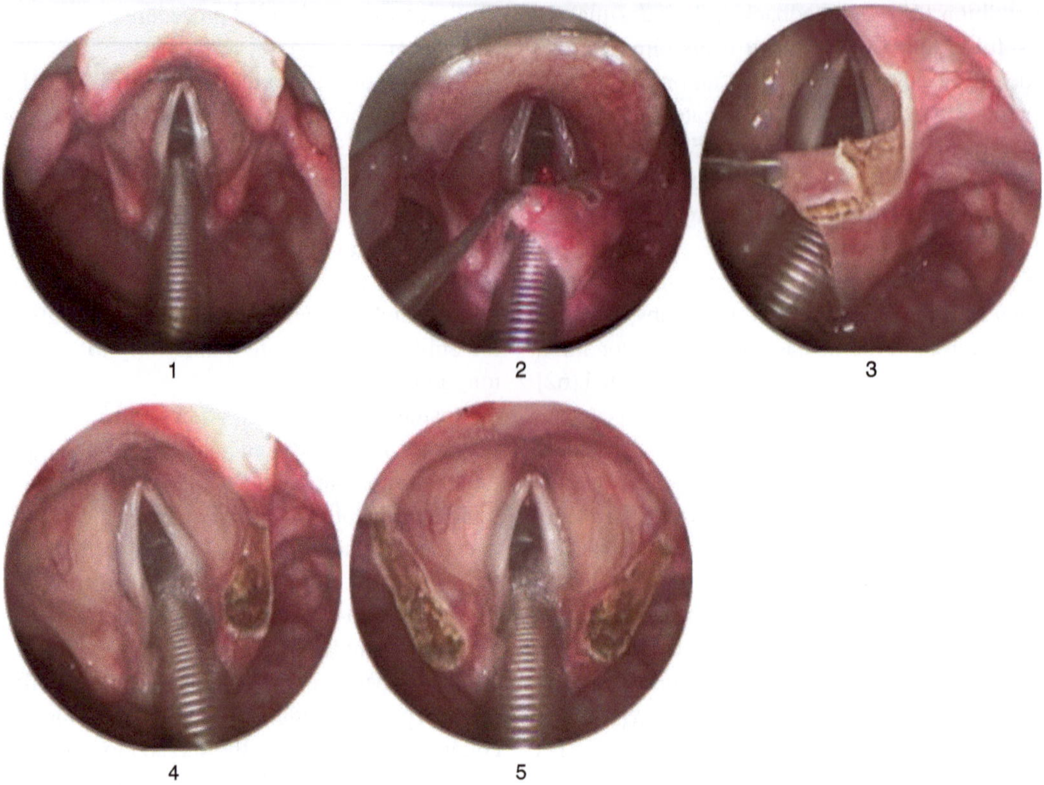

Fig. 11.4 Laryngoplasty. The different steps in a laryngoplasty operation. For more details and description, see text

commissure and the piriform sinus with wet tissue cloths, before applying the laser.

2. Grasp the aryepiglottic fold at the cuneiform tubercle with micro laryngeal forceps and pull slightly forward and medially stretching the aryepiglottic fold, revealing the amount of abundant tissue and the location of the cuneiform tubercle in the tissue.
3. The aryepiglottic fold is split anteriorly downward (tiny fibers of musculus aryepiglotticus can sometimes be observed) approaching the cranial margin of plica ventricularis. Next, tissue around the top of the cuneiform cartilage is removed in a circular pattern, creating a triangular-shaped excision. In cases where the cuneiform tubercles are pointy and exposed in the excision, presenting parts of this cartilage may be included.
4. Perform the same procedure on both sides.

Note: Reduction of excessive tissue on the aryepiglottic folds, fixation of the epiglottis, or reduction of its size may be included in the operative procedure. In cases of peri-operative edema of the laryngeal mucosa, corticosteroids are administrated to prevent laryngeal edema postoperatively. Normally, no antibiotic prophylaxis is required.

11.2.3 Effect of Surgical Treatment

Recent reports show that surgery generally has positive effects on symptoms caused by supraglottic EILO. Comparisons of pre- and postoperative CLE tests reveal the effect of surgery in several reports (Table 11.1). Siewers and coworkers performed a systematic literature review and found 11 published studies on the surgical treatment of EILO, including 75 patients all together. The authors concluded that the procedure is safe and indicates a favorable clinical response, but the heterogeneity of study methodologies and level of evidence preclude definitive recommendations for or against supraglottoplasty. The authors therefore recommend prospective

Table 11.1 Overview laryngoplasty reports. Reports on surgical treatment of exercise-induced laryngeal obstruction

Authors	Year	Number of patients	Examination
Smith et al.	1995	1	Exercise and laryngoscopy
Bent et al.	1996	2	Exercise and laryngoscopy
Björnsdottir et al.	2000	2	Exercise and laryngoscopy
Chemery et al.	2002	1	Exercise simultaneous laryngoscopy
Mandell et al.	2003	1	Laryngoscopy and spirometry
Richter et al.	2008	3	Exercise laryngoscopy
McNally et al.	2010	1	Exercise simultaneous laryngoscopy
Maat et al.	2011	23	
Dion et al.	2015	1	Exercise simultaneous laryngoscopy
Hilland et al.	2013	3	Exercise simultaneous laryngoscopy
Orbelo et al.	2014	1	
Norlander et al.	2015	14	Exercise simultaneous laryngoscopy
Mehlum et al.	2016	17	Exercise simultaneous laryngoscopy
Sandnes et al.	2019	45	Exercise simultaneous laryngoscopy
Famokunwa et al.	2020	19	Exercise simultaneous laryngoscopy
Total number of operated patients		134	

Based on previous published reports including systematic search identifying studies describing surgical treatment of EILO patients (for more details, see text and reference list)

and more methodological robust studies in order to sort this out [71]. After this review, Sandnes and co-workers reported a study on 45 surgically treated patients with EILO of whom 38 reported less symptoms post-operatively, while CLE scores decreased in all. Notably, 21/45 (47%) also improved at the glottic level [64]. Furthermore, Famokunwa and co-workers reported on 19 cases with positive outcome [68]. Based on experience from more than 120 reported patients treated with supraglottoplasty for EILO, it is reasonable to conclude that the procedure is safe with effects lasting for several years. Patients who are treated surgically seem to continue their physical activity longer than untreated patients do. This can be due to a selection bias for surgery in patients with strong motivation for athletic activity.

Still, being a new treatment, little is known about potential long-term complications like aspiration in late adulthood. Surgery is not successful in all cases, and some patients experience post-operative discomfort and lack of efficacy. Authors therefore emphasize that surgery should be recommended only in strictly selected cases [58, 67]. The number of published procedures so far is limited, and it is therefore not possible to give an estimate as to surgical risk. The authors of this chapter emphasize the importance of documenting potential side effects to surgery in order to find reliable estimations of complications.

It is recommended that every patient is carefully evaluated with exercise-induced asthma (EIA) test as well as a CLE test if supraglottoplasty is being considered as a treatment option [58]. The symptoms should be severe, the supraglottic EILO should be significant, and finally the patient should be motivated for surgery after information of potential effects and risk factors. Surgery aims at correcting severe supraglottic collapse; if obstruction is observed at the glottic level, there is a risk that the surgical procedure is ineffective; and surgery should be deprecated.

11.3 Important Results

EILO is an important differential diagnosis to EIA [21].

Larynx obstruction occurs at the glottic as well as at the supraglottic and simultaneously at both laryngeal levels in EILO patients [10].

Dyspnea is the most frequent symptom of EILO, and it normalizes quickly after exercise has stopped [11].

The prevalence of EILO among adolescents is approximately 6% [15].

The continuous laryngoscopy exercise (CLE) test is the gold standard for EILO evaluation [17].

Diversity in test situations, subjective observer decisions included in EILO grading schemes, and variable tolerability for EILO in patients can affect diagnostic decisions [66].

Supraglottoplasty is effective in severe cases of supraglottic subtype of EILO [66, 70].

11.4 Definition

The 2013 international consensus conference on nomenclature defined inducible laryngeal obstructions causing breathing problems and suggested an umbrella term inducible laryngeal obstructions (Ilo). According to this consensus, predefined descriptive terms should include inducer(s)[1] of the single attack and sub-categories[2] based on laryngoscopic findings:

Take-Home Messages
- EILO is relatively common among young athletes.
- Typical symptoms are respiratory distress, noise on inspiration, or stridor.
- Although EILO symptoms are different to those of EIA, the conditions are often not distinguished.
- The diagnostic procedure is important in order to observe the laryngeal function during exercise.
- Classification of the condition made from endoscopy findings is the basis for treatment decisions:
  - Severe supraglottic EILO can be treated effectively by surgery in selected cases.
  - Glottic type of EILO can be treated by different methods, e.g., inspiratory muscle strength training or respiratory maneuvers guided by a speech therapist.

[1] If the inducer is exercise, the suggested term is exercise-induced laryngeal obstruction (EILO).

[2] The circumstances for the diagnostic laryngoscopy should be described and findings reported in detail for sub-categorization, e.g., laryngeal level of obstruction (supraglottic, glottic, or a combination of both).

References

1. Olin JT, et al. Inducible laryngeal obstruction during exercise: moving beyond vocal cords with new insights. Phys Sportsmed. 2015;43(1):13–21.
2. Dunglison R. The practice of medicine a treatise on special pathology and therapeutics, vol. 2. Philadelphia: Lea & Blanchard; 1844.
3. Patterson R, Schatz M, Horton M. Munchausen's stridor: non-organic laryngeal obstruction. Clin Allergy. 1974;4(3):307–10.
4. Christopher KL, et al. Vocal-cord dysfunction presenting as asthma. N Engl J Med. 1983;308(26):1566–70.
5. Kellman RM, Leopold DA. Paradoxical vocal cord motion: an important cause of stridor. Laryngoscope. 1982;92(1):58–60.
6. Christensen PM, et al. ERS/ELS/ACCP 2013 international consensus conference nomenclature on inducible laryngeal obstructions. Eur Respir Rev. 2015;24(137):445–50.
7. England SJ, Bartlett D Jr. Changes in respiratory movements of the human vocal cords during hyperpnea. J Appl Physiol Respir Environ Exerc Physiol. 1982;52(3):780–5.
8. Belmont JR, Grundfast K. Congenital laryngeal stridor (laryngomalacia): etiologic factors and associated disorders. Ann Otol Rhinol Laryngol. 1984;93(5 Pt 1):430–7.
9. Liyanagedera S, McLeod R, Elhassan HA. Exercise induced laryngeal obstruction: a review of diagnosis and management. Eur Arch Otorhinolaryngol. 2017;274(4):1781–9.
10. Røksund OD, et al. Larynx during exercise: the unexplored bottleneck of the airways. Eur Arch Otorhinolaryngol. 2015;272(9):2101–9.
11. Morris MJ, Christopher KL. Diagnostic criteria for the classification of vocal cord dysfunction. Chest. 2010;138(5):1213–23.
12. Shembel AC, et al. Perceptual clinical features in exercise-induced laryngeal obstruction (EILO): toward improved diagnostic approaches. J Voice. 2019;33(6):880–93.
13. Anderson SD, et al. Exercise-induced asthma. Br J Dis Chest. 1975;69(1):1–39.
14. Griffin SA, Walsted ES, Hull JH. Infographic. The breathless athlete: EILO. Br J Sports Med. 2019;53(10):616–7.
15. Johansson H, et al. Prevalence of exercise-induced bronchoconstriction and exercise-induced laryngeal obstruction in a general adolescent population. Thorax. 2015;70(1):57–63.
16. McFadden ER Jr, Zawadski DK. Vocal cord dysfunction masquerading as exercise-induced asthma. A physiologic cause for "choking" during athletic activities. Am J Respir Crit Care Med. 1996;153(3):942–7.
17. Hull JH, et al. Feasibility of portable continuous laryngoscopy during exercise testing. ERJ Open Res. 2019;5(1):00219–2018.

18. Heimdal JH, et al. Continuous laryngoscopy exercise test: a method for visualizing laryngeal dysfunction during exercise. Laryngoscope. 2006;116(1):52–7.
19. Bent JP III, et al. Pediatric exercise-induced laryngomalacia. Ann Otol Rhinol Laryngol. 1996;105(3):169–75.
20. Weinberger M, Abu-Hasan M. Pseudo-asthma: when cough, wheezing, and dyspnea are not asthma. Pediatrics. 2007;120(4):855–64.
21. McArdle WD, Katch FI, Katch VL. Exercise physiology. Philadelphia: Lippincott Williams & Wilkins; 1995. p. 217–32.
22. Panchasara B, et al. Lesson of the month: rowing-induced laryngeal obstruction: a novel cause of exertional dyspnoea: characterised by direct laryngoscopy. Thorax. 2015;70(1):95–7.
23. Walsted ES, et al. Laryngoscopy during swimming: a novel diagnostic technique to characterize swimming-induced laryngeal obstruction. Laryngoscope. 2017;127(10):2298–301.
24. Maat RC, et al. Audiovisual assessment of exercise-induced laryngeal obstruction: reliability and validity of observations. Eur Arch Otorhinolaryngol. 2009;266(12):1929–36.
25. Christensen P, et al. Exercise-induced laryngeal obstructions objectively assessed using EILOMEA. Eur Arch Otorhinolaryngol. 2010;267(3):401–7.
26. Norlander K, et al. Differences in laryngeal movements during exercise in healthy and dyspnoeic adolescents. Int J Pediatr Otorhinolaryngol. 2020;129:109765.
27. Fretheim-Kelly Z, et al. Feasibility and tolerability of measuring translaryngeal pressure during exercise. Laryngoscope. 2019;129(12):2748–53.
28. Christensen PM, et al. Exercise-induced laryngeal obstructions: prevalence and symptoms in the general public. Eur Arch Otorhinolaryngol. 2011;268(9):1313–9.
29. Halvorsen T, et al. Inducible laryngeal obstruction: an official joint European Respiratory Society and European Laryngological Society statement. Eur Respir J. 2017;50(3):1602221.
30. Nonomura N, et al. Acquired airway obstruction caused by hypertrophic mucosa of the arytenoids and aryepiglottic folds. Am J Otolaryngol. 1996;17(1):71–4.
31. Logemann JA, et al. Closure mechanisms of laryngeal vestibule during swallow. Am J Physiol. 1992;262(2 Pt 1):G338–44.
32. Reidenbach MM. Aryepiglottic fold: normal topography and clinical implications. Clin Anat. 1998;11(4):223–35.
33. Smith RJ, et al. Exercise-induced laryngomalacia. Ann Otol Rhinol Laryngol. 1995;104(7):537–41.
34. Hilland M, et al. Congenital laryngomalacia is related to exercise-induced laryngeal obstruction in adolescence. Arch Dis Child. 2016;101(5):443–8.
35. Arora R, Gal TJ, Hagan LL. An unusual case of laryngomalacia presenting as asthma refractory to therapy. Ann Allergy Asthma Immunol. 2005;95(6):607–11.
36. Peron DL, Graffino DB, Zenker DO. The redundant aryepiglottic fold: report of a new cause of stridor. Laryngoscope. 1988;98(6 Pt 1):659–63.
37. Ayres JG, Gabbott PL. Vocal cord dysfunction and laryngeal hyperresponsiveness: a function of altered autonomic balance? Thorax. 2002;57(4): 284–5.
38. Shiba K, Isono S, Nakazawa K. Paradoxical vocal cord motion: a review focused on multiple system atrophy. Auris Nasus Larynx. 2007;34(4): 443–52.
39. Petcu LG, Sasaki CT. Laryngeal anatomy and physiology. Clin Chest Med. 1991;12(3):415–23.
40. Perkner JJ, et al. Irritant-associated vocal cord dysfunction. J Occup Environ Med. 1998;40(2): 136–43.
41. Thompson DM. Abnormal sensorimotor integrative function of the larynx in congenital laryngomalacia: a new theory of etiology. Laryngoscope. 2007;117(6 Pt 2 Suppl 114):1–33.
42. Sinclair CF, Téllez MJ, Ulkatan S. Human laryngeal sensory receptor mapping illuminates the mechanisms of laryngeal adductor reflex control. Laryngoscope. 2018;128(11):E365–e370.
43. Strohl KP, Butler JP, Malhotra A. Mechanical properties of the upper airway. Compr Physiol. 2012;2(3):1853–72.
44. Gimenez LM, Zafra H. Vocal cord dysfunction: an update. Ann Allergy Asthma Immunol. 2011;106(4):267–74; quiz 275.
45. Taramarcaz P, et al. Transient postviral vocal cord dysfunction. J Allergy Clin Immunol. 2004;114(6):1471–2.
46. Kenn K, Balkissoon R. Vocal cord dysfunction: what do we know? Eur Respir J. 2011;37(1):194–200.
47. Ibrahim WH, et al. Paradoxical vocal cord motion disorder: past, present and future. Postgrad Med J. 2007;83(977):164–72.
48. Andreatta RD, et al. Mucosal afferents mediate laryngeal adductor responses in the cat. J Appl Physiol (1985). 2002;93(5):1622–9.
49. Rundell KW, Spiering BA. Inspiratory stridor in elite athletes. Chest. 2003;123(2):468–74.
50. Koufman JA, Block C. Differential diagnosis of paradoxical vocal fold movement. Am J Speech Lang Pathol. 2008;17(4):327–34.
51. Maschka DA, et al. A classification scheme for paradoxical vocal cord motion. Laryngoscope. 1997;107(11 Pt 1):1429–35.
52. McFadden ER Jr. Glottic function and dysfunction. J Allergy Clin Immunol. 1987;79(5):707–10.
53. Fink BR. Folding mechanism of the human larynx. Acta Otolaryngol. 1974;78(1–2):124–8.
54. Beaty MM, Wilson JS, Smith RJ. Laryngeal motion during exercise. Laryngoscope. 1999;109(1):136–9.
55. Røksund OD, et al. Exercise induced dyspnea in the young. Larynx as the bottleneck of the airways. Respir Med. 2009;103(12):1911–8.
56. Haines J, Hull JH, Fowler SJ. Clinical presentation, assessment, and management of inducible laryngeal

obstruction. Curr Opin Otolaryngol Head Neck Surg. 2018;26(3):174–9.
57. Hull JH. Multidisciplinary team working for vocal cord dysfunction: now it's GO time. Respirology. 2019;24(8):714–5.
58. Maat RC, et al. Exercise-induced laryngeal obstruction: natural history and effect of surgical treatment. Eur Arch Otorhinolaryngol. 2011;268(10):1485–92.
59. Olin JT, et al. Therapeutic laryngoscopy during exercise: a novel non-surgical therapy for refractory EILO. Pediatr Pulmonol. 2017;52(6):813–9.
60. Boris M, Goldblatt A, Krigsman A. Laryngeal dysfunction: a common cause of respiratory distress, often misdiagnosed as asthma and responsive to antireflux therapy. Allergy Asthma Proc. 2002;23(2):133–9.
61. Woolnough K, et al. Acid suppression does not reduce symptoms from vocal cord dysfunction, where gastrolaryngeal reflux is a known trigger. Respirology. 2013;18(3):553–4.
62. Guglani L, et al. A systematic review of psychological interventions for adult and pediatric patients with vocal cord dysfunction. Front Pediatr. 2014;2:82.
63. Shaffer M, et al. Speech-language pathology as a primary treatment for exercise-induced laryngeal obstruction. Immunol Allergy Clin N Am. 2018;38(2):293–302.
64. Sandnes A, et al. Exercise-induced laryngeal obstruction in athletes treated with inspiratory muscle training. BMJ Open Sport Exerc Med. 2019;5(1):e000436.
65. Maat RC, et al. Surgical treatment of exercise-induced laryngeal dysfunction. Eur Arch Otorhinolaryngol. 2007;264(4):401–7.
66. Norlander K, et al. Surgical treatment is effective in severe cases of exercise-induced laryngeal obstruction: a follow-up study. Acta Otolaryngol. 2015;135(11):1152–9.
67. Mehlum CS, et al. Supraglottoplasty as treatment of exercise induced laryngeal obstruction (EILO). Eur Arch Otorhinolaryngol. 2016;273(4):945–51.
68. Famokunwa B, Sandhu G, Hull JH. Surgical intervention for exercise-induced laryngeal obstruction: a UK perspective. Laryngoscope. 2020;130:E667–73.
69. Sidell DR, et al. Pediatric exercise stress laryngoscopy following laryngotracheoplasty: a comparative review. Otolaryngol Head Neck Surg. 2014;150(6):1056–61.
70. Heimdal JH, Maat R, Nordang L. Surgical intervention for exercise-induced laryngeal obstruction. Immunol Allergy Clin N Am. 2018;38(2):317–24.
71. Siewers K, Backer V, Walsted ES. A systematic review of surgical treatment for supraglottic exercise-induced laryngeal obstruction. Laryngoscope Investig Otolaryngol. 2019;4(2):227–33.

Office-Based Procedures 12

Markus M. Hess and Susanne Fleischer

Key Points

- Office-based diagnostic examinations and interventions lower risks for patients, decrease costs, and improve comfort and convenience in manifold cases where highest precision like in microlaryngoscopy is not mandatory.
- Injections, biopsies, and laser procedures become more frequent as the latest endoscopes provide high-resolution imaging and further information from spectral imaging features.
- Trans*nasal* flexible surgery is taking over trans*oral* approaches, although transoral interventions still play an important role in office-based interventions.
- Unsedated transnasal esophagoscopy (TNE) and transnasal tracheoscopy (TNT) extend the endoscopic spectrum for diagnosis and treatment.

12.1 Introduction

Indirect laryngeal interventions are known since far more than 130 years. However, there is a renaissance of indirect, office-based interventions noticeable in the last time [1–20]. Within the last 10 years, office-based procedures have boomed worldwide. There are many reasons for this development. Imaging has improved with new camera systems like chip-on-tip technology, and refined image resolution with high-definition (HD) cameras is available. Flexible endoscopes are nowadays thinner, enabling easy nasal passage without too much of a limitation in image quality.

Many patients appreciate rapid interventions using topical anesthesia, which also is encouraging for laryngologists when surgery can be performed in shorter time, including faster patient-to-patient turnover time. For voice surgery, it cannot be stressed enough how advantageous the immediate testing of voice outcome in the awake patient is. Furthermore, it should not be forgotten that general anesthesia-related safety concerns can be bypassed with topical anesthesia. Health insurance companies indirectly encourage laryngologists by monetary incentives to avoid general anesthesia surgery and to use more office-based interventions within ambulatory settings.

The aim of this chapter is to briefly sketch the spectrum of office-based procedures, keeping in

M. M. Hess (✉) · S. Fleischer
Medical Voice Center, Hamburg, Germany
e-mail: hess@mevoc.de; fleischer@mevoc.de
http://www.mevoc.de

M. Remacle, H. E. Eckel (eds.), *Textbook of Surgery of Larynx and Trachea*,
https://doi.org/10.1007/978-3-031-09621-1_12

mind that only a few procedures can be covered in more detail. It should be mentioned at this point that all statements made in this chapter represent the authors' opinion and are based on 25 years' experience in performing indirect surgery at various clinics.

12.2 Possible Interventions in Office-Based Phonosurgery

Laryngeal procedures through suspension microlaryngoscopic techniques are referred to as "direct" techniques. "Direct" indicates that the optical axis of the microscope is in a direct line when visualizing the larynx. Thus, the term "indirect" refers to all other ways of imaging of the larynx (mirrors, angled rigid endoscopes, flexible endoscopes with glass fibers, or chip-on-tip cameras). In a generalized sense, "indirect" is also taken as a synonym for office-based or in-office procedures.

12.2.1 Biopsy/Excision

The classic indirect intervention in laryngology is taking a biopsy from an endolaryngeal site via transoral access. The "workhorse" instrument for this is the cupped forceps, which is turned to one side (left/right or rotatable). When more than a biopsy is taken and a lesion is removed completely, the surgery is called excision. With good surgical skills, excisions, for instance, of nodules and polyps are doable in indirect transoral techniques. The abovementioned procedures can also be performed with instruments passed through the channel of a flexible, transnasally routed endoscope, although this approach is different in using smaller instruments (a disadvantage), but accessibility might be easier (an advantage).

Dissections are not a domain of indirect phonosurgery, since most indirect office-based interventions are one-handed instrument procedures, making dissections almost impossible within this setting.

12.2.2 Injection

Injections are mostly used for intramuscular application of botulinum toxin, subepithelial steroid injection, hydrodissection of Reinke's space, intralesional infiltration of cidofovir or bevacizumab in papilloma, etc. Injections can be performed through transoral, transnasal, and percutaneous approaches.

12.2.3 Augmentation

A rapidly emerging field is the injection augmentation with fillers for vocal fold medialization (syn. "injection laryngoplasty"). Different ways to insert the cannula can be chosen: (a) transorally, (b) transnasally, or (c) percutaneously via a transcartilaginous, cricothyroid, or thyrohyoid approach. No matter which approach is chosen for positioning the cannula tip into the vocal fold, it is a straightforward procedure making augmentation an immediately rewarding intervention. Explanation of injection laryngoplasty and associated issues cannot be presented comprehensively in this chapter.

12.2.4 Laser

Laser treatment within office-based surgery requires a set of prerequisites and additionally specific safety conditions. Nowadays, we essentially have two different laser techniques which take advantage of different tissue energy absorption properties.

First, tissue coagulation, carbonization, vaporization, and ablation, i.e., many kinds of tissue destruction, are possible with all fiber-guided lasers (e.g., CO_2-, diode-, thulium-, and neodym-YAG lasers). With the introduction of hollow fibers as beam delivery system, the use of CO_2 lasers may make this kind of office-based intervention even more feasible, since CO_2 lasers are available at almost all ENT clinics worldwide.

Second, photoangiolytic lasers like pulse dye laser (PDL) and kalium-titanyl-phosphate (KTP) laser as well as the newer-generation blue laser (BL) are more and more popular for local therapy of selected laryngeal lesions. Papilloma, Reinke's edema, polyps, contact granuloma, ectatic vessels, leukoplakia, dysplasia, and other lesions with a red or brown chromophore are a domain of these selective "photoangiolytic" lasers. In some cases, these photoangiolytic lasers are the first choice of treatment. Laser surgery can be performed through transoral, transnasal, and percutaneous approaches.

12.2.5 Arytenoid Mobility Test

Office-based assessment of arytenoid mobility is a very helpful diagnostic transoral procedure to exclude arytenoid dislocation, (sub)luxation, or fixation. With topical anesthesia and use of a transorally routed blunt cotton-coated probe, arytenoid mobility testing is a rapid, safe, and easy method for the differential diagnosis of arytenoid immobility. From our experience, passive mobility could be proven in almost all cases of endoscopically visualized arytenoid immobility—showing us that arytenoid (sub)luxation and joint fixation could be ruled out in the vast majority of cases and suggesting that recurrent nerve paresis and paralysis were most likely.

12.2.6 EMG

Laryngeal electromyography (LEMG) is a classic office-based procedure. However, LEMG is still an underestimated diagnostic method for laryngeal examination. Electrophysiologic examination of selected laryngeal muscles with precise needle positioning in awake patients is an indispensable diagnostic tool to assess neuromuscular laryngeal function. Trained skills for the exact placement of EMG needles and routine analysis of biosignals are mandatory for meaningful neuromuscular function testing. We recommend that it should become a routine method in all professional voice centers. LEMG needle positioning, for example, for botulinum toxin injections, may be combined with other endoscopic procedures such as transnasal percutaneous injections. LEMG can be performed through transoral and percutaneous approaches.

12.2.7 Varia

Within this chapter, we can only mention other surgery-related fields of laryngology like stroboscopy, videokymography, high-speed imaging, narrow-band imaging (NBI) illumination, transnasal tracheoscopy (TNT), transnasal esophagoscopy (TNE), etc. These techniques and procedures are of great importance and certainly play an important role in a laryngology department, where outpatient comprehensive assessment and office-based therapy are offered. The reader is kindly referred to the great body of literature for more information on these topics.

12.3 Setting

In awake patient surgery, the appropriate setting is of crucial importance. Since the patient knows that "an operation" is performed, anxiety, discomfort, and nervousness are quite frequent. Confidence and trust are essential, and reassurance must be mediated by all staff members, resulting in a high level of patient compliance and finally making the operation successful. The patient should feel well cared for at all steps of the operation (Fig. 12.1).

12.3.1 Corona Virus and Protective Measures

The 2020 corona virus pandemic has changed a lot in terms of protective measures and equipment. Aerosol-generating procedures (AGPs),

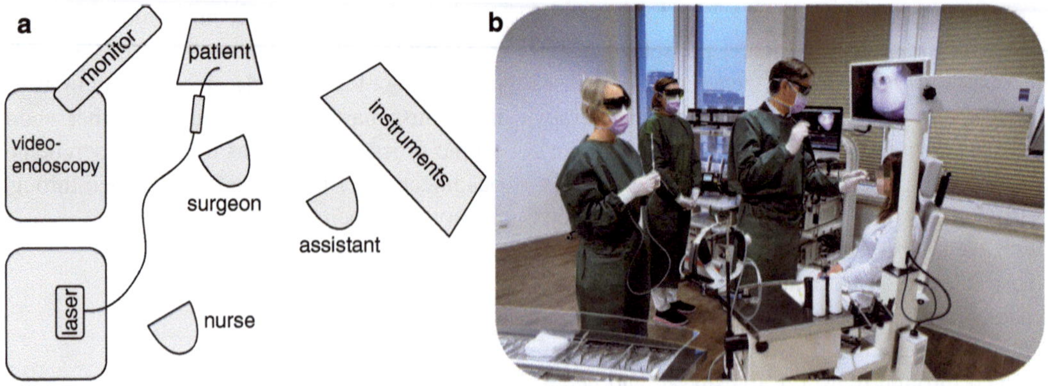

Fig. 12.1 (**a**) Sketch of examination room. (**b**) Examination room with enough space for the patient, examiner, assistant, and nurse. Endoscope equipment and ENT instruments within reach of the surgeon and assistant. Light is dimmable. Monitor position permits the surgeon to observe the patient and view the screen. Assistant supports with anesthesia, instruments, and suctioning

which include rigid laryngoscopies, but much more transnasal flexible endoscopies, are highly likely aerosol generating and increase the risks of infection for surgical staff. Furthermore, laser surgery of the larynx is definitely producing more aerosols when tissues are evaporated. Vegetative reactions such as coughing, throat clearing, as well as sneezing are accompanied with in-office procedures producing droplets and aerosols. Thus, they can jeopardize the surgeon when standing directly in front of the patient. Powered air purifying respirator (PAPR) usage or at least FFP2/3 (or N95) masks, gowns, and gloves are mandatory in potentially infectious patients. Adequate room ventilation is key to avoid infections due to increased room air aerosol concentration. In sum, surgeons and medical staff need to protect themselves with adequate personal protective equipment (PPE) according to regulations (Figs. 12.2 and 12.3).

12.3.2 Patient Position

For transoral operations, the patient is sitting in front of the surgeon. Patients are asked to hold their tongue with a gauze square. In transnasal and percutaneous operations, patients can sit, lean back in an angled position, or lie supine on the back.

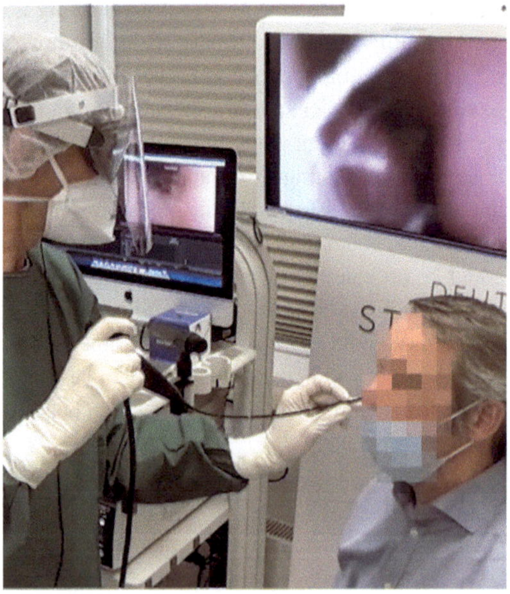

Fig. 12.2 Adequate personal protective equipment (PPE) according to regulations. Room ventilation is mandatory in potentially infectious patients in times of corona pandemic. Here, usage of FFP2/3 (or N95) masks, gowns, and gloves for laryngoscopy is shown

12.3.3 One Surgeon or Two Surgeons?

Transoral surgery mostly means that there is one surgeon holding the endoscope with one hand and keeping the other hand for interventions.

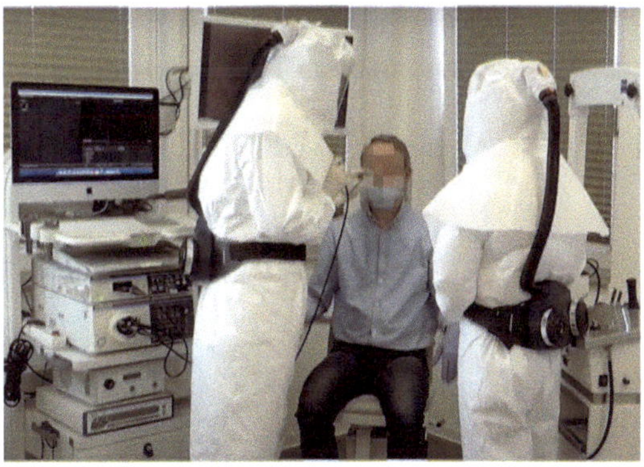

Fig. 12.3 Powered air purifying respirator (PAPR) usage for increased aerosol-producing office-based procedures such as transnasal laser operation

Transoral surgery is prototypical for one surgeon using one instrument. Transnasal and percutaneous operations mostly need two persons (surgeon and assistant). In these cases, the patient may be sitting or lying in an angled position or on a plinth in supine position, with one person on each side. Typically, the surgeon should focus on the surgical intervention itself. The assistant focuses on laryngeal imaging via flexible endoscopy. When transnasal laser operations are performed, the surgeon almost always needs an assistant.

12.3.4 Instrumentation

Special instruments are mandatory for each kind of approach, whether it is performed transorally or transnasally.

Transoral surgery requires curved instruments following the curvature of the upper airways. Preferably, instruments should be long enough for tall male patients with low larynx position, and rigidity of the intracorporal part of the instrument should be high enough to resist counterpressure from the tongue. In the authors' opinion, angled, cupped forceps are the most useful instruments. Palpation, pinching-like and pointed tissue pull, gripping of larger tissue areas, and biopsing are possible with this one instrument. A curved, large-bore, hollow cannula for delivery of flexible needles (for injection) and routing of glass fibers (for laser operations) is also very valuable. A small number of customized instruments are available on the market nowadays.

Transnasal interventions need instruments that can be passed through an instrument channel of a flexible endoscope, limiting the maximum instrument diameter to the diameter of the instrument channel (mostly 2 mm). Alternatively, with two flexible endoscopes, subsequently two instruments can be utilized—enhancing the interventional options.

12.3.5 Combined Methods

Of course, theoretically any combination of transoral/transnasal visualization and instrument routing can be used. When combined techniques are used and transnasal and transoral passages are chosen, predominantly transnasal fibroscopic visualization is selected for monitoring the endolarynx, while the surgical instrument is routed transorally or percutaneously, providing more degrees of freedom for lateral instrument movements and furthermore allowing to pass thicker instruments into the larynx.

12.4 Medication and Anesthesia

12.4.1 Medication

Sedation is needed only very rarely. Sedation can be achieved by 3.5–7 mg midazolam per oral 2 h before operation. Anti-cough medication (e.g., 30 drops of codeine) has proven advisable for some patients. Antibiotics are not administered in most cases; steroids are given for patients with augmentation or major manipulation within the larynx (e.g., 100 mg prednisolone per oral after surgery and same dosage the day after surgery). For food and beverage intake prior to surgery, we consider 2 h fasting (nil per os - nothing by mouth) as sufficient. Some patients who were fasting for more than 2 h seemed to have a nervousness level that was disadvantageous for indirect surgery. Besides pharmacological anesthetization, sufficient "verbal anesthesia" with reassuring the patient during the entire

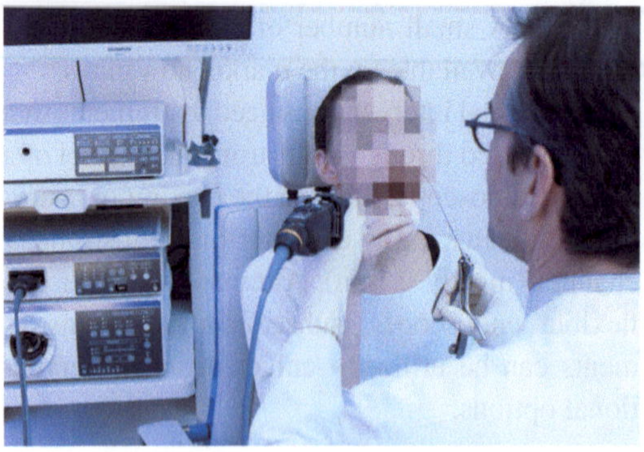

Fig. 12.4 Setting for transoral indirect surgery via rigid video endoscope. Topical anesthesia, no sedation required. Patient holds own tongue with gauze square. Operation is followed on screen and is simultaneously recorded. Instructional photo shown without PPE for surgeon

procedure is of utmost importance for successful office-based larynx surgery (Fig. 12.4).

12.4.2 Monitoring

Vital signs are checked pre- and postoperatively in most cases: blood pressure, heart beat rate, and pulse oximetry. Throughout the entire surgery, a pulse oximeter monitors heart beat rate and oxygen saturation. Normally, up to 2 h of postoperative monitoring of vital signs is sufficient. According to the type of intervention, a postoperative laryngoscopic check is advisable to rule out complications. In cases of patient sedation (definitively when midazolam was administered), the monitoring may have to be extended from 1 up to 8 h (especially in elderly patients). National medical and legal aspects apply and may differ widely from country to country.

12.4.3 "Verbal" Anesthesia

Patients appointed to office-based surgery have a strong sensibility is better for all circumstances related to "their" surgery. It was already pointed out that confidence, trust, and reassurance must be accomplished. "Verbal anesthesia" in a trustworthy environment significantly comforts patients, reduces gag response, and helps to calm the patients down—making interventions of all kinds easier for the surgeon.

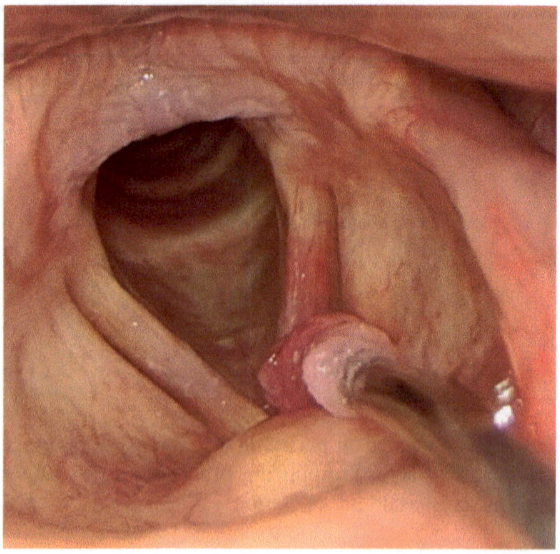

Fig. 12.5 After intraoral anesthesia, endolaryngeal anesthesia can be performed transorally with a cotton swab, soaked with lidocaine. In this case, the larynx was monitored with a rigid 70° rigid endoscope

12.4.4 Intranasal Anesthesia

Lidocaine 4% topically instilled onto lower and/or middle turbinates is very effective (1–2 cc). In rare cases, nasal decongestants and packages with topical anesthesia are used (Fig. 12.5).

12.4.5 Intraoral Anesthesia

For transoral (and in parts also for transnasal) approaches, topical anesthesia is usually administered: under the tongue, bilaterally at faucial arches, base of tongue, posterior wall of mesopharynx, and lateral side of epiglottis. Lidocaine (2%, 4%, or even 10%) can be applied with spray, by dripping the anesthetic, or topically with a blunt, soaked cotton swab. The swab has the advantage of testing "touch sensitivity," training the patient in getting acquainted to the new touch sensations during transoral operation and also predicting tolerance of further instrumental intervention. Tetracaine is also a very useful

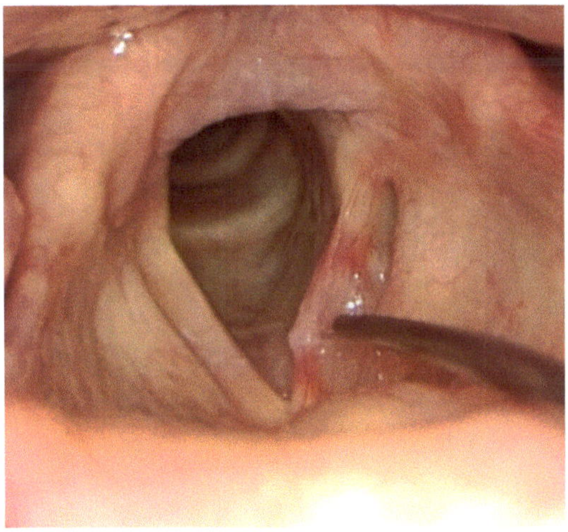

Fig. 12.6 Transoral injection of triamcinolone into the vocal fold with curved cannula with a 25-G tip. Here, left vocal fold with "bamboo node" is injected

anesthetic. Some authors use cocaine, which is one of the most potent substances, for topical anesthesia. However, such drugs have drawbacks and can be avoided (Fig. 12.6).

12.4.6 Anesthesia of the Pharynx and Larynx

As soon as topical anesthesia is applied onto the surfaces of the oral cavity and mesopharynx, the surgeon should—without losing time—move on with the procedure and administer lidocaine into the pharynx and larynx. Spraying should be avoided because of (corona) protection purposes as it is an AGP. The supralarynx, false vocal folds, and vocal folds can be anesthetized transorally with a lidocaine-soaked cotton swab. Touching of surfaces with the swab is helpful in checking the effect of sufficient numbing. The easier a reflex is elicited, the more numbing is needed. As a rule of thumb, the more posterior the endolaryngeal regions (toward the arytenoids), the more likely a gag response is elicited. Caveat: Fixation of the cotton wadding covering the tip of the curved cotton holder instrument (the "swab") must be checked by all means before intracorporal use, since slipping off of the cotton due to inappropriate fixation of the cotton would risk its aspiration.

For transnasally applied anesthesia, we prefer dripping lidocaine 4% directly into the endolarynx through the instrument channel or a small catheter while observing proper placement of the anesthetic. The patient is asked to produce a long gargle or to phonate so as to increase the contact time of the anesthetic in the endolarynx. Using this technique, we almost never need to apply topical anesthesia percutaneously.

Some colleagues prefer inhaled topical anesthesia, and some have the patients mouthwash with lidocaine for additional numbing. Subglottic and tracheal interventions require adequate numbing that can be achieved by flexible endoscopy (see above) or with percutaneous intraluminal injection of the anesthetic through the cricothyroid or thyrohyoid membrane.

12.5 Complications and Failures

In the past 30 years of performing office-based procedures, we have not encountered any serious complication. In the very rare cases of laryngospasm, which may occur, e.g., when too much lidocaine is suddenly applied in large amounts into the larynx, we interrupt the procedure and ask to cough effortfully, to swallow all secretions, and to breathe through the nose while closing the mouth. Although this last maneuver sounds paradox, it is clinical experience that transnasal breathing is a very good trigger for vocal fold abduction and results in widening the glottis. Of course, there are other causes for gag response or laryngospasm, e.g., when the mucosa wasn't anesthetized sufficiently or an instrument touches the mucosa too forcefully. This can easily happen in the posterior part of the larynx and anywhere at the arytenoid hump—a typical gag-triggering response area with high touch sensitivity.

In general, good topical anesthesia of the endolarynx should lead to sufficient numbing in more than 80% of cases. This anesthesia condition can be achieved in some patients in 2–3 min; in others, it takes 10 or more minutes. Approximately 5–10% of patients will not "allow" sufficient time or access for a complete surgery due to early onset of gagging, repetitive swallowing, and coughing. However, there are a habituation effect and a "learning curve" for most patients. Therefore, if a procedure doesn't work because of early onset of gagging, the same procedure might work at a second trial. Only about 5% of patients are by no means laryngeally accessible for indirect surgery. A last chance to get access into the larynx in cases with continuing gag response is to additionally infiltrate an anesthetic next to the interior branch of the superior laryngeal nerve (iSLN) via transcutaneous infiltration nerve block (e.g., lidocaine with epinephrine 1%) in the region of the inferior part of the thyrohyoid membrane. This injection is not as easily performed as it sounds, because precise positioning of injection in the desired region may be quite difficult in patients with thicker necks.

12.6 Transoral Surgery

The transoral technique is the oldest approach to the larynx and was used since more than 140 years. Before performing the intervention, one should always touch the larynx with a lidocaine-soaked cotton swab during anesthesia and carefully "map" the individual gag trigger zones for response levels. The lateral laryngeal approach, i.e., passing the instrument over the aryepiglottic fold and avoiding touching of the tip of the epiglottis as well as the arytenoid hump, makes this pathway most favorable. In some cases, midline passage over the median part of the tongue base and sliding over the tip of the epiglottis is easier than the lateral laryngeal approach. However, in the authors' opinion, the lateral pathway is the first choice (Fig. 12.7).

Whatever is planned for surgery, it should be performed in a speedy, but not rushed, manner. Fortunately, in many patients, pathologic lesions are located at the midmembranous part of the vocal folds, which is—luckily!—not very sensitive to manipulation, making interventions easy when the most sensitive gag response-triggering zones of the supralarynx are passed by the instrument.

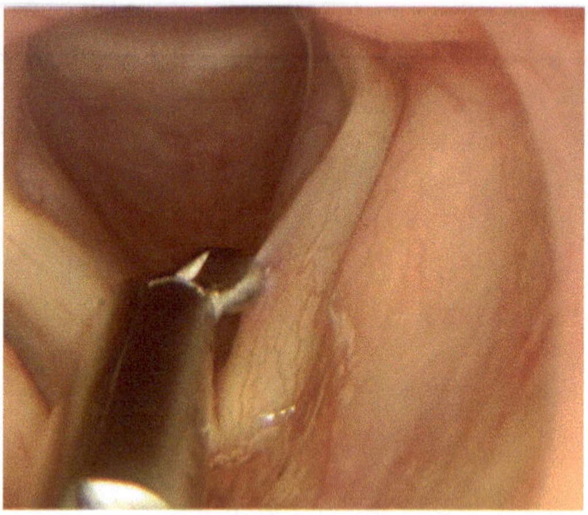

Fig. 12.7 Transoral excision: Curved forceps allow for precise palpation and grasping of tissue. Here, benign mass lesion of left vocal fold, before excision by tearing in longitudinal direction (anteriorly and posteriorly)

12.6.1 Palpation-Biopsy-Excision

Many interventions can be performed with an angled cupped forceps. The operation is started with the cotton swab, which anticipates all movements that will follow during intervention. This imitation of the movements gives a good feedback to the patient (immediate tolerance learning curve!) and also to the surgeon on how the procedure might be tolerated. Once the basic movements are tolerated, the cotton swab is laid aside, and the instrument is introduced in the same manner and position as the swab. When using cupped forceps, they should be introduced in closed position, avoiding scratching of mucosa in cases of sudden, unexpected movements. Again, brief palpation of the vocal folds, the lesion, and adjacent tissue immediately before grasping gives an impression of how much the following movements will be tolerated.

Superficial lesions of the vocal folds are checked for pliability in an inferior-superior (up and down) and posterior-anterior (back and forth) palpation movement.

In patients with a soft vocal fold polyp, we suggest to proceed as follows: First, take a gentle grasp of the lesion by not closing the forceps completely. Then make two predetermined epithelial notches at the anterior and posterior margins of the lesion by pinching and tearing the marginal epithelium carefully. These two epithelial discontinuities (notches) will help to avoid inadvertent de-epithelialization of adjacent and healthy mucosa by undesired stripping during instrumental pull on the body of the lesion. Second, grasp the polyp with a delicate squeeze, let loose, and check the new tissue indentation marks for how much tissue you would have excised if you would have punched it out. If your grasp was placed correctly, continue with the third step, i.e., grasp the entire polyp and remove it with the identical tissue grip. The pulling direction of the instrument is preferably from anterior to posterior, and the vector is almost in parallel with the longitudinal axis of the vocal fold. Every medial pull is unfavorable, because with medial pull unpredictable tear and stripping of adjacent, normal epithelium would be very likely. The anterior-to-posterior pull will tear the epithelium at the anterior notch and will stop at the posterior notch. Finally, straighten edge for epithelial "corners" at the notches, the so-called dog's ears, by grasping with the tip of the cupped forceps (Figs. 12.8 and 12.9).

Hemorrhage by capillary bleeding can follow—and it shouldn't frighten the surgeon when some drops of blood spread intralaryngeally. The surgeon shouldn't worry about the red-colored endolarynx when a few blood drops are spread by swallowing or throat clear, since blood is very effective in coloring saliva. The authors have never experienced a severe bleeding after many hundreds of interventions. After a short soft (!) throat clear or wiping of the vocal fold with the closed forceps (still containing the tissue specimen) directly after the excision while the instrument is in the larynx, the surgeon will get an occasion to visualize the vocal fold and decide whether it is straight or if additional trimming is needed. For the assessment of voice function, it would be most favorable to immediately switch over and use videolaryngostroboscopy to assess vibratory behavior and phonation, with the endoscope and instrument still in place, before lamina propria swelling begins.

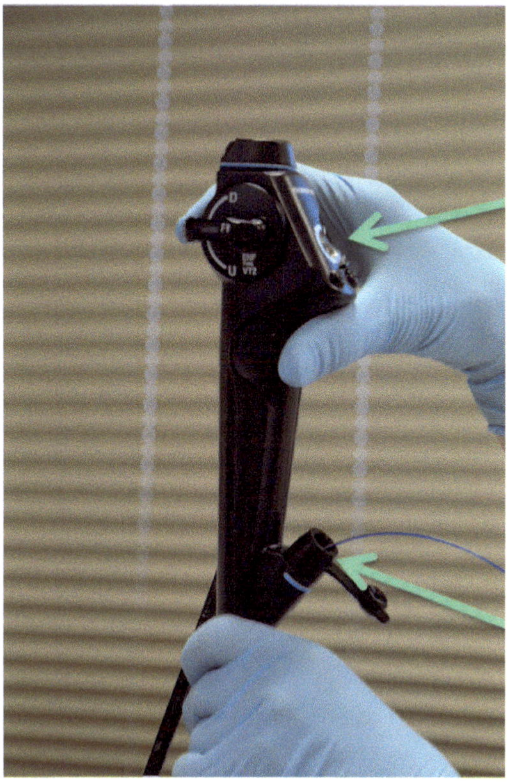

Fig. 12.8 Flexible endoscope with working channel, two openings (see arrows) for inlet and outlet (suction, medication, and instruments)

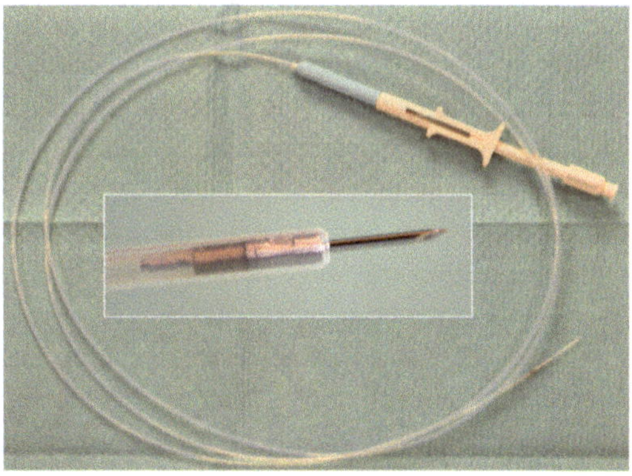

Fig. 12.9 Flexible, single-use catheter with a 25 G cannula for injections via working channel. The cannula is sheathed and can be advanced by an assistant with the external handpiece (white)

12.6.2 Injection and Augmentation

Again, as with indirect transoral excisions, the patient is transorally anesthetized with a cotton swab soaked with local anesthetic (see above). Wherever the injection is planned to be placed, it may be advisable to perform several pushing maneuvers onto the tissue with the blunt swab and inform the patient that this is what it feels like when the cannula is going to be inserted in a couple of seconds. Once the movements are tolerated, the cotton swab is laid aside, and the instrument with the curved cannula is taken. Make sure that, before you inject, the injectable is already advanced through the cannula lumen (so-called priming)—cannulas occasionally can have a lumen up to almost 0.5 cc, which means that before priming there is air instead of medication or implant inside the lumen. Also, a big lumen is a significant source of expensive implant loss. The curved cannula follows the same pathway as the swab. Advancement of the cannula requires visual control, avoiding pricking of the uvula, tonsils, tongue, epiglottis, and posterior oropharyngeal mucosa. In the beginning of insertion, the cannula is seen directly. As soon as the cannula passes the isthmus faucium, the cannula tip position may be visually controlled indirectly by rigid endoscopy. The injection itself can last up to 1 min, giving time for intracordal spread of the injectable. After withdrawal of the cannula, watch the injection site and check for bleeding or swelling.

Special points: Occasionally, the exact cannula tip position can only be found out during injection augmentation when watching the ballooning of the vocal fold. As a rule of thumb, the injection for augmentation should be interrupted when 0.2 cc do not show any effect of tissue augmentation (no matter which injection technique was chosen). Videostroboscopy with the optics in place can help in making decisions if additional augmentation is needed. In vocal fold augmentation, slight overcorrection is almost always advisable because of later filler distribution within the vocal fold. Depending on the implant material and technique used, overcorrection goes up to 50% (e.g., for some hyaluronic acid augmentations). In selected cases, molding of the vocal fold with a blunt instrument or with a cotton swab can help to mold the vocal fold in a favorable manner, mostly by straightening out a rounded, convex fold surface by soft massaging. Because vocal fold augmentation encompasses many special aspects, this topic actually needs to be covered in a separate chapter.

Botulinum toxin injections for the treatment of spasmodic dysphonia of adductor type (ADSD) are placed into the thyroarytenoid muscle or lateral cricoarytenoid muscle, i.e., always lateral to Reinke's space, or into the posterior cricoarytenoid muscle. Injections may also be advisable into the ventricular folds. Botulinum toxin injections can also alleviate vocal tremor; therefore, several intra- and extralaryngeal muscles may be targeted.

Steroids may be injected in patients with vocal fold scars, Reinke's edema, nodules, chronic cough, or granuloma. Intralesional steroid injections (ISI) may also help when endolaryngeal scars at any region are present. Choice of pharmacological formulation of the steroid depends on surgeon's choice, for instance, if long-lasting drugs are desired (crystalline suspension—triamcinolone) or short-term (water-based—dexamethasone) solutions. We very often use triamcinolone 10%, sometimes triamcinolone 40%.

Hematoma and bleeding may follow injections, but need not. Even in patients under anticoagulation therapy, bleeding after lateral paraglottic injection of augmentation material (hyaluronic acid, calcium hydroxylapatite) is mostly limited to some drops of blood.

12.6.3 Laser Surgery

Transoral glass fiber-guided laser application is a very favorable procedure when combined with rigid transoral or transnasal laryngoscopy. The transoral rigid laryngoscopy with a 70° video endoscope allows to take advantage of separation of optical axis and instrument positioning. It is one more—and significantly advantageous—degree of freedom when compared with the transnasal technique.

Nowadays, papilloma, edema, polyps, and many more lesions can be treated with photoangiolytic laser surgery (blue laser, KTP laser, PDL).

12.7 Transnasal Surgery

Almost all abovementioned transoral techniques can also be performed through a transnasal approach. However, while transoral techniques separate visualization and surgical instrument handling, this is not the case in transnasal (single) endoscope techniques. When a flexible endoscope with instrument channel is used, it must be kept in mind that endoscope movements (for better visualization of the endolarynx) inevitably result in movements of the instrument that is routed through the instrument channel. If a flexible endoscope with instrument channel is not available, a channeled single-use sheath can be used to cover the endoscope and deliver an instrument through the paralleled channel adjacent to the endoscope. Although it sounds that transnasal approaches are more disadvantageous, the advantages outweigh. Transnasal flexible procedures are far more tolerable to most patients. Some surgeon colleagues prefer that imaging and instrument movement is actually coupled in channeled fibroscopic approaches. Furthermore, the possibility of getting very close to target by dipping and rotating the flexible endoscope gives easier access to the inferior aspect of the vocal folds and also for Morgagni's ventricle.

Most transnasal procedures need an assistant. As soon as two persons work together, coordinated and concerted actions have to be trained before a harmonized intervention can be performed.

An exemplary team approach was realized by Ricci-Maccharini, de Rossi, and Borragan. These colleagues pushed their office-based, transnasal intervention techniques to a very high level of expertise (even when not all interventions are true in-office procedures because some of them require analgo-sedation, which is provided by an anesthesiologist in the operating room).

12.7.1 Palpation-Biopsy-Excision

Before surgery, the surgeon might want to palpate the targeted tissues. One can touch the surface with an instrument for assessing the pliability and softness (or rigidity) of the tissue. We mostly use the catheter of the (still shielded) injection cannula routed through the working channel, or we palpate with the closed biopsy forceps. When patients tolerate endolaryngeal interventions, one can also use the stiffness of a 400 μm laser glass fiber for superficial palpation. These palpatory procedures are also recommended before surgery to check whether the patient tolerates an intervention. Indentation and shearing gives a lot of information of the covering tissues, definitely useful on the surfaces of the vocal folds. Sometimes we also use this technique to search for a sulcus vocalis, to move pediculated mass lesions, and to scratch off coagulated tissues during laser procedures (Figs. 12.10 and 12.11).

For a biopsy or excision, it is important to be able to rotate the forceps within the working channel until you have the two cups in an advantageous angle for the tissue to be grasped. Palpation in between with closed forceps is also possible. As the next step, one can hold the tissue with very little closing pressure and move it to get more information, e.g., pedunculated polyp or not (communicate this with the assistant). After excision, some bleeding may follow. Sometimes, the tearing of the tissue is easier when one combines pulling and endoscope rotation. The bleeding will of course usually stop by itself, but it disturbs the visibility of the surfaces. Depending on how big the specimen is after excision, one can remove only the forceps through the channel or, in most cases better, the endo-

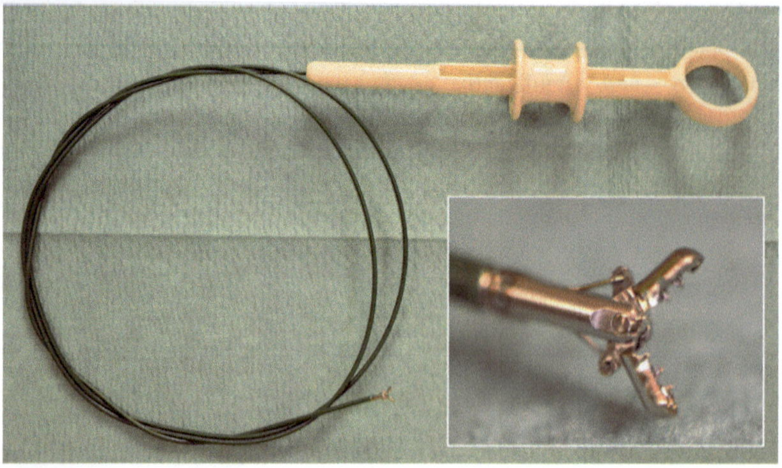

Fig. 12.10 Transnasal biopsy forceps for excisions via working channel. The forceps can be opened and closed by an assistant with the external handpiece (white)

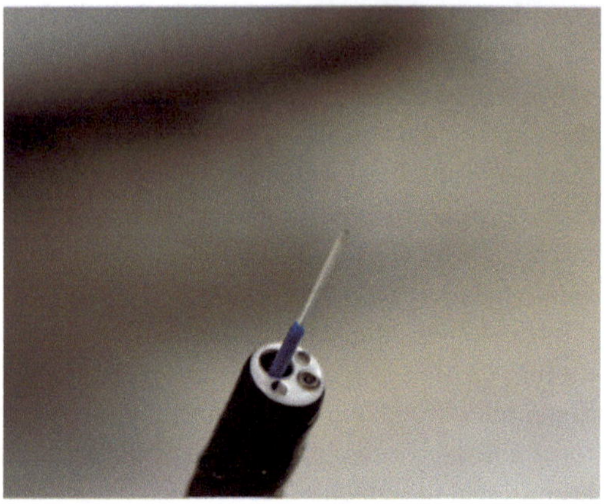

Fig. 12.11 Transnasal laser glass fiber in working channel. 400 μm fibers can easily pass the channel with 2 mm diameter. The glass fiber should ideally be inserted before endoscopy when the endoscope is hanging straight

scope with the specimen within the forceps' cups but still outside of the working channel so to not shear off parts of the specimen.

12.7.2 Injection and Augmentation Laryngoplasty

An easy way of injecting fluids with very low viscosity (steroids, botulinum toxin, cidofovir, bevacizumab, etc.) into the vocal folds is the transnasal technique through the working channel. We prefer to use a long, flexible, single-use catheter with a 25 G cannula. The cannula is sheathed and can be advanced externally through the handpiece by the assistant. For all injections, one therefore needs an assistant.

A typical indication is the injection of botulinum toxin for treating adductor-type spasmodic dysphonia. Compared with the percutaneous approach, one has the advantage of getting access to the false vocal folds as well—which shows good results with less side effects. Another common indication is the injection of steroids for treating scars on the surface, for instance, of the vocal folds. The injection must be done with precision to administer a few drops exactly into the superficial lamina propria.

Paraglottic injection augmentation of a vocal fold is more challenging. Of course, when the patient's preference is to receive a rapid treatment in the office once the diagnosis of, say, unilateral vocal fold paresis/paralysis is made and general anesthesia should be avoided, this is a significant advantage. Furthermore, there is a big advantage in monitoring the voice during the procedure as well as seeing how the filler medializes the vocal fold with normal muscle tone, when compared to surgery in general anesthesia. One of the drawbacks is that vocal folds cannot be easily molded once the filler is in the paraglottic space. Injecting a filler through the catheter routed through a flexible scope is probably not feasible because of the viscosity of most fillers. However, transoral or transnasal laryngoscopy combined with percutaneous augmentation is easier (Figs. 12.12, 12.13, and 12.14).

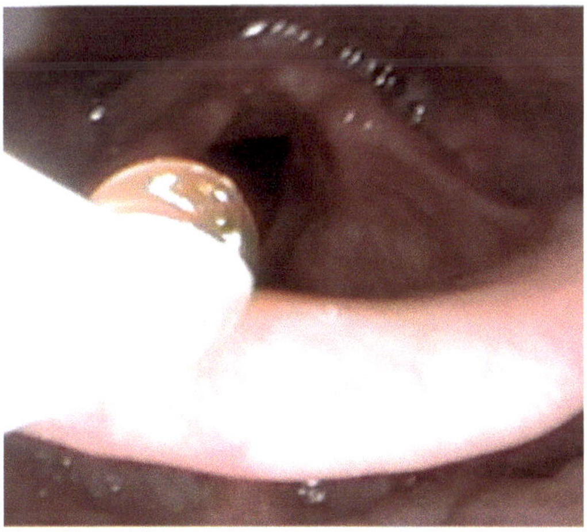

Fig. 12.12 Transnasal topical anesthesia for the pharynx and endolarynx. Here, lidocaine is instilled with a single-use catheter for injections (25 G cannula)

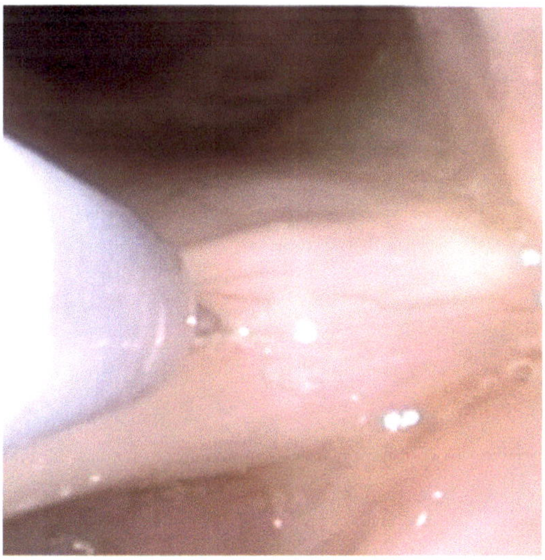

Fig. 12.13 Transnasal injection into the lamina propria of the vocal fold. Here, application of steroid into the right vocal fold for the treatment of scar

12.7.3 Laser Surgery

Glass fiber-guided laser application via a transnasal approach is an easily performed procedure. With a 400 μm glass fiber routed through the working channel, one can approach many areas within the hypopharynx and larynx. In combination with the dipping maneuver and rotation

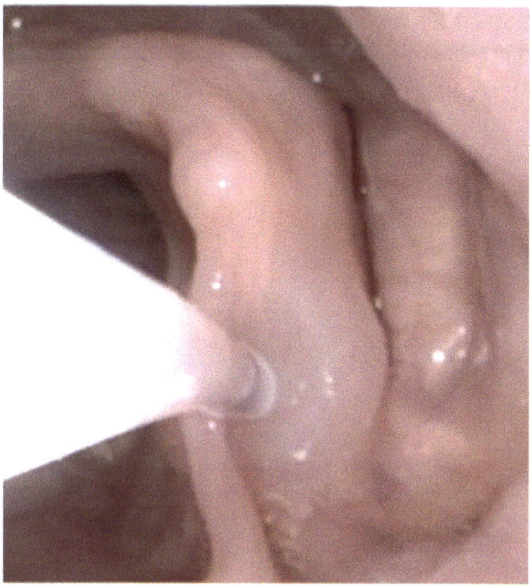

Fig. 12.14 Transnasal injection of steroid and local anesthetic into left aryepiglottic fold (region of iSLN) for cough suppression

laryngoscopy, the surgeon has access also to Morgagni's ventricle and the inferior aspect of the vocal fold. With the use of a four-way direction flexible fiberscope tip, maneuvering of the glass fiber is even more facilitated. With sufficient anesthesia, procedures can be performed up to 30 min duration. Skilled handling of the endoscope with the laser glass fiber and appropriate choice of laser settings are mandatory and should be trained in endoscopy courses. Laser safety measures are extremely important. Special attention should be addressed for the correct selection of appropriate laser light filtering eye wear. Indications for laser surgery can be manifold from debulking of masses (granuloma, cysts, polyps, papilloma, edema) down to small lesions like hemangioma and vascular ectasias. The debulking laser procedures can be done with all fiber-guided lasers. Biofilm ("photodisinfection"), leukoplakia, dysplasia, and small cancers can also be treated in the office, and preferably photoangiolytic lasers are chosen for these indications (e.g., PDL, KTP, BL).

Technically, laser in-office procedures are performed by a surgeon with an assistant. Support is needed for suctioning, changing of laser settings, and activating and deactivating the laser and since the corona pandemic changed hygiene requirements making donning and doffing more cumbersome—so any assistance is very helpful (Figs. 12.15, 12.16, 12.17, and 12.18).

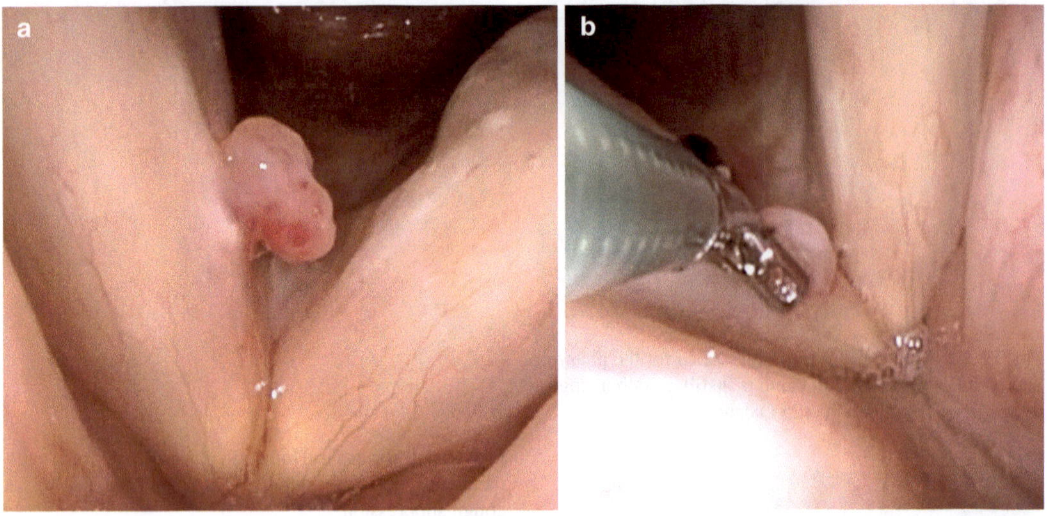

Fig. 12.15 Transnasal biopsy of polyp at the right vocal fold: (**a**) before surgery and (**b**) during surgery just before grasping the polyp with forceps via working channel

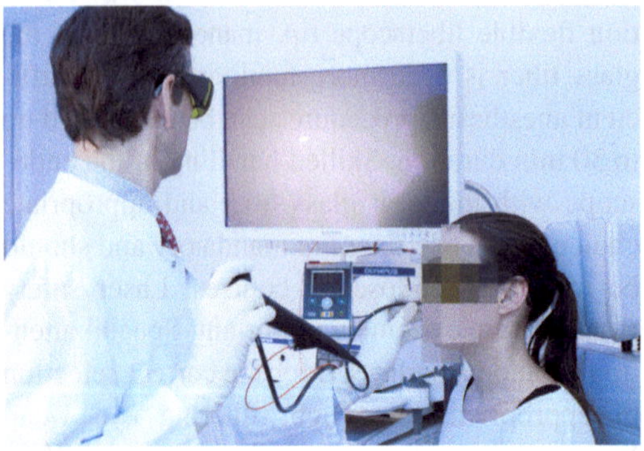

Fig. 12.16 Endoscope handling during transnasal laser surgery. Protective glasses for patient and surgeon. Instructional photo without PPE. Assistance needed for laser procedure

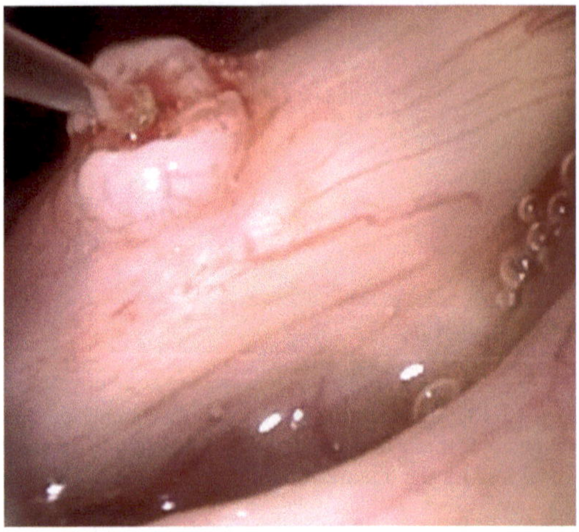

Fig. 12.17 Transnasal laser surgery: Laser surgery of the right vocal fold tumor using a laser glass fiber routed through the working channel. The distal end of the glass fiber can be seen. Direction of laser glass fiber is determined by the movement of flexible endoscope

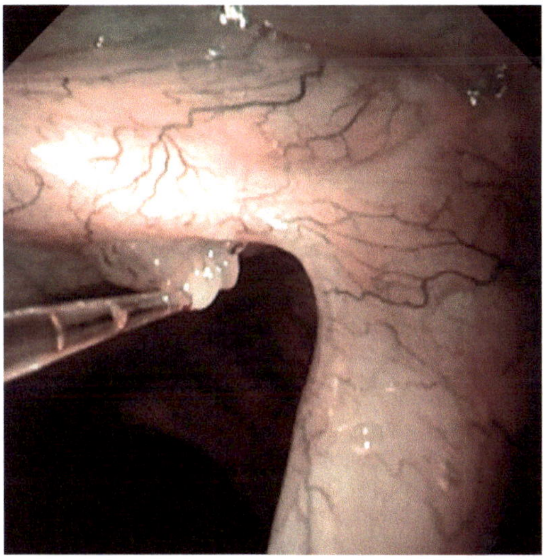

Fig. 12.18 Transnasal laser surgery: Here, anterior-inferior left vocal fold with papilloma directly before laser surgery, shown with NBI illumination and rotation of endoscope (synechia was pre-existing)

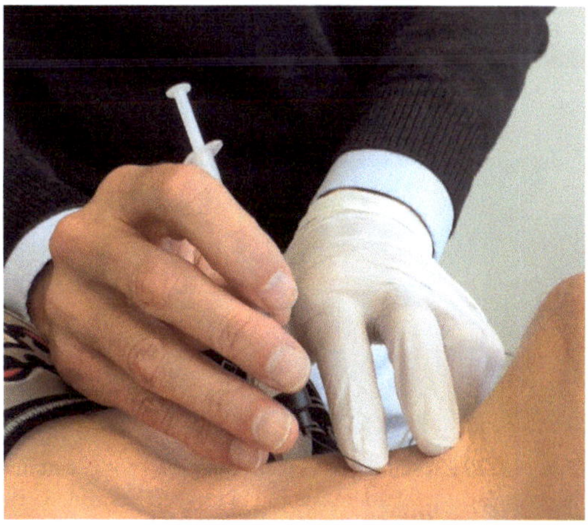

Fig. 12.19 Percutaneous injection of botulinum toxin, controlled by EMG monitoring. Patient supine with head reclined

12.8 Percutaneous Procedures

The percutaneous approach is defined by the route of instrument passed through the skin of the anterior neck. It is combined with laryngoscopy, e.g., in cases of augmentation, or without endolaryngeal visualization, e.g., for botulinum toxin injections. Laser procedures can also be pone via this approach, but is only performed in selected cases.

12.8.1 Injections

Mostly, injection cannulas and laryngeal EMG needles are passed percutaneously. Three main pathways can be chosen: trans-cricothyroid, trans-cartilage (thyroid ala), and trans-thyrohyoid. The most easy way is the cricothyroid technique for passing an EMG needle, e.g., a 25 G botulinum toxin cannula, or a 20–25 G and >30-mm-long cannula for vocal fold augmentation. The posterior cricoarytenoid muscle can be reached by a median trans-cricothyroid membrane and transcartilaginous (cricoid) approach or from lateral behind the larynx. All this is preferably done in combination with LEMG (Fig. 12.19).

To bypass a cough reflex, the needle/cannula may be inserted ipsilaterally and approx. 5 mm paramedian, avoiding intraluminal passage. It is the endolaryngeal epithelium that is most sensitive to all kinds of intervention by eliciting a sudden cough, swallow reflex, or gag response. It may help to apply topical anesthesia, sprayed onto the mucosa through the upper airways, or intraluminally applied onto the laryngeal mucosa through a percutaneously and medially inserted cannula.

12.8.2 Vocal Fold Medialization

The percutaneous approach for vocal fold medialization is a rewarding procedure in office-based phonosurgery. In principle, the augmentation procedure resembles the transoral technique. But in percutaneous augmentation, the visualization is provided by an assistant handling a flexible endoscope, while injections are performed by the

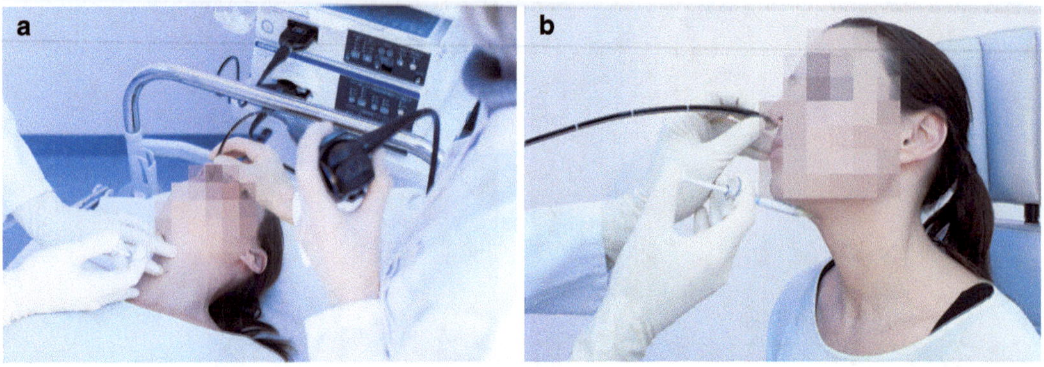

Fig. 12.20 Percutaneous augmentation with calcium hydroxylapatite. Patient supine with head reclined. (**a**) Surgeon passes a 20 G needle through the cricothyroid membrane, controlling the effect of augmentation on monitor. Assistant provides continuous visualization of vocal fold with transnasal flexible laryngoscopy. (**b**) Percutaneous augmentation via thyrohyoid approach. Again, an assistant is needed for monitoring the injection (assistant not shown)

surgeon through the abovementioned percutaneous approaches. The authors prefer having the patient supine with the head overextended, but the patient can also sit. The cricothyroid approach with a 40-mm-long cannula (20–25 G), angled up 45°, is good for (mostly higher) female larynges. Thinner needles (e.g., 25 G) may be too flexible for some male patients. However, we now favor the trans-thyrohyoid approach with a 23 G 60 mm cannula, sometimes additionally bent, to better reach the vocal folds. This works in males and females; however, in low larynx positions, it is easier (mostly males). Monitoring of correct cannula placement is ensured via transnasal endoscopy (Fig. 12.20).

12.8.3 Percutaneous Endolaryngeal Laser Surgery

In patients with difficult-to-expose larynges in suspension microlaryngoscopy, an office laser approach with percutaneous laser technique may be another alternative to avoid open neck surgery. Endolaryngeal laser surgery (and endolaryngeal injections) can be performed through a percutaneously routed cannula. A 60-mm-long 20-G cannula can be inserted in a thyrohyoid approach as a guiding instrument for a 300 μm laser glass fiber advanced into the endolaryngeal lumen. Joystick-like movements of the outer cannula part allow for directing the glass fiber tip to all endoluminally visible surfaces. Surgery is monitored with a flexible laryngoscope. Since there are many fiber-guided lasers utilizable for endolaryngeal surgery (KTP, BL, argon, neodym-YAG, diode, etc.), this approach extends our armamentarium for laryngeal surgery.

12.8.4 Transnasal Esophagoscopy (TNE)

Transnasal esophagoscopy in the office is possible with the use of transnasal flexible endoscopes. Patients with dysphagia, reflux disease, head and neck cancer, and many other diseases and disorders related to this area can be diagnosed unsedated without being examined in general anesthesia. Therapeutically, biopsies can be taken, injections can be applied, and furthermore small laser surgery and balloon dilation of the esophagus can be performed. TNE provides various advantages over conventional endoscopy with equivalent clinical results. Some of the advantages are patient's convenience, comfort, personal preference, and last but not least improved safety with decreased costs (Fig. 12.21).

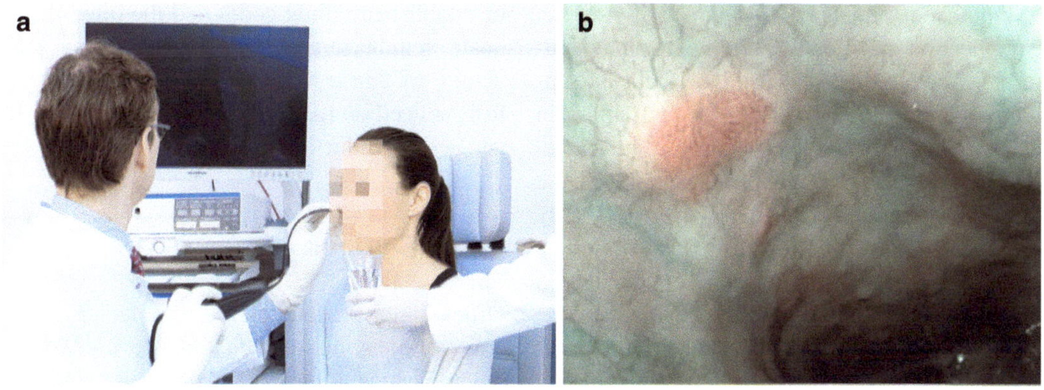

Fig. 12.21 (**a**) Transnasal esophagoscopy (TNE) can easily be performed when the patient swallows approx. ten sips of water without breathing, thus "swallowing the endoscope." (**b**) TNE enables endoluminal visualization of the esophagus. NBI illumination for higher contrast. Lesion on the upper left side (red). Biopsy could also be taken through channeled endoscope

12.8.5 Transnasal Tracheoscopy (TNT)

Transnasal tracheoscopy in the office is one step further to "dipping" into the endolarynx. Adequate endolaryngeal and endotracheal topical anesthesia, delivered via inhalation, via dripping through the endoscope working channel, or administered via cannula percutaneously, allows for the advancement of the flexible endoscope into the trachea and performing interventions like intralesional steroid injections, biopsies, or even laser surgery. TNT as a diagnostic procedure provides various advantages over conventional endoscopy and is easy to perform—however, the techniques according to Killian and Türck (for rigid endoscope) or the "dipping maneuver" for flexible endoscopy should be followed for best imaging results (Fig. 12.22).

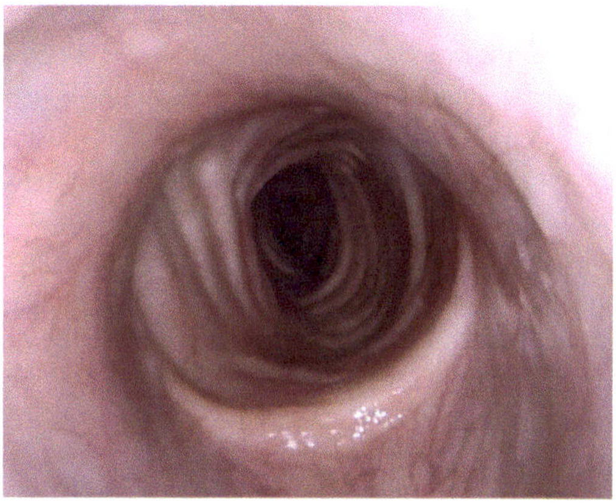

Fig. 12.22 Transnasal (flexible) tracheoscopy (TNT): In most patients, this is possible when topical anesthesia is administered. TNT is facilitated by using the "dipping maneuver" (dip endoscope into the larynx and trachea during extremely prolonged inspiration)

12.9 Possible Complications

In the authors' view, it is felt that the likelihood for severe complications in office-based surgery may be most frequently associated with inadequate technique within injection laryngoplasty (augmentation), so that special attention is needed for these interventions. Within injection laryngoplasty, no matter which approach is chosen (transnasal, transoral, or percutaneous), the highest risk is to inject into the wrong layer, i.e., too superficially (Reinke's space!), or to inject too much. Whatever leads to misplacement of the injectable, e.g., movement of patient, gag response, limited visualization, unexpected migration within the paraglottic space, filling of Reinke's space, etc.—only step-by-step learning will lead to high professionality. Thus, if in doubt, injecting less material and having a wait-and-see attitude is advisable. One can start with more "forgiving" fillers such as resorbable hyaluronic acid injections.

Another extremely rare, but potentially severe, complication may be intra-fold hematoma, hemorrhage, or bleeding which might occur by rupturing superficial capillaries or a small artery in deeper vocal fold tissues followed by rapid, potentially airway occluding swelling of the vocal fold. Therefore, it is advisable to strongly reconsider the indication for in-office augmentation in patients with anticoagulation and also to take all measures to control patients intra- and postoperatively. Choosing the thinnest cannula possible to perform augmentations is always a good choice. However, after many hundreds of augmentations in the office, we did not encounter any severe complications.

In more than 30 years of performing office-based procedures, no severe cardiovascular reaction nor bradycardia has appeared. Very few cases with vasovagal reactions of lesser degree could be handled by supine positioning—legs up! Very few short-lasting laryngospasms encountered in the office were self-limiting and were treated rapidly and effectively with reassurance and breathing techniques (see above). Since many years, we do not administer atropine anymore. Finally, except in one case of a patient with panic attacks, we do not sedate patients anymore.

12.10 Disinfection and Hygiene

There is no office-based intervention without handling the instrument reprocessing with greatest care. We are aware of the fact that regulations and guidelines may differ enormously from country to country. Thus, local regulations and guidelines for the decontamination, cleaning, disinfection, and reprocessing of instruments, for rigid and for flexible endoscopes, and especially for those with a working channel apply and have to be checked. Cleaning costs could be a major problem as well as the turnover time for flexible endoscopes which can limit the number of interventions in a laryngology unit. These additional limitations may be difficult to bear, given the lack of established billing codes and the often inadequate reimbursement. Since the corona pandemic, we see a worldwide change in usage of PPE as well as room hygiene including droplet and aerosol reduction.

12.11 Outlook

Office-based procedures are now facing a new era—for many reasons. First, we have new technology which is versatile with better imaging while using instruments through a working channel. Diagnostic time pressures force us to get a rapid and reliable diagnosis, especially when malignancy might be present. With less availability of performing surgery in general anesthesia and a focus on patient centeredness in an outpatient clinical setting, we now are able to perform one-stop treatments with diagnostics and therapy in one session. Outpatient procedures can be done with topical anesthesia only, the patient sitting and communicating with the surgeon, avoiding high risks for general anesthesia, and also having shorter postoperative recovery time. This includes unsedated injections, biopsies, augmentations, and laser procedures in the pharynx, larynx, as well as transnasal esophagus. Therefore, it is not only a highly effective but also an efficient alternative. The outlook on the improvement of our healthcare services will go along with significant cost savings when in-office procedures with latest technology and competencies, surgical skills, and knowledge come together.

The indication for office-based surgery is always based on multiple factors and is essentially the result of the patient's and surgeon's decision-making process. In general, it is always beneficial having access to office-based surgery techniques to broaden one's spectrum of surgical procedural choices. In the authors' opinion, office-based interventions will play a significant role in the future of laryngology. They will not replace interventions in general anesthesia, but surely give more and more alternatives for diagnostics and therapeutical interventions.

References

1. Bastian RW, Delsupehe KG. Indirect larynx and pharynx surgery: a replacement for direct laryngoscopy. Laryngoscope. 1996;106:1280–6.
2. Fleischer S, Pflug C, Hess M. Dipping and rotating: two maneuvers to achieve maximum magnification during indirect transnasal laryngoscopy. Eur Arch Otorhinolaryngol. 2020;277(5):1545–9.
3. Friedrich G, Remacle M, Birchall M, Marie JP, Arens C. Defining phonosurgery: a proposal for classification and nomenclature by the Phonosurgery Committee of the European Laryngological Society (ELS). Eur Arch Otorhinolaryngol. 2007;264(10): 1191–200.
4. Hess MM, Fleischer S, Ernstberger M. New 445 nm blue laser for laryngeal surgery combines photoangiolytic and cutting properties. Eur Arch Otorhinolaryngol. 2018;275(6):1557–67.
5. Koufman JA, Rees CJ, Frazier WD, et al. Office-based laryngeal laser surgery: a review of 443 cases using three wavelengths. Otolaryngol Head Neck Surg. 2007;137:146–51.
6. Mahieu HF, Dikkers FG. Indirect microlaryngostroboscopic surgery. Arch Otolaryngol Head Neck Surg. 1992;118:21–4.
7. Mallur PS, Johns MM III, Amin MR, Rosen CA. Proposed classification system for reporting 532-nm pulsed potassium titanyl phosphate laser treatment effects on vocal fold lesions. Laryngoscope. 2014;124(5):1170–5.
8. Remacle M, Ricci-Maccarini A, Matar N, Lawson G, Pieri F, Bachy V, Nollevaux MC. Reliability and efficacy of a new CO_2 laser hollow fiber: a prospective study of 39 patients. Eur Arch Otorhinolaryngol. 2012;269(3):917–21.
9. Rosen CA, Amin MR, Sulica L, Simpson CB, Merati AL, Courey MS, Johns MM III, Postma GN. Advances in office-based diagnosis and treatment in laryngology. Laryngoscope. 2009;119(Suppl 2): S185–212.
10. Shoffel-Havakuk H, Sadoughi B, Sulica L, Johns MM III. In-office procedures for the treatment of benign vocal fold lesions in the awake patient: a contemporary review. Laryngoscope. 2019;129(9):2131–8.
11. Volk GF, Hagen R, Pototschnig C, Friedrich G, Nawka T, Arens C, Mueller A, Foerster G, Finkensieper M, Lang-Roth R, Sittel C, Storck C, Grosheva M, Kotby MN, Klingner CM, Guntinas-Lichius O. Laryngeal electromyography: a proposal for guidelines of the European Laryngological Society. Eur Arch Otorhinolaryngol. 2012;269(10):2227–45.
12. Von Bruns V. Die erste Ausrottung eines Polypen in der Kehlkopfshöhle durch Zerschneiden ohne blutige Eröffnung der Luftwege nebst einer kurzen Anleitung zur Laryngoskopie. Tübingen: Laupp; 1862.
13. Von Bruns V. Die Laryngoskopie und die laryngoskopische Chirurgie. 2. Ausgabe. Tübingen: Laupp; 1873.
14. Wellenstein DJ, de Witt JK, Schutte HW, et al. Safety of flexible endoscopic biopsy of the pharynx and larynx under topical anesthesia. Eur Arch Otorhinolaryngol. 2017;274(9):3471–6.
15. Wellenstein DJ, Schutte HW, Takes RP, Honings J, Marres HAM, Burns JA, van den Broek GB. Office-based procedures for the diagnosis and treatment of laryngeal pathology. J Voice. 2018;32(4):502–13.
16. Williams GT, Farquharson IM, Anthony J. Fibreoptic laryngoscopy in the assessment of laryngeal disorders. J Laryngol Otol. 1975;89:299–316.
17. Woo P. Office-based laryngeal procedures. Otolaryngol Clin N Am. 2006;39:111–33.
18. Young VN, Smith LJ, Sulica L, et al. Patient tolerance of awake, in-office laryngeal procedures: a multiinstitutional perspective. Laryngoscope. 2012;122:315–21.
19. Zeitels SM, Burns JA. Laser applications in laryngology: past, present, and future. Otolaryngol Clin N Am. 2006;39:159–72.
20. Zeitler DM, Amin MR. The thyrohyoid approach to in-office injection augmentation of the vocal fold. Curr Opin Otolaryngol Head Neck Surg. 2007;15:412–6.

13 Laryngeal Surgery in Children

Bronagh Lang, Rania Mehanna, and John Russell

Key Points

- Laryngeal surgery in children differs from adults in many respects but particularly in relation to the anatomy, the assessment and the distinct pathological disorders.
- Diagnostic procedures vary with age. The older child can tolerate videostroboscopy and voice analysis, whereas the infant and younger child will often need assessment under general anaesthesia.
- Modern paediatric anaesthesia is critical in order to provide a safe and tubeless surgical field to work in.
- A multidisciplinary team approach is essential for the best outcome and includes a paediatric otolaryngologist, anaesthetist, intensivist, radiologist, paediatrician, neonatologist and speech pathologist working in a designated paediatric institution.
- Most paediatric laryngeal disorders can be managed surgically with an endoscopic minimally invasive technique.
- Speech therapy is the therapeutic treatment of choice for vocal cord nodules.
- Only 10% of children with laryngomalacia require a supraglottoplasty.
- Injection medialisation laryngoplasty is the primary treatment of unilateral vocal cord paralysis.
- Fifty percent of children with bilateral vocal cord paralysis will have spontaneous resolution in the first 24 months.
- The most popular endoscopic treatment of subglottic stenosis is balloon dilation after scar division with or without local steroid injection.
- Endoscopic marsupialisation of subglottic cysts is the most common surgical treatment.
- Symptomatic type 1, type 2 and some type 3 laryngeal clefts can be repaired endoscopically using an endoscopic suture repair.
- Beta-blockers are the first-line treatment for subglottic haemangiomas.
- Endoscopic marsupialisation of vallecular cysts is the first-line treatment for the majority of cases.
- Laser photoreduction of sarcoidosis of the supraglottis can be useful to avoid a

B. Lang · R. Mehanna · J. Russell (✉)
Department of Paediatric Otolaryngology, Children's Health Ireland - Crumlin, Dublin, Ireland
e-mail: john@drjrussellent.com

M. Remacle, H. E. Eckel (eds.), *Textbook of Surgery of Larynx and Trachea*,
https://doi.org/10.1007/978-3-031-09621-1_13

tracheostomy in cases unresponsive to systemic steroids.
- Granulomatosis with polyangiitis (GPA) with involvement of the subglottis can be surgically managed with the removal of granulation, balloon dilatation and intralesional corticosteroid injection.
- Subtotal endoscopic excision is the main treatment for neurofibroma of the larynx.

13.1 Introduction

Laryngeal surgery in children is different in many respects to that of adults. The last two centuries have witnessed significant advances in laryngoscopy and bronchoscopy with the development of new instrumentation, fibre optics, light sources, video electronics and advanced anaesthesia techniques.

The anatomy of a child's airway has unique features that may pose a challenge for airway management. Unique features include a prominent occiput resulting in neck flexion, large tongue, adenotonsillar hypertrophy, superior laryngeal position and lower functional residual capacity with higher oxygen metabolism resulting in more rapid desaturations in the presence of apnoea.

Diagnostic procedures will vary with age. The older child can tolerate investigations such as stroboscopy and voice analysis. However, the infant and younger child will often need assessment under general anaesthesia.

The diagnosis and surgical management of laryngeal disorders in children require a skilled paediatric anaesthetist, the objective being to provide a safe tubeless field for endoscopy and surgical management on the smaller larynx. Endotracheal tubes obstruct the view and limit the surgical access. Modern techniques used are inhalational anaesthesia, total intravenous anaesthesia (TIVA) or a combination with oxygenation provided via a nasopharyngeal tube or high flow oxygen techniques such as AIRVO.

A wide range of paediatric surgical instrumentation are required such as laryngoscopes, endoscopes, bronchoscopes, cold steel microsurgical instruments, lasers, microdebriders and high-pressure balloons.

A spectrum of pathologies are different to those seen in adults and vary from neonates to infants to young and older children. Paediatric otolaryngologists manage such conditions as vocal cord nodules, laryngomalacia, subglottic stenosis and cysts, vocal cord paralysis and recurrent respiratory papillomatosis. On the other hand, adult otolaryngologists frequently encounter laryngitis, muscle tension dysphonia, spasmodic dysphonia, vocal cord paralysis, vocal cord polyps, nodules or cysts (non-cancerous lesions) and pre-cancerous and cancerous lesions.

A multidisciplinary approach is essential and includes paediatric otolaryngologists, anaesthetists and intensivists, radiologists, paediatricians and neonatologists, speech and swallow therapists and specialist nurses in a designated paediatric institution.

It is fair to say that most paediatric laryngeal disorders can be treated endoscopically apart from severe subglottic/glottic stenosis which requires open surgery and will be discussed in detail in Chap. 16.

13.2 Laryngeal Assessment

Neonate, infant and young child The most common symptom necessitating an ENT referral in a neonate is stridor. History should include onset and diurnal variation of stridor, antenatal and perinatal events, previous intubation or intensive care, underlying genetic conditions, feeding difficulties, failure to thrive, chronic cough and history of apnoea or cyanosis.

Examination should assess for the inspiratory versus expiratory nature of the stridor, tachypnoea, grunting, inward retractions of the chest wall, nasal flaring, central cyanosis and a weak cry.

Other features which should be noted include haemangiomas in the beard distribution, lymphatic malformations, evidence of craniofacial abnormalities or neuromuscular disease, congenital abnormalities, dysmorphic features, micrognathia, patency of the nasal apertures and macroglossia.

Flexible laryngoscopy is now widely used in the assessment of neonatal stridor and involves the use of a small 2.2 mm fiberoptic endoscope. The procedure is well tolerated and gives a good view of the supraglottis and vocal cords and allows dynamic assessment of the airway in an awake child. In addition, during the procedure, the paediatric otolaryngologist will be able to assess for stridor or a weak cry. Flexible laryngoscopy however, does not allow visualisation of the subglottis and trachea. Therefore, most children with stridor other than mild and moderate laryngomalacia still require microlaryngoscopy and bronchoscopy (MLB) under general anaesthesia. MLB is the gold standard for assessing the paediatric airway.

An additional investigation useful when assessing neonates with airway obstruction is polysomnography. Many babies with airway obstruction will suffer with sleep apnoea as the upper airway musculature relaxes during sleep. Polysomnography can therefore be a useful tool when investigating these neonates and deciding upon operative management [1].

Lateral neck X-ray and Cincinnati views show the subglottis, oropharynx and nasopharynx and allow the identification of subglottic stenosis or rare space-occupying lesions.

The main indications for computed tomography or magnetic resonance angiogram are to confirm the presence of external airway compression when suspected following a microlaryngoscopy and bronchoscopy, for example, innominate artery compression, a double aortic arch or a pulmonary artery sling.

Modified barium swallow (MBS) and fiberoptic endoscopic evaluation of swallowing (FEES) can be used to assess the child's swallow. FEES uses a fiberoptic scope with real-time observation of the hypopharynx and larynx during swallowing. It is advantageous in that it does not expose the child to radiation. However, MBS can also assess the oral and pharyngeal phases of swallowing, and the patient does not need to cooperate like with FEES.

Laryngeal ultrasound is a safe, non-invasive alternative to flexible nasendoscopy to evaluate vocal cord mobility in neonates [2].

Laryngeal EMG can provide prognostic information on patients with unilateral or bilateral vocal cord paralysis. It may also assess the potential for recovery and can be useful prior to considering a reinnervation procedure. It, however, must be performed under general anaesthesia in children, and its reliability is highly dependent on the placement of electrodes by the otolaryngologist and the interpretation of the data by an experienced electroneurophysiologist.

Young child/teenager Hoarseness is the most common presenting symptom of laryngeal pathology in the older child. Dedicated paediatric voice clinics include an assessment with a paediatric otolaryngologist and a paediatric speech and language therapist. Assessment includes fiberoptic laryngoscopy and stroboscopy in the older child. Speech and language therapists assess voice using a number of parameters as recommended by the European Laryngological Society including perceptual evaluation of voice using a standardised voice evaluation tool, acoustic analysis of voice, evaluation of aerodynamic support for voicing and subjective rating of impact using parent questionnaires [3].

- Videolaryngostroboscopy is the main clinical tool for the aetiological diagnosis of voice disorders and should be recorded in order to assess the effectiveness of treatment. It can be carried out using a flexible nasendoscopy or a rigid telescope. Transoral examination using a 70-degree reverse angle sinus scope or a 70-degree Hopkins rod allows for excellent visualisation of vocal fold lesions and is surprisingly well tolerated [4].

- Basic parameters assessed are glottal closure, mucosal wave and symmetry of the mucosal waves.
- For perceptual-auditory vocal analysis, the GRB scale has been used worldwide. This scale evaluates the general degree of vocal alteration (G-grade), the irregular vibrations of the glottal cycle (R-roughness) and the turbulent air leakage through an insufficient glottic closure (B-breathiness). For reporting purposes, a 4-point grading scale is convenient (0, normal; 1, slight deviance; 2, moderate deviance; 3, severe deviance), but it is also possible to score on a visual analogue scale.
- Acoustic analysis provides objective quantitative values to measure vocal function. Currently, acoustic parameters most commonly used include the fundamental frequency (Fo), jitter, shimmer and noise-to-harmonic ratio.
- The simplest aerodynamic parameter of voicing is the maximum phonation time (MPT) in seconds. Another useful measure is the mean air flow rate which is equal to the vital capacity (mL)/MPT (s). It can also be calculated using a pneumotachograph. This device provides a direct measurement of the mean airflow rate (mL/s) for sustained phonation over a comfortable duration, usually 2–3 s, at the habitual pitch and intensity level and following inspiration of a habitual kind. There is a large overlapping range of values in normal and dysphonic children, and this limits its value for diagnostic purposes [5].
- The use of quality-of-life protocols for the voice has been greatly valued, since they allow the quantification of the clinical improvement of vocal symptoms in the daily activity of children. One of the most used protocols is the paediatric voice handicap index (pVHI) which includes ten open-ended questions regarding the impact of the child's voice quality on overall communication, development, education and social and family life [5].

13.3 Equipment and Theatre Setup

See Figs. 13.1 and 13.2; Table 13.1.

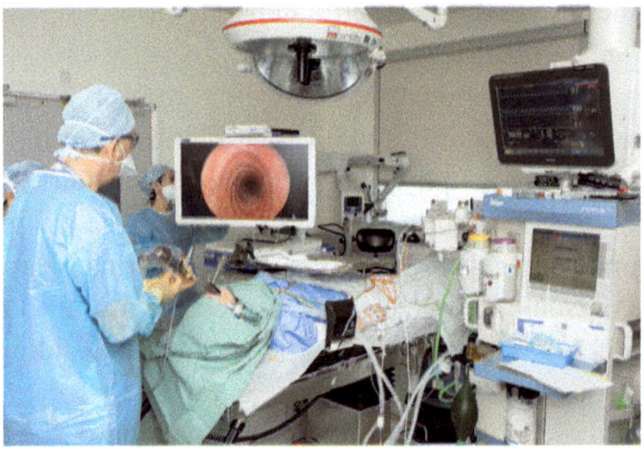

Fig. 13.1 Theatre setup for microlaryngoscopy and bronchoscopy

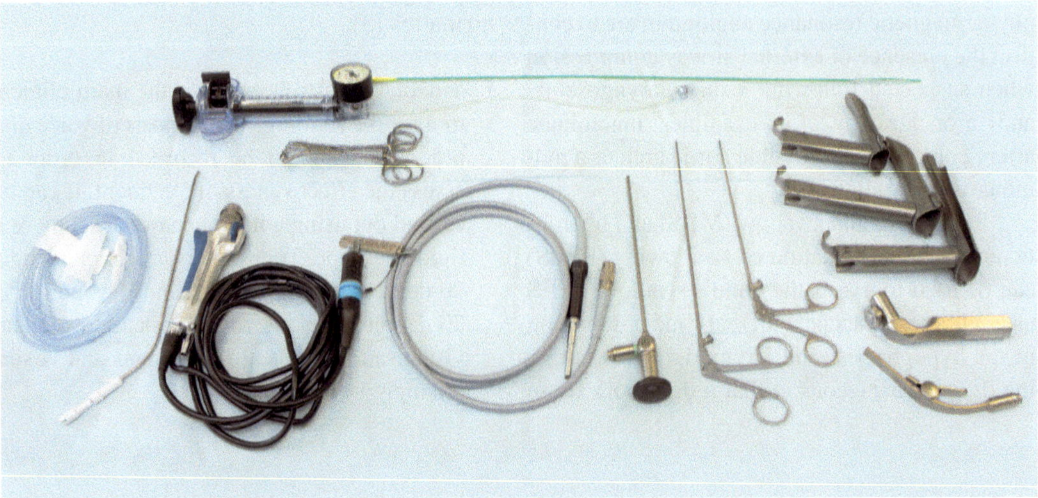

Fig. 13.2 Equipment for microlaryngoscopy and bronchoscopy

Table 13.1 List of instruments for microlaryngoscopy and bronchoscopy

Lindholm laryngoscope
Benjamin laryngoscope
Benjamin-Havas clip
Rigid bronchoscopes
Hopkins rod telescopes 0 30
Microdebrider/laryngeal blades
Microlaryngeal instruments
Coblator
High-pressure balloons
CO_2/pulse dye/KTP lasers
Light lead
Suction

13.4 Paediatric Anaesthetic Considerations

Anaesthesia for paediatric airway surgery requires training, experience and good communication between the anaesthetist and surgeon to determine the most appropriate mode of anaesthesia.

Traditionally, the classic inhalational anaesthesia was the most common anaesthesia technique during airway surgery; however, in recent years, total intravenous anaesthesia (TIVA) has become more and more popular. TIVA has many advantages in paediatric airway procedures which include reduced airway reactivity, reduced episodes of hypoxia, reduced laryngospasm and bronchospasm and there is no reliance on the inhalation route for administration of anaesthesia [6].

Preoperatively, an oral sedative can be useful in the anxious child provided there are no signs of imminent airway obstruction. Monitoring includes pulse oximetry, electrocardiography (ECG), non-invasive blood pressure and capnography (carbon dioxide measurement). A difficult intubation trolley should always be immediately available and stocked with a variety of laryngoscope blades, supraglottic airways, tracheal tube guides, oral and nasal airways and fiberoptic and videolaryngoscopic instruments.

In children, anaesthetic induction can be achieved using inhalation agents, total intravenous anaesthesia (TIVA) or a hybrid technique with a combination of inhalation and TIVA. Sevoflurane is the pharmacologic agent of choice for inhalation induction. Spontaneous ventilation is recommended although occasionally it might be necessary to assist ventilation with gentle mask ventilation. After induction, a cannula should be sited, if it has not been sited prior to induction. Intravenous anaesthetics such as propofol, dexmedetomidine, ketamine and/or remifentanil are used for anaesthesia maintenance as they provide a reliable level of anaesthesia. The correct balance of these agents is essential for effective and safe management in paediatric airway procedures, and this requires a good understanding of their respective and combined pharmacokinetics and pharmacodynamics [6]. When the child is deeply anaesthetised, laryngoscopy should be performed, and the larynx and trachea sprayed with 4% lignocaine (maximum dose 4 mg/kg). The laryngoscope is withdrawn and oxygenation is maintained. Once adequate depth of anaesthesia is achieved, the ENT surgeon re-exposes the larynx, and the child is placed on suspension. Supplemental oxygen is provided through a nasopharyngeal tube with the tip in the oropharynx or via high flow nasal oxygen such as AIRVO [7, 8].

A T-piece circuit can be attached to the side-arm of a ventilating bronchoscope to allow delivery of oxygen and anaesthetic gases during the procedure.

Despite the plan to have the patient spontaneously breathing, a set of appropriately sized endotracheal tubes should be available both for airway sizing and for intermittent intubation if needed.

13.5 Disorders of the Larynx in Children and Their Surgical Management

13.5.1 Laryngomalacia

13.5.1.1 Introduction

Laryngomalacia is the most common cause of stridor in infants and children. Dynamic obstruction of the supraglottic area during inspiration causes stridor, but the pathophysiological mechanism is still debated. The exact aetiology is unknown, but the most popular theory is that laryngomalacia is caused by hypotonia due to abnormal sensorimotor integrative function. This hypotonia allows for prolapse of the supraglottic airway which leads to obstructive airway symptoms. Gastrooesophageal reflux disease plays a role, although it is not fully understood. One theory is that the airway obstruction as a result of laryngomalacia generates negative intrathoracic pressure which promotes gastric acid reflux, which in turn results in supraglottic oedema and further obstruction [9].

13.5.1.2 Clinical Features

Typical symptoms of laryngomalacia include inspiratory stridor that worsens with feeding, crying, supine positioning and agitation. Symptoms typically begin within the first weeks of life, peak at a few months of age and commonly resolve on their own within 12–24 months. Infants with laryngomalacia may have a difficult time coordinating the suck-swallow-breath sequence needed for feeding as a result of their airway obstruction. The increased metabolic demand of coordinating eating and breathing against the obstruction can be so severe that it results in weight loss and failure to thrive. In severe cases, apnoea and cyanosis may occur.

13.5.1.3 Diagnosis

Diagnosis is suspected on clinical history and can be confirmed with flexible nasendoscopy. Once diagnosed, laryngomalacia can be classified as mild, moderate or severe depending on the associated feeding and obstructive symptoms. In mild cases, the baby will have inspiratory stridor without any feeding difficulties or apnoea. In moderate cases, the baby will have stridor with associated feeding difficulties, while in severe cases, which account for 10–20% of cases, there is significant airway obstruction as well as feeding difficulties and failure to thrive (FTT).

13.5.1.4 Management

In 1999, *Olney* et al. classified laryngomalacia based on the site of the obstruction. Type 1 which is the most common is secondary to prolapse of the mucosa overlying the arytenoid cartilage. Type 2 is secondary to short aryepiglottic folds. Type 3 occurs due to posterior displacement of the epiglottis [10]. Children who present with mild disease are managed conservatively and should be reviewed 6 weeks following diagnosis to ensure symptoms are improving. Those children with moderate laryngomalacia are initially managed in conjunction with the speech and swallow therapists with feeding modification techniques such as thickened formula, bottle pacing and upright position for feeding as well as acid suppression treatment. Babies with severe laryngomalacia should be admitted to hospital and managed within a multidisciplinary team including otolaryngologists, paediatricians, respiratory physicians, speech and swallow therapists and dieticians. Investigations will include a paediatric review to exclude any underlying genetic, neurologic or cardiac abnormalities, a feeding assessment such as a videofluoroscopic swallowing study (VFSS) or fiberoptic endoscopic evaluation of swallowing (FEES) as well as a sleep study [11].

13.5.1.5 Surgery

Approximately 10% of children with laryngomalacia will have severe symptoms which require surgical intervention in the form of a supraglottoplasty.

Supraglottoplasty has a success rate of greater than 90%. The most common type involves debulking of the arytenoids using graspers and microscissors or the microdebrider as well as division of the aryepiglottic (AE) folds with microscissors.

This can also be done using laser, but it is thought that cold steel is less painful and causes less damage to the sensory nerves of the supraglottis. It is very important to avoid traumatising the mucosa on the medial surface of the arytenoid in order to prevent interarytenoid scarring and supraglottic stenosis. Most cases are successfully treated by the above procedure. Occasionally, for a type 3 laryngomalacia, a different type of supraglottoplasty (epiglottopexy) is required. This involves resection of mucosa with diathermy, laser or coblation to the lingual surface of the epiglottis and base of the tongue in order to encourage scar/adhesion formation as well as suturing of the epiglottis to tongue base [12].

Following supraglottoplasty, patients are often fed via nasogastric tube for 24–48 h. Children are commenced on proton pump inhibitors for 1 month postoperatively in order to break the cycle of oedema resulting in obstruction, increased negative pressure, worsening reflux and increasing oedema [13] (Fig. 13.3).

Approximately 10% of children with laryngomalacia will have severe symptoms which require surgical intervention in the form of a supraglottoplasty.

13.5.2 Vocal Cord Paralysis

13.5.2.1 Introduction

Vocal cord paralysis (VCP) is the second most common cause of neonatal stridor after laryngomalacia. It accounts for approximately 10% of congenital laryngeal lesions. Unilateral vocal cord paralysis (UVCP) and bilateral vocal cord paralysis (BVCP) are different entities with varying presenting symptoms, causes and treatment. The most common causes of VCP are neurologic, traumatic, iatrogenic or idiopathic. The Arnold-Chiari (Chiari II) malformation is the most common neurologic finding in BVCP. Intubation and birth trauma related to breach or vertex delivery or the use of forceps can lead to compression or stretching of the recurrent laryngeal nerve in the neck. Cardiothoracic surgery, in particular, patent ductus arteriosus repair, is most often implicated as a cause of iatrogenic UVCP [14].

13.5.2.2 Unilateral Vocal Cord Paralysis

Clinical Features

Although stridor is the most common presenting symptom, children may also present with an abnormal cry, dysphonia and feeding difficulties.

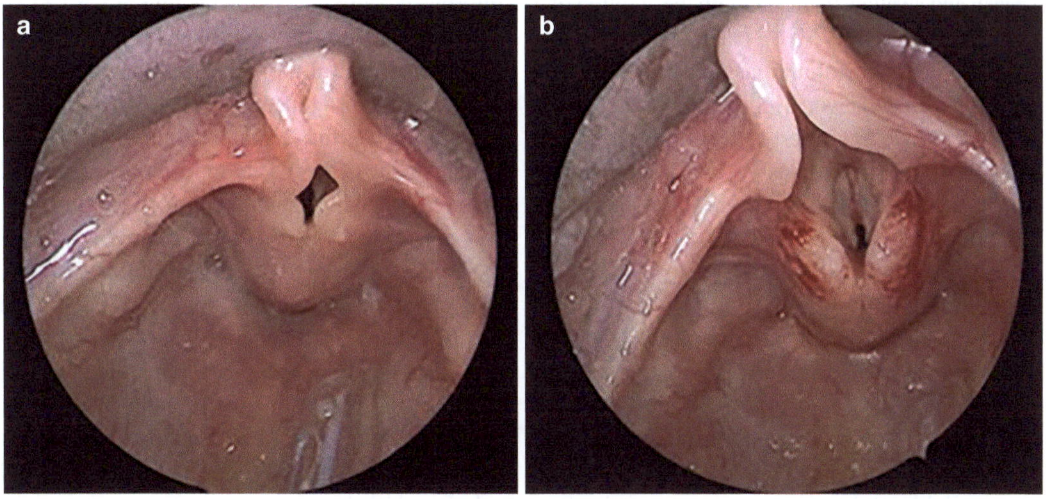

Fig. 13.3 Severe laryngomalacia (**a**) before and (**b**) after supraglottoplasty

Diagnosis

Unilateral vocal cord paralysis (UVCP) can be confirmed on dynamic assessment of the larynx with a flexible fiberoptic endoscopy; however, this does have its challenges. Difficulty in visualising the larynx can occur due to increased respiratory rate, floppy supraglottic structures, secretions and a narrowed epiglottis.

Because of these difficulties, other methods have been proposed to evaluate the neonatal larynx.

Ultrasonography of the larynx is a useful noninvasive and reliable adjunctive examination.

MLB under general anaesthesia is often carried out if the diagnosis is unclear after awake flexible laryngoscopy or if a secondary airway lesion is suspected.

The role of laryngeal electromyography (EMG) in contributing to the diagnosis and prognosis of vocal cord immobility in children has been debated. This test assesses for the presence and morphology of motor unit action potentials (MUAPs) in the denervated muscles. EMG is not routinely used except in a limited number of institutions [15].

Management

The treatment of unilateral vocal cord paralysis is determined by a patient's symptoms, and in many instances, there is effective compensation from the contralateral vocal cord, and no surgical intervention is required. All children are assessed by a speech and swallow therapist, with the addition of a swallow study such as VFSS or FEES if necessary.

Multiple treatment options are currently available for unilateral vocal cord paralysis, but the three most common procedures are injection medialisation laryngoplasty (IML), thyroplasty and ansa cervicalis to recurrent laryngeal nerve (RLN) reinnervation procedures.

Surgery

Injection medialisation laryngoplasty (IML) is the mainstay of treatment for unilateral vocal cord paralysis. Glottic closure is improved by injecting the thyroarytenoid muscle in the paralysed cord. A number of injectable substances are available and are currently categorised as temporary such as carboxymethyl cellulose or long term such as calcium hydroxyapatite. The decision regarding what substance to use is based on the duration of the paralysis as well as the indication for the procedure. Carboxymethyl cellulose is the most commonly used temporary material and is useful in providing temporary results if return of vocal function is possible or while deciding whether to proceed with a more permanent procedure such as injection with calcium hydroxyapatite or reinnervation [16].

In thyroplasty, the paralysed vocal cord is medialised permanently with an implant positioned by an external neck incision. It remains a common intervention in adults; however, in paediatrics, it is generally reserved for adolescents who are able to tolerate the procedure while awake so that intraoperative phonation can be tested for optimal vocal cord positioning.

Nonselective laryngeal reinnervation using the ansa cervicalis to the recurrent laryngeal nerve has gained tremendous popularity in the past decade. The goal of laryngeal reinnervation is to provide bulk and tone to the denervated vocal fold not to restore mobility. Reinnervation is a permanent intervention that does not affect laryngeal development or framework. Reinnervation typically takes 4–6 months for evidence of effect; therefore, clinicians will often perform concomitant IML with a resorbable implant material to temporarily provide bulk and improve closure during the healing process [17].

Preoperatively, laryngeal electromyography (EMG) is a useful tool to better understand and anticipate the prognosis.

A key issue that remains controversial in the management of UVCP is the timing of surgical intervention. This should be guided by symptom severity, knowledge of UVCP natural history and the effect of dysphonia on the child. Children who experience aspiration due to UVCP should be offered at least a temporary surgical intervention. For the first few years after diagnosis of UVCP, conservative measures and/or temporary measures should be offered, whereas thyroplasty and reinnervation are two long-term surgical solutions [18, 19].

Injection medialisation laryngoplasty (IML) is the mainstay of treatment of unilateral vocal cord palsy.

13.5.2.3 Bilateral VCP

Clinical Features

In patients with BVCP, as opposed to UVCP, their voice is often normal as the vocal cords are usually in a paramedian position with abductor paralysis. Stridor, cyanosis, apnoeic episodes and respiratory distress are more likely to occur in patients with BVCP.

Diagnosis

BVCP can be confirmed on flexible nasendoscopy. Children should undergo an MRI of the brain to outrule any central nervous system or brainstem cause.

Management

Management options for BVCP depend primarily on the degree of airway compromise. It varies from watchful waiting, non-invasive positive pressure ventilation (NIPPV), endoscopic surgery such as anterior and posterior cricoid split, cordotomy, suture lateralisation, posterior cricoid split with endoscopic insertion of cartilage grafts or tracheostomy [20, 21].

Endoscopic Surgery

More than 50% of children with BVCP will have spontaneous resolution in the first 24 months of life; therefore, any procedure to establish a safe airway should have minimal impact on the ability to phonate and swallow for the child and carers. Historically, tracheostomy was performed on the majority of patients with BVCP, and although the majority of children will be decannulated, it is associated with significant morbidity and lengthy hospital stays. As a result, several procedures have been described as an alternative to tracheostomy, but there is no one operation that is clearly superior than others [22].

1. Endoscopic Percutaneous Suture Lateralisation

   Suture laterofixation has been a treatment modality for BVCP for several decades in adults. Several different techniques have been described in recent years to modify this technique for use in neonates. Suture lateralisation provides a stable, long-lasting and wide airway that is potentially reversible as the anatomical structures are not significantly disturbed.

   Reversal needs to be carefully considered, because reinnervation of the two vocal cords does not necessarily occur simultaneously. This decision will be based on clinical symptoms such as aspiration and dysphonia. Potentially in the future, this decision could be considered if endoscopic and/or laryngeal electromyographic examinations confirm the reinnervations [23].
2. Cordotomy

   Endoscopic cordotomy consists of an incision in the posterior third of the true vocal fold. The technique enlarges the posterior part of glottis, while the vocal folds still have a good contact on the anterior commissure. While this technique may have a lesser impact on voice and swallowing, it does require an irreversible alteration of the larynx.
3. Anterior and Posterior Cricoid Split (APCS)

   The anterior and posterior cricoid split was first described in 2017. As governed by Poiseuille's law, a small increase in the radius of the airway will exponentially increase airflow through the larynx. They proposed that by achieving a modest increase in intraluminal diameter without making permanent or potentially destructive changes to the glottic structures, tracheostomy could be avoided in some children. The biggest disadvantage of anterior posterior cricoid split is its irreversible alteration of the laryngeal skeleton, and the long-term sequelae to phonation are unknown. Early results are promising, but the duration of intubation post-procedure is variable and not clearly defined [20].

4. Endoscopic Posterior Cricoid Split with Graft

   Endoscopic posterior cricoid split with rib cartilage graft is a relatively new technique used for bilateral VCP. Previously, posterior cricoid grafting with costal cartilage was used for children with subglottic or posterior glottic stenosis, but Inglis has described its success in children with bilateral VCP [24].

   The CO_2 laser or cold steel is used to perform the posterior cricoid split. Measurements of the width and length of the split are taken and recorded. The rib cartilage graft is harvested from the fourth or fifth rib on the right side with a horizontal incision and shaped to distract the free edges of the cricoid. The graft is snapped into place under direct microscopic visualisation, and no sutures are used to fix the graft in place.

   The advantages of endoscopic posterior cricoid split with rib cartilage graft are that it avoids injury to the vocal cords and in theory is reversible in the event of recovery of function [23]. The disadvantage is that it is not suitable for neonates or infants with BVCP.

5. Selective Laryngeal Reinnervation

   Selective laryngeal reinnervation aims to restore the physiological function of the vocal cords by reinnervating both the laryngeal abductors and adductors. The main advantage of this procedure is that unlike the above-described static glottic enlargement procedures, reinnervation does not permanently compromise voice quality as patients can regain considerable abduction but also adduction [25]. The technique has been modified and honed by Professor Jean Marie and recently has been described in children. Branches of the phrenic nerve and hypoglossal nerve are most commonly used. Careful patient selection is essential as this procedure is not suitable for small babies or young children or those with severe underlying cardiorespiratory disorders due to the long duration of surgery required [26] (Fig. 13.4).

Fifty percent of children with BVCP will have spontaneous resolution in the first 24 months of life; therefore, any procedure to establish a safe airway should have minimal impact on the ability to phonate and swallow long term.

13.5.3 Subglottic Stenosis

13.5.3.1 Introduction

Subglottic stenosis (SGS) can be congenital or acquired, and our focus in this chapter is on the endoscopic management of the less severe grades

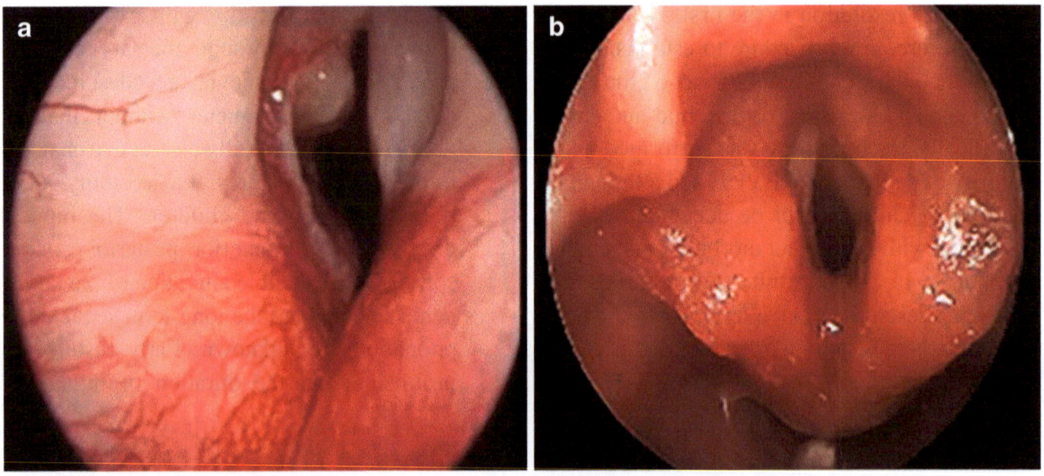

Fig. 13.4 (**a**) Post-left cordotomy and (**b**) post-right suture lateralisation for bilateral vocal cord paralysis

of acquired SGS. Laryngotracheal stenosis will be discussed in detail in Chap. 16.

The severity of subglottic stenosis is determined as per the Cotton-Myer grading system: Grade I, up to 50% stenosis; Grade II, 51–70% stenosis; Grade III, 71–99% stenosis; and Grade IV, 100% stenosis [27].

Congenital SGS forms as a result of failure of recanalisation of the airway which usually occurs by the tenth week of gestation. Congenital subglottic stenosis varies from mild narrowing to complete laryngeal atresia depending on the severity of incomplete cricoid recanalisation. It is often associated with syndromes, such as trisomy 21, CHARGE and 22q11 deletion.

Acquired SGS is most commonly associated with post-intubation injury in 90% of cases. Leung and Berkowitz described the incidence of severe acquired SGS requiring surgical intervention as 0.005%. While an exact incidence of acquired SGS is difficult to determine, it is clear that a trend towards a decreased incidence is evident, most likely due to advances in neonatal care. The two main advances have been the use of surfactant and the avoidance of intubation due to the increased use of non-invasive ventilation in very premature babies [28]. Other factors that are suspected to play a role include the size and type of the endotracheal tube, duration of intubation, traumatic intubation, number of intubations, presence of an infection while intubated and possibly gastrooesophageal reflux disease [29].

13.5.3.2 Clinical Features and Diagnosis

The presentation of subglottic stenosis depends on the degree of narrowing. Mild SGS may go undiagnosed for years only to manifest as recurrent croup during childhood. Severe SGS may present immediately with inspiratory or biphasic stridor, respiratory distress and difficulty with intubation. Flexible fiberoptic laryngoscopy is important to assess for possible concurrent laryngomalacia and vocal fold immobility. However, a rigid direct laryngoscopy and bronchoscopy under general anaesthesia is required to formally evaluate the airway distal to the level of the vocal cords. The airway should be sized by placing a series of increasing sized endotracheal tubes (ET) through the laryngeal inlet and observing for leak, evidenced by air bubbles around the ET tube at the level of the cords at less than 20 cm of water pressure.

Plain film X-ray may reveal a characteristic narrowed appearance, similar to that seen in croup, known as the steeple sign.

Multidisciplinary paediatric workup is required in particular an assessment of the patients' swallow function, and if there are any concerns, a functional evaluation of swallowing (FEES) is useful. The cardiac, respiratory, neurological and nutritional status of the child are important factors in deciding what type of surgery is needed.

13.5.3.3 Surgery

Surgical techniques are broadly grouped into either endoscopic or open procedures. Open procedures are not discussed here; see Chap. 16.

13.5.3.4 Endoscopic

Indications for endoscopic techniques include Cotton-Myer Grade II and less severe Grade III, membranous stenosis with adequate cartilaginous support and craniocaudal extension of stenosis no longer than 1 cm.

The mainstay of endoscopic treatment of subglottic stenosis is high-pressure balloon dilatation after scar division with or without steroid injection. In endoscopic balloon dilatation, the balloon is inserted into the airway and gently inflated, applying radial pressure circumferentially to the stricture. Recently, new balloons pioneered by Professor Rutter at Cincinnati Children's Hospital have been introduced. These are designed so that on initial inflation, two hubs appear distally and proximally on the balloon. This locks the balloon in place over the stricture and prevents it from sliding proximally or distally on inflation. Balloon dilatation is also useful as an adjunct to open surgery either preoperatively or postoperatively. Scar division can be useful for patients with thicker stenosis refractory to dilatation and can be done prior to dilatation. Typically, three radial incisions are carried out in a "Mercedes-Benz" configuration with a Blitzer knife or laser. This creates weak points in the stenosis, allowing dilation to produce controlled tears through the scar tissue.

13.5.3.5 Medical

Adjuvant topical treatments include intralesional steroids and topical mitomycin C. Steroids, such as triamcinolone, are particularly beneficial if an underlying inflammatory disorder is suspected [30]. Mitomycin C is an antibiotic and an antineoplastic agent that inhibits the proliferation of fibroblasts and has been used topically with the aim of preventing restenosis. Its use is controversial as it is a potential carcinogen with a lack of evidence of effectiveness and has therefore fallen out of favour recently [31].

13.5.3.6 Open Surgery

Open surgical techniques are reserved for patients with more severe grades of subglottic stenosis, patients with multilevel disease or those who fail repeated endoscopic balloon dilatations [32, 33] (Fig. 13.5).

The mainstay of endoscopic treatment of subglottic stenosis is balloon dilatation after scar division +/– local steroid injection.

13.5.4 Subglottic Cysts

13.5.4.1 Introduction

Subglottic cysts are a rare but increasingly recognised cause of respiratory complications in neonates. From all previous reports in the literature, it seems likely that subglottic cysts are usually acquired lesions since all reported infants with subglottic cysts have a prior history of intubation [34].

The pathogenesis of subglottic cysts is likely to involve mucosal damage, fibrosis, obstruction of mucous glands and subsequent mucus retention cyst formation [35].

13.5.4.2 Clinical Presentation and Diagnosis

The most common presenting symptom is biphasic stridor. Other symptoms include apnoea, recurrent croup and feeding difficulties. Children may present with acute airway obstruction or may present a more indolent course as the cyst progressively enlarges.

Direct laryngoscopy and bronchoscopy is the gold standard for diagnosis.

13.5.4.3 Surgery

Management options include observation and endoscopic or open surgical approaches.

Endoscopic treatment of cysts mostly consists of marsupialisation of the cysts using laser, cold steel or the microdebrider.

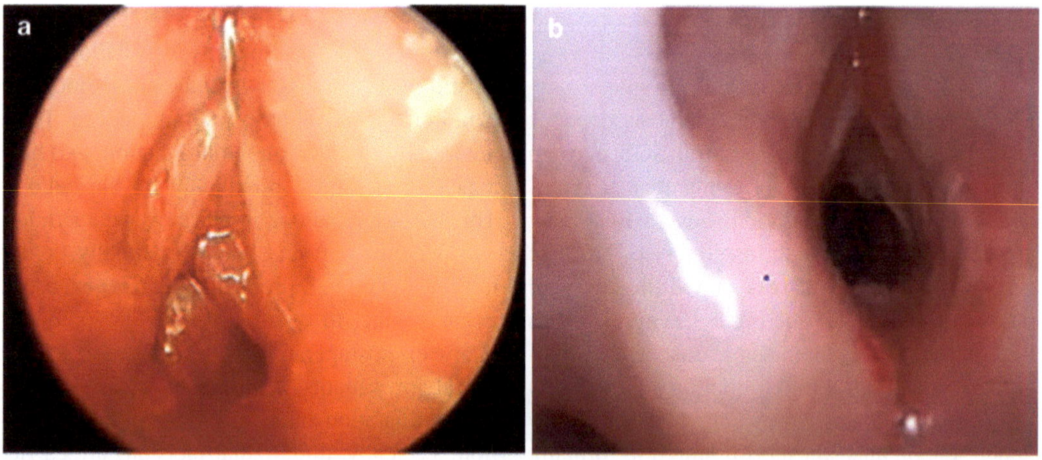

Fig. 13.5 (**a**) Early subglottic stenosis; (**b**) 1-week post-cricoid split and balloon dilatation

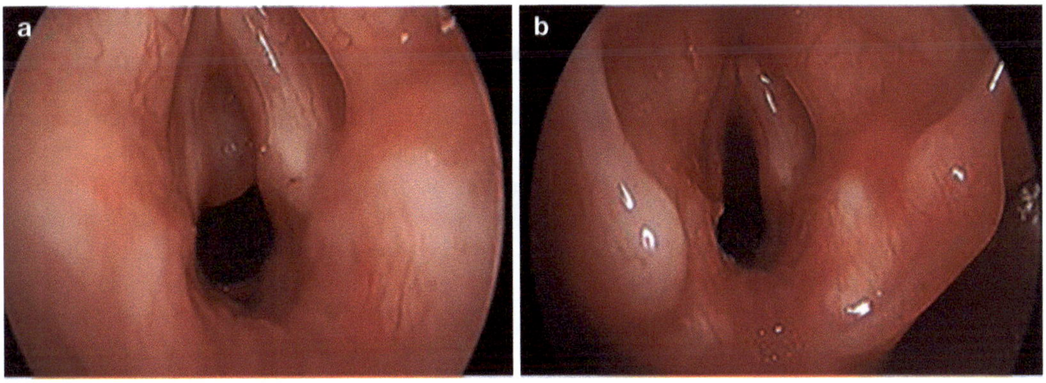

Fig. 13.6 (**a**) Subglottic cyst; (**b**) following excision with microdebrider

Patients who have had subglottic cysts treated should have a follow-up assessment as there is a tendency for these cysts to recur (Fig. 13.6).

Endoscopic treatment of cysts mostly consists of marsupialisation of the cysts using laser, cold steel or the microdebrider.

13.5.5 Recurrent Respiratory Papillomatosis

13.5.5.1 Introduction

Recurrent respiratory papillomatosis (RRP) is discussed in more detail in Chap. 14, and our focus in this chapter is on the management of juvenile-onset RRP in children who present with more severe disease.

Recurrent respiratory papillomatosis (RRP) is the most common benign neoplasm of the larynx in children with an estimated incidence of 4.3 per 100,000 children. The juvenile-onset form of RRP usually develops in early childhood with a mean age of diagnosis between 3 and 4 years. It is caused by human papillomavirus, and subtypes 6 and 11 are thought to be responsible for more than 85% of cases. Transmission of the virus is thought to occur through the birth canal, and there is a 200-fold increased risk for RRP if the mother has active condyloma at the time of delivery. The majority of patients, however, delivered to HPV-positive mothers will not develop RRP, and caesarean section delivery does not completely prevent the disease; hence, much is still unknown about HPV transmission in utero and peripartum [36].

13.5.5.2 Natural History

The natural history varies significantly and is difficult to predict. Some children experience minor symptoms with spontaneous and complete remission at puberty, while others require multiple surgeries throughout childhood. In rare situations, the disease may transform into malignant lesions or, in 1–3% of cases, may spread to the lower respiratory tract, entailing high mortality.

Worldwide with increasing vaccination rates, the incidence of juvenile RRP should theoretically decrease overall [37].

13.5.5.3 Clinical Features

The most common presenting symptoms are progressive hoarseness, stridor and respiratory distress.

13.5.5.4 Diagnosis

RRP is diagnosed on flexible nasendoscopy and confirmed on direct microlaryngoscopy and bronchoscopy. At the time of the diagnostic MLB, a sample should be sent for pathological analysis, while many institutions will also perform DNA analysis by PCR to determine the viral subtype which may help to predict the aggressiveness of the lesions [38].

The most common staging systems are the Derkay score and the modified Wiatrak score which can be used to document severity and facilitate surveillance [39, 40].

13.5.5.5 Surgery

Although multiple treatment options exist, there is no cure, and surgical debulking remains the mainstay of therapy along with a variety of topical, intralesional and systemic adjuvant therapies. Laryngeal microdebrider is the most popular technique, but other options include the CO_2 laser, KTP (potassium titanyl phosphate) laser, pulsed dye laser, cold steel and radiofrequency ablation. The aim of surgery is to remove the papillomas while preserving anatomic structures, and care should be taken to avoid opposing raw surfaces which could result in scarring, webbing and/or stenosis [36].

13.5.5.6 Adjuvant Therapy

Several intralesional adjuvant therapies have been described. Cidofovir and bevacizumab are the most widely used although they remain off-label use.

Growing evidence exists in support of vascular endothelial growth factor (VEGF) as an important factor in the development of RRP, and bevacizumab is a recombinant monoclonal antibody designed to bind VEGF and inhibit the VEGF receptor. It has been used in the past systemically to treat metastatic carcinoma and topically to treat hereditary haemorrhagic telangiectasia. Zietells et al. were the first to report its use intralesionally in RRP in adults in 2009. Doses used sublesionally are far lower than those required for systemic treatment with reduced potential for adverse side effects which would include coagulopathy, poor wound healing and gastrointestinal perforation. Bevacizumab has been shown to reduce disease recurrence and disease severity.

Cidofovir is an antiviral that selectively inhibits viral DNA polymerase, which prevents viral replication and transcription. Its use remains off-label and controversial. There are known side effects such as nephrotoxicity; however, the potential carcinogenicity in vitro of cidofovir has caused widespread concern about its use. A Cochrane review in 2012 reported no benefit with its use, and as such, its use has fallen out of favour [41].

Novel adjuvant systemic therapy may be considered in those patients who require more than four procedures per year, have disease present in locations difficult to treat with standard surgical interventions or have rapid regrowth with airway compromise. Bevacizumab is the most promising systemic treatment, but its use remains off-label. Other systemic treatments include the HPV recombinant vaccine, interferon and systemic antivirals [38].

RRP requires ongoing surveillance as there is no known cure and the clinical course can vary from spontaneous regression to rapidly progressive fatal disease.

Complications of surgery in RRP are in general secondary to overaggressive resections resulting in granulation tissue, fibrosis, scarring and stenosis. These complications can end up being more troublesome than the initial disease and often are harder to treat. Special care should be taken at the anterior and posterior commissure to prevent webbing [36] (Fig. 13.7).

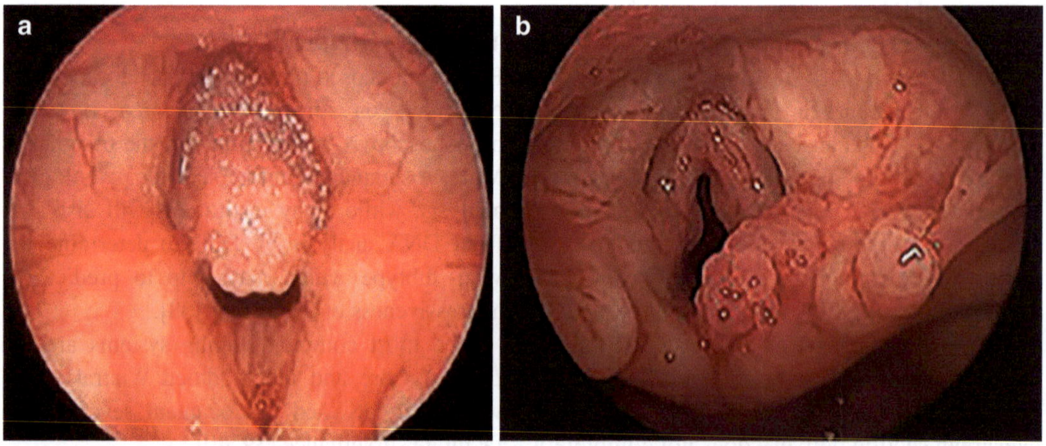

Fig. 13.7 Recurrent respiratory papillomas: (**a**) glottic and (**b**) supraglottic and glottic

Although multiple treatment options exist, there is no cure, and surgical debulking remains the mainstay of therapy along with a variety of topical, intralesional and systemic adjuvant therapies.

13.5.6 Vocal Cord Nodules

13.5.6.1 Introduction

Vocal fold nodules (VFNs) are benign lesions usually occurring at the junction of the anterior and middle third of the vocal folds. They develop as a result of trauma due to contact between opposing surfaces of the vocal folds, often associated with repeated vocal abuse. Many factors, including gastrooesophageal reflux, allergies, sinusitis, postnasal discharge and chronic cough, can be effective in creating a more favourable environment for VFN formation [42].

13.5.6.2 Clinical Features and Diagnosis

The most common symptom in patients with VFNs is dysphonia. Diagnosis can be achieved with flexible nasendoscopy, direct laryngoscopy and bronchoscopy or laryngeal stroboscopy.

Speech and language therapists will assess a number of parameters such as perceptual evaluation of voice (grade, roughness, breathiness, strain), acoustic analysis and aerodynamics [43].

13.5.6.3 Management

Speech therapy is the therapeutic cornerstone for paediatric vocal fold nodules. Intervention must be tailored not only to the pathology but also to a child's willingness to engage. Generally, if the child is bothered by their voice, they will be motivated to change it, whereas if the child is not troubled, they are unlikely to comply with voice hygiene or cessation of vocally abusive behaviours.

Indirect therapy or voice hygiene typically includes education about healthy voice care, increased hydration and elimination of abusive habits. Direct voice therapy encompasses a variety of behavioural techniques including progressive relaxation, laryngeal massage, vocal intensity reduction and pitch elevation. Both direct and indirect voice therapy approaches appear to improve voice-related quality of life although there doesn't appear to be a significant difference between the two forms of therapy [44–46].

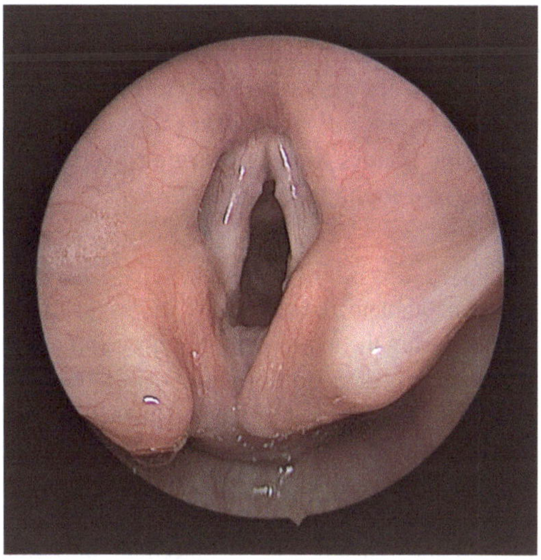

Fig. 13.8 Vocal cord nodules

In addition to speech therapy, any exacerbating factors such as allergic rhinitis or gastrooesophageal reflux should be addressed.

13.5.6.4 Surgery

Laryngeal microsurgery is reserved for cases where significant vocal limitations remain despite optimal behavioural management (Fig. 13.8).

13.5.7 Anterior Glottic Web

13.5.7.1 Introduction

Glottic webs are characterised by the formation of abnormal, epithelium-covered fibrous tissue between the vocal folds. The anterior glottis is the most common site of involvement. Glottic webs may be congenital or acquired. Acquired anterior glottic webs are more common and typically occur from a traumatic injury to the larynx such as intubation, laryngeal trauma or surgery close to the anterior commissure. Congenital webs result

Speech therapy is the therapeutic treatment of choice for paediatric vocal fold nodules as well as treating any exacerbating factors such as allergic rhinitis or gastrooesophageal reflux.

from incomplete recanalisation of the primitive larynx during the tenth week of embryogenesis.

A variety of conditions are associated with congenital anterior glottic webs. The incidence of 22q11 microdeletion (DiGeorge syndrome) in patients presenting laryngeal webs is reported to be as high as 65%.

Laryngeal webs can be classified into four subtypes proposed by Cohen. Type I membranes consist of less than or equal to 35% of glottic involvement and do not extend to the subglottic region. Type II webs have 35–50% of glottic involvement and may present with concomitant isolated subglottic stenosis. Type III webs have a 50–75% glottic involvement, are thick and potentially have a cartilaginous involvement of the adjacent subglottic region. Type IV webs are uniformly thick and involve from 75% to 90% of the glottic area with cartilaginous subglottic extension [47].

13.5.7.2 Clinical Features

Clinical manifestations vary according to the extent of glottic involvement. Large webs are usually identified at birth presenting with biphasic stridor. Smaller webs may not be identified until later in life and can present with dysphonia, hoarseness, recurrent croup and impaired exercise tolerance.

13.5.7.3 Diagnosis

Microlaryngoscopy and bronchoscopy (MLB) under general anaesthesia is imperative to evaluate extension of the web to the subglottic area, size the airway and exclude other concomitant airway anomalies.

13.5.7.4 Management

Management of laryngeal webs consists of conservative, endoscopic and open approaches.

13.5.7.5 Surgery

Endoscopic approaches include division of the web with either cold knife instruments or laser. Mucosal flaps and/or keel placement may be used in order to prevent web reformation by separating the divided mucosa at the anterior commissure.

Mitomycin C has been used in the past, but for reasons discussed earlier, it has fallen out of favour [48].

Open surgery is seldom required nowadays and is reserved for patient with Cohen grade 3 or 4 webs with significant subglottic extension which cannot be managed endoscopically [48] (Fig. 13.9).

Less extensive anterior glottic webs can be managed endoscopically.

13.5.8 Laryngeal Cleft

13.5.8.1 Introduction

Laryngotracheal clefts (LC) are congenital malformations of the upper aerodigestive tract resulting from a failure of posterior fusion of the larynx and trachea. This deformity creates an inappropriate communication between the larynx and oesophagus [49].

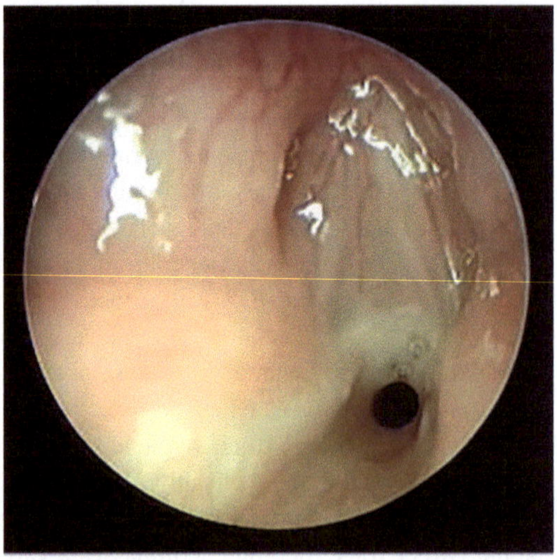

Fig. 13.9 Anterior glottic web

In 1989, Benjamin-Inglis classified laryngeal clefts into four types:

- Type 1 is an interarytenoid cleft that extends no further than the level of the true vocal cords.
- Type 2 is a partial defect of the cricoid cartilage.
- Type 3 is a complete defect of the cricoid cartilage extending into the cervical trachea.
- Type 4 is a defect involving the thoracic trachea which can be subdivided into type 4a (extension to the carina) and type 4b (extension into one of main bronchi) [50].

Estimates of the incidence of laryngeal clefts are challenging because type 1 clefts often go misdiagnosed for long periods or are asymptomatic.

Laryngeal clefts are associated with a number of syndromes including Opitz-Frias syndrome, Pallister-Hall syndrome, VACTERL syndrome and CHARGE syndrome. Approximately 12% of patients with LC have a concurrent tracheoesophageal fistula [51].

13.5.8.2 Clinical Features

The presenting symptoms of LC are varied, but generally the severity of the symptoms correlates with the severity of the cleft.

Patients with type 3 and 4 LC may present at birth with respiratory distress, cyanosis, stridor with feeds and florid aspiration. In contrast, the diagnosis of type 1 and 2 LC is frequently delayed due to non-specific signs and symptoms. Stridor, feeding difficulties, chronic cough, chronic aspiration and choking with feeds are commonly reported symptoms.

13.5.8.3 Diagnosis

The gold standard for diagnosis is direct laryngoscopy and bronchoscopy with palpation of the interarytenoid area.

Both modified barium swallow (MBS) and fiberoptic endoscopic evaluation of swallowing (FEES) can be used to diagnose laryngeal aspiration, while persistent chronic aspiration may be seen on chest X-rays.

13.5.8.4 Medical Management

The first-line treatment of children with symptomatic type 1 clefts is conservative management strategies with feeding therapy and anti-reflux medication. The goal is to achieve adequate nutrition while preventing pulmonary complications [52].

13.5.8.5 Surgery

Surgery should be considered for those patients with type 1 laryngeal clefts who do not respond to medical treatment as well as all type 2, 3 and 4 clefts.

13.5.8.6 Endoscopic

Type 1, type 2 and some type 3 laryngeal clefts can be repaired endoscopically with a suture repair. The endoscopic surgical technique involves removing the opposing mucosa of the cleft with laser or cold steel and then using absorbable sutures with an interrupted one- or two-layer closure.

Some patients may require concurrent supraglottoplasty to prevent postoperative obstruction.

13.5.8.7 Open

Some type 3 and all type 4 clefts require open surgery which often necessitates extracorporeal membrane oxygenation (ECMO) or cardiopulmonary bypass [52] (Fig. 13.10).

> **Symptomatic type 1, type 2 and some type 3 laryngeal clefts can be repaired endoscopically using an endoscopic suture repair.**

13.5.9 Subglottic Haemangioma

13.5.9.1 Introduction

Infantile haemangiomas (IH) are the most common tumours of the head and neck, affecting

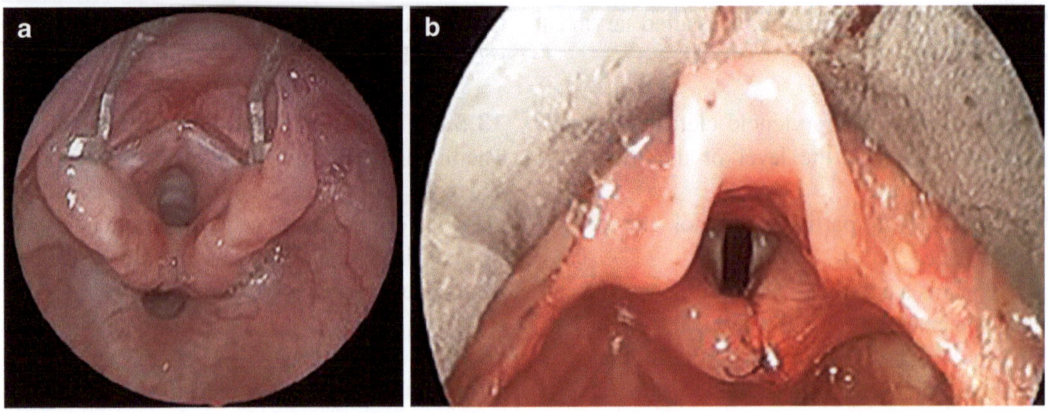

Fig. 13.10 (**a**) Type 2 laryngeal cleft pre-op; (**b**) post-endoscopic suture repair

4–5% of the paediatric population. For reasons unknown, they affect females more than males and occur more commonly on the left side of the subglottis [13]. They are benign vascular tumours which can occur anywhere in the body. Classically, they develop in the first few months of life and grow rapidly for 3–6 months. This proliferative phase is then followed by an involution phase with regression of the lesion over a few years. Involvement of the subglottic region is rare but can lead to life-threatening airway obstruction. Children with a haemangioma in the beard distribution have a much higher incidence of subglottic haemangiomas. Approximately one-half of infants diagnosed with an airway IH also have a cutaneous IH, although only 1–2% of children with cutaneous IHs also have airway IHs.

Children with both subglottic and cutaneous facial haemangiomas are at significant risk for PHACE syndrome (posterior fossa malformation, haemangiomas, arterial anomalies, coarctation of the aorta/cardiac defects and eye abnormalities).

13.5.9.2 Clinical Features

The primary presenting symptom is biphasic stridor which often begins during the proliferation phase usually at 6–12 weeks old. Subglottic haemangiomas are often mistaken as croup especially because they typically worsen in the presence of an upper respiratory illness. Physicians should have a high index of suspicion in children with a beard distribution cutaneous haemangioma and respiratory symptoms.

13.5.9.3 Diagnosis

The diagnosis of IH can be made on direct visualisation with laryngoscopy and bronchoscopy. Characteristically, a smooth, rounded, vascular-appearing submucosal lesion in the left posterolateral subglottis is seen [13]. In the past, an asymmetrical subglottic narrowing seen on X-ray was considered pathognomonic of a subglottic haemangioma.

Computed tomography (CT) and magnetic resonance imaging (MRI) can provide more information on the degree of luminal narrowing and can differentiate the haemangioma from other vascular anomalies by demonstrating the internal architecture of the lesion.

Definitive diagnosis of PHACE syndrome requires MRI and MRA imaging of the head and neck, echocardiogram including the aortic arch and an ophthalmologic evaluation [53].

13.5.9.4 Management

Treatments for subglottic haemangiomas have evolved over time.

13.5.9.5 Medical Treatment

In 2008, Dr. Leaute-Labreze, a dermatologist from Bordeaux in France, accidentally discovered that propranolol, a nonselective beta-blocker, drastically reduced the size of cutaneous haemangiomas in an infant who had developed hypertrophic obstructive cardiomyopathy as a complication of the child's initial systemic steroid treatment. Steroid therapy was the first-line treatment of haemangiomas at that time [54].

This discovery has revolutionised the management of haemangiomas and is now the first-line treatment. Side effects of propranolol are rare, but may include bradycardia, hypotension, bronchospasm, hyperkalaemia and hypoglycaemia [55].

Steroids may be helpful in refractory cases, but long-term steroid use carries a significant risk of complications such as severe gastrooesophageal reflux disease, hypertension, hyperglycaemia, osteoporosis and avascular joint necrosis.

13.5.9.6 Surgery

Surgical interventions may be required in children who are resistant to propranolol or in children with PHACE syndrome who are not suitable for propranolol due to the possible increased risk of stroke.

Operative interventions include intralesional injection of corticosteroids, partial ablation of the IH with laser or complete open resection with laryngotracheal reconstruction [56] (Fig. 13.11).

Beta-blockers have revolutionised the management of haemangiomas and are now the first-line treatment.

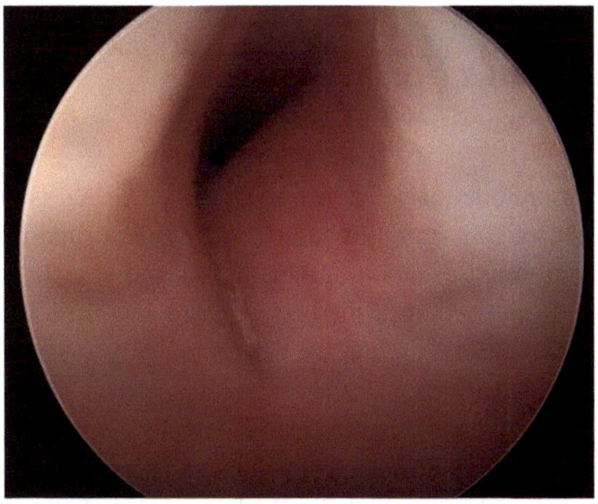

Fig. 13.11 Subglottic haemangioma

13.5.10 Vallecular Cysts

13.5.10.1 Introduction

Congenital vallecular cysts are a rare cause of stridor in newborn infants. Numerous mucus glands line the vallecula, and ductal obstruction may lead to the formation of a mucous-filled vallecula cyst.

True vallecular cysts have an internal mucosal lining of nonkeratinising squamous or respiratory epithelium and a fibrous wall. Extralaryngeal extension into the neck through the thyrohyoid or cricothyroid membrane has been described [13].

13.5.10.2 Clinical Presentation

Clinical presentation includes stridor, feeding difficulties, failure to thrive and, in some cases, cyanotic episodes. The timing and severity of presentation of vallecular cysts are dependent on the size of cyst and its impact on airway.

13.5.10.3 Diagnosis

The gold standard for diagnosis is direct laryngoscopy under general anaesthesia.

A vallecular cyst may be diagnosed on flexible nasendoscopy although this can be challenging and the vallecula may not be visualised due to the presence of co-existing laryngomalacia.

A lateral airway radiograph may show an alteration in the airway contour in support of the diagnosis, while preoperative CT and MRI can help to determine the size, location and anatomic dimensions of a cyst and to plan for surgical resection.

13.5.10.4 Surgery

Endoscopic marsupialisation is the first-line treatment for the majority. Microlaryngeal scissors or a laser can be used to deroof the cyst.

Simple aspiration of the cyst carries a high risk of recurrence and is not recommended [57].

Rarely, an open approach is required for cases of recurrent cysts or cysts with extensive extralaryngeal extension (Fig. 13.12).

Endoscopic marsupialisation of vallecular cysts is the first-line treatment for the majority.

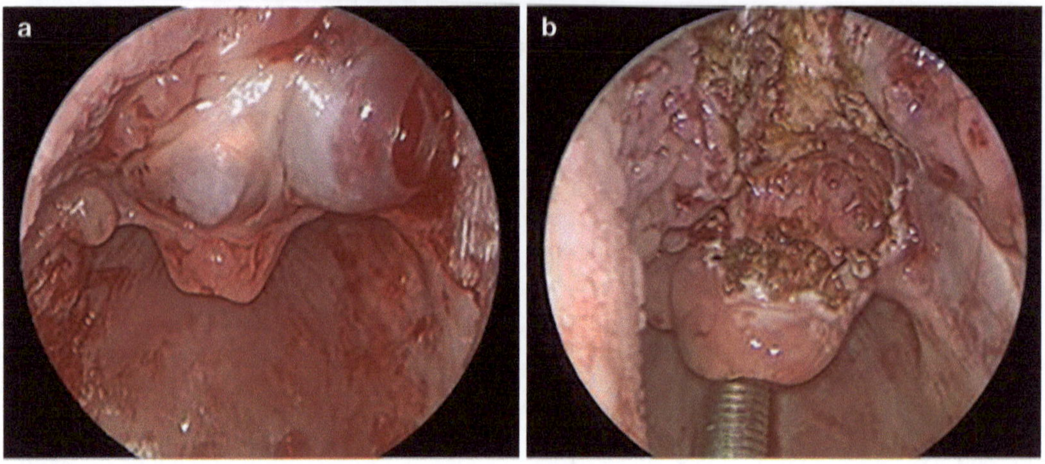

Fig. 13.12 (**a**) Vallecular cyst; (**b**) post-CO_2 laser excision of vallecular cyst

13.5.11 Laryngeal Manifestations of Systemic Diseases

13.5.11.1 Laryngeal Sarcoidosis

Laryngeal involvement is uncommon in sarcoidosis. Obstruction is most often supraglottic, due to preferential involvement of the arytenoids, epiglottis and aryepiglottic folds. This is thought to result from a comparatively rich lymphatic supply to this tissue.

First-line therapy remains corticosteroids. Treatment options that have been used with variable success in cases resistant to corticosteroid therapy include immunosuppressive agents such as methotrexate, azathioprine, cyclosporine, hydroxychloroquine, sirolimus and biological agents such as infliximab.

Surgery

Surgical options such as endoscopic laser photoreduction using carbon dioxide laser are useful in patients with significant airway compromise in order to avoid tracheostomy or in patients unresponsive to steroids [58]. Other approaches that have been used successfully include intralesional steroids, external beam radiotherapy and surgery. Spontaneous resolution of laryngeal sarcoidosis can occur, so watchful waiting is a reasonable strategy for asymptomatic or minimally symptomatic patients [59] (Fig. 13.13).

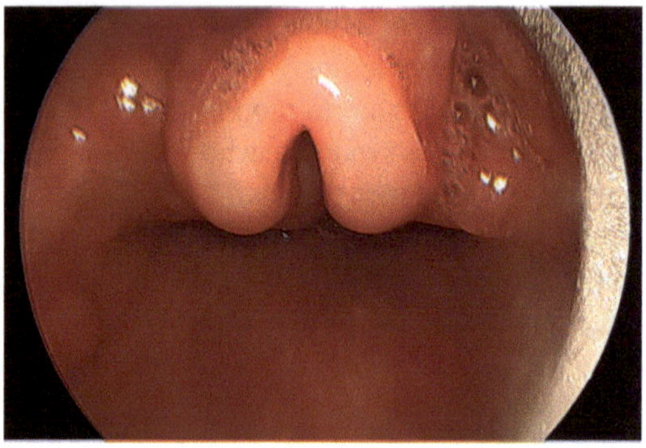

Fig. 13.13 Laryngeal sarcoidosis

First-line therapy is systemic corticosteroids.

13.5.11.2 Granulomatosis with Polyangiitis of the Larynx

Granulomatosis with polyangiitis (GPA) is a necrotising granulomatous vasculitis primarily affecting the small- and medium-sized vessels.

Any portion of the body may be involved, but most commonly, the upper and lower respiratory tract are affected, with eventual renal involvement. Head and neck manifestations are present in up to 84% at diagnosis, and as such, otolaryngologists need to have a high level of suspicion. Patients may present in adolescence with subglottic stenosis or multilevel obstruction. The course of the disease tends to be relapsing and remitting, but in untreated instances, it can become rapidly fatal.

Treatment for GPA involves steroids as well as immunosuppressants and more recently monoclonal antibodies such as rituximab. Rituximab is a monoclonal anti-CD20 chimeric antibody that was originally used to treat B-cell lymphoma. The therapy depletes B cells as well as the anti-neutrophil cytoplasmic antibodies (ANCAs).

Surgery

Surgical approaches include removal of granulation and scar tissue, balloon dilatation and intralesional corticosteroid injections [60] (Fig. 13.14).

> **Surgical approaches include removal of granulation and scar tissue, balloon dilatation and intralesional corticosteroid injections.**

13.5.11.3 Neurofibromas of the Larynx

Neurofibromas are benign proliferations of Schwann cells, perineurial cells and fibroblasts. They may occur in isolation, but more commonly, they are associated with neurofibromatosis type 1 or 2. The most common sites of laryngeal involvement include the aryepiglottic folds and the arytenoids, areas of the larynx rich in terminal nerve plexuses.

Neurofibromas may be classified as plexiform (expanding pre-existing nerves), diffuse (growing as a nodule) or both based on their pattern of growth.

Owing to its slow growth and variability of location and size, laryngeal neurofibroma can remain symptom-free for years or become symptomatic at birth.

Further evaluation with CT and MRI can help determine the extent of the lesion.

Surgery

Choice of treatment for neurofibroma of the larynx is based on the location, extension and severity of symptoms. A conservative approach is advisable when total resection is not possible and the patient has minimal symptoms. Subtotal excision has been the mainstay of therapy because of the propensity for diffuse involvement and poor margin control. Endoscopic laser excision is recommended for patients who present with a small, localised lesion that is accessible via suspension laryngoscopy. Complete resection of laryngeal neurofibroma and preservation of laryngeal functions are often impossible owing to the lesion's infiltrative nature [61].

> **Subtotal endoscopic excision has been the mainstay of therapy because of the propensity for diffuse involvement and poor margin control.**

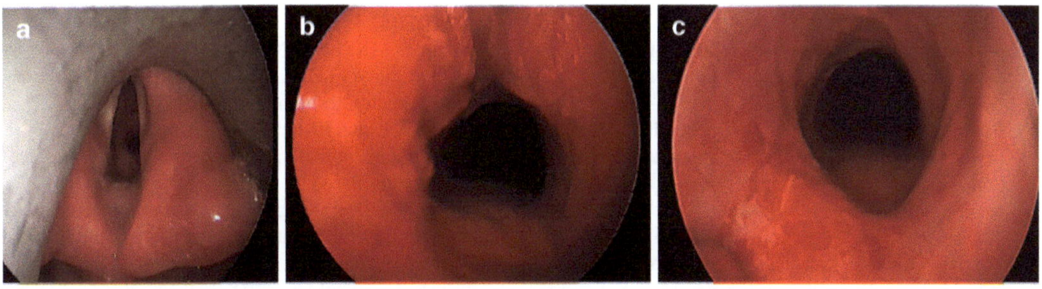

Fig. 13.14 (**a**) GPA with subglottic stenosis, (**b**) immediately post-balloon dilatation and steroid injection, and (**c**) 1-month post-procedure

References

1. Daniel M, Cheng A. Neonatal stridor. Int J Pediatr. 2012;2012:859104.
2. Ongkasuwan J, et al. Laryngeal ultrasound and vocal fold movement in the pediatric cardiovascular intensive care unit. Laryngoscope. 2017;127(1):167–72.
3. Smillie I, et al. The paediatric voice clinic. Arch Dis Child. 2014;99(10):912–5.
4. Ongkasuwan J, et al. Transoral rigid 70-degree laryngoscopy in a pediatric voice clinic. Laryngoscope. 2019;129(7):1657–9.
5. Zur KB, et al. Pediatric Voice Handicap Index (pVHI): a new tool for evaluating pediatric dysphonia. Int J Pediatr Otorhinolaryngol. 2007;71(1):77–82.
6. Lauder G, et al. Volatiles or TIVA: which is the standard of care for pediatric airway procedures? A procon discussion. Pediatr Anesth. 2020;30(3):209–20.
7. Londino A, Jagannathan N. Anesthesia in diagnostic and therapeutic pediatric bronchoscopy. Otolaryngol Clin N Am. 2019;52(6):1037–48.
8. Karsli C. Managing the challenging pediatric airway: continuing professional development. Can J Anesth. 2015;62(9):1000–16.
9. Landry A, Thompson D. Laryngomalacia: disease presentation, spectrum, and management. Int J Pediatr. 2012;2012:1–6.
10. Olney D, et al. Laryngomalacia and its treatment. Laryngoscope. 1999;109(11):1770–5.
11. Carter J, et al. International Pediatric ORL Group (IPOG) laryngomalacia consensus recommendations. Int J Pediatr Otorhinolaryngol. 2016;86:256–61.
12. Del Do M, et al. Supraglottoplasty surgery types 1–3: a practical classification system for laryngomalacia surgery. Int J Pediatr Otorhinolaryngol. 2018;111:69–74.
13. Parkes W, Propst E. Advances in the diagnosis, management, and treatment of neonates with laryngeal disorders. Semin Fetal Neonatal Med. 2016;21(4):270–6.
14. Daya H, et al. Pediatric vocal fold paralysis. Arch Otolaryngol Head Neck Surg. 2000;126(1):21.
15. Lesnik M, et al. Idiopathic bilateral vocal cord paralysis in infants: case series and literature review. Laryngoscope. 2014;125(7):1724–8.
16. Cohen J, Benyamini L. Voice outcome after vocal fold injection augmentation with carboxymethyl cellulose versus calcium hydroxyapatite. J Laryngol Otol. 2020;134(3):263–9.
17. Marie JP, et al. Nonselective reinnervation as a primary or salvage treatment of unilateral vocal fold palsy. Laryngoscope. 2020;130(7):1756–63.
18. Bouhabel S, Hartnick CJ. Current trends in practices in the treatment of pediatric unilateral vocal fold immobility: a survey on injections, thyroplasty and nerve reinnervation. Int J Pediatr Otorhinolaryngol. 2018;109:115–8.
19. Butskiy O, et al. Surgical interventions for pediatric unilateral vocal cord paralysis: a systematic review. JAMA Otolaryngol Head Neck Surg. 2015;141(7):654–60.
20. Rutter M, et al. Endoscopic anterior-posterior cricoid split for pediatric bilateral vocal fold paralysis. Laryngoscope. 2017;128(1):257–63.
21. Dahl J, et al. Endoscopic posterior cricoid split with costal cartilage graft: a fifteen-year experience. Laryngoscope. 2016;127(1):252–7.
22. Funk R, et al. Factors associated with tracheotomy and decannulation in pediatric bilateral vocal fold immobility. Int J Pediatr Otorhinolaryngol. 2015;79(6):895–9.
23. Montague GL, Bly RA, Nadaraja GS, Conrad DE, Parikh SR, Chan DK. Endoscopic percutaneous suture lateralization for neonatal bilateral vocal fold immobility. Int J Pediatr Otorhinolaryngol. 2018;108:120–4.
24. Chen E, Inglis A. Bilateral vocal cord paralysis in children. Otolaryngol Clin N Am. 2008;41(5):889–901.
25. Lee J, et al. Bilateral selective laryngeal reinnervation for bilateral vocal fold paralysis in children. JAMA Otolaryngol Head Neck Surg. 2020;146(5):401.
26. Marina M, et al. Laryngeal reinnervation for bilateral vocal fold paralysis. Curr Opin Otolaryngol Head Neck Surg. 2011;19(6):434–8.
27. Myer CM III, et al. Proposed grading system for subglottic stenosis based on endotracheal tube sizes. Ann Otol Rhinol Laryngol. 1994;103(4):319–23.
28. Leung R, Berkowitz RG. Incidence of severe acquired subglottic stenosis in newborns. Int J Pediatr Otorhinolaryngol. 2007;71(5):763–8.
29. Rutter M, Kuo I. Predicting and managing the development of subglottic stenosis following intubation in children. J Pediatr. 2020;96(1):1–3.
30. Sekioka A, et al. Serial intralesional triamcinolone acetonide injections for acquired subglottic stenosis in premature infants. Pediatr Surg Int. 2018;34(10):1047–52.
31. Yung KC, et al. A randomized controlled trial of adjuvant mitomycin-c in endoscopic surgery for laryngotracheal stenosis. Laryngoscope. 2020;130(3):706–11.
32. Bakthavachalam S, McClay JE. Endoscopic management of subglottic stenosis. Otolaryngol Head Neck Surg. 2008;139(4):551–9.
33. George M, et al. Management of severe pediatric subglottic stenosis with glottic involvement. J Thorac Cardiovasc Surg. 2010;139(2):411–7.
34. Lim J, et al. Subglottic cysts: the Great Ormond street experience. Int J Pediatr Otorhinolaryngol. 2003;67(5):461–5.
35. Steehler MK, et al. Management of subglottic cysts with Mitomycin-C—a case series and literature review. Int J Pediatr Otorhinolaryngol. 2011;75(3):360–3.
36. Hoff SR, Koltai PJ. Operative management of juvenile-onset recurrent respiratory papillomatosis. Oper Tech Otolaryngol Head Neck Surg. 2012;23(2):117–23.
37. Novakovic D, et al. A prospective study of the incidence of juvenile-onset recurrent respiratory papillomatosis after implementation of a national HPV vaccination program. J Infect Dis. 2018;217(2):208–12.
38. Lawlor C, et al. International Pediatric Otolaryngology Group (IPOG): juvenile-onset recurrent respiratory

papillomatosis consensus recommendations. Int J Pediatr Otorhinolaryngol. 2020;128:109697.
39. Derkay CS, et al. A staging system for assessing severity of disease and response to therapy in recurrent respiratory papillomatosis. Laryngoscope. 1998;108(6):935–7.
40. Wiatrak BJ, et al. Recurrent respiratory papillomatosis: a longitudinal study comparing severity associated with human papilloma viral types 6 and 11 and other risk factors in a large pediatric population. Laryngoscope. 2004;114(S104):1–23.
41. Chadha NK, James A. Adjuvant antiviral therapy for recurrent respiratory papillomatosis. Cochrane Database Syst Rev. 2010;12(12):CD005053.
42. Birchall MA, Carding P. Vocal nodules management. Clin Otolaryngol. 2019;44(4):497–501.
43. Cohen W, et al. Development of a minimum protocol for assessment in the paediatric voice clinic. Part 1: Evaluating vocal function. Logopedics Phoniatrics Vocol. 2012;37(1):33–8.
44. Ongkasuwan J, Friedman EM. Is voice therapy effective in the management of vocal fold nodules in children? Laryngoscope. 2013;123(12):2930–1.
45. Martins RHG, et al. Clinical practice: vocal nodules in dysphonic children. Eur J Pediatr. 2013;172(9):1161–5.
46. Hartnick C, et al. Indirect vs direct voice therapy for children with vocal nodules: a randomized clinical trial. JAMA Otolaryngol Head Neck Surg. 2018;144(2):156–63.
47. Avelino MAG, et al. Congenital laryngeal webs: from diagnosis to surgical outcomes. Braz J Otorhinolaryngol. 2020; https://doi.org/10.1016/j.bjorl.2020.06.018.
48. Fussey JM, et al. Surgical management of acquired anterior glottic web: a systematic review. J Laryngol Otol. 2019;133(10):867–74.
49. Chiang T, et al. Surgical management of type I and II laryngeal cleft in the pediatric population. Int J Pediatr Otorhinolaryngol. 2014;78(12):2244–9.
50. Yeung JC, et al. International Pediatric Otolaryngology Group: consensus guidelines on the diagnosis and management of type I laryngeal clefts. Int J Pediatr Otorhinolaryngol. 2017;101:51–6.
51. Fraga JC, et al. The association between laryngeal cleft and tracheoesophageal fistula: myth or reality? Laryngoscope. 2015;125(2):469–74.
52. Johnston DR, et al. Laryngeal cleft: evaluation and management. Int J Pediatr Otorhinolaryngol. 2014;78(6):905–11.
53. Raol N, et al. Propranolol for the treatment of subglottic hemangiomas. Int J Pediatr Otorhinolaryngol. 2011;75(12):1510–4.
54. Léauté-Labrèze C, et al. Propranolol for severe hemangiomas of infancy. N Engl J Med. 2008;358(24):2649–51.
55. Hardison S, et al. The use of propranolol in the treatment of subglottic hemangiomas: a literature review and meta-analysis. Int J Pediatr Otorhinolaryngol. 2016;90:175–80.
56. Darrow DH. Management of infantile hemangiomas of the airway. Otolaryngol Clin N Am. 2018;51(1):133–46.
57. Li Y, et al. Vallecular cyst in the pediatric population: evaluation and management. Int J Pediatr Otorhinolaryngol. 2018;113:198–203.
58. Butler CR, et al. Endoscopic airway management of laryngeal sarcoidosis. Arch Otolaryngol Head Neck Surg. 2010;136(3):251–5.
59. Kelleher KJ, et al. Treatment-recalcitrant laryngeal sarcoidosis responsive to sirolimus. BMJ Case Rep. 2020;13(8):e235372.
60. Eustaquio ME, et al. Multilevel airway involvement in children with Wegener's granulomatosis: clinical course and the utility of a multidisciplinary approach. Arch Otolaryngol Head Neck Surg. 2011;137(5):480–5.
61. Rahbar R, et al. The biology and management of laryngeal neurofibroma. Arch Otolaryngol Head Neck Surg. 2004;130(12):1400–6.

Recurrent Respiratory Papillomatosis

14

Frederik G. Dikkers, Riaz Y. Seedat, and Michel R. M. San Giorgi

Key Points
- Recurrent respiratory papillomatosis (RRP) is a condition induced by human papillomavirus (HPV), characterized by recurrent growths of intraluminal papillomas in the airway.
- Patients present with dysphonia (both roughness and breathiness), coughing, and eventually airway obstruction.
- The disease can occur in both children and adults.
- The most common causative HPV types are HPV6 and HPV11.
- In the absence of a curative treatment, patients have to undergo frequent surgical treatment.
- Due to the debilitating and progressive nature of the disease, early recognition and treatment of the disorder are necessary.
- Introducing prophylactic vaccination against HPV6 and HPV11, as implemented in many countries, is critical to reduce the incidence of RRP.

F. G. Dikkers (✉)
Department of Otorhinolaryngology, Amsterdam University Medical Centers, University of Amsterdam, Amsterdam, The Netherlands
e-mail: f.g.dikkers@amsterdamumc.nl

R. Y. Seedat
Department of Otorhinolaryngology, Faculty of Health Sciences, University of the Free State, Bloemfontein, South Africa
e-mail: seedatry@ufs.ac.za

M. R. M. San Giorgi
Department of Otorhinolaryngology, Head and Neck Surgery, University Medical Center Groningen, Groningen, The Netherlands
e-mail: m.r.m.san.giorgi@umcg.nl

14.1 Introduction

Recurrent respiratory papillomatosis (RRP) is a human papillomavirus (HPV)-induced disease characterized by recurrent growth of respiratory papillomas, mainly in the larynx. The most frequent causative types are HPV6 and HPV11. The condition can cause significant morbidity, can affect quality of life, and can be life-threatening. Correct diagnosis and treatment are therefore of great importance.

14.2 Epidemiology

There are two clinical presentations: juvenile-onset RRP (JoRRP), where the onset of disease is below the age of 12 years, and adult-onset RRP

M. Remacle, H. E. Eckel (eds.), *Textbook of Surgery of Larynx and Trachea*,
https://doi.org/10.1007/978-3-031-09621-1_14

(AoRRP). These two types mainly differ in severity, with JoRRP being more aggressive.

The overall incidence and prevalence of RRP are similar in Europe, Africa, and South America (Table 14.1). AoRRP predominates in Europe, North America, and South America, as opposed to sub-Saharan Africa where JoRRP predominates (Tables 14.2 and 14.3) [1–18]. In Europe, there are three peaks in the incidence of the disease, at around 7, 35, and 64 years [19]. In sub-Saharan Africa, the last peak of AoRRP is absent, with a large peak at around 5 years and a smaller peak at around 45 years [3].

The incidence and prevalence of JoRRP in developing countries are similar to or slightly higher than that in developed countries (Table 14.2), but these data are probably underestimated for developing countries as patients often have symptoms that are not sufficiently severe to present or demise due to upper airway obstruc-

Table 14.1 Incidence and prevalence of recurrent respiratory papillomatosis

Region	Incidence per 100,000 population	Prevalence per 100,000 population per year
Funen and Jutland, Denmark (1965–1984) [1]	0.38	
United Kingdom (2014–2015) [2]		1.42
Free State, South Africa (2011–2015) [3]	0.51	1.39
São Paulo State, Brazil [6]	0.50	0.97

Table 14.2 Incidence and prevalence of juvenile-onset recurrent respiratory papillomatosis (JoRRP)

Region	Incidence per 100,000 children	Prevalence per 100,000 children per year
Funen and Jutland, Denmark (1965–1984) [1]	0.36	
Copenhagen, Denmark (1980–1983) [7]	0.6	0.8
Denmark (1974–1993) [11]	0.35	
Norway (1987–2009) [4]	0.17	
USA (1993–1994) [8]	4.3	
Atlanta and Seattle, USA (1996) [5]	0.12–2.13	1.00–3.97
USA (2006) [9]	0.51–1.03	1.45–2.93
Canada (1994–2007) [12]	0.24	1.11
Free State, South Africa (2011–2015) [3]	1.34	3.88
Lesotho (2011–2013) [10]	0.49	1.04
Japan [16]	0.1	
Thailand [16]	2.8	
Republic of Korea (2002–2015) [17]	0.3	
Australia (1998–2008) [15]		0.6–1.1
Australia (2000–2013) [13]		0.81
Australia (2012–2016) [14]	0.068	

Table 14.3 Incidence and prevalence of adult-onset recurrent respiratory papillomatosis (AoRRP)

Region	Incidence per 100,000 adults	Prevalence per 100,000 adults per year
Funen and Jutland, Denmark (1965–1984) [1]	0.39	
Copenhagen, Denmark (1980–1983) [18]	0.8	2.3
Norway (1987–2009) [4]	0.54	
USA [8]	1.8	
Free State, South Africa (2011–2015) [3]	0.18	0.38

tion prior to presentation. In Australia, the prevalence of JoRRP is lower than in other parts of the world, with an incidence that is declining following introduction of a HPV vaccination program including coverage of HPV6 and HPV11 [14].

14.3 Human Papillomavirus

Human papillomaviruses are non-enveloped DNA viruses that belong to the family *Papillomaviridae* [20]. The virion particle consists of a circular double-stranded DNA genome of approximately 8000 base pairs [20]. The HPV genome is divided into three regions, the long control region (LCR), early region (E1, E2, E4, E5, E6, and E7), and late region (L1 and L2) [20]. Expression and replication of the viral genes are controlled by E1 and E2 genes, while the E6 and E7 genes induce cellular proliferation, downregulate the tumor suppressors p53 and pRb, and influence the immune response by affecting several immunological pathways.

Classification of HPVs is based on the nucleotide sequence of the L1 gene, the most conserved region of the viral genome, with the L1 gene of different HPV types having less than 90% similarity [21]. Over 220 human papillomavirus (HPV) types have been identified [22]. RRP is caused mainly by HPV6 and/or HPV11 [14, 16, 23–33], the same HPV types that cause genital warts, although other types have been implicated in some studies [28, 32–34].

Variants of an HPV type have less than 2% similarity in the L1 gene [21]. Intratypic variants of HPV6 and HPV11 vary by geographic area but are not as geographically restricted as high-risk types [35–37].

14.4 Immune Response

HPV interferes with innate immunity and skews the adaptive immune response to a Th2-like or T-regulatory cell phenotype, instead of a more effective Th1-like response [38]. The change in immune response causes a virus-friendly cell environment, which allows the virus to evade normal clearance. Patients with RRP seem to be more prone to this change in immune responsiveness. HLA gene patterns and innate immune cell receptor expression have shown to differ between the general population and patients with RRP [39].

14.5 Etiology

HPV transmission in JoRRP is believed to occur during birth as the fetus passes through an infected birth canal. Primigravidae are more likely to have a long second stage of labor with prolonged exposure of the baby to HPV in the birth canal, leading to a higher chance of infection in the first-born child. While a minority of mothers of children with RRP have a history of genital condylomata, most have histological evidence of HPV infection [40].

In AoRRP, HPV infection is believed to be sexually transmitted, but may also be as a result of infection acquired at birth remaining latent until adulthood [41]. Activation of latent viral infection as a result of age-associated loss of immunity has been suggested for the last age group [19].

Papillomata occur mainly at sites at which ciliated and squamous epithelia are juxtaposed [42]. Squamous metaplasia following surgical trauma results in new iatrogenic squamociliary junctions being created. Tracheotomy also causes iatrogenic squamociliary junctions and often results in papillomata surrounding the tracheotomy opening and tip of the cannula.

14.6 Clinical Presentation

Patients with JoRRP usually present between the ages of 2 and 9 years, but cases with papillomata in the neonatal period have been described, and some patients may present as teenagers with symptoms for many years [3–5, 11–14, 32, 43, 44]. Boys and girls are equally affected.

The first symptom is progressive dysphonia, followed by stridor and difficulty with breathing. Recurrent upper respiratory tract infections, chronic cough, and hemoptysis are other symptoms that may occur. Patients are frequently misdiagnosed as having asthma, laryngotracheobronchitis, foreign body aspiration, or laryngomalacia. In developing countries, patients often present with a history of hoarseness for many years and upper airway obstruction as a result of the poor availability and accessibility of healthcare services. In rare cases, pulmonary hypertension and cor pulmonale may occur as a complication of chronic upper airway obstruction [45].

Patients with AoRRP usually present with progressive dysphonia (both roughness and breathiness) or cough and rarely with dyspnea. In rare cases, sore throat is an initial symptom.

Patients from the first adult peak usually present in their late twenties to thirties. Often there is persistent dysphonia after a specific provoking incident. The second peak of AoRRP is in the early sixties. These patients often have no provoking incident. RRP may even be an incidental finding during intubation, without the patient having any complaints. Males are more commonly affected than females [4, 41].

The larynx is the most frequently affected site, with the trachea being the most common site of extralaryngeal involvement. Other extralaryngeal sites that may be involved include the nose, nasopharynx, oral cavity, oropharynx, and lungs. Extralaryngeal spread is significantly more common in patients with HPV11 disease [46]. Malignant transformation is rare but may occur in both laryngeal and pulmonary papillomas. The absence of HPV in the papillomata has been associated with malignant transformation with AoRRP [47].

14.7 Diagnosis

All patients with progressive or persistent hoarseness, stridor, and/or respiratory distress should undergo flexible laryngoscopy or direct laryngoscopy and biopsy [48]. The papillomata are recognizable as exophytic, pedunculated, or lobulated masses which may be single or multiple (Fig. 14.1). Histologically, the papillomata are exophytic finger-like protrusions of keratinized squamous epithelium overlying a layer of connective tissue stroma, with basal cell layer hyperplasia and abnormal keratinization (Fig. 14.2). Inspection of the airway should be extended up to the carina during the first surgery so that distant extension of papillomata can be found early and treated. Use of narrow-band imaging (NBI) can be very helpful in discerning the lesions (Fig. 14.3) [49]. Tumor evaporation by laser is not recommended at the first surgical

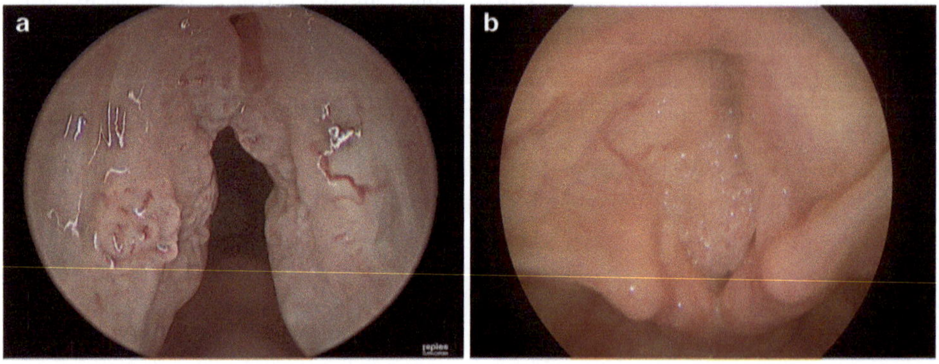

Fig. 14.1 Variety of perioperative laryngeal images of patients suffering from recurrent respiratory papillomatosis, with papilloma growth in different (supra)glottic locations and severity. Age and gender of patients shown in figure. (**a**) A 9-year-old female. (**b**) A 10-year-old female. (**c**) An 18-year-old female. (**d**) A 25-year-old female. (**e**) A 45-year-old female. (**f**) An 11-year-old male. (**g**) A 15-year-old male. (**h**) A 16-year-old male. (**i**) An 18-year-old male. (**j**) A 29-year-old male. (**k**) A 33-year-old male. (**l**) A 48-year-old male. (**m**) A 61-year-old male. (**n**) A 66-year-old male

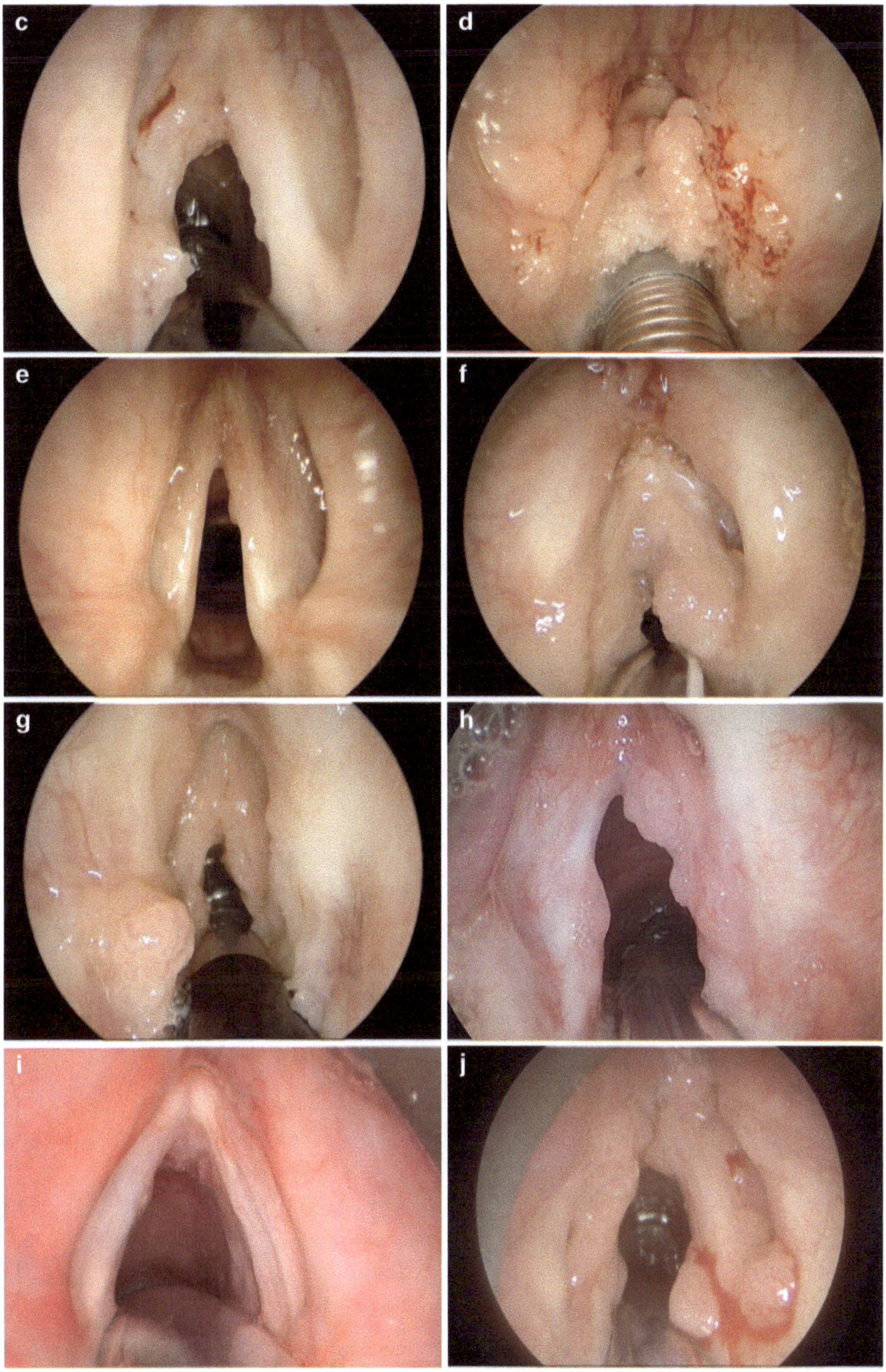

Fig. 14.1 (continued)

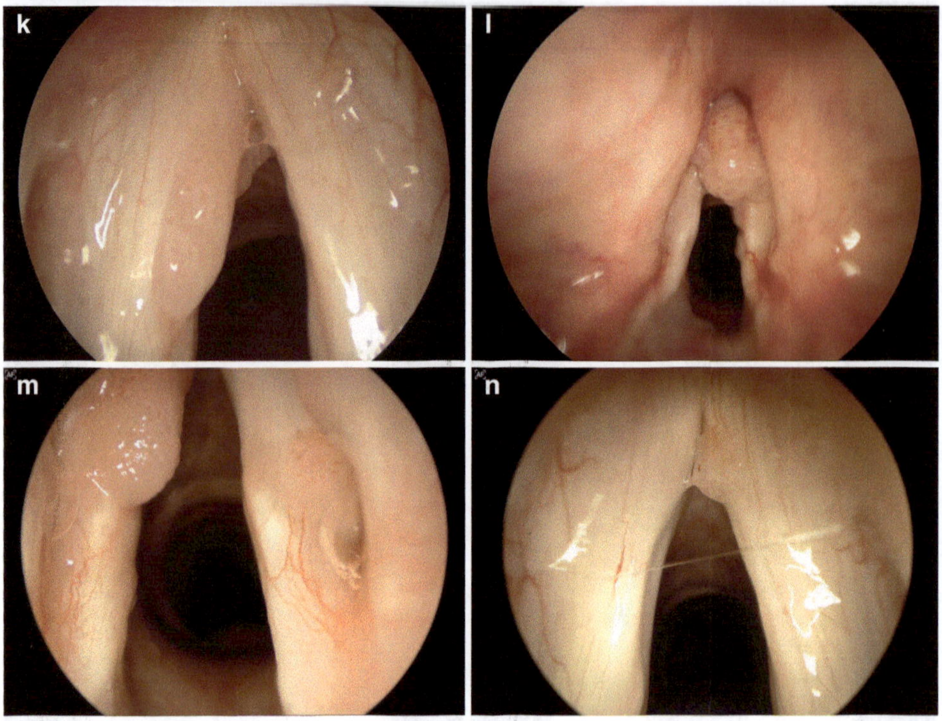

Fig. 14.1 (continued)

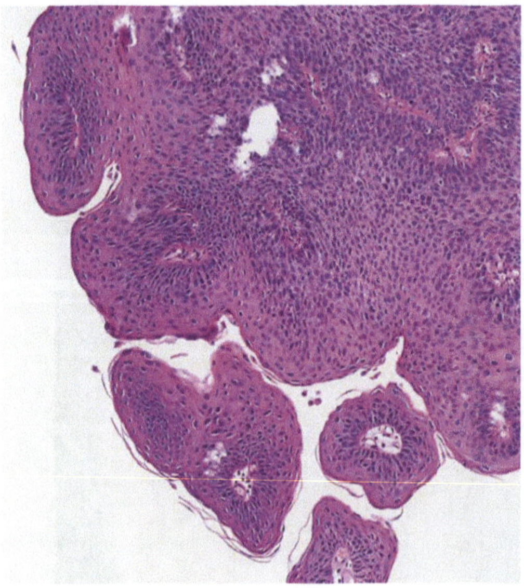

Fig. 14.2 Histological section (HE staining, original magnification 100×) of biopsy of recurrent respiratory papilloma of right true vocal cord. There are conspicuous finger-shaped protrusions that are cut transversely

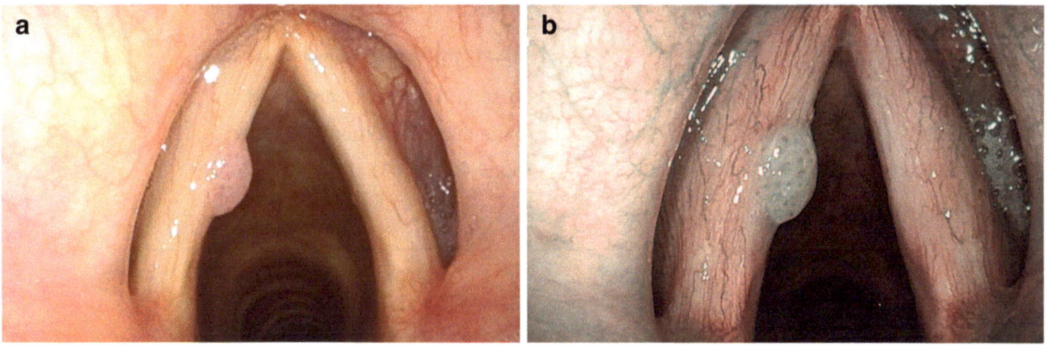

Fig. 14.3 Laryngeal papilloma (**a**) without narrow-band imaging and (**b**) with narrow-band imaging

procedure as tissue should be collected for histological examination and HPV typing. An early laryngeal carcinoma may macroscopically appear similar to papilloma. Chest imaging by either chest X-ray or CT scan should be performed in patients with pulmonary symptoms or signs, although CT scanning in all patients is being advocated [50].

14.8 Clinical Course

The clinical behavior of RRP is variable and unpredictable. In most patients, the frequency of surgery decreases over time, but in about one-third of cases, the surgical frequency remains constant or increases [11, 12, 15, 26, 46, 48, 51]. Although the disease eventually goes into remission in the most patients, some may have active RRP for many years. Recurrence may occur after many years of remission as the latent viral infection persists in the laryngeal tissue [46]. At least 50% of children with RRP require more than ten surgical procedures to control their disease, and 4–7% of all patients undergo more than a hundred procedures in their lifetime [46].

14.9 Quality of Life

The recurrent and persistent nature of the disease, need for frequent surgery, and dysphonia adversely affect the quality of life (QoL) of patients and place a significant social burden on the families of affected children [27, 52, 53]. In comparison with controls, adult RRP patients have more voice problems and a lower general health perception and are anxious [52]. Although all patients are more prone than average to depression and anxiety, older women suffer the most. Voice handicap has been found to be associated with smoking [52]. Screening for RRP-related psychosocial, practical, and medical problems that might be overlooked in normal outpatient clinic visits has been shown to significantly improve distress [54].

14.10 Staging

Several disease scoring systems have been proposed [25, 55, 56]. The most commonly used scoring system is the Derkay scoring system (Fig. 14.4) [56]. This system encompasses both a functional assessment of the patient, in which the severity of the hoarseness and degree of airway obstruction are assessed, and an anatomical assessment of the extent of disease. The respiratory tract, including the larynx, is divided into anatomical subsites, and all areas are scored based on the size of the papillomata on a scale 0–3. Scoring is difficult to carry out retrospectively as symptoms and extralaryngeal papillomata are also scored, but this staging system is widely used on a prospective basis.

Clinical score:

Describe the patient's voice today:	Normal(0) / Abnormal(1) / Aphonic(2)
Describe the patient's stridor today:	Absent(0) / With activity(1) / At rest(2)
Describe the urgency of today's intervention:	Scheduled(0) / Urgent(1) / Emergent(2)
Describe today's level of respiratory distress:	None(0) / Mild(1) / Moderate(2) / Severe(3) / Extreme(4)

Total clinical score:________

Anatomical score:

For each site, score as: 0=None, 1=Surface lesion, 2=Raised lesion, 3=Bulky lesion

Larynx:

Epiglottis	Lingual surface:_____	Laryngeal surface:_____
Aryepiglottic folds	Left:_____	Right:_____
Arytenoids	Left:_____	Right:_____
True Vocal Cords	Left:_____	Right:_____
False Vocal Cords	Left:_____	Right:_____

Anterior commissure:_____

Posterior commissure:_____

Subglottis:_____

Trachea:

Upper one-third:_____

Middle one-third:_____

Lower one-third:_____

Bronchi	Left:_____	Right:_____

Tracheostomy stoma:_____

Other:

Nose:_____

Palate:_____

Pharynx:_____

Oesophagus:_____

Lungs:_____

Other:_____

Total anatomical score:_______

Total score (Total clinical score + Total anatomical score):_______

Fig. 14.4 The Derkay staging system for recurrent respiratory papillomatosis [56]

14.11 Disease Severity

Involvement of multiple levels of the larynx or, specifically, of the subglottis at initial presentation is associated with more severe disease [57]. Histologically, the presence of atypical mitoses and of mitoses above the basal cell layer of the epithelium has been associated with more severe disease, but no such association has been found with the degree of dysplasia [58].

Most studies have found that patients with HPV11-induced RRP have more aggressive disease than those with HPV6-induced RRP [25–28, 46]. HPV typing is therefore a possible tool to detect disease aggressiveness [46, 59]. However, younger age at diagnosis is also associated with more aggressive disease and has been found to be a more significant marker of aggressiveness than HPV type [30, 46].

The possible role of intratypic variants in differences in severity of respiratory papillomatosis is unclear. Although functional differences have been found between intratypic variants of HPV6 and HPV11 [60, 61], there does not appear to be a difference in disease aggressiveness between variants of a particular HPV type [62].

A maternal history of condyloma acuminata appears to be associated with more aggressive JoRRP [30, 40]. Gastroesophageal reflux disease and asthma have previously been suspected to be associated with aggressive disease, but this has not been shown to be the case [46, 63].

14.12 Surgery

As there is no cure, treatment consists of repeated microlaryngoscopic procedures to remove the papillomata while maintaining the normal laryngeal tissue until the patient goes into remission. The goal of surgical interventions should not be to remove all visible papillomata. Even if they are all removed, the disease is expected to recur as HPV DNA is found in the adjacent macroscopically uninvolved laryngeal tissue and other adjacent anatomical sites. Removal of the papillomata is performed using various methods, such as cold steel instruments, microdebrider, laser (CO_2, KTP, or pulse dye laser), or coblation, depending on surgeon's preference and availability of equipment [48]. The use of a laser or microdebrider has not been associated with a longer intersurgical interval, while treatment with the microdebrider may result in a better voice outcome compared with the CO_2 laser [64].

It may be necessary to stage surgical interventions, in order to prevent synechia formation in the anterior commissure. In the authors' experience, a 6-week interval between surgeries on the two sides of the anterior commissure seems to be sufficient.

Further procedures are performed based on the severity of the disease of an individual patient. A watchful waiting policy should be considered in the absence of voice or airway complaints.

Laryngeal complications such as anterior commissure synechiae, scarring of superficial vocal cord epithelium on the underlying layers, ventral glottic stenosis, dorsal glottic stenosis, and granuloma formation from repeated surgical procedures are common [31]. These complications result in abnormal voice quality in the long term, with a higher number of surgical procedures correlating with the development of complications and poorer voice quality [15, 64, 65].

A tracheotomy may be required for patients with airway obstruction. The presence of a tracheotomy has been associated with possible spread of papillomata to the trachea and lower airways, but this view is controversial. Tracheotomies are usually for patients with the most aggressive disease, who may develop distal spread regardless of whether or not they had a tracheotomy [31, 48]. The tracheotomy rate in developed countries is generally low, but is much higher in developing countries, mainly because the expertise to manage patients with RRP is not as readily available.

14.13 Adjuvant Treatment

Adjuvant treatments that have been used in RRP include indole-3-carbinol, mumps vaccination, MMR vaccination, HPV vaccination, interferon-α, bevacizumab, cidofovir, programmed cell death protein 1 (PD-1 inhibitors), and celecoxib. The highly variable disease course makes it difficult to determine the effectiveness of these treatments. Use of programmed cell death protein 1 (PD-1), celecoxib, and heat shock protein E7 is no longer recommended in the treatment of JoRRP [48].

Cidofovir and bevacizumab are mainly used as intralesional therapies. Cidofovir is a cytosine nucleotide analog that blocks DNA virus replication by inhibiting viral DNA polymerase. Several uncontrolled and retrospective studies have shown that intralesional cidofovir is effective for RRP with about 40–50% of patients achieving remission [55, 66]. However, a systematic review of adjuvant antiviral therapy for the treatment of RRP identified only one randomized, double-blind, placebo-controlled trial of intralesional cidofovir administered at the time of surgical debulking that showed significant clinical improvements in both the cidofovir and placebo groups and no significant difference between the two groups [66, 67]. It would be extremely difficult to perform a large prospective randomized trial of intralesional cidofovir because of the small number of patients.

Bevacizumab is a recombinant human monoclonal antibody that blocks angiogenesis by binding to human vascular endothelial growth factor A (VEGF-A) [68]. Intralesional bevacizumab has been shown to extend the intersurgical interval in small series, while systemic bevacizumab has been shown to be of benefit in case studies of patients with severe RRP [68, 69]. However, systemic use of bevacizumab might become the treatment of first choice [70, 71].

Of the three HPV vaccines available in 2022, the bivalent vaccine (Cervarix®), the quadrivalent vaccine (Gardasil®), and the nonavalent vaccine (Gardasil® 9), two (Gardasil® and Gardasil® 9) protect against HPV6 and HPV11. In Australia, a significant decrease in the incidence of JoRRP was observed following the introduction of a national vaccination program with a high uptake using the quadrivalent HPV vaccine in 2007 [14]. This is probably due to the decreased prevalence of HPV6 and HPV11 genital infection in the Australian population resulting in a reduction of intrapartum transmission of the virus [14]. There were no new cases of JoRRP reported in Australia in 2018 and 2019 [72]. The introduction of vaccines that are protective against HPV6 and HPV11 would probably have a greater impact in regions with a higher incidence of JoRRP.

Although these are prophylactic vaccines, they have also been used as adjuvant therapy for patients with RRP, mainly in adults. There are two proposed mechanisms of action: inhibition of latent HPV infection in the mucosa surrounding the surgical site by antibodies produced in response to the vaccine and activation of the cell-mediated response by the vaccine. A systematic review and meta-analysis found a statistically significant reduction in the mean number of surgical procedures per month after use of the HPV vaccine as a therapeutic agent [73].

14.14 Speech Therapy

Most patients have poor voice quality that can range from mild hoarseness to aphonia [52, 65]. While speech therapy can be used for most benign vocal cord abnormalities, surgery is the treatment of choice for dysphonia due to RRP. Speech therapy can be considered as complementary to surgery or if surgical options for a scarred larynx are not considered feasible.

14.15 Conclusion

RRP is a condition that initially manifests itself as hoarseness, but can lead to life-threatening obstruction of the upper airway. Treatment requires repeated surgical procedures as there is no cure.

References

1. Lindeberg H, Elbrønd O. Laryngeal papillomas: the epidemiology in a Danish subpopulation 1965–1984. Clin Otolaryngol Allied Sci. 1990;15:125–31.
2. Donne AJ, Keltie K, Cole H, Sims AJ, Patrick H, Powell S. Prevalence and management of recurrent

respiratory papillomatosis (RRP) in the UK: cross-sectional study. Clin Otolaryngol. 2017;42:86–91.
3. Seedat RY, Schall R. Age of diagnosis, incidence and prevalence of recurrent respiratory papillomatosis-a South African perspective. Clin Otolaryngol. 2018;43:533–7.
4. Omland T, Akre H, Vårdal M, Brøndbo K. Epidemiological aspects of recurrent respiratory papillomatosis: a population-based study. Laryngoscope. 2012;122:1595–9.
5. Armstrong LR, Preston EJ, Reichert M, Phillips DL, Nisenbaum R, Todd NW, et al. Incidence and prevalence of recurrent respiratory papillomatosis among children in Atlanta and Seattle. Clin Infect Dis. 2000;31:107–9.
6. Mercuri G, Rodrigues SA, Martins RHG. An estimate of the incidence and prevalence of laryngeal papillomatosis in São Paulo State (Brasil). Rev Assoc Médica Bras. 2020;66:1247–51.
7. Bomholt A. Juvenile laryngeal papillomatosis. An epidemiological study from the Copenhagen region. Acta Otolaryngol (Stockh). 1988;105:367–71.
8. Derkay CS. Task force on recurrent respiratory papillomas: a preliminary report. Arch Otolaryngol Head Neck Surg. 1995;121:1386–91.
9. Marsico M, Mehta V, Chastek B, Liaw K-L, Derkay C. Estimating the incidence and prevalence of juvenile-onset recurrent respiratory papillomatosis in publicly and privately insured claims databases in the United States. Sex Transm Dis. 2014;41:300–5.
10. Seedat RY. The incidence and prevalence of juvenile-onset recurrent respiratory papillomatosis in the Free State province of South Africa and Lesotho. Int J Pediatr Otorhinolaryngol. 2014;78:2113–5.
11. Silverberg MJ, Thorsen P, Lindeberg H, Ahdieh-Grant L, Shah KV. Clinical course of recurrent respiratory papillomatosis in Danish children. Arch Otolaryngol Head Neck Surg. 2004;130:711–6.
12. Campisi P, Hawkes M, Simpson K. The epidemiology of juvenile onset recurrent respiratory papillomatosis derived from a population level national database. Laryngoscope. 2010;120:1233–45.
13. Novakovic D, Cheng ATL, Baguley K, Walker P, Harrison H, Soma M, et al. Juvenile recurrent respiratory papillomatosis: 10-year audit and Australian prevalence estimates. Laryngoscope. 2016;126:2827–32.
14. Novakovic D, Cheng ATL, Zurynski Y, Booy R, Walker PJ, Berkowitz R, et al. A prospective study of the incidence of juvenile-onset recurrent respiratory papillomatosis after implementation of a National HPV Vaccination Program. J Infect Dis. 2018;217:208–12.
15. Novakovic D, Cheng ATL, Cope DH, Brotherton JML. Estimating the prevalence of and treatment patterns for juvenile onset recurrent respiratory papillomatosis in Australia pre-vaccination: a pilot study. Sex Health. 2010;7:253–61.
16. Ushikai M, Fujiyoshi T, Kono M, Antrasena S, Oda H, Yoshida H, et al. Detection and cloning of human papillomavirus DNA associated with recurrent respiratory papillomatosis in Thailand. Jpn J Cancer Res. 1994;85:699–703.
17. Oh JK, Choi HY, Han M, Jung YS, Lee SJ, Ki M. Estimated incidence of juvenile-onset recurrent respiratory papillomatosis in Korea. Epidemiol Health. 2021;43:e2021019.
18. Bomholt A. Laryngeal papillomas with adult onset. An epidemiological study from the Copenhagen region. Acta Otolaryngol (Stockh). 1988;106:140–4.
19. San Giorgi MRM, van den Heuvel ER, Tjon Pian Gi REA, Brunings JW, Chirila M, Friedrich G, et al. Age of onset of recurrent respiratory papillomatosis: a distribution analysis. Clin Otolaryngol. 2016;41:448–53.
20. IARC Working Group on the Evaluation of Carcinogenic Risks to Humans. IARC monographs on the evaluation of carcinogenic risks to humans, Vol. 100B. A review of human carcinogens. Part B: Biological agents. International Agency for Research on Cancer: Lyon, France; 2012.
21. de Villiers E-M, Fauquet C, Broker TR, Bernard H-U, zur Hausen H. Classification of papillomaviruses. Virology. 2004;324:17–27.
22. Mühr LSA, Eklund C, Dillner J. Towards quality and order in human papillomavirus research. Virology. 2018;519:74–6.
23. Abramson AL, Steinberg BM, Winkler B. Laryngeal papillomatosis: clinical, histopathologic and molecular studies. Laryngoscope. 1987;97:678–85.
24. Komloš KF, Kocjan BJ, Košorok P, Luzar B, Meglič L, Potočnik M, et al. Tumor-specific and gender-specific pre-vaccination distribution of human papillomavirus types 6 and 11 in anogenital warts and laryngeal papillomas: a study on 574 tissue specimens. J Med Virol. 2012;84:1233–41.
25. Wiatrak BJ, Wiatrak DW, Broker TR, Lewis L. Recurrent respiratory papillomatosis: a longitudinal study comparing severity associated with human papilloma viral types 6 and 11 and other risk factors in a large pediatric population. Laryngoscope. 2004;114:1–23.
26. Seedat RY, Thukane M, Jansen AC, Rossouw I, Goedhals D, Burt FJ. HPV types causing juvenile recurrent laryngeal papillomatosis in South Africa. Int J Pediatr Otorhinolaryngol. 2010;74:255–9.
27. Montaño-Velázquez BB, Nolasco-Renero J, Parada-Bañuelos JE, Garcia-Vázquez F, Flores-Medina S, García-Romero CS, et al. Quality of life of young patients with recurrent respiratory papillomatosis. J Laryngol Otol. 2017;131:425–8.
28. Pou AM, Rimell FL, Jordan JA, Shoemaker DL, Johnson JT, Barua P, et al. Adult respiratory papillomatosis: human papillomavirus type and viral coinfections as predictors of prognosis. Ann Otol Rhinol Laryngol. 1995;104:758–62.
29. Kocjan BJ, Gale N, Hocevar Boltezar I, Seme K, Fujs Komlos K, Hosnjak L, et al. Identical human papillomavirus (HPV) genomic variants persist in recurrent respiratory papillomatosis for up to 22 years. J Infect Dis. 2013;207(4):583–7.

30. Buchinsky FJ, Valentino WL, Ruszkay N, Powell E, Derkay CS, Seedat RY, et al. Age at diagnosis, but not HPV type, is strongly associated with clinical course in recurrent respiratory papillomatosis. PLoS One. 2019;14:e0216697.
31. Soldatski IL, Onufrieva EK, Steklov AM, Schepin NV. Tracheal, bronchial, and pulmonary papillomatosis in children. Laryngoscope. 2005;115:1848–54.
32. Sanchez GI, Jaramillo R, Cuello G, Quintero K, Baena A, O'Byrne A, et al. Human papillomavirus genotype detection in recurrent respiratory papillomatosis (RRP) in Colombia. Head Neck. 2013;35(2):229–34.
33. Gerein V, Rastorguev E, Gerein J, Draf W, Schirren J. Incidence, age at onset, and potential reasons of malignant transformation in recurrent respiratory papillomatosis patients: 20 years experience. Otolaryngol Neck Surg. 2005;132:392–4.
34. Peñaloza-Plascencia M, Montoya-Fuentes H, Flores-Martínez SE, Fierro-Velasco FJ, Peñaloza-González JM, Sánchez-Corona J. Molecular identification of 7 human papillomavirus types in recurrent respiratory papillomatosis. Arch Otolaryngol Head Neck Surg. 2000;126:1119–23.
35. Combrinck CE, Seedat RY, Randall C, Roodt Y, Burt FJ. Novel HPV-6 variants of human papillomavirus causing recurrent respiratory papillomatosis in southern Africa. Epidemiol Infect. 2012;140:1095–101.
36. Jelen MM, Chen Z, Kocjan BJ, Burt FJ, Chan PKS, Chouhy D, et al. Global genomic diversity of human papillomavirus 6 based on 724 isolates and 190 complete genome sequences. J Virol. 2014;88:7307–16.
37. Jelen MM, Chen Z, Kocjan BJ, Hošnjak L, Burt FJ, Chan PKS, et al. Global genomic diversity of human papillomavirus 11 based on 433 isolates and 78 complete genome sequences. J Virol. 2016;90:5503–13.
38. Ivancic R, Iqbal H, deSilva B, Pan Q, Matrka L. Immunological tolerance of low-risk HPV in recurrent respiratory papillomatosis. Clin Exp Immunol. 2020;199:131–42.
39. Bonagura VR, Du Z, Ashouri E, Luo L, Hatam LJ, DeVoti JA, et al. Activating killer cell immunoglobulin-like receptors 3DS1 and 2DS1 protect against developing the severe form of recurrent respiratory papillomatosis. Hum Immunol. 2010;71:212–9.
40. Gerein V, Schmandt S, Babkina N, Barysik N, Coerdt W, Pfister H. Human papilloma virus (HPV)-associated gynecological alteration in mothers of children with recurrent respiratory papillomatosis during long-term observation. Cancer Detect Prev. 2007;31:276–81.
41. Kashima HK, Shah F, Lyles A, Glackin R, Muhammad N, Turner L, et al. A comparison of risk factors in juvenile-onset and adult-onset recurrent respiratory papillomatosis. Laryngoscope. 1992;102:9–13.
42. Kashima H, Mounts P, Leventhal B, Hruban RH. Sites of predilection in recurrent respiratory papillomatosis. Ann Otol Rhinol Laryngol. 1993;102:580–3.
43. Armstrong LR, Derkay CS, Reeves WC. Initial results from the national registry for juvenile-onset recurrent respiratory papillomatosis. RRP Task Force. Arch Otolaryngol Head Neck Surg. 1999;125:743–8.
44. Lindeberg H, Elbrønd O. Laryngeal papillomas: clinical aspects in a series of 231 patients. Clin Otolaryngol. 1989;14:333–42.
45. Grobbelaar J, Seedat RY, Brown S, Claassen AJ. Pulmonary hypertension due to recurrent juvenile laryngeal papillomatosis. Int J Pediatr Otorhinolaryngol. 2005;69:1279–82.
46. Tjon Pian Gi REA, San Giorgi MRM, Slagter-Menkema L, van Hemel BM, van der Laan BFAM, van den Heuvel ER, et al. Clinical course of recurrent respiratory papillomatosis: comparison between aggressiveness of human papillomavirus-6 and human papillomavirus-11. Head Neck. 2015;37:1625–32.
47. Omland T, Lie KA, Akre H, Sandlie LE, Jebsen P, Sandvik L, et al. Recurrent respiratory papillomatosis: HPV genotypes and risk of high-grade laryngeal neoplasia. PLoS One. 2014;9:e99114.
48. Lawlor C, Balakrishnan K, Bottero S, Boudewyns A, Campisi P, Carter J, et al. International Pediatric Otolaryngology Group (IPOG): juvenile-onset recurrent respiratory papillomatosis consensus recommendations. Int J Pediatr Otorhinolaryngol. 2020;128:109697.
49. Zwakenberg M, Plaat B. A photographic atlas of lesions in the pharynx and larynx: conventional white light imaging versus narrow band imaging. Groningen: Olympus OEKG/University Medical Center Groningen (UMCG); 2019.
50. Pai SI, Wasserman I, Ji YD, Gilman M, Hung YP, Faquin WC, Mino-Kenudson M, Muniappan A. Pulmonary manifestations of chronic HPV infection in patients with recurrent respiratory papillomatosis. Lancet Respir Med. 2022;18:S2213-2600(22)00008-X.
51. Ongkasuwan J, Friedman EM. Juvenile recurrent respiratory papilloma: variable intersurgical intervals. Laryngoscope. 2012;122:2844–9.
52. San Giorgi MRM, Aaltonen L-M, Rihkanen H, Tjon Pian Gi REA, van der Laan BFAM, Hoekstra-Weebers JEHM, et al. Quality of life of patients with recurrent respiratory papillomatosis. Laryngoscope. 2017;127:1826–31.
53. Chadha NK, Allegro J, Barton M, Hawkes M, Harlock H, Campisi P. The quality of life and health utility burden of recurrent respiratory papillomatosis in children. Otolaryngol Head Neck Surg. 2010;143:685–90.
54. San Giorgi MRM, Aaltonen L-M, Rihkanen H, Tjon Pian Gi REA, van der Laan BFAM, Hoekstra-Weebers JEHM, et al. Validation of the distress thermometer and problem list in patients with recurrent respiratory papillomatosis. Otolaryngol Head Neck Surg. 2017;156:180–8.
55. Dikkers FG. Treatment of recurrent respiratory papillomatosis with microsurgery in combination with intralesional cidofovir—a prospective study. Eur Arch Otorhinolaryngol. 2006;263:440–3.

56. Derkay CS, Malis DJ, Zalzal G, Wiatrak BJ, Kashima HK, Coltrera MD. A staging system for assessing severity of disease and response to therapy in recurrent respiratory papillomatosis. Laryngoscope. 1998;108:935–7.
57. Moreddu E, Lambert E, Kacmarynski D, Nicollas R, Triglia J-M, Smith RJ. Risk factors for severity of juvenile-onset recurrent respiratory papillomatosis at first endoscopy. Eur Ann Otorhinolaryngol Head Neck Dis. 2019;136:25–8.
58. El Achkar VNR, Duarte A, Carlos R, León JE, Ribeiro-Silva A, Pignatari SSN, et al. Histopathological features of juvenile-onset laryngeal papillomatosis related to severity. Head Neck. 2019;41:1412–7.
59. Combrinck CE, Seedat RY, Burt FJ. FRET-based detection and genotyping of HPV-6 and HPV-11 causing recurrent respiratory papillomatosis. J Virol Methods. 2013;189:271–6.
60. Seedat RY, Combrinck CE, Bester PA, Lee J-Y, Burt FJ. Determination of the complete genome and functional analysis of HPV6 isolate VBD19/10 from a patient with aggressive recurrent respiratory papillomatosis. Epidemiol Infect. 2016;144:2128–35.
61. Measso do Bonfim C, Simão Sobrinho J, Lacerda Nogueira R, Salgado Kupper D, Cardoso Pereira Valera F, Lacerda Nogueira M, et al. Differences in transcriptional activity of human papillomavirus type 6 molecular variants in recurrent respiratory papillomatosis. PLoS One. 2015;10:e0132325.
62. Sichero L, Ferreira S, López RVM, Mello BP, Costa V, El-Achkar VNR, Carlos R, Ribeiro-Silva A, Pignatari S, Kaminagakura E, Villa LL. Prevalence of human papillomavirus 6 and 11 variants in recurrent respiratory papillomatosis. J Med Virol. 2021;93(6):3835–40.
63. San Giorgi MRM, Helder HM, Lindeman R-JS, de Bock GH, Dikkers FG. The association between gastroesophageal reflux disease and recurrent respiratory papillomatosis: a systematic review. Laryngoscope. 2016;126:2330–9.
64. Holler T, Allegro J, Chadha NK, Hawkes M, Harrison RV, Forte V, et al. Voice outcomes following repeated surgical resection of laryngeal papillomata in children. Otolaryngol Head Neck Surg. 2009;141:522–6.
65. Ilmarinen T, Nissilä H, Rihkanen H, Roine RP, Pietarinen-Runtti P, Pitkäranta A, et al. Clinical features, health-related quality of life, and adult voice in juvenile-onset recurrent respiratory papillomatosis. Laryngoscope. 2011;121:846–51.
66. McMurray JS, Connor N, Ford CN. Cidofovir efficacy in recurrent respiratory papillomatosis: a randomized, double-blind, placebo-controlled study. Ann Otol Rhinol Laryngol. 2008;117:477–83.
67. Chadha NK, James A. Adjuvant antiviral therapy for recurrent respiratory papillomatosis. Cochrane Database Syst Rev. 2012;12:CD005053.
68. Maturo S, Hartnick CJ. Use of 532-nm pulsed potassium titanyl phosphate laser and adjuvant intralesional bevacizumab for aggressive respiratory papillomatosis in children: initial experience. Arch Otolaryngol Head Neck Surg. 2010;136:561–5.
69. Ryan MA, Leu GR, Upchurch PA, Tunkel DE, Walsh JM, Boss EF. Systemic Bevacizumab (Avastin) for Juvenile-Onset Recurrent Respiratory Papillomatosis: A Systematic Review. Laryngoscope. 2021;131(5):1138–46.
70. Pogoda L, Ziylan F, Smeeing DPJ, Dikkers FG, Rinkel RNPM. Bevacizumab as treatment option for recurrent respiratory papillomatosis: a systematic review. Eur Arch Otorhinolaryngol. 2022. https://doi.org/10.1007/s00405-022-07388-6.
71. Derkay CS, Wikner EE, Pransky S, Best SR, Zur K, Sidell DR, Klein A, Rosen C, Dikkers FG, Johnson R. Systemic Use of Bevacizumab for Recurrent Respiratory Papillomatosis: Who, What, Where, When, and Why? Laryngoscope. 2022. https://doi.org/10.1002/lary.30180.
72. Teutsch SM, Nunez CA, Morris A, Booy R, McGregor S, King J, et al. Australian Paediatric Surveillance Unit (APSU) annual surveillance report 2019. Commun Dis Intell. 2020;44:1–20.
73. Rosenberg T, Philipsen BB, Mehlum CS, Dyrvig A-K, Wehberg S, Chirilă M, et al. Therapeutic use of the human papillomavirus vaccine on recurrent respiratory papillomatosis: a systematic review and meta-analysis. J Infect Dis. 2019;219:1016–25.

15 Laryngotracheal Blunt Trauma

Ferhan Öz and M. Barış Karakullukçu

Key Points

- The incidence of laryngotracheal trauma is probably underestimated because the consequence of a laryngotracheal trauma can range from mild hoarseness to complete airway compromise.
- Narrowing of the airway results in breathing difficulty. These are the patients registered in emergency archives. Among these patients, complications such as chronic stenosis and voice changes are as common as 15–25%. The team in charge of the patient has to keep in mind that the airway will become worse with time as the edema increases.
- The elasticity of the cartilage framework contributes to its recoil, saving the airway even if the external pressure or blow is strong enough to exceed the resistance of this structure.
- The larynx and trachea are vulnerable only to direct blows to the anterior of the neck. The object of contact has to approach the larynx in a horizontal manner. If the object is in vertical position relative to the body, the impact will be blocked by the facial skeleton and/or sternum and clavicle heads.
- Fiberoptic laryngoscopy has become the initial evaluation tool. In case the endolarynx cannot be assessed with flexible laryngoscopy due to laryngeal edema, direct laryngoscopy should be carried out under general anesthesia. All of the upper aerodigestive tract mucosa should be examined.
- Cartilage frame fractures are extremely rare in pediatric age group, while soft tissue edema and hematoma are more common. In elderly people, the cartilage framework is usually calcified and underwent osseous transformation. The laryngotracheal fractures in this age group are more common and usually more severe.
- Posterior or lateral dislocations of the arytenoids may occur at this stage when the thyroid cartilage is pressed against the vertebra by external pressure. Posterior dislocation of the arytenoids is reported to be more common; however,

F. Öz (✉)
Department of Otorhinolaryngology, Acıbadem Bakırköy Hospital, Istanbul, Turkey

M. B. Karakullukçu
Department of Head and Neck Surgery and Oncology, Antoni van Leeuwenhoek Hospital, The Netherlands Cancer Institute, Amsterdam, The Netherlands
e-mail: b.karakullukcu@nki.nl

M. Remacle, H. E. Eckel (eds.), *Textbook of Surgery of Larynx and Trachea*,
https://doi.org/10.1007/978-3-031-09621-1_15

this is usually associated with a traumatic orotracheal intubation trauma rather than an external trauma. Dislocations can be confused with vocal cord paralysis. EMG is an important tool to differentiate the two conditions.

- In case of complete disruption between the cricoid cartilage and the trachea, the strap muscles and the surrounding fascia can rarely serve as a temporary airway until the patient is managed by intubation or tracheotomy.
- Once the injuries are addressed and the patient is stabilized and assessed, surgical repair of the larynx and cervical trauma should be done as soon as possible. A patient with minimal soft tissue edema, mobile vocal cords, and no difficulty with breathing can be observed closely.

Laryngotracheal trauma including blunt and penetrating traumas is one of the common reasons of airway compromise. The incidence of this type of injury is probably underestimated because the consequence of a laryngotracheal trauma can range from mild hoarseness to complete airway compromise. In the USA, 1 in 14,000 to 30,000 of emergency room visits is due to laryngotracheal trauma [1, 2]. Many more are unnoticed because the injured person doesn't take mild hoarseness seriously and doesn't apply to the emergency department.

The most common causes are motor vehicle accidents and sports injuries [3, 4]. A decrease in the incidence of laryngotracheal injury was observed, thanks to the safety belt and increased safety features of motor vehicles. The introduction of airbags should eliminate sudden and savage blow of the anterior neck trauma caused with the steering wheel or other hardware on the dashboard as well as injuries caused by misplaced safety belts. However, there is no objective study demonstrating this beneficial effect.

Laryngotracheal trauma due to sports injuries is not uncommon in contact sports like football, basketball, baseball, and soccer. One of the common causes of blunt larynx trauma is biking or traffic accidents, where the larynx is hit against steering bar of the bicycle or the steering wheel of the car.

The degree of injury may vary from mild soft tissue edema to severe laryngeal framework fractures and to complete separation between the larynx and trachea. Mild injuries that result in temporary voice changes or throat pain probably go unregistered in medical archives. This degree of injury is only temporary due to the extreme flexibility and resistance of the laryngotracheal framework. More severe trauma may cause injury to the framework and severe soft tissue edema or hematoma. Narrowing of the airway results in breathing difficulty. These are the patients registered in emergency archives. Among these patients, complication rates are as high as 15–25% [5, 6]. Complications include chronic airway obstruction and chronic voice changes. Injury to the laryngotracheal structure can be lethal because of airway compromise. Severe injuries with complete airway obstruction necessitate immediate airway management either with orotracheal intubation or more commonly with emergency tracheotomy. Some of these patients may not survive the time interval between the accident and arrival of medical assistance. Mortality rates are reported to be 2–35% among the severe laryngotracheal injuries [5, 6]. The principles of immediate airway management as well as long-term management of complications will be discussed in this chapter.

15.1 Injury of the Cartilage Framework of the Larynx and Cervical Trachea

The airway is well protected as it passes through the neck. Thyroid cartilage and tracheal rings provide a framework that prevents the airway from external compression. The elasticity of the cartilage framework contributes to its recoil, saving the airway even if the external pressure or blow is strong enough to exceed the resistance of this structure. The larynx and more pronouncedly trachea can almost completely be compressed and can recoil to the original structure once the external pressure subsides. The optimal balance of strength and elasticity of the cartilage network is achieved at early adulthood. During childhood, the cartilage is much more elastic and lacks the structural strength. At this period in life, the airway is more vulnerable to external pressure resulting in complete obstruction of airway. However, the recoil effect is more pronounced as well. Once the external pressure is removed, the recoil is almost complete. Therefore, cartilage frame fractures are extremely rare in pediatric age group, while soft tissue edema and hematoma are more common [7, 8]. In elderly people, the cartilage framework is usually calcified and underwent osseous transformation. The airway is more resistant to external pressure. This increased resistance doesn't necessarily serve the airway protection. Loss of elasticity results in fractures with less forceful blows. The laryngotracheal fractures in this age group are more common and usually more severe [6, 8].

Surrounding the cartilage framework are the strap muscles, the subcutaneous fat, and the skin. These extralaryngeal soft tissues offer a buffer between the impact and laryngotracheal cartilage framework. Sternocleidomastoid muscles protect the larynx from lateral blows. The mandible often blocks the impact that comes from a superior to inferior angle. Likewise, the clavicles and sternum may block the impact that comes from an inferior direction. The larynx and trachea are vulnerable only to direct blows to the anterior of the neck. The object of contact whether it be a bat, a steering wheel, a dashboard, or a rope has to approach the larynx in a horizontal manner. If the object is in vertical position relative to the body, the impact will be blocked by the facial skeleton and/or sternum and clavicle heads [8].

The most common blunt trauma to the larynx and cervical trachea is caused by motor vehicle accidents. The steering wheel and dashboards are located at the correct angle to produce an injury to the larynx and trachea. Collision of the vehicle causes a sudden deceleration throwing the body into the steering wheel and dashboards. Safety belts help to slow the velocity of the impact, whereas airbags may help to prevent the contact totally. In the case where no seatbelt and airbag are present, the upper body is thrown violently against the steering wheel and dashboard. Even at this situation, the head is usually flexed, and the mandible serves to protect the larynx. If the larynx comes into contact with a hardware, the first impact is taken by the thyroid prominence, and the thyroid cartilage is compressed against the vertebra, displacing the thyroid alas laterally. When the point of maximal compressibility is reached, the thyroid cartilage fractures in vertical axis either medially or more commonly paramedially [8, 9] (Figs. 15.1, 15.2, and 15.3). The point of maximal compressibility varies greatly with age and from person to person. Younger victims may experience a single line of fracture, while older people may have multiple fractures.

If the impact is more inferior, the cricoid cartilage may be affected (Fig. 15.4). The cricoid cartilage is a complete cartilage ring with more rigidity compared to the tracheal rings and the thyroid cartilage. While the thyroid alas can spread laterally with the advantage of being not a completely circular structure, the cricoid cartilage cannot displace laterally but rather gets compressed into an oval shape [8]. This can result in a median fracture. More severe blows can cause the fragmentation of the cricoid cartilage and the loss of airway (Fig. 15.5). This fragmentation can also cause the injury to one or both the recurrent laryngeal nerves at the region of the cricothyroid joint with subsequent vocal cord paralysis and further narrowing of the airway.

If the impact is lower than the cricoid cartilage, a complete separation of the larynx and trachea may occur. The usual site of separation is between the cricoid cartilage and first tracheal ring [10] (Fig. 15.6). The separation can be accompanied by a cricoid cartilage fracture or

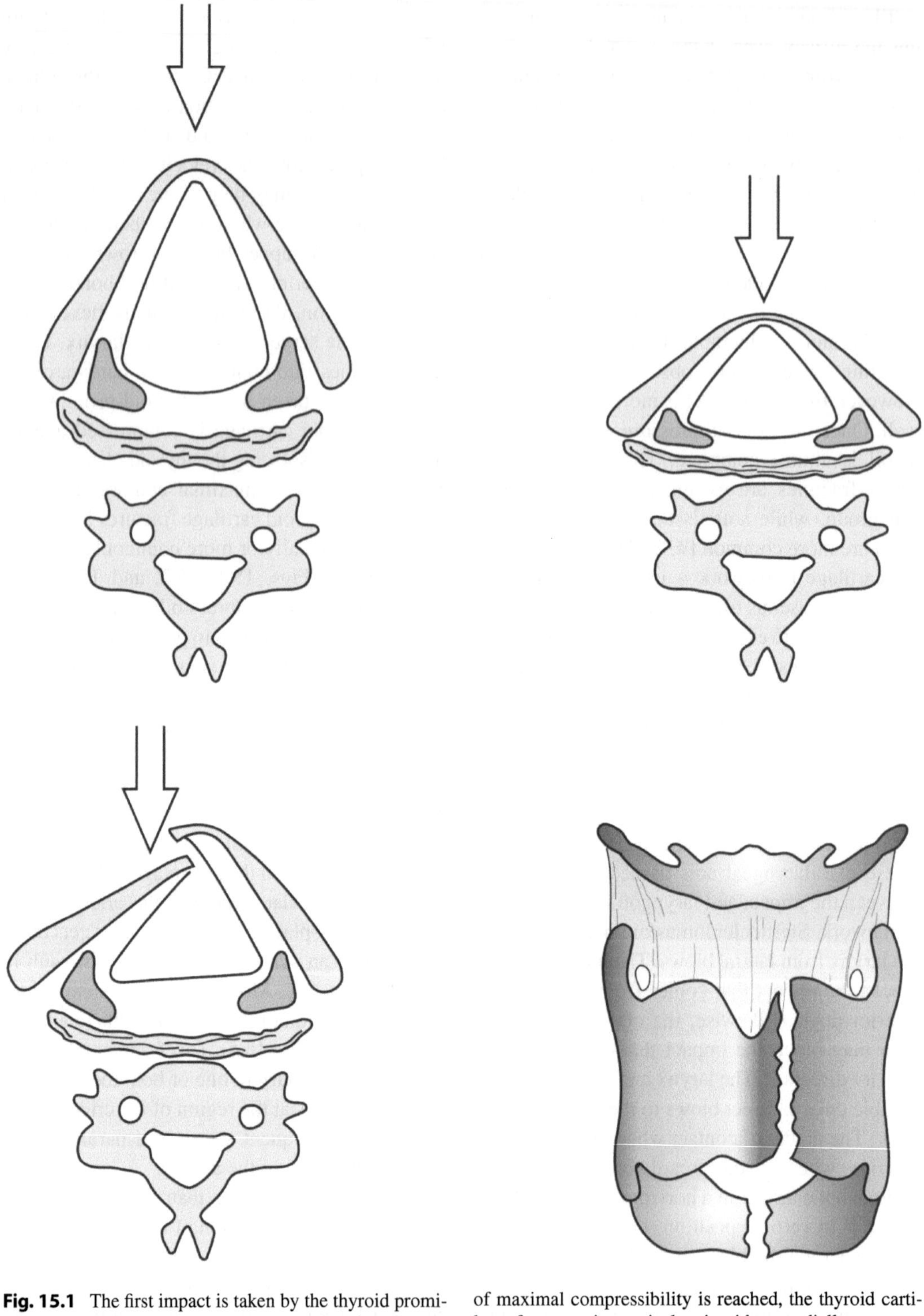

Fig. 15.1 The first impact is taken by the thyroid prominence, and thyroid cartilage is compressed against the vertebra, displacing the thyroid alas laterally. When the point of maximal compressibility is reached, the thyroid cartilage fractures in vertical axis either medially or more commonly paramedially

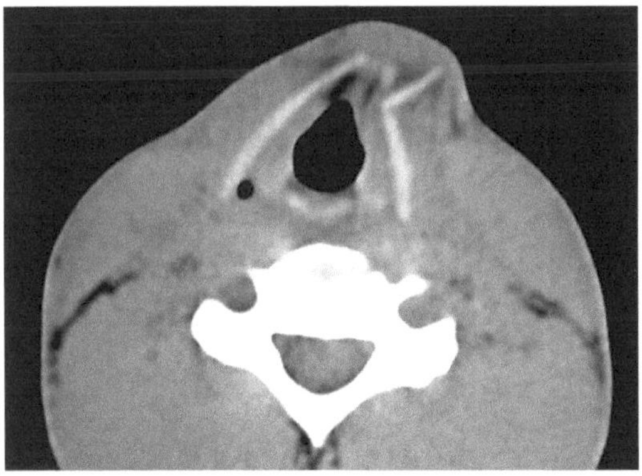

Fig. 15.2 CT image of a patient with paramedian fracture of the thyroid cartilage. A fragment of cartilage is displaced laterally. The airway appears to be patent

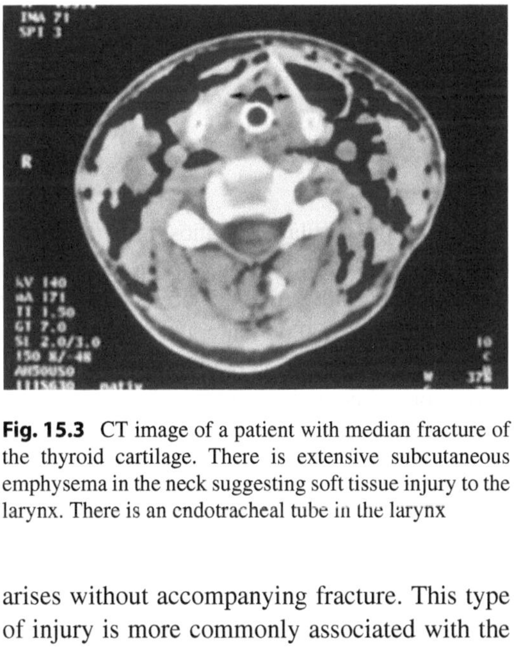

Fig. 15.3 CT image of a patient with median fracture of the thyroid cartilage. There is extensive subcutaneous emphysema in the neck suggesting soft tissue injury to the larynx. There is an endotracheal tube in the larynx

arises without accompanying fracture. This type of injury is more commonly associated with the neck coming into contact with a fixed cable or rope while riding a motorbike, jet ski, snowmobile, and similar vehicles where the neck is not protected against outside objects.

There are two vectors of force causing the laryngotracheal separation. The first one is the compression of the cricoid cartilage and the trachea against the vertebral bodies as described above. The second vector is the "telescoping effect." When the neck comes into contact with a fixed wire or a rope while traveling fast, the neck comes to a complete stop, while the body still moves forward. This induces a pulling of the tra-

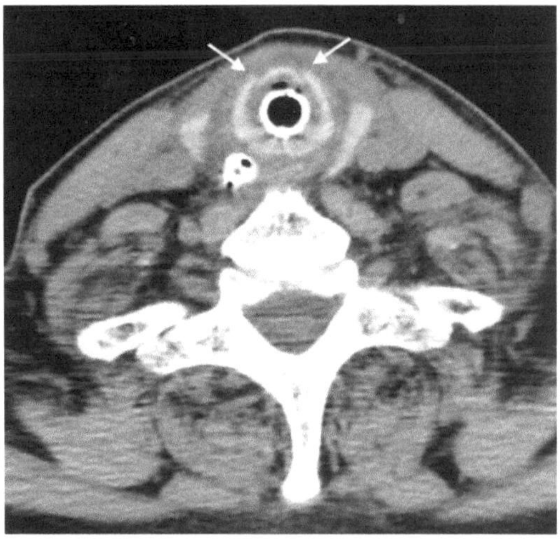

Fig. 15.4 CT image of patient with cricoid fracture. The cricoid cartilage is fractured in two places. There is an endotracheal tube in the airway

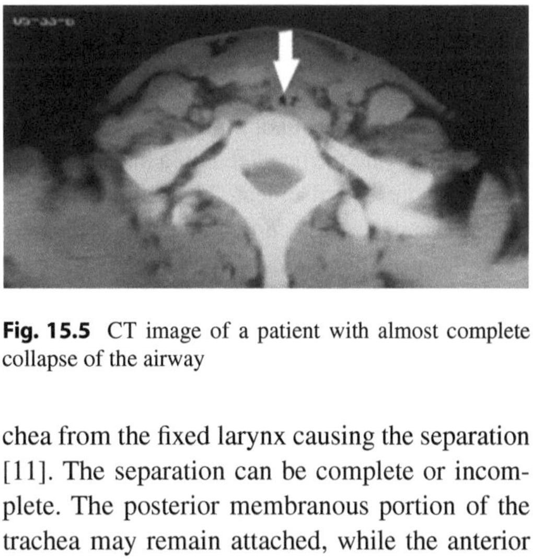

Fig. 15.5 CT image of a patient with almost complete collapse of the airway

chea from the fixed larynx causing the separation [11]. The separation can be complete or incomplete. The posterior membranous portion of the trachea may remain attached, while the anterior cartilaginous trachea is separated from the larynx. In that case, the trachea doesn't retract completely into the chest. An intubation or a tracheotomy is easier in case of incomplete separation airway, the posterior wall serving as a guide for airway management.

If the trachea is completely separated from the larynx, it retracts into the chest. This will most often result in complete and sudden loss of airway, which is fatal. The strap muscles and the surrounding fascia can rarely serve as a temporary airway until the patient is managed by intubation or tracheotomy.

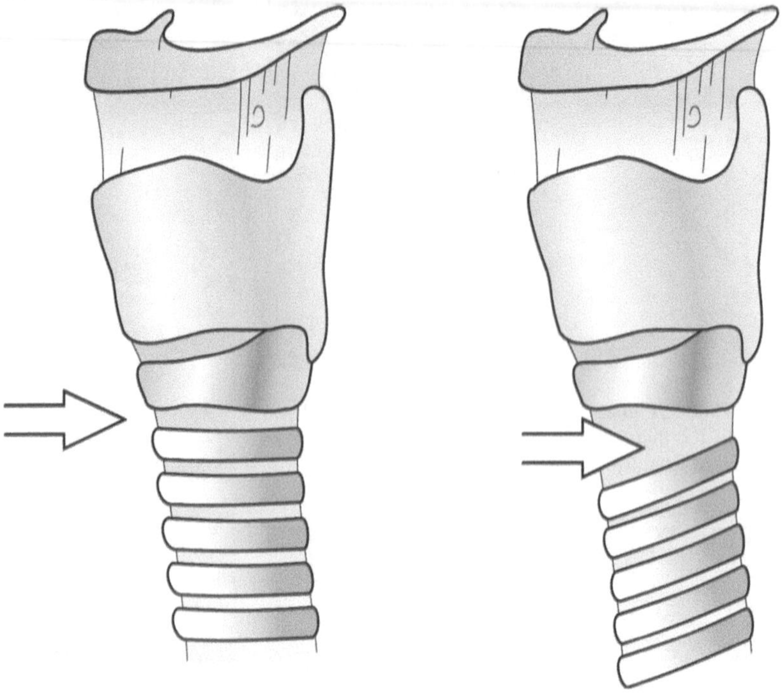

Fig. 15.6 A horizontal trauma at the level of cricoid and first thyroid cartilage usually results in cricotracheal separation. Posterior tracheal wall may still be attached

Another mechanism of injury is caused by children falling onto the handlebar of a bicycle or onto any horizontal hard object. This kind of impact may cause the cricoid cartilage to displace superiorly under the thyroid cartilage [12, 13]. This can cause a doubling of the soft tissues onto themselves and a severe soft tissue edema. Frequently, this injury happens in younger children with flexible cartilages. Fractures don't occur with this kind of trauma in younger children. Adults who experience this kind of impact present with cricoid fractures. This displacement may cause injury to one or both the recurrent laryngeal nerves with subsequent vocal cord paralysis [11–14].

15.2 Injury of the Cricoarytenoid Joint

Arytenoid cartilages are in relation with the cricoid cartilage via a joint and with the thyroid cartilage via the vocal ligament and the thyroarytenoid muscle. Arytenoid cartilages are located deep to the thyroid cartilage and the hyoid bone. In case of external laryngeal trauma, the fracture of arytenoid cartilages is prevented by the thyroid cartilage, but most importantly the extreme mobility of the cricoarytenoid joint [15]. When the thyroid cartilage is pressed against the vertebra by external pressure, the arytenoid cartilages are displaced laterally and posteriorly. Posterior or lateral dislocations of the arytenoids may occur at this stage. With the sudden release of pressure, the thyroid cartilage springs back to its original shape. This sudden springing motion pulls the arytenoid cartilages by its muscular attachments anteriorly to the thyroid cartilage [9, 16]. This motion may result in anterior luxation or subluxation of the arytenoid cartilages. Posterior dislocation of the arytenoids is reported to be more common; however, this is usually associated with a traumatic orotracheal intubation trauma rather than an external trauma [16]. Dislocations of the arytenoid cartilages are usually associated with severe soft tissue trauma. Soft tissue trauma can cause an edema masking the larynx and making the diagnosis of dislocation difficult [17]. Dislocation of the cricoarytenoid joint impairs vocal cord movement. Dislocations can be confused with vocal cord paralysis. EMG is an important tool to differentiate the two conditions. EMG would detect the muscle contraction potentials in case of an arytenoid dislocation. These potentials would be absent in case of vocal cord paralysis.

15.3 Laryngeal Soft Tissue Injury

External blunt trauma to the larynx almost always results in soft tissue injury. The loose submucosal connective tissue is very prone to fluid collection and edema. Even the mildest trauma results in some degree of swelling of the endolarynx. This may manifest as change in voice or more seriously as breathing difficulty. As the impact of trauma increases, the likelihood of having a mucosal laceration increases as well. Lacerations may cause bleeding and contribute to airway problems. Laryngeal framework fractures are usually associated with mucosal injuries [9]. Mucosal injury may range from mild tissue edema to large lacerations. Mucosa can be crushed or caught between cartilage fragments. In case of laryngotracheal separation, the mucosa cannot withstand the pulling forces and separate as well. Large laceration of the mucosa may cause an emphysema by air leakage into the soft tissues of the neck. Air can accumulate around the strap muscles as well as in the subcutaneous plane. Extensive ecchymosis and crepitation of the skin make the diagnosis of emphysema easily recognizable. Soft tissue emphysema may contribute to airway compromise (Figs. 15.7 and 15.8). After

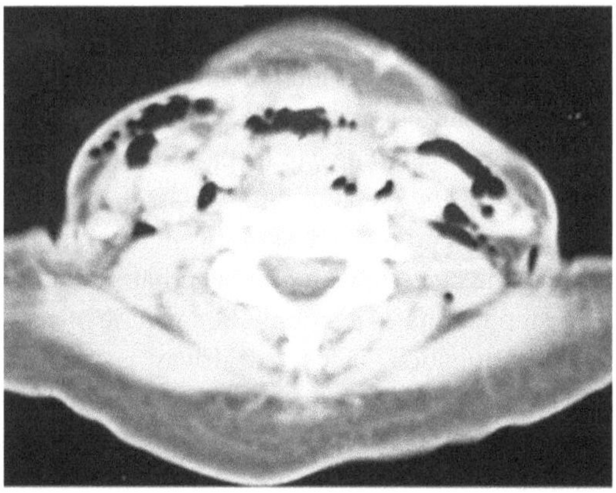

Fig. 15.7 In this CT scan, there is extensive subcutaneous emphysema, and the airway cannot be identified

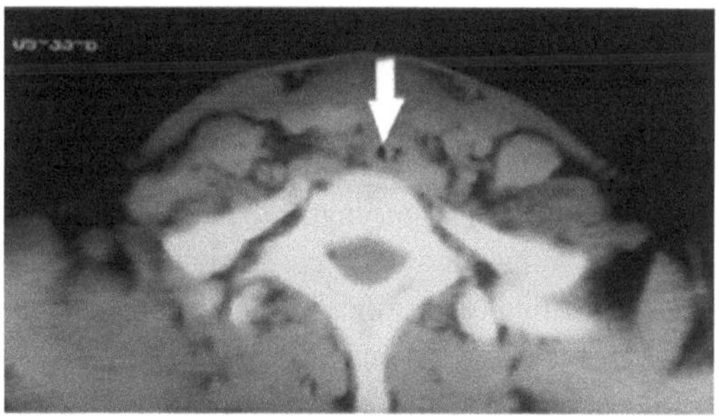

Fig. 15.8 CT scan at the level of the hyoid bone demonstrating subcutaneous emphysema. The airway can only be identified by the presence of an endotracheal tube

repair of the larynx, air in the soft tissues is gradually resorbed.

A distinct soft tissue injury is the rupture of thyroarytenoid muscle and ligament. As the thyroid cartilage is pressed against the vertebra and springs back, the muscle and the ligament relax and undergo a tension in a very short time period. This may result in rupture or detachment of the ligament from the thyroid cartilage at the level of the anterior commissure. As the ligament detaches from the anterior commissure, usually a small piece of cartilage also detaches. Rupture or detachment result in bunching of the vocal cord and narrowing of the airway. The injury is always accompanied by a severe edema of Reinke's space. Dislocation of the arytenoid cartilage may also accompany the injury [15].

Suicidal or accidental hanging causes trauma to the supraglottic larynx. The rope around the neck tightens at the level of the thyrohyoid membrane [18]. The external pressure causes the preepiglottic space to move posteriorly pushing the epiglottis against the arytenoid cartilages. This causes a complete obstruction of the airway. If the person survives the impact, the subsequent injury is a severe supraglottic edema. The thyrohyoid membrane may rupture, and the preepiglottic fat tissue may herniate into the airway. Hyoid bone fractures occur rarely if the rope tightens at the level of the hyoid bone [19]. Hyoid bone fractures don't have any clinical implications unless a fragment is tearing through the airway mucosa. Thyroid and cricoid cartilages can also be fractured. Laryngotracheal separation is reported to occur with hanging injuries [20].

15.4 Emergency Management of Laryngotracheal Blunt Trauma

Blunt trauma to the laryngotracheal area can be an airway emergency. All cases should be managed according to the emergency airway management protocol of the managing institute regardless of the degree and place of the trauma. Loss of precious time can be lethal in case of laryngotracheal injuries. Elaborate examination and imaging should be left for later. Management of the airway is the primary objective. If the patient is not breathing at the time of initial management, cardiopulmonary resuscitation should be carried out immediately. Many of these patients have accompanying cervical spine injuries. Care should be taken not to move the cervical spine. Unless proven otherwise, all patients should be assumed to have cervical spine injury. Endolaryngeal edema develops immediately after the laryngotracheal trauma. If the emergency team arrives soon after the trauma, orotracheal intubation may be successful. After a certain period of time, the edema is present, and an intubation may be extremely difficult necessitating a tracheotomy [1, 21]. The team in charge of the patient has to keep in mind that the airway will become worse with time as the edema increases. In case of extensive laryngotracheal trauma, intubation should be considered even if the patient is able to breathe sufficiently. As mentioned before, intubation could be difficult if not impossible as time passes. Orotracheal intubation can be achieved even in case of laryngotracheal separation. Laryngotracheal separation usually occurs in the anterior wall of the trachea between the cricoid and first tracheal rings, with the posterior wall of the trachea staying intact. If the endotracheal tube is advanced with the guidance of the posterior tracheal wall, intubation of the separated tracheal segment can be achieved. Even if the complete separation occurs, the surrounding soft tissues don't collapse immediately and can serve as a guide for intubation [1, 21] (Fig. 15.9). If orotracheal intubation can be achieved, the endotracheal tube serves as a stent preventing a possible synechia of the endolaryngeal mucosa and thus making further airway management easier. If intubation cannot be achieved after a few trials, no time should be lost before attempting the tracheotomy.

The level of tracheotomy should be decided according to the level of the trauma. For a high laryngeal injury like a hanging case, the fastest and easiest way would be a cricothyrotomy. However, if the thyroid cartilage and/or cricoid cartilage is fractured, a lower tracheotomy is necessary. The level of injury can be determined by palpation of the neck under emergency conditions. Fragments of cartilage and/or depressions in the laryngotracheal framework show the site of injury. However, the edema and hematomas developing in the soft tissues of the neck can make this examination difficult. In this case, the mechanism of injury gives clues about the injury site. As said before, the most common laryngotracheal injuries are caused by steering wheel and dashboard impacts in motor vehicle accidents, inducing an injury at the level of thyroid and cricoid cartilages. Bicycle and sports accidents also cause an injury at the same level. In this case, the best level for tracheotomy is two tracheal rings below the injury site [1, 21] (Fig. 15.9). Tracheotomy should be realized below the third tracheal ring. Laryngotracheal separation is likely in case of a jet ski or snowmobile accident where the neck comes into contact with a fixed object like a rope. Laryngotracheal separation is the hardest injury to manage in terms of airway. The airway can be secured by neck exploration and identification of the separated tracheal segment low in the neck or thorax. The endotracheal tube can be passed into the trachea from the separation. Tracheal segment should be secured to the skin incision and to the head of the clavicle with non-absorbable sutures. This step facilitates a reintubation in case of accidental extubation. Once the airway is secured, other life-threatening injuries should be addressed before any attempt to repair the laryngotracheal damages.

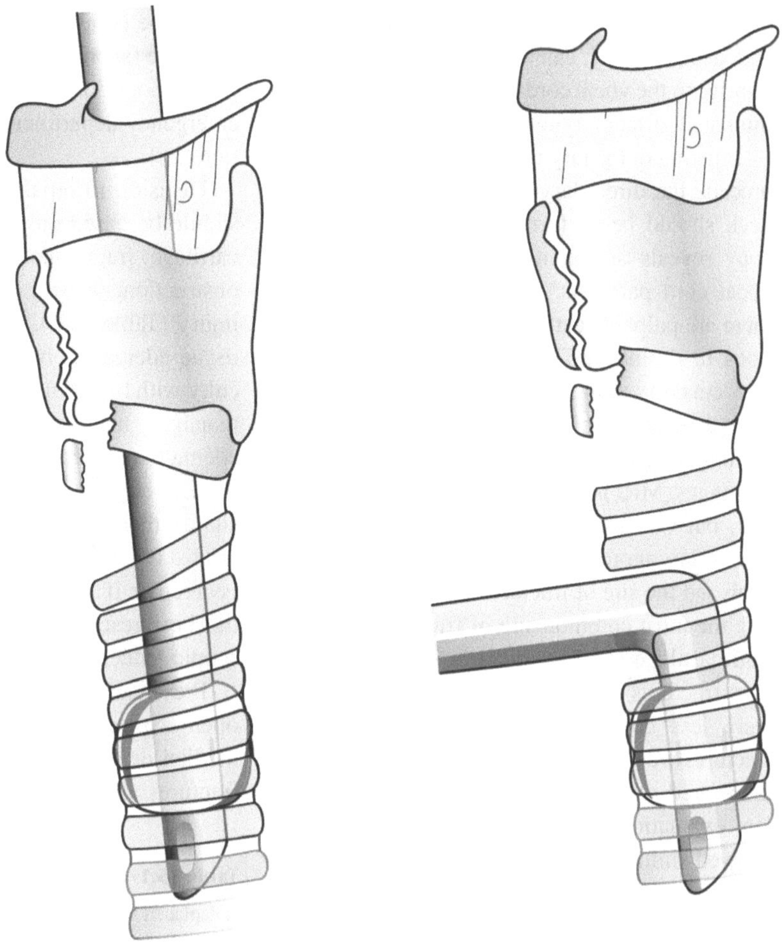

Fig. 15.9 The first option for airway management is endotracheal intubation. Posterior tracheal wall can guide the endotracheal tube in the airway even if the distant airway cannot be visualized. The second option is to perform a tracheotomy. The best place to perform a tracheotomy is two tracheal rings below the site of injury

15.5 Evaluation of Laryngotracheal Injury

Once the patient is stabilized, evaluation of damages should be done.

Endoscopic assessment is the next step. Today, fiberoptic laryngoscopy has become the initial evaluation tool. Fiberoptic laryngoscopy is less traumatic and much more comfortable for the patient. Checking the airway patency and any potential causes that might impair the airway is the first priority. Tracheotomy should be performed in case of increasing edema or hematoma. If the airway patency is adequate, the site and degree of damage should be evaluated. Mucosal lacerations, location of arytenoids, and vocal cord mobility must be assessed.

Supraglottic edema may prevent examination of glottic and subglottic areas [22]. In case the endolarynx cannot be assessed with flexible laryngoscopy due to laryngeal edema, direct laryngoscopy should be carried out under general anesthesia. All of the upper aerodigestive tract mucosa should be examined. Mobility of the arytenoid cartilages should be tested with a blunt instrument, such as a velvet tip suction or cup forceps with the tip in closed position. Additional trauma to the laryngeal mucosa should be avoided.

Bronchoscopy can also be performed to assess the trachea. The downside of direct laryngoscopy is the inability to assess the function properly.

Esophagoscopy should be carried out as well. Esophageal trauma as a result of an impact to the neck is not infrequent. Videostroboscopy is a valuable tool to assess vocal cord injuries. Videostroboscopy can reveal even very subtle injuries to the vocal cords. If the patient is already intubated, direct laryngoscopy is indicated.

Imaging of the laryngotracheal framework can precede the direct laryngoscopy. CT scan of the neck should be performed if flexible laryngoscopy reveals an extensive soft tissue injury, a vocal cord paralysis, and a bare cartilage or if there are palpable cartilage fractures and crepitations in the neck. The CT scan should include fine cuts through the larynx. Special attention should be given to thyroid, cricoid, and tracheal cartilages, as well as the localization of arytenoid cartilages. MRI is better to assess soft tissue injuries, but CT remains the imaging of choice to assess laryngotracheal framework. Buch et al. analyzed the site of fractures on CT and reported that the most common site of fracture is the thyroid cartilage (45/55 patients), followed by cricoid fractures in 13/55 patients. Hyoid fractures were less common (8/55 patients). Multi-site fractures were observed in 12/55 patients usually associated with severe edema [23]. A postmortem evaluation of 284 cases with neck trauma showed similar injury rates with 40% fracture of the superior horn of the thyroid cartilage and 20% hyoid bone fracture [24]. Laryngeal EMG is very important to assess nerve injuries. Superior laryngeal nerve is usually not disturbed by external trauma to the larynx. However, recurrent laryngeal nerve may frequently be affected by injury involving the cricoid cartilage and laryngotracheal separation. EMG can detect contraction potentials and resting potentials even in unconscious patients.

If observation is decided, repeated fibroscopies or direct laryngoscopies can be done at 24, 48, and 72 h after surgery to monitor the endolaryngeal edema.

15.5.1 Laryngotracheal Trauma Repair

Once the lethal injuries are addressed and the patient is stabilized and assessed, if indicated, surgical repair of the larynx and cervical trauma should be done as soon as possible. Early repair has more favorable results compared to late repair [25]. About 50% of the patients reporting to the emergency department require surgical intervention [26].

Decision to repair the laryngotracheal injury should be based on the presence and severity of cartilage fragmentation, the degree of airway obstruction, and a recurrent laryngeal nerve injury (Table 15.1). A patient with minimal soft tissue edema, mobile vocal cords, and no difficulty with breathing can be observed closely. The managing team should remember that soft tissue edema may worsen with time. Close observation is necessary. Extensive soft tissue injuries necessitate either endoscopic or open repair. Table 15.2 is a list of endoscopic findings that indicate laryngeal repair. If an arytenoid dislocation is observed, the best results are obtained with early endoscopic reduction.

Presence of cartilage fractures usually requires open exploration, repair, and fixation. Single median or paramedian vertical thyroid cartilage fractures are the most common fractures. Close

Table 15.1 Indications for open surgery

Displaced single fracture of the laryngotracheal framework
Multiple fractures of the laryngotracheal framework (including non-displaced fractures)
Laryngotracheal separation
Thyroarytenoid muscle and ligament tear or detachment
Esophageal tears
Arytenoid dislocation that cannot be reduced endoscopically
Hematoma that is obstructing the airway
Denuded cartilage

Table 15.2 Endoscopic findings that require surgery

Exposed cartilage
Depressions in airway that suggest cartilage fracture
Laryngotracheal separation
Mucosal fragments that obstruct airway
Injury to the free edge of vocal cords
Cricoarytenoid dislocation
Displacement of the epiglottis
Herniation of preepiglottic contents
Thyroarytenoid muscle or ligament injury

observation can be an option if the fracture is single and not displaced, without extensive soft tissue injury or detachment of the thyroarytenoid muscle. However, fixation of the framework by an external approach is the safe alternative because the fragments of cartilage can be displaced afterward, obstructing the airway.

Penetrating tears of the esophagus should be addressed with an open neck exploration.

If there is no indication for open approach (see Table 15.1), repair can be carried out with rigid laryngoscopy. Mucosal flaps that obstruct the airway or interfere with phonation should be removed. Obtaining straight free edges of vocal cords is essential. Mucosal flaps on the free edge of the vocal cord should be positioned back in place or removed. Cold steel instruments, powered instruments, or laser can be used for removal. If the preepiglottic space contents are herniated into the airway without accompanying fractures, these tissues should be removed. In case of epiglottis obstructing the airway, part of or the entire epiglottis can be resected. This can be achieved with laser or powered instruments.

In case of cricoarytenoid luxation, repositioning of the arytenoid cartilage should be attempted. Early reduction has better results, because ankylosis will be organized in about a week. Posterior dislocation can be reduced by applying a medial and anterior force with an instrument placed posterior to the dislocated arytenoid. Laryngoscope can be used to force the arytenoids anteriorly. Anterior dislocations can be reduced by placing the rigid laryngoscope just anterior to the displaced arytenoids and applying posterior pressure. In anterior dislocations, there is a tendency of the arytenoid to displace inferiorly. In that case, a blunt right angle instrument such as a blunt hook can be placed anteriorly and inferiorly to the arytenoid, and the arytenoid can be lifted and pushed posteriorly. The maneuvers have to be very gentle. Vocal process can be fractured with forceful movements resulting in poor-quality voice after the reduction.

In some occasions, endoscopic repair can be combined with an open neck approach. Open surgery is done through a horizontal incision in a skin crease or close to the thyroid cartilage. Subplatysmal flaps are elevated; strap muscles are divided in midline and retracted laterally. Adequate exposure of the thyroid and cricoid cartilages is essential. Care should be taken not to injure the external branches of the superior laryngeal nerves or the recurrent nerves. If there is a vertical thyroid cartilage fracture, the larynx can be entered through the fracture line. Mucosal incision should preferentially be made at the midline across the anterior commissure to prevent further mucosal injury. If there is a horizontal fracture, the opening can be achieved with a midline vertical laryngofissure.

Mucosal injury should be assessed when the exposure is achieved. Reconstruction of the deep structures is the first step. Arytenoid cartilages should be restored to their original positions. Thyroarytenoid muscle or ligament tears should be repaired with sutures. If there is a thyroarytenoid muscle detachment, a strong suture can be passed through the vocal ligament and fixed to the cartilage segment corresponding to the original position of the anterior commissure (Fig. 15.10). Incorrect positioning of the vocal ligament results in poor voice quality. Once the deeper architecture is restored, the mucosal tears can be considered. The goal is to cover the entire endolaryngeal surface with mucosa to facilitate the wound healing and prevent the granuloma formation. Irreparable mucosal fragments should be removed. Remaining mucosa should be aligned and sutured with fine absorbable sutures. If there isn't enough mucosa to cover the all larynx, priority should be given to the glottic area and especially the anterior commissure. Anterior commissure is indeed the most common site of scar and synechia formation. Keels can be used to prevent web formation as well. The second important area is the arytenoid cartilages. Adequate covering of arytenoids will prevent the ankylosis of the joint by scar formation. Local mucosal flaps can be raised to facilitate the mucosal redraping. Laterally based piriform sinus flaps and posteriorly based postcricoid flaps can be used to cover the arytenoid region. Epiglottic flaps can be used to cover the anterior commissure. If there is an extensive mucosal and cartilage fragmentation in the anterior commissure,

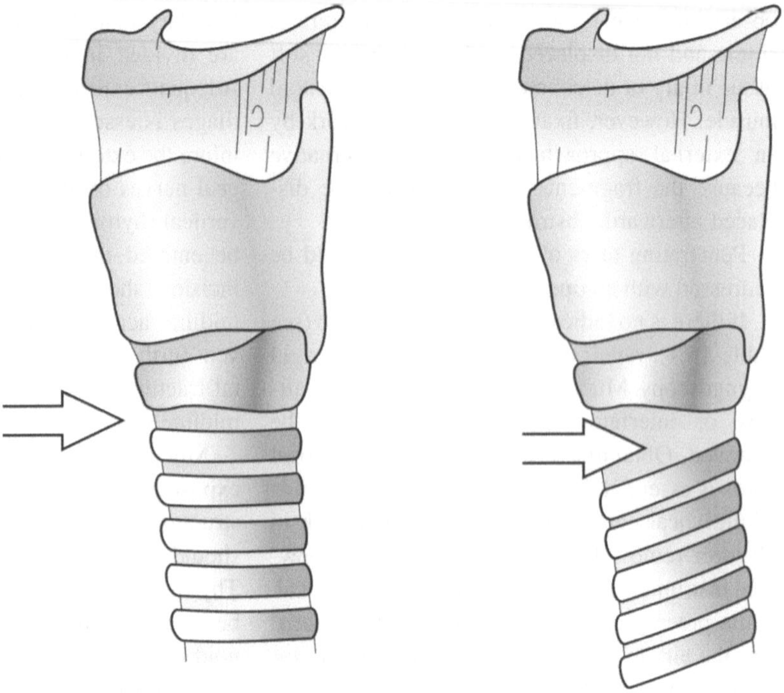

Fig. 15.10 In the case of detachment of anterior commissure, the vocal ligaments should be suspended to the cartilage fragment that corresponds to the cartilage potion of the anterior commissure with non-absorbable sutures

the epiglottic cartilage can be mobilized from its anterior attachments and pulled inferiorly to cover both the mucosal and cartilage defects.

In case of epiglottis displacement and herniation of the preepiglottic contents, these epiglottic contents should be removed and the epiglottis tracted anteriorly and fixed to the hyoid bone with strong absorbable sutures. Removal of part of the epiglottis should be considered if the traction cannot be achieved.

When the endolaryngeal repairing is achieved, it must be decided to put a stent or not. Stents are useful in preventing synechia. If there are an extensive mucosal injury and the likelihood of synechia formation, a stent should be placed. There are several commercially available stents. A custom-made stent can be constructed from a finger of a surgical glove or a Penrose drain filled with sponge and tied at both ends with silk sutures. Stents should be fixed to the neck skin to prevent any dislocation. Strong silk sutures are passed through the stent and brought to the neck skin and tied on a button to prevent the pulling on the sutures and the irritation of the neck skin. Stents can be taken out endoscopically after 3–5 weeks. In case of anterior commissure injury, a keel should be placed and secured to the skin (see Chap. 12b—Lichtenberger—anterior commissure).

The next step is the reconstruction of the laryngotracheal framework. Each cartilage fragment has to be identified and positioned in the correct alignment. The perfusion of the cartilage is through the perichondrium. Free cartilage fragments can still be used as free grafts as long as they are covered with well-perfused tissue. Comminuted pieces that cannot be fixed should be removed. A complete reconstruction of the cartilage frame is not necessary as long as the three-dimensional shape of the larynx can be achieved. Miniplates and recently introduced absorbable plates are the best materials to join the cartilage fragments (Fig. 15.11). Single fractures that assume the natural shape once brought together can be repaired with wire or sutures, but miniplates should be used if they are available. Miniplates of 1.0–1.4 mm thickness should be preferred because they are easy to shape and their thinner profile is not visible through the skin. If the remaining cartilage is not sufficient to reconstruct the framework, free cartilage grafts, such as nasal septal cartilage and costal cartilage, can be used. The epiglottis is another source of carti-

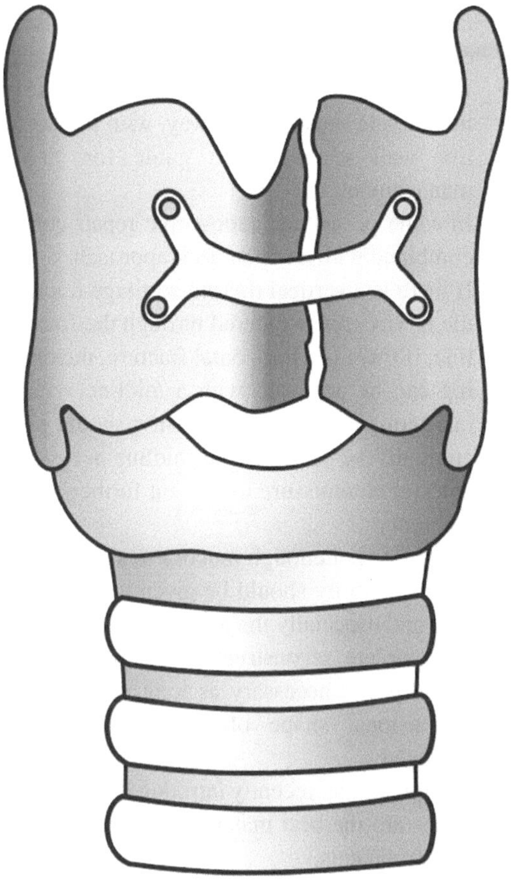

Fig. 15.11 External fixation of the tracheal cartilage with miniplates gives excellent reconstructive results

lage and has the advantage of providing a pedicled flap. Correct placement of the vocal ligaments is essential to obtain a good-quality voice after reconstruction. The cartilage fragment attached to the vocal ligaments must be exactly positioned at the level of a normal anterior commissure. If one of the vocal ligaments is detached, it has to be reattached at exactly the same level of the contralateral ligament with a sturdy suture. If the vocal ligament cannot be attached to a cartilage fragment, the suture can be tied on a plate. In this case, a non-absorbable suture and plate should be preferred to avoid any detachment.

Laryngotracheal separation is repaired by end-to-end anastomosis. If the tracheotomy tube is placed in the tracheal segment, it has to be removed and placed through a tracheotomy incision 2–3 rings below the avulsed site as the first step of reconstruction. If the tracheal ring is severed, it should be removed.

The tracheal ring should be suspended to the cricoid ring with sturdy absorbable sutures that are as much as possible outside. Ideally, the stitches are also extra-mucosal. The reason for these precautions is the prevention of granuloma and stenosis. If the end-to-end anastomosis cannot perfectly be performed and if the larynx reconstruction is not stable, a T-tube is put in place to serve as a stent, allowing voice production and breathing. According to the trauma and the reconstruction, this tube can stay in place from 3 weeks to 3–4 months.

All additional neck injuries should be addressed as the neck is being explored. Esophageal tears should be repaired as soon as possible. Leak from the esophagus may have life-threatening consequences, like a mediastinitis. Tears should be closed in a watertight fashion. We currently prefer absorbable sutures placed in a running mattress style. A second layer of muscle should be closed over the suture line. A nasogastric feeding tube can be placed during surgery to allow postoperative feeding.

If a recurrent nerve injury is observed, an attempt to find the separated segments should be made. It might be difficult to find both ends of the recurrent laryngeal nerve in the trauma field. The nerve might part intralaryngeally or more frequently right where it enters the larynx. If both ends of the nerve are found, end-to-end anastomosis should be done. Primary repair of the recurrent laryngeal nerve doesn't have favorable results. Abduction and adduction functions may not return. However, if tonus to the vocal cord is achieved, vocal rehabilitation is easier.

Additional repairs may be necessary after the initial surgical repair. Laryngotracheal separation has a high stenosis rate after primary anastomosis. Anterior commissure injuries are associated with anterior web formation. Synechiae and granulomas may develop after extensive soft tissue injuries. The secondary repairs are beyond the scope of this chapter and are addressed in different chapters. Unilateral vocal cord paralysis can be treated by vocal cord injection or medialization thyroplasty.

15.6 Postoperative Management

Last but not least, postoperative care is crucial. Voice rest and adequate humidification help the healing process. Antibiotics are administered to prevent chondritis. Antireflux medications should be administered. Steroids may be used to limit endolaryngeal edema in patients without tracheotomies. However, patients with tracheotomy should not receive steroids, as they might impair tissue healing. Stents and keels are usually removed 3–5 weeks after placement.

Closing of tracheotomy should be delayed until the tissue edema disappears and the patient becomes able to clear secretions adequately. Permanent tracheotomy may be necessary with some patients, in case of severe stenosis or bilateral vocal cord paralysis. Speech therapy is an important part of postoperative care. Speech therapy should be started as soon as the tissue edema disappears.

15.7 Tips and Pearls

- The level of injury can be determined by palpation of the neck under emergency conditions. Fragments of cartilage and/or depressions in the laryngotracheal framework show the site of injury. However, the edema and hematomas developing in the soft tissues of the neck can make this examination difficult. In this case, the mechanism of injury gives clues about the injury site.
- Suicidal or accidental hanging causes trauma to the supraglottic larynx. The most common laryngotracheal injuries are caused by steering wheel and dashboard impacts in motor vehicle accidents, inducing an injury at the level of thyroid and cricoid cartilages. Bicycle and sports accidents also cause an injury at the same level. Laryngotracheal separation is likely in case of a jet ski or snowmobile accident where the neck comes into contact with a fixed object like a rope.
- Large laceration of the mucosa may cause emphysema by air leakage into the soft tissues of the neck. Extensive ecchymosis and crepitation of the skin make the diagnosis of emphysema easily recognizable.
- Intubation or tracheotomy is easier in case of incomplete separation airway, with the posterior wall serving as a guide for airway management.
- In some occasions, endoscopic repair can be combined with an open neck approach.
- If there is a vertical thyroid cartilage fracture, the larynx can be entered through the fracture line. If there is a horizontal fracture, the opening can be achieved with a midline vertical laryngofissure. Mucosal incision should preferentially be made at the midline across the anterior commissure to prevent further mucosal injury.
- If there is not enough mucosa to cover the all larynx, priority should be given to the glottic area and especially the anterior commissure.
- A complete reconstruction of the cartilage frame is not necessary as long as the three-dimensional shape of the larynx can be achieved.
- Miniplates and recently introduced absorbable plates are the best materials to join the cartilage fragments.
- If the reconstruction is not stable, a T-tube is put in place to serve as a stent, allowing voice production and breathing.

References

1. Bent JP, Silver JR, Porubsky ES. Acute laryngeal trauma: a review of 77 patients. Otolaryngol Head Neck Surg. 1993;109:441–9.
2. Schafer SD. The treatment of acute external laryngeal injuries. Arch Otolaryngol Head Neck Surg. 1991;117:35–9.
3. Komisar A, Blaugrund SM, Camins M. Head and neck trauma in taxicabs. Arch Otolaryngol Head Neck Surg. 1991;117:442–5.
4. Angood PB, Attia EL, Brown RA, Mudder DS. Extrinsic civilian trauma to the larynx and cervical trachea - important predictors of long term morbidity. J Trauma. 1986;26(10):869–73.
5. Minard G, Kudsk KA, Croce MA, Butts JA. Laryngotracheal trauma. Am Surg. 1992;58:181–7.
6. Jewett BS, Schocley WW, Rutledge r. External laryngeal trauma: analysis of 392 patients. Arch Otolaryngol Head Neck Surg. 1999;125:877–80.

7. Hollinger PH, Schild JA. Pharyngeal, tracheal and laryngeal injuries in the pediatric age group. Ann Otol Rhinol Laryngol. 1972;81(4):538–45.
8. Travis LW, Olson NR, Melvin JW, Snyder RG. Static and dynamic impact trauma of the human larynx. Am Acad Ophthalmol Otolaryngol. 1975;80:382–90.
9. Pennington CL. External trauma of the larynx and trachea: immediate treatment and management. Ann Otol Rhinol Laryngol. 1972;81:546–54.
10. Ashbaugh DG, Gordon JH. Traumatic avulsion of the trachea associated with cricoid fracture. J Thorac Cardiovasc Surg. 1975;69:800–3.
11. Ford HR, Gardner MJ, Lynch JM. Laryngotracheal disruption from blunt pediatric neck injuries: impact of early recognition and intervention on outcome. J Pediatr Surg. 1995;30:331–4.
12. Gold SM, Gerber MF, Shott SR, Myer CM III. Blunt laryngotracheal trauma in children. Arch Otolaryngol Head Neck Surg. 1997;123:83–7.
13. Alonso WA, Caruso VG, Roncace EA. Minibikes, a new factor in laryngotracheal trauma. Ann Otol Rhinol Laryngol. 1973;82:800–4.
14. Myer CM, Orobello P, Cottor RT, Bratcher GO. Blunt laryngeal trauma in children. Laryngoscope. 1987;97:1043–8.
15. Dillon JP, Gallagher R, Smyth D. Arytenoid subluxation. Ir J Med Sci. 2003;172(4):206.
16. Bryce DP. Current management of laryngotracheal injury. Adv Otorhinolaryngol. 1983;29:27–38.
17. Rubin AD, Hawkshaw MJ, Moyer CA, Dean CM, Sataloff RT. Arytenoid cartilage dislocation: a 20-year experience. J Voice. 2005;19(4):687–701.
18. Khokhlov VD. Injuries to the hyoid bone and laryngeal cartilages: effectiveness of different methods of medico-legal investigation. Forensic Sci Int. 1997;88(3):173–83.
19. DiMaio VJ. Homicidal asphyxia. Am J Forensic Med Pathol. 2000;21(1):1–4.
20. Borowski DW, Mehrotra P, Tennant D, El Badawey MR, Cameron DS. Unusual presentation of blunt laryngeal injury with cricotracheal disruption by attempted hanging: a case report. Am J Otolaryngol. 2004;25(3):195–8.
21. Schaeffer SD. The treatment of acute external laryngeal injuries. Arch Otolaryngol Head Neck Surg. 1991;117:35–9.
22. Schaefer SD, Close LG. Acute management of laryngeal trauma. Ann Otol Rhinol Laryngol. 1989;98:98–104.
23. Buch K, Takumi K, Curtin HD, Sakai O. CT-based assessment of laryngeal fracture patterns and associated soft tissue abnormality. Eur Radiol. 2021;31(7):5212–21.
24. de Bakker HM, Warmbrunn MV, van den Biggelaar P, Soerdjbalie-Maikoe V, de Bakker BS. Fracture patterns of the hyoid-larynx complex after fatal trauma on the neck: retrospective radiological post-mortem analysis of 284 cases. Int J Legal Med. 2020;134(4):1465–73.
25. Leopold DA. Laryngeal trauma: a historical comparison of treatment methods. Arch Otolaryngol. 1983;109:106–12.
26. DePorre AR, Schechtman SA, Hogikyan ND, Thompson A, Westman AJ, Sargent RA, Rosko AJ, Bauer A, Shanks AM, Kupfer RA, Healy DW. Airway management and clinical outcomes in external laryngeal trauma: a case series. Anesth Analg. 2019;129(2):e52–4.

16 Glottic Airway Stenosis

Maral J. Rouhani and Guri Sandhu

Key Points

- There are a wide-ranging number of conditions that cause and contribute to glottic airway stenosis.
- Thorough assessment is essential to guide diagnosis and management options.
- There are a number of medical and surgical options available to treat the varying severities of this condition.
- In doing so, a balance must be sought with the effects on the other fundamental functions of the larynx.

16.1 Introduction

In the spectrum of laryngotracheal stenosis disease, management of glottic airway compromise is the most challenging. Glottic stenosis describes impaired vocal cord movement or narrowing of the upper airway at the level of the glottis. It is caused by a heterogeneous group of diseases and differing patterns of injury, which can affect airflow and mucociliary clearance, as well as cause voice and swallowing difficulties. This chapter describes the various aetiologies and the different approaches to managing this condition.

M. J. Rouhani
Department of ENT, Charing Cross Hospital, London, UK

G. Sandhu (✉)
National Centre for Airway Reconstruction, Charing Cross Hospital, Imperial College Healthcare NHS Trust, London, UK

16.2 Anatomy of the Glottis

The upper limit of the glottis, and inferior boundary of the supraglottis, is defined as the horizontal plane passing through the apex of the laryngeal ventricle [1, 2]. The lower limit of the glottis is defined by the UICC as 1 cm below the most medial part of the vocal fold [1] and in the USA is defined by the AJCC as the horizontal plane 1 cm below apex of the laryngeal ventricle [2]. The glottis thus comprises the vocal folds, including the anterior and posterior commissure; however, this is problematic as the AJCC description of the posterior commissure is potentially inclusive of both the supraglottic structures (arytenoid) and the glottis itself [3].

There is much debate regarding terminology of the use of 'true' vocal cord (Fig. 16.1) or vocal fold [3]; in this chapter, the term 'vocal fold' will be used throughout.

M. Remacle, H. E. Eckel (eds.), *Textbook of Surgery of Larynx and Trachea*,
https://doi.org/10.1007/978-3-031-09621-1_16

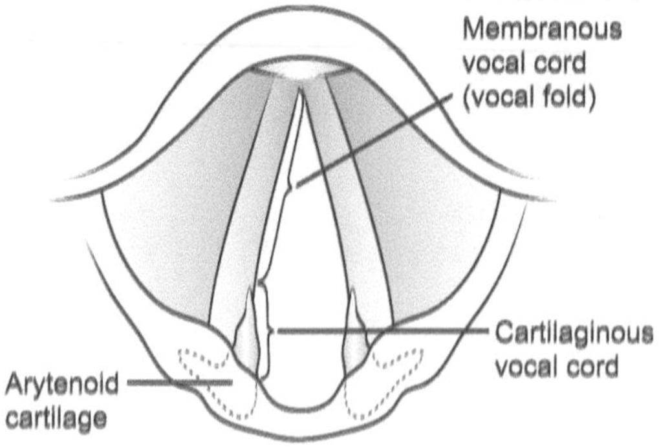

Fig. 16.1 Anatomy of the glottis

16.3 Relevant Embryology

The larynx develops from the laryngotracheal groove, within the respiratory diverticulum (which develops from the primitive foregut), between gestational weeks 5 and 6. It then develops as an anterior and two lateral laryngeal swellings, which surround the primordial glottis [4]. The anterior portion develops into the epiglottis, whilst the lateral swellings develop into the arytenoid cartilages. By the tenth week of gestation, a structure called the epithelial lamina obliterates the lumen of the primitive larynx [5]; this is then followed by recanalisation, leading to a pair of laryngeal ventricles. The ventricles are bound cranially and caudally by the vestibular and vocal folds, respectively. In the absence of recanalisation, congenital laryngeal atresia results. Partial and incomplete recanalisation may lead to a spectrum of stenosis or webbing [6, 7].

16.4 Physiology of the Glottis

The larynx itself serves three main physiological roles in order of priority: airway protection, respiration and phonation [8]. An appreciation of laryngeal evolution provides an understanding of its functional priorities [9, 10].

In other mammals, the larynx occupies a high-riding position, such that the soft palate overlaps the epiglottis; this allows these animals to breathe and feed simultaneously. Conversely in humans, the larynx sits in a lower and more precarious position in the neck, sharing a common passageway with the upper digestive system; this complicates the sphincter protection of the laryngeal airway and also results in compromised respiration [10]. It is felt that the reason for this evolutionary change, to allow phonation, is due to our complex communication needs [11, 12]. This does, however, mean that humans are at high risk of aspiration. Indeed, confounded by the fact that the glottis is the narrowest segment of the upper airway, injury to the glottis can severely compromise phonation, swallowing and breathing.

The vocal folds abduct during an in-breath, and the degree of abduction increases with exertion or exercise. Additionally, the maximal airflow through the larynx occurs at the posterior glottis (Fig. 16.2), which also represents the largest cross-sectional area; this has implications when considering the different approaches to management.

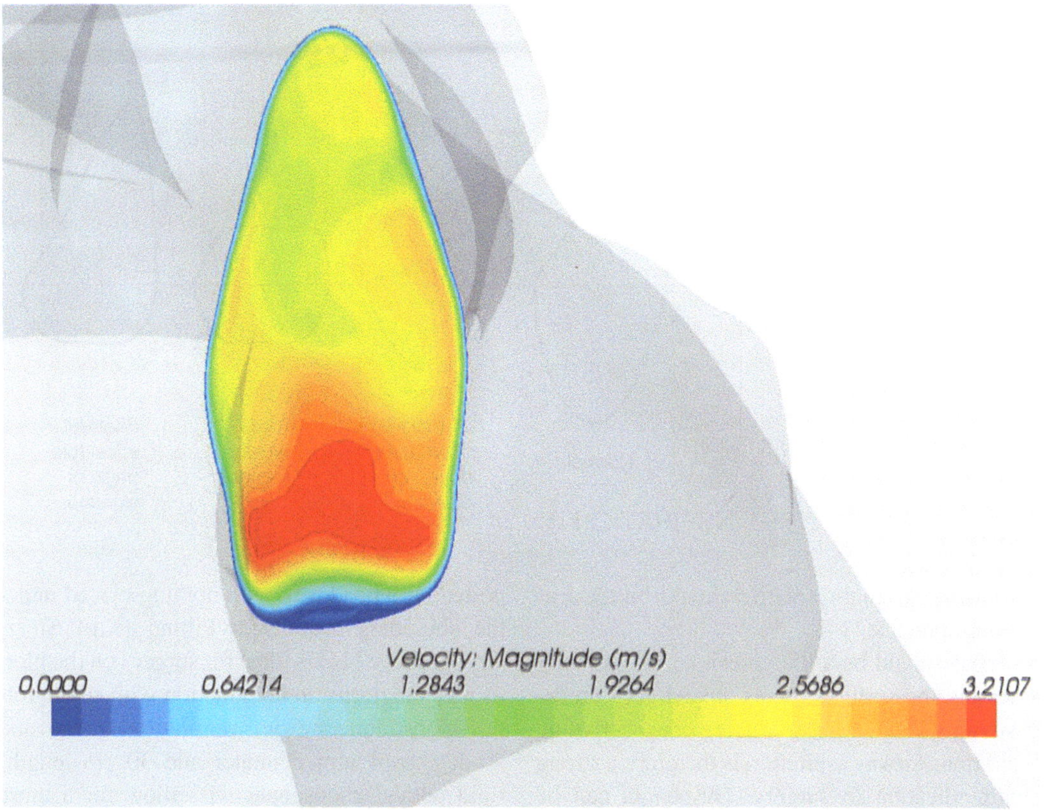

Fig. 16.2 Modelling of airflow studies through the glottis demonstrating maximum airflow between the arytenoids. (Courtesy of Professor Denis Doorly at Imperial College London)

16.5 Clinical Assessment

When first consulting with a patient, a clinical history will determine the extent to which the voice, airway and swallowing are impacted. Questions about previous airway intubation, neck surgery, systemic inflammatory disorders, previous infections, external trauma, neurological conditions and laryngeal radiotherapy are important. A general head and neck examination should be performed, followed by flexible nasal endoscopy. Careful observation of the vocal folds needs to be made, identifying scars, webs and any other lesions. Asking the patient to repeatedly say 'eeee', followed by a powerful nasal sniff, allows for estimates of the degree of abduction of each vocal fold. If the vocal folds are immobile, observations should be made of adjacent muscle activity, which, if present, could imply fixed cricoarytenoid joints. Excessive secretions around the larynx and pharynx may be an indication of swallowing problems.

Airway-specific investigations should include a high-definition computer tomographic (CT) scan of the larynx and trachea. As well as the chest, this scan should extend to include the entire neck and brainstem, if there is an unexplained vocal fold palsy. Imaging is usually not very helpful around the glottis but will help to identify other potential airway damage.

Spirometry with flow-volume loop testing is very useful for aiding diagnosis as well as assessing response to treatment. It has been shown that calculating the expiratory disproportion index (EDI; ratio of forced expiratory volume in 1 second, FEV1, to peak expiratory flow rate, PEFR) can reliably diagnose laryngotracheal stenosis [13]. The pattern of flow-volume loops will also give an indication of the nature of the glottic stenosis (Fig. 16.3).

In a dedicated airway service, patient-reported outcome measures on voice, swallowing,

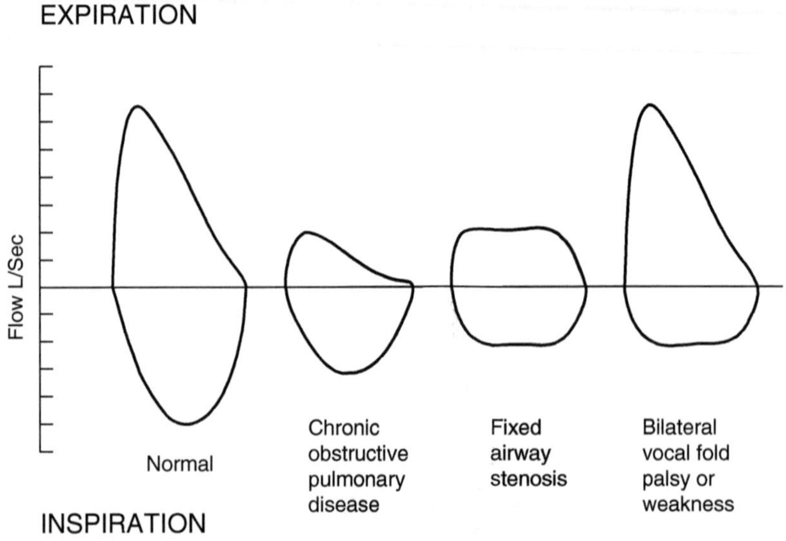

Fig. 16.3 If the stenosis is confined to the glottis, flow-volume loops can diagnose the nature of the problem

dyspnoea and quality of life should be used as standard practice [14].

There should be a low threshold for formally assessing the swallowing, as any surgery on the posterior glottis risks introducing or exacerbating aspiration. Airway aspiration is therefore a strong contraindication to surgery. Dysphagia can be assessed through fiberoptic endoscopic evaluation of swallowing (FEES) or videofluoroscopy (a modified barium swallow study).

Laryngeal electromyography (EMG) identifies muscle denervation or aberrant reinnervation and may have a role in the diagnosis and prognostication in bilateral vocal fold immobility (BVFI), in the absence of interarytenoid scarring or cricoarytenoid joint fixation. This will help in decision-making with respect to definitive surgical management, as well as in selecting the side of surgery [15].

Laboratory investigations for infection (WCC, CRP) and inflammatory markers (ESR, rheumatoid factor, ANCA, serum ACE) are useful both for screening and where there is uncertainty about the diagnosis.

Assessment of the airway under anaesthesia is useful for determining the site, extent and nature (inflammatory vs. mature scar) of glottic damage, and palpation of the cricoarytenoid joints aids in the diagnosis of recurrent laryngeal nerve palsies. Suspension laryngoscopy also allows for curative or palliative surgical interventions. For optimal surgical access, the patient's head should be supported on a head ring with nothing placed under the shoulders. The Dedo-Pilling (Karl Storz) laryngoscope [16] is ideal for surgery on the glottis and subglottis, in conjunction with supraglottic, high-frequency, jet ventilation. Zero- and 70-degree (4 mm diameter and 30 cm length) rigid optical endoscopes will allow for a more complete assessment. The Lindholm (Karl Storz) laryngoscope is better suited for operating on the glottis and supraglottis; however, in cases of glottic stenosis, a subglottic jetting catheter may be necessary.

Contraindications to surgery on the glottis should include laryngeal aspiration, but also comorbidities that preclude general anaesthesia. Glottic airway surgery under local anaesthesia is possible in some circumstances, but outcomes are very variable. Morbid obesity is a relative contraindication to airway surgery.

16.6 Anaesthesia for Glottic Airway Surgery

For both children and adults, general anaesthesia tends to be delivered totally intravenously. Children will usually have oxygen delivered via a nasopharyngeal tube as spontaneous breathing is maintained. Adults will require supraglottic or subglottic high-frequency jet ventilation, using 100% oxygen, as spontaneous breathing techniques are not reliable in this age group. If the patient has a tracheostomy, this can be removed or changed to a laser-safe airway tube during the surgery.

16.7 Causes of Glottic Stenosis

The cause of glottic stenosis can be congenital or acquired. Acquired causes are more common and encompass a wide number of aetiologies: iatrogenic, inflammatory, traumatic, infective, neoplastic and neurological causes.

Congenital glottic stenosis is rare and can range from a small anterior web to complete glottic stenosis. These conditions result from failure of normal recanalisation of the laryngotracheal tube during the third month of gestation.

16.7.1 Congenital Glottic Stenosis

Laryngeal atresia can cause complete airway obliteration through failure of recanalisation of the laryngeal lumen during embryogenesis and is usually part of a congenital high airway obstruction syndrome (CHAOS). The diagnosis may be made prenatally based on a pattern of ultrasonographic findings, including tracheal dilation and bilateral hypoechoic enlargement of the foetal lung fields, which suggest foetal upper airway obstruction [5, 17]. With early diagnosis, it is possible to bypass the airway obstruction, via a tracheostomy, and establish adequate ventilation during an EXIT (ex utero intrapartum treatment) procedure, whilst the foetus is still connected to the placenta.

Laryngeal webs account for 5% of congenital laryngeal anomalies [18] and most commonly occur at the anterior commissure. They can occur in isolation, but as many as 65% of patients with anterior glottic webs have an associated 22q11.2 deletion [19, 20] as seen in velo-cardio-facial (Shprintzen) and DiGeorge syndrome [17]. Cohen's classification (Fig. 16.4) [21] describes four grades of anterior laryngeal webs [22]: Type 1 webs are thin and involve 35% or less of the

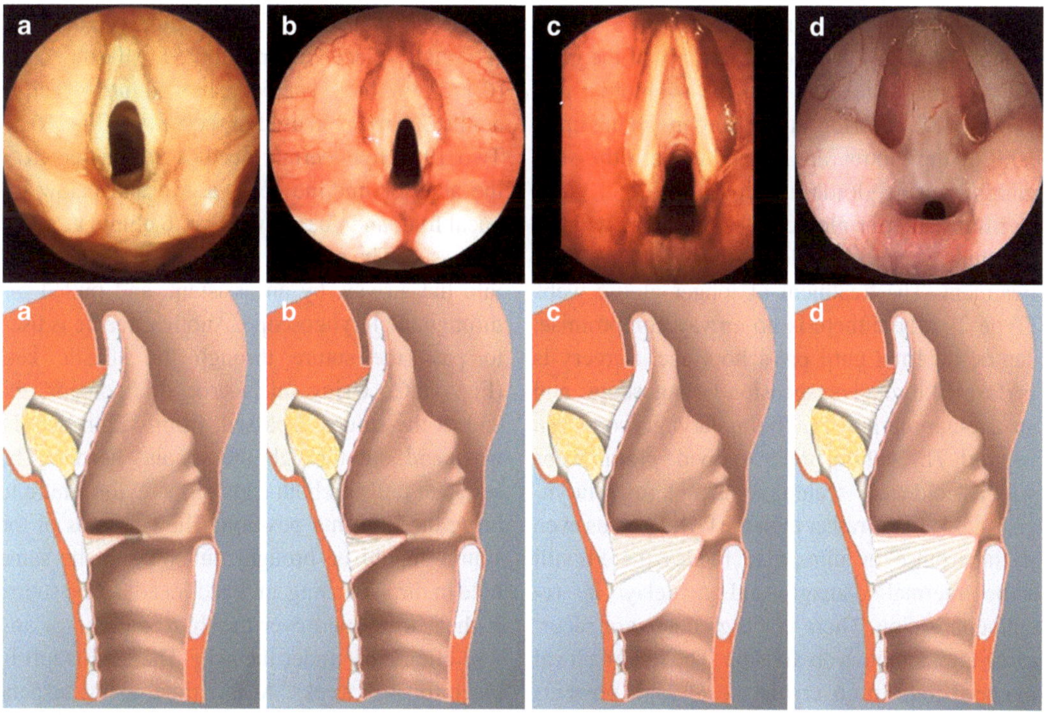

Fig. 16.4 Cohen's classification of glottic webs. Type 1, <35% of glottic length (**a**); Type 2, 35–50% + minimal subglottic extension (**b**); Type 3, 50–75% glottic length + anterior subglottic extension (**c**); and Type 4, 75–90% glottic length + severe subglottic extension + cartilage involvement (**d**) [21]

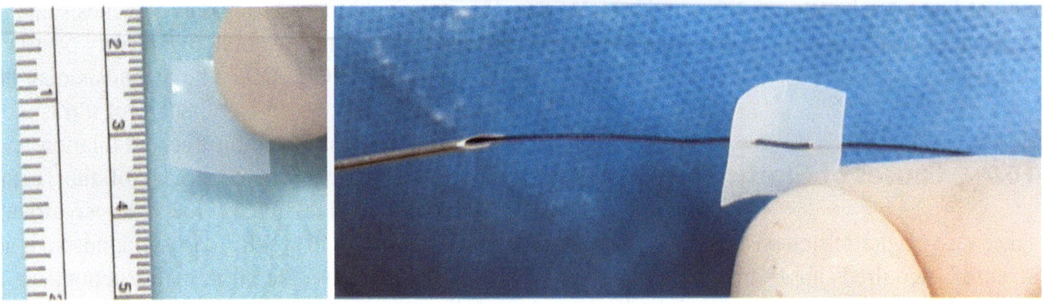

Fig. 16.5 The keel is fashioned from a sheet of 0.175-mm-thick reinforced silastic sheet (left). A 2/0 nylon suture is used to secure it (right)

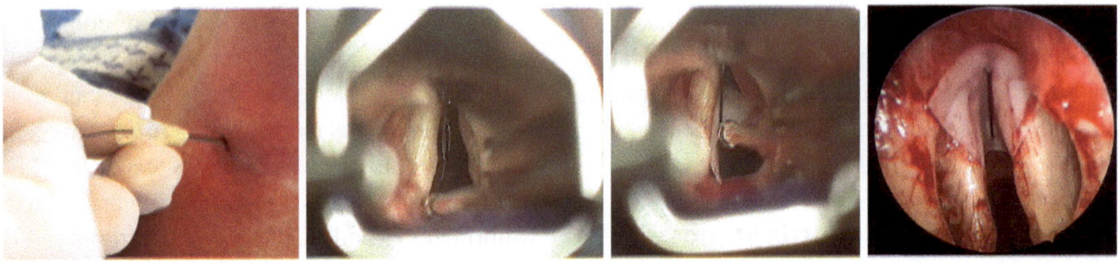

Fig. 16.6 Following suspension laryngoscopy, a 19-G needle is used to pass a 2/0 nylon suture just below the vocal folds (left). The suture is withdrawn out of the laryngoscope (centre left) and passed through the silastic keel as shown in Fig. 16.5. A second needle is passed into the larynx above the vocal folds, and the nylon suture is passed through it from within to the skin (centre right and right). A knot is tied externally to secure the keel (see text)

glottis; Type 2 webs involved 35–50% of the glottis; Type 3 webs involve 50–75% of the glottis, typically extending into the subglottis; and Type 4 webs describe a thick web involving up to 90% of the glottis, and extending into the subglottis, causing glottic fusion.

Minor anterior glottic webs (Type 1), with no breathing or voice problems, do not always need treatment. The treatment of longer glottic webs (Type 2), where there is no airway compromise, can be deferred until pre-school age. Surgery is performed through suspension laryngoscopy, and an age-appropriate Lindholm laryngoscope can be used. The authors prefer to divide glottic webs with a 'cold steel' technique using a microlaryngeal sickle blade rather than the CO_2 laser, as even in 'superpulse' or 'ultrapulse' modes, there is still some thermal damage and a delay in re-epithelialisation. There is a high degree of recurrence after simple web division. The use of a local mucosal flap, to cover one vocal fold, prevents two opposing raw surfaces and reduces the chance of the web reforming [23, 24]. However, this has a greater risk of lifelong dysphonia. The alternative is the placement of a keel after web division. A small piece of reinforced silastic sheet (0.175 mm thick) can be fashioned into a keel. In adults, 2/0 nylon is used to secure this (Fig. 16.5). Two 19-G hypodermic needles are passed from the anterior midline neck, above and below the vocal fold, and flushed with air to eliminate cored out tissue. The nylon is passed through the needle into the airway, by an assistant, and pulled out through the laryngoscope. Another needle is used to pass the suture through the silastic keel (Fig. 16.6). Using micro-crocodile forceps, the end of the suture is passed, from within the airway, and out through the second needle. The assistant pulls on both ends of the nylon suture to bring the keel into position. The two ends of the suture should be brought out through the same hole in the skin using an 'eyed' needle. The suture is then firmly tied over the thyroid cartilage and will often bury under the skin. The keel is left in place for 4–6 weeks. At this time, using suspension laryngoscopy, the suture is cut internally, and the keel removed. The suture material is removed with a small skin puncture over the knot.

This technique can also be used for acquired anterior glottic webs. These often result from extensive endolaryngeal surgery, particularly in patients who have required multiple procedures, as in recurrent respiratory papillomatosis (RRP). Anterior webs appear in situations where both sides of the anterior commissure or contiguous areas of both vocal folds have been traumatised or denuded of epithelium [25]. Preserving a strip of mucosa anteriorly on one vocal fold may mean leaving some disease, and necessitating repeat surgery, but it does reduce the chance of webbing and stenosis [26].

Open keel placement is virtually obsolete and reserved for repeated failure of the endoscopic approach. One approach in revision surgery is to suture a superficial skin graft to the keel (epidermis against silastic) before insertion (Fig. 16.7). This encourages early re-epithelialisation. Keels may also fail if there is an unidentified subglottic stenosis in association with the web.

Type 3 webs with respiratory symptoms may necessitate a tracheostomy and surgical repair within the first 2 years of life. If the web is thick and associated with subglottic narrowing, then an open laryngotracheal reconstruction (LTR) is indicated. A full laryngofissure is performed extending to the second tracheal ring. Submucosal

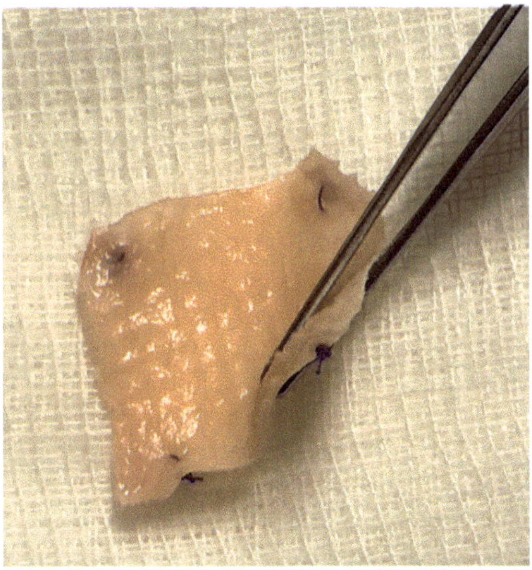

Fig. 16.7 A superficial skin graft sutured to the keel (epidermis against silastic)

resection of the anterior subglottic scar is carried out avoiding damage to the anterior commissure. The anterior subglottis is expanded with a 'boat-shaped' piece of cartilage sutured in place over an endoluminal stent. The graft must not expand the anterior commissure as this will lead to lifelong voice problems. The stent is removed 3–4 weeks later, followed by a trial of decannulation when the airway is stable.

Type 4 webs and complete laryngeal atresia will require an LTR with anterior and posterior grafting using rib cartilage and stenting. Alternatively, in the most severe cases, an extended cricotracheal resection (CTR) and stenting have been described [27].

Congenital bilateral vocal fold paralysis can result from traumatic delivery, neurological conditions and an Arnold-Chiari malformation; however, many are idiopathic in nature [17, 28]. Spontaneous recovery may be seen in 50% of cases after a period of months to years, suggesting a degree of neurological immaturity.

There are a number of management options for congenital bilateral vocal fold paralysis, ranging from watchful waiting to early tracheostomy [13], which is estimated to be required in more than 50% of patients [29]. Botulinum toxin, injected into the cricothyroid muscles, can also be useful in increasing airway patency in these patients [30]. Endoscopic surgical options include unilateral or bilateral cordotomy, laser arytenoidectomy and suture lateralisation. It has been argued that suture lateralisation is advantageous, as it is a more conservative surgical option, in situations where spontaneous recovery of bilateral vocal fold paralysis is the most likely outcome [31, 32]. This high rate of spontaneous recovery is the reason many advocate waiting at least 12 months, with or without a tracheostomy, before offering a destructive surgical procedure [29, 33]. Open approaches such as external arytenoidopexy and arytenoidectomy have been shown to be successful as measured by tracheostomy decannulation rates. Posterior cricoid split and costal cartilage placement, performed as an open or endoscopic procedure, are used in revision cases [29]. To date, no study has demonstrated superiority of one treatment over another [34].

16.7.2 Acquired Causes of Bilateral Impaired Vocal Fold Function

The causes of bilateral vocal fold mobility impairment (BVFI) can be subdivided into:

1. Bilateral recurrent laryngeal nerve (RLN) injury.
2. Bilateral cricoarytenoid joint (CAJ) fixation.
3. Interarytenoid scarring.

Surgery conducted along the course of both recurrent laryngeal nerves (RLN) can risk bilateral vocal fold palsy. Most commonly, this follows thyroid surgery, bilateral carotid endarterectomy or sometimes cardiac surgery [35].

Idiopathic bilateral vocal fold immobility (BVFI) in adults requires a thorough history and examination, in conjunction with imaging such as computed tomography (CT), to follow the tenth cranial and recurrent laryngeal nerves and an MRI of the brain to exclude central neurological causes. In a series of 61 patients with BVFI, both adult and paediatric, up to 39% were found to be idiopathic [36]. A more recent study of nine adult patients with idiopathic BVFI found that one-third of the cohort experienced eventual and spontaneous recovery of vocal fold motion and the authors advocate waiting at least 1 year from onset for signs of return of motion [37]. Careful examination, EMG and follow-up are important so as not to over-diagnose idiopathic BVFI, as paradoxical vocal cord motion and some forms of progressive laryngeal dystonia may mimic the condition.

Paradoxical vocal fold motion (PVFM), a type of vocal cord dysfunction, is a disorder in which the vocal cords inappropriately adduct during inspiration, which can lead to dyspnoea and even stridor, and is often misdiagnosed as asthma. Patients may present repeatedly to the emergency medical services. There is controversy around the causes of this condition, and psychological, neurological and environmental irritants and even gastro-oesophageal reflux (GORD) have been postulated [38]. The treatment of PVFM should be multidisciplinary and include ENT and respiratory physicians, as well as a speech therapy, clinical psychology and respiratory physiotherapy. In the more resistant cases, botulinum toxin injection into the thyroarytenoid muscle [39] is used, but the results are not reliable, and there may be a large 'placebo effect'. In only the most severe cases should tracheostomy be offered, as it provides an identifiable label of 'ill-health' for the patient.

Vocal cord dysfunction can be a feature of neurodegenerative disorders such as multiple sclerosis (MS) and amyotrophic lateral sclerosis (ALS) [40]. It is estimated that up to 30% of patients with bulbar-onset ALS suffer with bilateral vocal cord abductor paresis [41] due to both infranuclear and supranuclear mechanisms. Apparent PVFM can also be seen in advanced cases of ALS [42]. Vocal cord abductor paresis has been described in multi-system atrophy (MSA), due to atrophy of the posterior cricoarytenoid muscle, and more rarely in Parkinson's disease. Patients typically present in the late stages of these diseases. The vocal folds are bowed and paramedian, and there is characteristic inspiratory stridor due to 'drawing in' of the folds through the Bernoulli effect. Reduced muscle tone means laser procedures, in isolation, will make this stridor worse and disproportionately impact voice and swallowing. When the alternative is a tracheostomy, the senior author has bought time by performing a cricothyroid approximation and at the same time a small laser arytenoidectomy. This tensions the cords to improve the voice by reducing the 'laxity', but without the arytenoidectomy, the breathing would be worse. Any decisions regarding a tracheostomy require multidisciplinary input.

Rheumatoid arthritis can involve the cricoarytenoid joints, leading to ankylosis and joint fixation [43, 44]; eventually, this may result in BVFI [45]. This is estimated to occur in up to 25% of patients with rheumatoid arthritis [25]. Other inflammatory conditions that have been found to cause cricoarytenoid arthritis with subsequent BVFI include ankylosing spondylitis [46], sys-

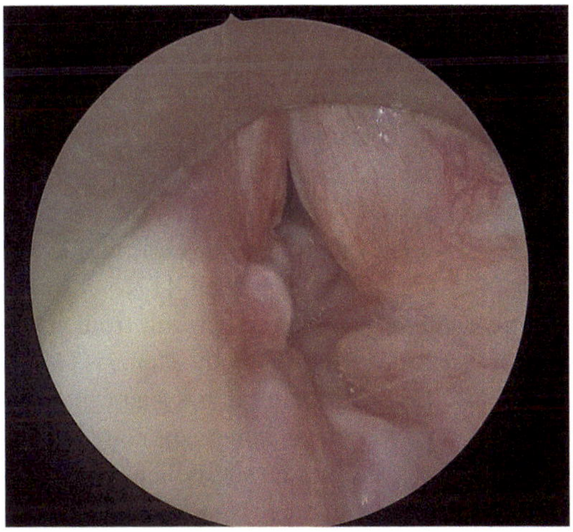

Fig. 16.8 Posterior glottic inflammation and granulation following extubation

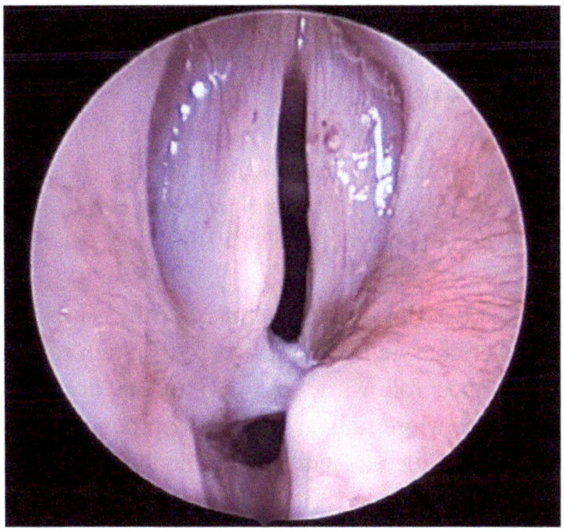

Fig. 16.9 Bogdasarian classification Type I

temic lupus erythematous (SLE) [47] and relapsing polychondritis (RP) [48].

The most common cause of posterior glottic stenosis is endotracheal intubation [49]. In these cases, at extubation, there are inflammation and granulation of the posterior glottis due to pressure necrosis (Fig. 16.8), which can then progress to dense interarytenoid scarring and subsequent vocal fold fixation [50].

Bilateral cricoarytenoid joint fixation, if not treated early, will lead to permanent ankylosis of these joints. Risk factors for post-intubation stenosis include lengthy intubation, large endotracheal tube size, repeated motion of the patient or endotracheal tube and gastro-oesophageal reflux [25]. Patients with aggressive healing biology in their airway are more likely to heal with scarring.

It is also important to avoid injury to the posterior commissure during any kind of laryngeal or airway procedure, as scar formation and webs in this area can impair vocal fold movement. Endoscopic approaches to manage this type of injury tend to have poor outcomes, and the best that can be hoped for is a compromise between voice, airway and swallowing.

The Bogdasarian classification of posterior glottic stenosis is widely used to stratify treatment options:

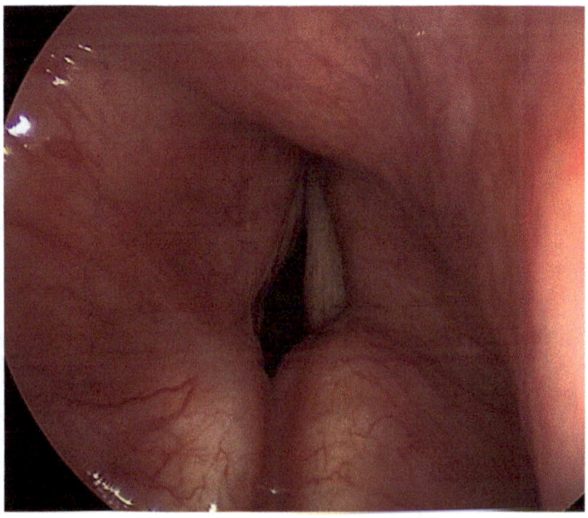

Fig. 16.10 Bogdasarian classification Type II

Type I involves an interarytenoid scar band between the vocal folds that is anterior and separate from the posterior interarytenoid mucosa (Fig. 16.9). If identified, early division of this band and balloon dilatation will restore normal function. However, delaying treatment will lead to ankylosis of the cricoarytenoid joints.

Type II stenosis involves scarring of the mucosa or musculature of the posterior interarytenoid area (Fig. 16.10). If identified early, 'cold steel' division, balloon dilatation and steroid injection may restore function. The procedure may need to be repeated at 2–4 weeks. If unsuccessful, then the approach for *type IV* stenosis should be considered.

Type III stenosis is described as unilateral cricoarytenoid joint fixation (Fig. 16.11).

Type IV describes bilateral cricoarytenoid joint fixation (Fig. 16.12).

In posterior glottis stenosis with associated fixed cricoarytenoid joints, there is a high rate of recurrence following scar division or arytenoidectomy. More radical surgical approaches need to be considered and are detailed later in this chapter.

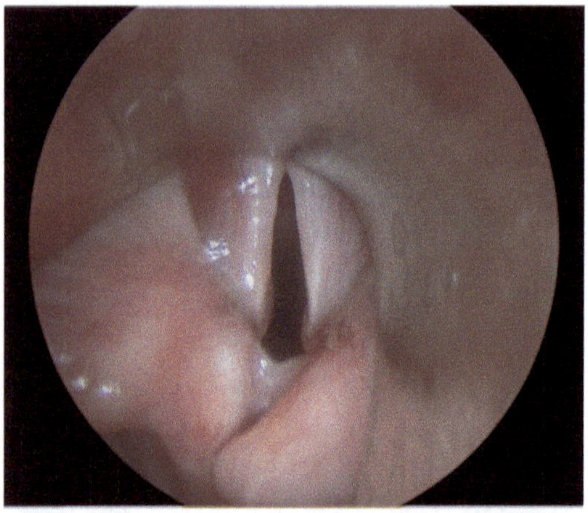

Fig. 16.11 Bogdasarian classification Type III

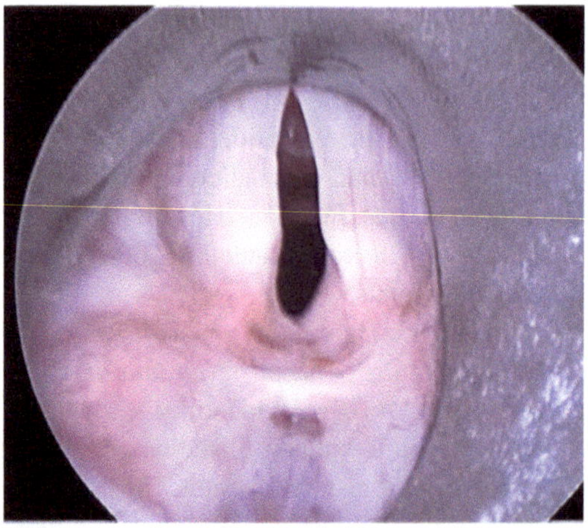

Fig. 16.12 Bogdasarian classification Type IV

16.7.3 Systemic Causes of Glottic Stenosis

Granulomatosis with polyangiitis (GPA, previously Wegener's granulomatosis) is a systemic autoimmune ANCA-positive vasculitis that typically affects the subglottis; however, glottic stenosis has also been described [17]. Posterior glottic stenosis may indirectly result from proximal progression of the subglottic stenosis [51].

Sarcoidosis, a chronic multi-system granulomatous condition of unknown aetiology, affects the larynx in 1% of cases and typically involves the supraglottis (Fig. 16.13). As the disease has a predilection for the lymphatic system, the glottis is rarely involved. Secondary dysfunction can occur due to fixation of the vocal folds usually as a result of gross distortion of normal anatomy or through a peripheral neuropathy involving the recurrent laryngeal nerves [52].

Management of the condition is medical and beyond the scope of this chapter; however, the airway surgeon can assist in maintaining a patent airway until the disease is under control. The technique is to inject the supraglottic tissue, throughout its three-dimensional extent, with a sustained-release steroid such as methylprednisolone or triamcinolone (40 mg/mL). Up to 3 mL can be used. Using the steroid injection alone temporarily expands the appar-

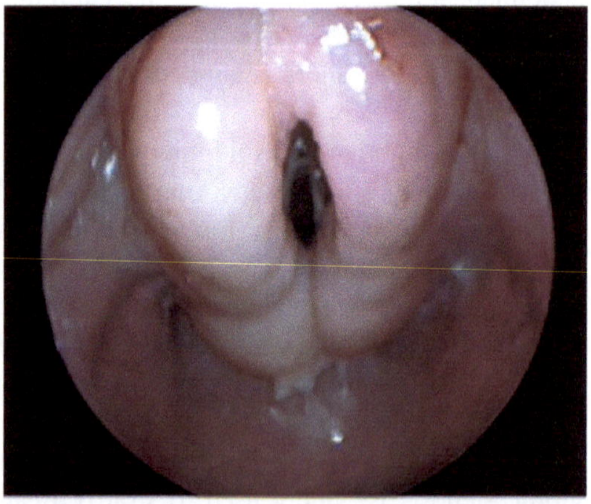

Fig. 16.13 Appearance of laryngeal sarcoidosis with submucosal swelling over the arytenoids, aryepiglottic folds and epiglottis as well as narrowing of the airway

ent bulk of the disease and narrows the airway further, and the patient wakes up with greater stridor. The aim is to reduce disease bulk without causing circumferential scar within the laryngeal inlet. The 'pepper-pot technique' was developed to solve this problem [53]. The CO_2 laser is set at 10 W power, finely focussed spot size and superpulse or ultrapulse mode in a continuous delivery. The laser is fired in one spot over the disease, for 2–4 s, to cause a deep interstitial burn. This is repeated again and again with the spots separated by 1–2 mm (Fig. 16.14). This, combined with the steroid injection, will reduce disease bulk and should be repeated every 4 weeks, until there is no evidence of disease regrowth. Sometimes, the technique needs to be combined with radial cuts through the aryepiglottic folds and/or balloon dilatation to obtain an adequate airway so that the patient can safely recover from anaesthesia.

Laryngeal amyloidosis accounts for 1% of all benign laryngeal lesions [54]. Amyloid deposits typically are found in the supraglottis; however, the glottis can also be affected [55–57]. IgG4-related disease, a systemic immune-mediated condition characterised by a lymphoplasmacytic infiltrate rich in IgG4-positive plasma cells [58, 59], is similarly rare, but there have also been reports of glottic stenosis secondary to bilateral vocal fold immobility, due to fibrosis [60], as well as more extensive disease extending from the supraglottis down to the trachea [61].

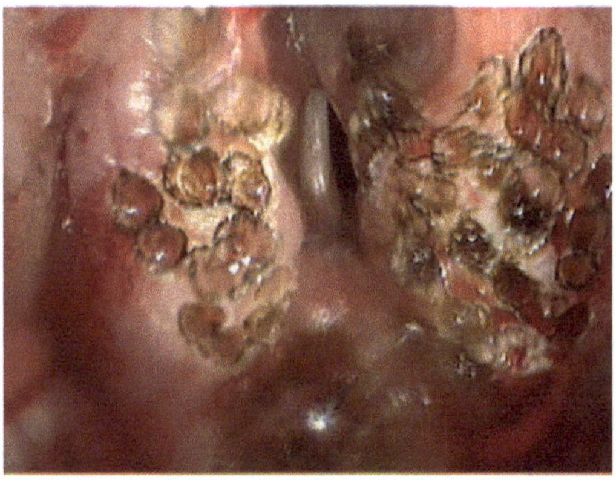

Fig. 16.14 'Pepper-pot' CO_2 laser technique to treat laryngeal amyloidosis (see text for details)

Additionally, both diseases could conceivably cause BVFI through direct infiltration [62] or mechanical compression at the skull base [63] or mediastinum [63, 64] at the tenth cranial or recurrent laryngeal nerves.

Cicatricial pemphigoid, also known as mucous membrane pemphigoid and characterised by widespread scarring, can result in glottic/supraglottic stenosis [65] and even total laryngeal stenosis [66].

Acromegaly can impair vocal cord mobility bilaterally and has been described in a handful of cases in the literature [67]. Grotting and Pemberton have previously postulated four potential mechanisms: arthritis of the cricoarytenoid joint, cartilaginous enlargement causing impaired mobility of the cricoarytenoid joint, stretching of the recurrent laryngeal nerves by laryngeal enlargement or recurrent laryngeal nerve injury by thyroid enlargement [68]. Other potential pathophysiological mechanisms include mass effect from thickened laryngeal structures causing vocal cord fixation as well as possible axonal demyelination as a direct result of acromegaly [69]. BVFI improvement has been observed in the successful treatment of acromegaly, giving more weight to reversible aetiologies, which should be considered when treating this condition.

16.7.4 Traumatic Causes of Glottic Stenosis

Penetrating trauma to the neck can cause immediate BVFI if both RLN are injured [70]. Blunt laryngeal trauma or even attempted strangulation can result in bilateral fold palsies; however, in most cases, recovery of one or both nerves can be expected, and the patient may need airway management with a temporary tracheostomy.

External laryngeal injuries can also result in mucosal tears and cartilaginous fractures, which disrupt the laryngeal framework (Fig. 16.15); timely treatment is required to prevent long-term glottic stenosis [71, 72]. Fractures into or haemarthrosis of the cricoarytenoid joints can also lead to immobility.

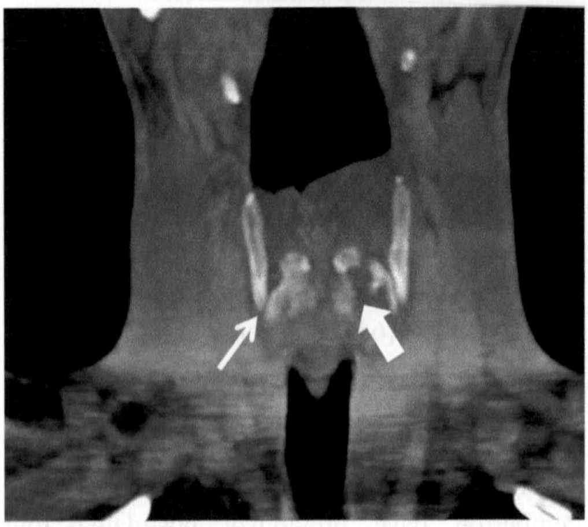

Fig. 16.15 Coronal maximum intensity projection (MIP) reconstruction demonstrating the widely separated fracture of the left posterior cricoid cartilage (block arrow) resulting in disruption of the cricoarytenoid joint. Note the normal right cricoarytenoid joint (arrow)

Endolaryngeal trauma, caused by caustic injection [73], foreign bodies [17] or thermal burns [74], can also result in glottic stenosis.

16.7.5 Infective Causes of Glottic Stenosis

Tuberculosis (TB) can affect the larynx, commonly at the posterior glottis as well as the arytenoid cartilages [75, 76], and may occur in isolation or alongside pulmonary TB. Other infective causes include leprosy, syphilis, diphtheria and rhinoscleroma [49]. The majority of bacterial and viral infections that affect the larynx do not result in long-term glottic stenosis. However, most upper respiratory tract infections are associated with a degree of laryngopharyngitis, and prolonged airway intubation during this inflammatory phase, as seen during the COVID-19 pandemic of 2020, can lead to both glottic injury and posterior glottic and subglottic stenosis [77].

16.7.6 Neoplastic Causes of Glottic Stenosis

Primary laryngeal cancer, the most common form of which is squamous cell carcinoma, can narrow the glottic airway and cause BVFI. Non-laryngeal malignancies include lung, thyroid, oesophageal and other mediastinal masses, e.g. enlarged lymph nodes, which can compress or invade the RLN in the tracheo-oesophageal groove [78].

Radiotherapy for laryngeal, pharyngo-oesophageal and thyroid cancers can cause glottic stenosis and impair vocal fold movement, weeks, months or years following completion of treatment [79–81]. Endoscopic airway surgery and laryngotracheal reconstruction have a high risk of failure in these patients due to poor healing, but also because of the negative impact on swallowing. A significant number of patients aspirate due to severely impaired laryngopharyngeal function, presenting up to 20 years after completion of radiotherapy [82, 83]. They risk death from respiratory complications through chronic aspiration. Tracheostomies and alternative routes for feeding only serve to buy time, and ultimately, a laryngectomy may need to be offered.

16.8 Management of Glottic Stenosis

It is important to include the patient and the multidisciplinary team in decision-making in the management of glottic stenosis. It should be emphasised that the aim of treatment is for an optimal balance between voice, swallowing and airway, and it must be understood that ongoing speech and swallowing therapy, as well as 'fine-tuning' surgical procedures, may be necessary. Attention must also be given to the likelihood of potential reversibility of BVFI, as this will influence the choice of treatment, particularly if a glottic resection is being considered. It must also be mentioned that in procedures where the airway is at risk, safety is paramount, and the possibility of a tracheostomy should be part of the consent process.

16.8.1 Laser Techniques

A simple anterior or posterior glottic scar can be divided endoscopically using cold steel instruments or the CO_2 laser, alongside intralesional steroid injection and balloon dilatation. Some recurrence of the scar is to be expected. Placement of an anterior keel at the time of scar division has been found to reduce recurrence [84] and is described above.

CO_2 laser arytenoidectomy and posterior cordotomy, now an established technique [85–87], were first described by Ossoff et al. in 1983 [88]. A good glottic airway may be achieved; however, it is important to perform a pre-operative swallow assessment in the form of fiberoptic endoscopic evaluation of swallowing (FEES) or videofluoroscopic swallow study (VFSS). The swallow can be compromised as a result of these procedures, leading to aspiration [89] and subsequent granulation and healing by scarring. In situations where there is a marginal impairment of swallowing, the authors advocate starting with a small partial CO_2 laser arytenoidectomy. The aim is to resect the posterior vocal process and medial arytenoid (Fig. 16.16) whilst preserving the outer rim and height of the arytenoid [49]. This resection can subsequently be enlarged, depending on the degree of airway improvement, the extent to which the voice and swallowing have been compromised and how much of the resection heals.

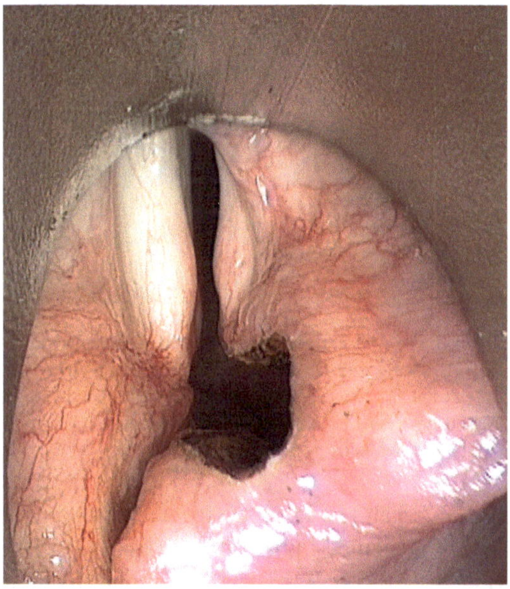

Fig. 16.16 Partial laser arytenoidectomy using the CO_2 laser

In cases of dense posterior glottic scar, the authors advocate a posterior cricoid split, via an open laryngofissure approach. Costal cartilage is then harvested and fashioned into a 'spacer' (Fig. 16.17). This procedure can also be performed endoscopically. Interarytenoid scar resection and reconstruction with a postcricoid mucosal advancement flap, first described by Montgomery [90], can be carried out as an open or endoscopic operation [91].

16.8.2 Suture Lateralisation

Suture lateralisation may be used as a temporary solution in situations where nerve function may recover and can be performed as an open or endoscopic procedure; most commonly, in recent years, it has been performed endoscopically.

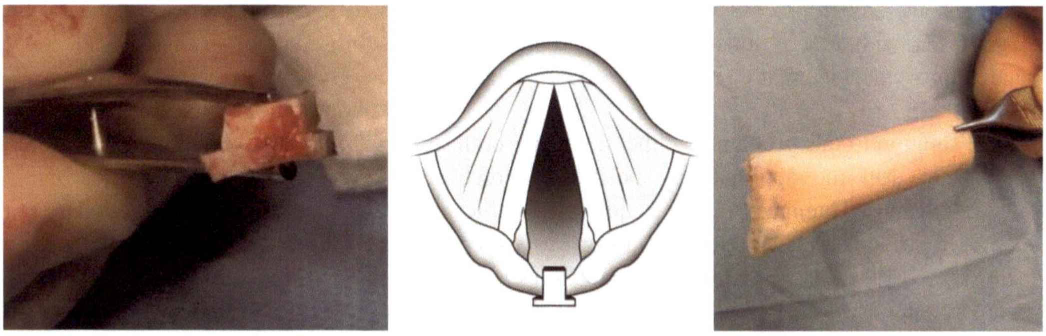

Fig. 16.17 A piece of costal cartilage is harvested from right fifth or sixth rib and carved with flanges as shown (left). Following a laryngofissure approach and a midline posterior cricoid split, this cartilage is placed as shown (centre). A closed laryngeal stent, created from the vertical limb of a suitably sized silastic T-tube and covered with a superficial skin graft, is stitched in place for 2 weeks (right). A covering tracheostomy is removed at 2 weeks, immediately following endoscopic removal of the stent

A number of early twentieth-century otolaryngologists described external approach suture lateralisation; Erwin Payr (Vienna) described a technique where the paralysed vocal folds are sutured to the thyroid alar. Rethi (Budapest) used a similar technique, opening the cricoarytenoid joint via a laryngofissure approach to then abduct the arytenoid and overlying mucosa, with a temporary suture tied over a rubber tube placed on the skin of the neck for 10 days [92]. These procedures were prone to infection.

Other methods include Schobel's technique, which preserves the posterior cricoarytenoid ligament as a hinge to allow lateral tilt of the arytenoid cartilage [93]; permanent retention sutures are used which run in the submucosa along the arytenoid cartilage and are fixed with burr holes on the posterior margin of the thyroid cartilage. Woodson and Weiss [94] described a similar technique in 2007, using a suture from the muscular process of the arytenoid to the inferior cornu of the thyroid cartilage.

As the use of rigid endoscopes, operating microscopes and surgical laser techniques developed in the twentieth century, endolaryngeal techniques have evolved using similar basic principles to the open methods of suture lateralisation.

Due to age-related changes, particularly in males, the thyroid lamina gradually calcifies starting at its posterior edge, making it difficult to insert a very posterior suture. This difficulty means that the suture tends to be placed more anterior than is desirable and the result is lateralisation of the vocal process of the arytenoid (Fig. 16.18), with a large impact on voice and a small improvement in breathing (as demonstrated in Fig. 16.2).

The solution to this problem is either a small incision to drill the appropriately positioned holes in the thyroid lamina or utilising equipment such as the endolaryngeal thread guide instrument (ETGI) [95], for an endoscopic abduction arytenoid lateropexy (EAAL). The ETGI uses a mobile integrated curved blade (Fig. 16.19) with a hole at the tip; this allows mounting of a suture, which is then passed between the external neck and internal laryngeal cavity, even through a highly calcified posterior thyroid cartilage (Fig. 16.20). In cricoarytenoid joint fixation, bilateral EAAL is advocated, whereas unilateral EAAL is performed in BVFI. Prior to suturing, where it is necessary, glottic scar tissue should first be divided, and the cricoarytenoid joint should be mobilised using an angled sickle knife, if it is fixed.

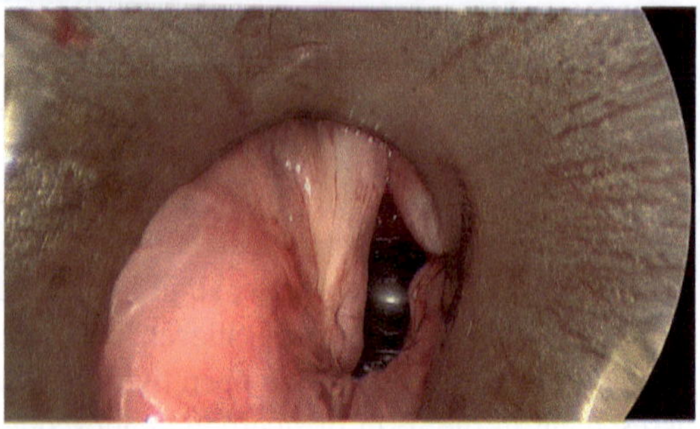

Fig. 16.18 Traditional suture lateralisation technique causes membranous vocal fold lateralisation as well, impacting the voice

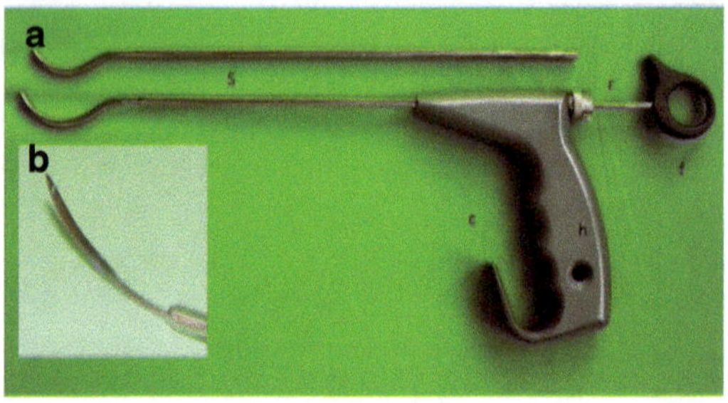

Fig. 16.19 The endolaryngeal thread guide instrument (ETGI) uses a mobile integrated curved blade (**b**) with a hole at the tip; this allows for mounting of a suture, to be passed between the external neck and internal laryngeal cavity and out again

The most common indication for suture lateralisation is bilateral vocal fold palsies, where recovery is expected, as it is said to be reversible. Advocates of this technique state that recovery can take 6–12 months and the only other option is a tracheostomy, because an arytenoidectomy would permanently damage and fix the cricoarytenoid joint. The reality is that most of these cases of bilateral palsies are seen post-thyroidectomy and the patient either is

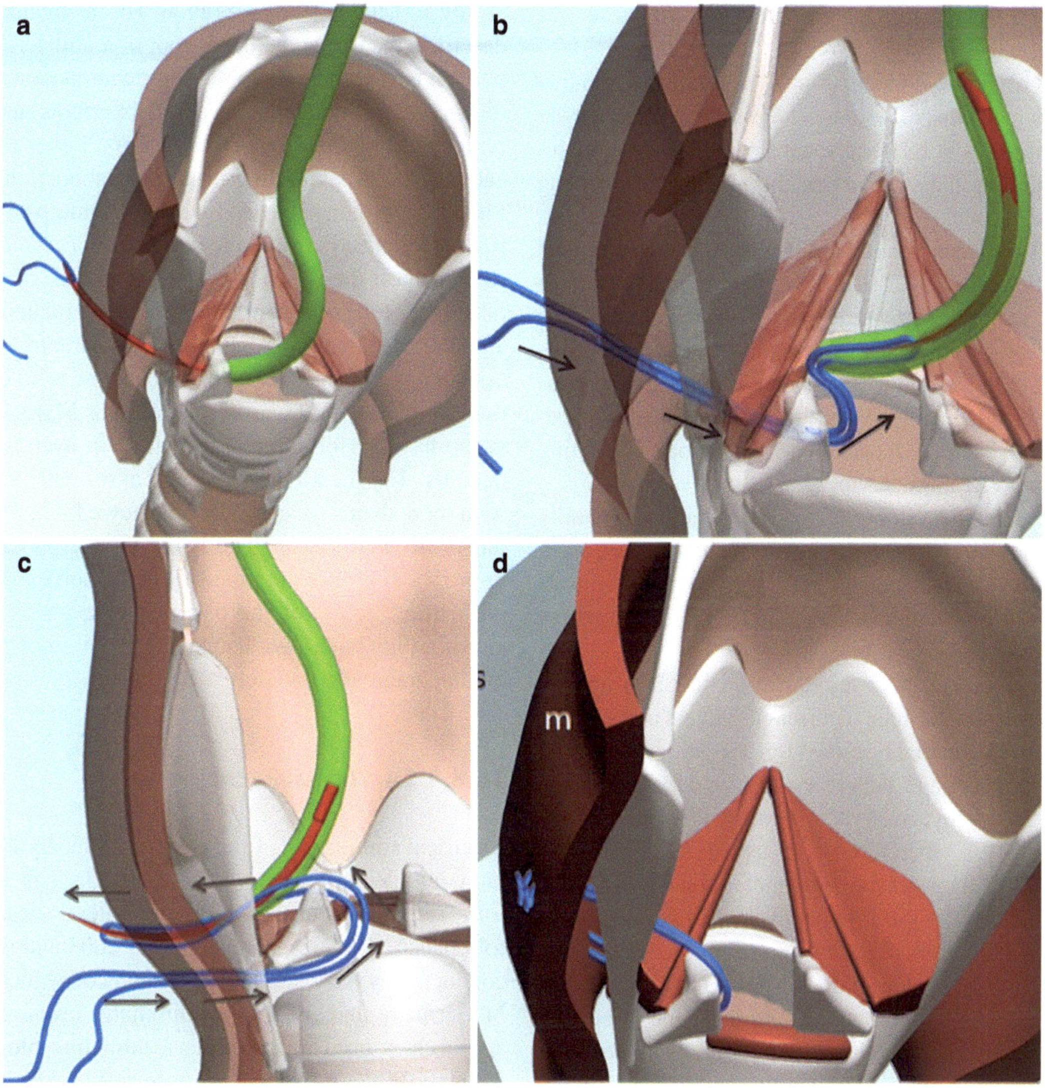

Fig. 16.20 The ETGI device is used during suspension laryngoscopy to pass its curved blade under the vocal process to the surface of the neck. A 1/0 nylon suture is laced through the hole at the tip of the needle. The double loop of suture is pulled into the airway (**a**) and pushed out over the thread above the vocal process (**b**) to the surface of the neck. The double folded thread is cut (**c**), and the ends of the suture are passed using the 'eye needle' to a common hole in the skin. The corresponding ends are knotted under the skin (**d**)

given a tracheostomy shortly after or manages with a partially compromised airway. If there is going to be useful return of airway function, it appears within a few days as oedema and swelling resolve or within a few weeks if the original injury was a neuropraxia. Recovery after many months is usually from a more significant nerve injury and is virtually always synkinetic. Classically, the patient starts off with a weak voice but only partially restricted breathing as the vocal folds lie in the paramedian position. Months later, the voice tends to become stronger and breathing gets worse, through aberrant and synkinetic reinnervation. The increased medial force can break or cause the suture to cut into the cartilage. Hence, there is a need for tracheostomy or revision surgery in 13–38% of EAAL [50].

16.8.3 Selective Reinnervation

Laryngeal reinnervation is a surgical technique which aims to restore nerve function to the larynx in cases of bilateral vocal fold palsy whilst maintaining the structure of the larynx and avoiding detrimental effects to the voice and swallow. These techniques are not suitable for mechanical fixation such as scar tissue or CAJ ankylosis; it is therefore prudent to have performed an examination under anaesthesia to assess CAJ mobility. Laryngeal reinnervation can be selective or non-selective, and the main target is the posterior cricoarytenoid muscle, the principal abducting muscle of the larynx.

Reinnervation can be performed unilaterally or bilaterally, and three main techniques are used: nerve implantation into the muscle, nerve-muscle pedicle implantation and selective nerve anastomosis.

Non-selective reinnervation involves anastomosis to the main recurrent laryngeal nerve trunk, which inevitably causes reinnervation of both the abductor and adductor intrinsic laryngeal muscles; recovery of vocal fold mobility and phonation is therefore not usually achieved in BVFI. Non-selective reinnervation has a role in unilateral vocal fold paralysis [96].

Selective reinnervation aims to separately reinnervate the abductor and adductor muscle groups to enable vocal fold mobility, to enlarge the glottis and to improve breathing whilst allowing adduction for phonation and airway protection. The phrenic and hypoglossal nerves are used most commonly, as they have similar properties to the recurrent laryngeal nerve in terms of function and success has been found in animal experiments.

In the 1980s, Tucker et al. described the nerve-muscle pedicle technique, using an ansa hypoglossi nerve with omohyoid to reinnervate the posterior cricoarytenoid muscle; in a case series of 202 patients, 74% demonstrated good outcomes; however, other surgeons have since not been able to replicate these results [97].

Professor Marie (Rouen, France) advocates the use of the phrenic nerve for selective reinnervation in BVFI due to its inherent physiological ability to activate for inspiration. His technique describes the use of the upper root of a unilateral phrenic nerve (to preserve the contralateral hemidiaphragm), to innervate the posterior cricoarytenoid muscles bilaterally in the form of a Y-shaped cable graft, thus initiating inspiratory abduction. Phonation is then achieved by using an interposition nerve graft between the nerve to thyrohyoid (a branch off the hypoglossal nerve) and the distal stump of the recurrent laryngeal nerve bilaterally. Pre-operative laryngeal electromyography is essential to the success of the procedure to rule out complete muscle atrophy. Professor Marie's group have performed this technique in over 50 patients. The most recent data, from 40 patients with more than 1-year follow-up, showed that 35 out of 40 were decannulated and the dyspnoea improved in 75% of the patients [50]. Importantly, the partial section of the phrenic nerve on one side does not have significant detrimental impact on diaphragmatic function.

16.8.4 Laryngeal Pacing

Electrical stimulation of the posterior cricoarytenoid muscle, known as laryngeal pacing, is a form of dynamic rehabilitation for bilateral vocal fold palsies. This research started in 2003 and is conducted by Andreas H. Mueller and colleagues in Germany and Austria. A minimally invasive approach is used to introduce a miniature biocompatible electrode into the posterior cricoarytenoid muscle; they have found this technique circumvents the previously encountered problems of post-operative scarring following an open approach. Additionally, they have improved the electrode to be able to withstand high electrical charge densities to reduce the risk of corrosion. They have used bipolar stimulation and optimal electrode geometry to reduce the risk of coactivation of the adductor muscles [98].

Laryngeal EMG was found to be important in identifying the synkinetic reinnervation of the internal laryngeal muscles in bilateral palsies. Patients in whom this synkinesis was approximately 85% were found to be good candidates for laryngeal pacing [50].

Mueller et al. started a prospective feasibility human study in 2012 in unilateral implantation of the stimulation electrode, in patients with persistent bilateral vocal fold palsies, present for at least 1 year. The initial results were published in 2016 [99] where they found an immediate and stable improvement in dyspnoea based on spirometry in nine patients, without negative effects on phonation. This demonstrates promise in this technique whilst highlighting the need for further research in larger patient cohorts.

References

1. Jea B, editor. Union for international cancer control TNM classification. 8th ed. Hoboken, NJ: Wiley-Blackwell; 2016. p. 31.
2. Compton CCBD, Garcia-Aguilar J, et al., editors. AJCC Cancer Staging Atlas: a companion to the seventh editions of the AJCC cancer staging manual and handbook. 2nd ed. New York, NY: Springer; 2012. p. 80.
3. Hall A, Cobb R, Kapoor K, Kuchai R, Sandhu G. The Instrument of voice: the "true" vocal cord or vocal fold? J Voice. 2017;31(2):133–4.
4. Nouraei SM. SARN. Anatomy of the larynx and trachea. In: Laryngeal and tracheobronchial stenosis. San Diego: Plural Publishing; 2016.
5. Landry AM, Rutter MJ. Airway anomalies. Clin Perinatol. 2018;45(4):597–607.
6. Wyatt ME, Hartley BE. Laryngotracheal reconstruction in congenital laryngeal webs and atresias. Otolaryngol Head Neck Surg. 2005;132(2):232–8.
7. Lungova V, Verheyden JM, Sun X, Thibeault SL. beta-Catenin signaling is essential for mammalian larynx recanalization and the establishment of vocal fold progenitor cells. Development. 2018;145(4):dev157677.
8. Negus V. The comparative anatomy of the larynx with particular reference to the functions of the organ in man. Lect Sci Basis Med. 1954;4:332–57.
9. Sasaki CT, Weaver EM. Physiology of the larynx. Am J Med. 1997;103(5A):9S–18S.
10. Sasaki CT. Anatomy and development and physiology of the larynx. GI Motility Online. 2016; https://doi.org/10.1038/gimo7.
11. Ghazanfar AA, Rendall D. Evolution of human vocal production. Curr Biol. 2008;18(11):R457–60.
12. Lieberman PH, Klatt DH, Wilson WH. Vocal tract limitations on the vowel repertoires of rhesus monkey and other nonhuman primates. Science. 1969;164(3884):1185–7.
13. Nouraei SA, Nouraei SM, Patel A, Murphy K, Giussani DA, Koury EF, et al. Diagnosis of laryngotracheal stenosis from routine pulmonary physiology using the expiratory disproportion index. Laryngoscope. 2013;123(12):3099–104.
14. Clunie GM, Roe JWG, Alexander C, Sandhu G, McGregor A. Voice and swallowing outcomes following airway reconstruction in adults: a systematic review. Laryngoscope. 2021;131(1):146–57.
15. Munin MC, Heman-Ackah YD, Rosen CA, Sulica L, Maronian N, Mandel S, et al. Consensus statement: using laryngeal electromyography for the diagnosis and treatment of vocal cord paralysis. Muscle Nerve. 2016;53(6):850–5.
16. Sandhu GS, Reza Nouraei SA. Laryngeal and tracheobronchial stenosis. San Diego: Plural Publishing; 2016.
17. Stephenson KA, Wyatt ME. Glottic stenosis. Semin Pediatr Surg. 2016;25(3):132–7.
18. Holinger PH, Brown WT. Congenital webs, cysts, laryngoceles and other anomalies of the larynx. Ann Otol Rhinol Laryngol. 1967;76(4):744–52.
19. Lawlor CM, Dombrowski ND, Nuss RC, Rahbar R, Choi SS. Laryngeal web in the pediatric population: evaluation and management. Otolaryngol Head Neck Surg. 2020;162(2):234–40.
20. Miyamoto RC, Cotton RT, Rope AF, Hopkin RJ, Cohen AP, Shott SR, et al. Association of anterior glottic webs with velocardiofacial syndrome (chromosome 22q11.2 deletion). Otolaryngol Head Neck Surg. 2004;130(4):415–7.
21. Monnier P. Pediatric airway surgery. Berlin: Springer; 2011. p. 127.
22. Cohen SR. Congenital glottic webs in children. A retrospective review of 51 patients. Ann Otol Rhinol Laryngol Suppl. 1985;121:2–16.
23. McGuirt WF, Salmon J, Blalock D. Normal speech for patients with laryngeal webs: an achievable goal. Laryngoscope. 1984;94(9):1176–9.
24. Edwards J, Tanna N, Bielamowicz SA. Endoscopic lysis of anterior glottic webs and silicone keel placement. Ann Otol Rhinol Laryngol. 2007;116(3):211–6.
25. Gardner GM. Posterior glottic stenosis and bilateral vocal fold immobility: diagnosis and treatment. Otolaryngol Clin N Am. 2000;33(4):855–78.
26. Ossoff RH, Werkhaven JA, Dere H. Soft-tissue complications of laser surgery for recurrent respiratory papillomatosis. Laryngoscope. 1991;101(11):1162–6.
27. Monnier P. Partial cricotracheal resection and extended cricotracheal resection for pediatric laryngotracheal stenosis. Thorac Surg Clin. 2018;28(2):177–87.
28. Lesnik M, Thierry B, Blanchard M, Glynn F, Denoyelle F, Couloigner V, et al. Idiopathic bilateral vocal cord paralysis in infants: case series and literature review. Laryngoscope. 2015;125(7):1724–8.
29. Brigger MT, Hartnick CJ. Surgery for pediatric vocal cord paralysis: a meta-analysis. Otolaryngol Head Neck Surg. 2002;126(4):349–55.
30. Daniel SJ, Cardona I. Cricothyroid onabotulinum toxin A injection to avert tracheostomy in bilateral vocal fold paralysis. JAMA Otolaryngol Head Neck Surg. 2014;140(9):867–9.

31. Mathur NN, Kumar S, Bothra R. Simple method of vocal cord lateralization in bilateral abductor cord paralysis in paediatric patients. Int J Pediatr Otorhinolaryngol. 2004;68(1):15–20.
32. Miyamoto RC, Parikh SR, Gellad W, Licameli GR. Bilateral congenital vocal cord paralysis: a 16-year institutional review. Otolaryngol Head Neck Surg. 2005;133(2):241–5.
33. Lee JW, Bon-Mardion N, Smith ME, Marie JP. Bilateral selective laryngeal reinnervation for bilateral vocal fold paralysis in children. JAMA Otolaryngol Head Neck Surg. 2020;146(5):401–7.
34. Thorpe RK, Kanotra SP. Surgical management of bilateral vocal fold paralysis in children: a systematic review and meta-analysis. Otolaryngol Head Neck Surg. 2020;2020:194599820944892.
35. Rosenthal LH, Benninger MS, Deeb RH. Vocal fold immobility: a longitudinal analysis of etiology over 20 years. Laryngoscope. 2007;117(10):1864–70.
36. Gupta AK, Mann SB, Nagarkar N. Surgical management of bilateral immobile vocal folds and long-term follow-up. J Laryngol Otol. 1997;111(5):474–7.
37. Abu Ghanem S, Junlapan A, Tsai SW, Shih LC, Sung CK, Damrose EJ. The clinical course of idiopathic bilateral vocal fold motion impairment in adults: case series and review of the literature. J Voice. 2020;34(3):465–70.
38. Vance D, Heyd C, Pier M, Alnouri G, Sataloff RT. Paradoxical vocal fold movement: a retrospective analysis. J Voice. 2020;35(6):927–9.
39. deSilva B, Crenshaw D, Matrka L, Forrest LA. Vocal fold botulinum toxin injection for refractory paradoxical vocal fold motion disorder. Laryngoscope. 2019;129(4):808–11.
40. van der Graaff MM, Grolman W, Westermann EJ, Boogaardt HC, Koelman H, van der Kooi AJ, et al. Vocal cord dysfunction in amyotrophic lateral sclerosis: four cases and a review of the literature. Arch Neurol. 2009;66(11):1329–33.
41. Hillel AD, Miller R. Bulbar amyotrophic lateral sclerosis: patterns of progression and clinical management. Head Neck. 1989;11(1):51–9.
42. Hillel A, Dray T, Miller R, Yorkston K, Konikow N, Strande E, et al. Presentation of ALS to the otolaryngologist/head and neck surgeon: getting to the neurologist. Neurology. 1999;53(8 Suppl 5):S22–5; discussion S35–6.
43. Copeman WS. Rheumatoid arthritis of the crico-arytenoid joints. Br Med J. 1957;1(5032):1398–9.
44. Copeman WS, Elkin AC, Pearce R. A case of rheumatoid arthritis with ankylosis of the crico-arytenoid joints. Br Med J. 1959;1(5137):1575.
45. Eckel HE, Wittekindt C, Klussmann JP, Schroeder U, Sittel C. Management of bilateral arytenoid cartilage fixation versus recurrent laryngeal nerve paralysis. Ann Otol Rhinol Laryngol. 2003;112(2):103–8.
46. Miller FR, Wanamaker JR, Hicks DM, Tucker HM. Cricoarytenoid arthritis and ankylosing spondylitis. Arch Otolaryngol Head Neck Surg. 1994;120(2):214–6.
47. Saluja S, Singh RR, Misra A, Gairola AK, Prasad K, Ahuja GK, et al. Bilateral recurrent laryngeal nerve palsy in systemic lupus erythematosus. Clin Exp Rheumatol. 1989;7(1):81–3.
48. Hussain SS. Relapsing polychondritis presenting with stridor from bilateral vocal cord palsy. J Laryngol Otol. 1991;105(11):961–3.
49. Lahav Y, Shoffel-Havakuk H, Halperin D. Acquired glottic stenosis-the ongoing challenge: a review of etiology, pathogenesis, and surgical management. J Voice. 2015;29(5):646.e1–e10.
50. Sandhu G, Nouraei SAR, Rovo L, Marie JP, Mueller AH, Castellanos PF. Bilateral impaired vocal cord mobility. In: Laryngeal and tracheobronchial stenosis. San Diego, CA: Plural Publishing; 2016. p. 195–7.
51. Dion GR, De la Chapa JS, Bettenhausen W, Dominguez LM, Simpson CB. Differing progression to posterior glottic stenosis in autoimmune and idiopathic subglottic stenosis. Laryngoscope. 2021;131(8):1816–20.
52. Dean CM, Sataloff RT, Hawkshaw MJ, Pribikin E. Laryngeal sarcoidosis. J Voice. 2002;16(2):283–8.
53. Butler CR, Nouraei SA, Mace AD, Khalil S, Sandhu SK, Sandhu GS. Endoscopic airway management of laryngeal sarcoidosis. Arch Otolaryngol Head Neck Surg. 2010;136(3):251–5.
54. Phillips NM, Matthews E, Altmann C, Agnew J, Burns H. Laryngeal amyloidosis: diagnosis, pathophysiology and management. J Laryngol Otol. 2017;131(S2):S41–S7.
55. Thompson LD, Derringer GA, Wenig BM. Amyloidosis of the larynx: a clinicopathologic study of 11 cases. Mod Pathol. 2000;13(5):528–35.
56. Hazenberg AJ, Hazenberg BP, Dikkers FG. Long-term follow-up after surgery in localized laryngeal amyloidosis. Eur Arch Otorhinolaryngol. 2016;273(9):2613–20.
57. Rudy SF, Jeffery CC, Damrose EJ. Clinical characteristics of laryngeal versus nonlaryngeal amyloidosis. Laryngoscope. 2018;128(3):670–4.
58. Bozzalla Cassione E, Stone JH. IgG4-related disease. Curr Opin Rheumatol. 2017;29(3):223–7.
59. Matsushima K, Ohira S, Matsui H, Fukuo A, Honma N, Wada K, et al. IgG4-related disease with pseudotumor formation in the larynx. Auris Nasus Larynx. 2020;47(2):305–8.
60. Shaib Y, Ton E, Goldschmeding R, Tekstra J. IgG4-related disease with atypical laryngeal presentation and Behcet/granulomatous polyangiitis mimicking features. BMJ Case Rep. 2013;2013:bcr2013009158.
61. Virk JS, Stamatoglou C, Kwame I, Salama A, Sandison A, Sandhu G. IgG4-sclerosing pseudotumor of the trachea: a case report and review of the literature. Arch Otolaryngol Head Neck Surg. 2012;138(9):864–6.
62. Pihtili A, Bingol Z, Durmus H, Parman Y, Kiyan E. Vocal cord paralysis and hypercapnic respiratory failure in a patient with familial amyloidotic polyneuropathy. Intern Med. 2016;55(13):1783–6.

63. Kosumi Y, Nakamura H, Watanabe R, Watanabe T, Horita T. Glossopharyngeal/vagus nerve disorder due to IgG4-related hypertrophic pachymeningitis. Rheumatology (Oxford). 2019; https://doi.org/10.1093/rheumatology/kez009.
64. Conaghan P, Chung D, Vaughan R. Recurrent laryngeal nerve palsy associated with mediastinal amyloidosis. Thorax. 2000;55(5):436–7.
65. Drenger B, Zidenbaum M, Reifen E, Leitersdorf E. Severe upper airway obstruction and difficult intubation in cicatricial pemphigoid. Anaesthesia. 1986;41(10):1029–31.
66. Ito H, Suzuki K, Hoshino T, Nozue M. Total laryngeal stenosis in cicatricial pemphigoid. Auris Nasus Larynx. 1991;18(2):163–7.
67. Cooper T, Dziegielewski PT, Singh P, Seemann R. Acromegaly presenting with bilateral vocal fold immobility: case report and review of the literature. J Voice. 2016;30(6):758.e13–6.
68. Grotting JK, Pemberton JD. Fixation of the vocal cords in acromegaly. AMA Arch Otolaryngol. 1950;52(4):608–17.
69. Murrant NJ, Gatland DJ. Respiratory problems in acromegaly. J Laryngol Otol. 1990;104(1):52–5.
70. Levine RJ, Sanders AB, LaMear WR. Bilateral vocal cord paralysis following blunt trauma to the neck. Ann Emerg Med. 1995;25(2):253–5.
71. Cheng J, Cooper M, Tracy E. Clinical considerations for blunt laryngotracheal trauma in children. J Pediatr Surg. 2017;52(5):874–80.
72. Danic D, Prgomet D, Sekelj A, Jakovina K, Danic A. External laryngotracheal trauma. Eur Arch Otorhinolaryngol. 2006;263(3):228–32.
73. Hillel AT, Karatayli-Ozgursoy S, Samad I, Best SR, Pandian V, Giraldez L, et al. Predictors of posterior glottic stenosis: a multi-institutional case-control study. Ann Otol Rhinol Laryngol. 2016;125(3):257–63.
74. Lowery AS, Dion G, Thompson C, Weavind L, Shinn J, McGrane S, et al. Incidence of laryngotracheal stenosis after thermal inhalation airway injury. J Burn Care Res. 2019;40(6):961–5.
75. Thaller SR, Gross JR, Pilch BZ, Goodman ML. Laryngeal tuberculosis as manifested in the decades 1963–1983. Laryngoscope. 1987;97(7 Pt 1):848–50.
76. Bailey CM, Windle-Taylor PC. Tuberculous laryngitis: a series of 37 patients. Laryngoscope. 1981;91(1):93–100.
77. Rouhani MJ, Clunie G, Thong G, Lovell L, Roe J, Ashcroft M, et al. A prospective study of voice, swallow and airway outcomes following tracheostomy for COVID-19. Laryngoscope. 2021;131(6):E1918–25.
78. Feehery JM, Pribitkin EA, Heffelfinger RN, Lacombe VG, Lee D, Lowry LD, et al. The evolving etiology of bilateral vocal fold immobility. J Voice. 2003;17(1):76–81.
79. Guimaraes AV, Dedivitis RA, Matos LL, Aires FT, Cernea CR. Comparison between transoral laser surgery and radiotherapy in the treatment of early glottic cancer: a systematic review and meta-analysis. Sci Rep. 2018;8(1):11900.
80. Eom JS, Kim B, Kim H, Jeon K, Um SW, Koh WJ, et al. Fibrotic airway stenosis following radiotherapy in patients with adenoid cystic carcinoma. Respirology. 2014;19(6):914–20.
81. Gallo A, Pagliuca G, Greco A, Martellucci S, Mascelli A, Fusconi M, et al. Laryngotracheal stenosis treated with multiple surgeries: experience, results and prognostic factors in 70 patients. Acta Otorhinolaryngol Ital. 2012;32(3):182–8.
82. Anschuetz L, Shelan M, Dematte M, Schubert AD, Giger R, Elicin O. Long-term functional outcome after laryngeal cancer treatment. Radiat Oncol. 2019;14(1):101.
83. Theunissen EA, Timmermans AJ, Zuur CL, Hamming-Vrieze O, Paul de Boer J, Hilgers FJ, et al. Total laryngectomy for a dysfunctional larynx after (chemo)radiotherapy. Arch Otolaryngol Head Neck Surg. 2012;138(6):548–55.
84. Langman AW, Lee KC, Dedo HH. The endoscopic Teflon keel for posterior and total glottic stenosis. Laryngoscope. 1989;99(6 Pt 1):571–7.
85. Bosley B, Rosen CA, Simpson CB, McMullin BT, Gartner-Schmidt JL. Medial arytenoidectomy versus transverse cordotomy as a treatment for bilateral vocal fold paralysis. Ann Otol Rhinol Laryngol. 2005;114(12):922–6.
86. Kashima HK. Bilateral vocal fold motion impairment: pathophysiology and management by transverse cordotomy. Ann Otol Rhinol Laryngol. 1991;100(9 Pt 1):717–21.
87. Lawson G, Remacle M, Hamoir M, Jamart J. Posterior cordectomy and subtotal arytenoidectomy for the treatment of bilateral vocal fold immobility: functional results. J Voice. 1996;10(3):314–9.
88. Ossoff RH, Karlan MS, Sisson GA. Endoscopic laser arytenoidectomy. Lasers Surg Med. 1983;2(4):293–9.
89. Yilmaz T, Suslu N, Atay G, Ozer S, Gunaydin RO, Bajin MD. Comparison of voice and swallowing parameters after endoscopic total and partial arytenoidectomy for bilateral abductor vocal fold paralysis: a randomized trial. JAMA Otolaryngol Head Neck Surg. 2013;139(7):712–8.
90. Montgomery WW. Posterior and complete laryngeal (glottic) stenosis. Arch Otolaryngol. 1973;98(3):170–5.
91. Goldberg AN. Endoscopic postcricoid advancement flap for posterior glottic stenosis. Laryngoscope. 2000;110(3 Pt 1):482–5.
92. Rethi A. Losung der bei der beiderseitigen Postikuslahmung bestehenden medianlage. Mschr Ohr Laryngorhinol. 1922;56:200–4.
93. Schobel H. [Dilatation of the glottis in bilateral vocal cord paralysis. Review of various surgical procedures and a report of personal experience using a functional lateral fixation surgical technic]. HNO. 1986;34(12):485–95.

94. Woodson G, Weiss T. Arytenoid abduction for dynamic rehabilitation of bilateral laryngeal paralysis. Ann Otol Rhinol Laryngol. 2007;116(7):483–90.
95. Rovo L, Madani S, Sztano B, Majoros V, Smehak G, Szakacs L, et al. A new thread guide instrument for endoscopic arytenoid lateropexy. Laryngoscope. 2010;120(10):2002–7.
96. Marie JP, Hansen K, Brami P, Marronnier A, Bon-Mardion N. Nonselective reinnervation as a primary or salvage treatment of unilateral vocal fold palsy. Laryngoscope. 2020;130(7):1756–63.
97. Tucker HM. Long-term results of nerve-muscle pedicle reinnervation for laryngeal paralysis. Ann Otol Rhinol Laryngol. 1989;98(9):674–6.
98. Mueller AH. Laryngeal pacing for bilateral vocal fold immobility. Curr Opin Otolaryngol Head Neck Surg. 2011;19(6):439–43.
99. Mueller AH, Hagen R, Pototschnig C, Foerster G, Grossmann W, Baumbusch K, et al. Laryngeal pacing for bilateral vocal fold paralysis: voice and respiratory aspects. Laryngoscope. 2017;127(8):1838–44.

Subglottic and Tracheal Stenosis 17

Pierre Guilcher and Kishore Sandu

Key Points

- Treatment of laryngotracheal stenosis (LTS) begins with precise diagnosis, and this includes performing a thorough patient evaluation and a detailed aerodigestive endoscopy. Airway dynamics and exact details of the stenosis are critical to know.
- It is important to recognize concomitant airway lesions and associated patient comorbidities and collect tracheobronchial secretions for microbiological culture and antibiotic studies. Remember, it is treatment of a **specific patient** with a **specific stenosis**—each having varying decannulation rates.
- Before a surgery, the patient must be optimally treated for airway infections and gastroesophageal reflux to avoid surgical failures.
- An airway surgeon must be well trained in endoscopic and all types of open interventions, and the treatment should not be biased as per his training.
- Prevention of LTS should include sharing information regarding the pathophysiology of its development with anesthesiology and intensive care colleagues and the nursing staff.
- The best results of LTS treatment lie in the first operation. Salvage in failed operations will have significant patient morbidity.
- The use of the new ELS classification for LTS reliably predicts outcomes, and its use is highly recommended in decision-making of the treatment. It should serve as a common language between various airway teams and as a base for future research.

P. Guilcher · K. Sandu (✉)
Airway Unit, Department of Otolaryngology-Head and Neck Surgery, University Hospital of Lausanne, Lausanne, Switzerland
e-mail: pierre.guilcher@chuv.ch; kishore.sandu@chuv.ch

M. Remacle, H. E. Eckel (eds.), *Textbook of Surgery of Larynx and Trachea*,
https://doi.org/10.1007/978-3-031-09621-1_17

17.1 Introduction

Intubation trauma due to faulty technique, inappropriate selection of endotracheal tube sizes, sub-optimal patient sedation, and nursing can cause severe laryngotracheal lesions, which in turn can evolve into full-fledged airway stenosis. Patient factors such as a difficult-to-intubate upper airway and neck anatomy, cardiopulmonary abnormalities affecting laryngotracheal mucosal perfusion, obesity, and obstructive sleep apnea are significant risk factors for the development of these lesions. Typical intubation lesions include ulcers, edema, granulations, cysts, cartilage exposure due to mucosal denudation, and stenosis. The commonest causes of tracheostomy in neonates, infants, and small children are (1) prolonged intubation due to prematurity and (2) congenital laryngotracheal anomalies (subglottic stenosis, bilateral vocal cord palsy, webs) and (3) for obstructive sleep apnea in children with craniofacial abnormalities [1]. In adults, the main indications for performing a tracheostomy are for pulmonary toilet and prolonged intubation [2]. Non-optimal treatment of the acute intubation lesions and tracheostomy itself could develop into various types and grades of laryngotracheal stenoses (LTS).

Treatment of LTS starts with performing an optimal aerodigestive endoscopy and includes endoscopic and various open airway operations. Management of LTS in infants and children is very challenging and allows little margin of error.

There is no established management algorithm for LTS, because of the heterogeneity in type and severity of subglottic and tracheal stenoses and because of the individual patient comorbidities and differences. Therefore, careful selection of the appropriate treatment must be tailored to each individual patient, with the help of standardized assessment tools and in collaboration with multidisciplinary teams.

17.2 Anatomy (Fig. 17.1)

The subglottis extends from the insertion of the conus elasticus into the vocal folds, at the transition from the stratified squamous epithelium to the respiratory epithelium, to the inferior margin of the cricoid. Due to the non-expandable rigid cricoid cartilage, it is the narrowest section of the upper airway and is smaller than the dynamically abducted glottis. It has an inverse dome shape; therefore, stents that are not shaped accordingly may induce iatrogenic lesions. The trachea, on the other hand, is supported by incomplete cartilaginous rings, the posterior membranous wall, and flexible cartilages allowing for posterior expansibility during the two respiratory phases. The anatomy and inner dimensions of the larynx and trachea are different in children and adults,

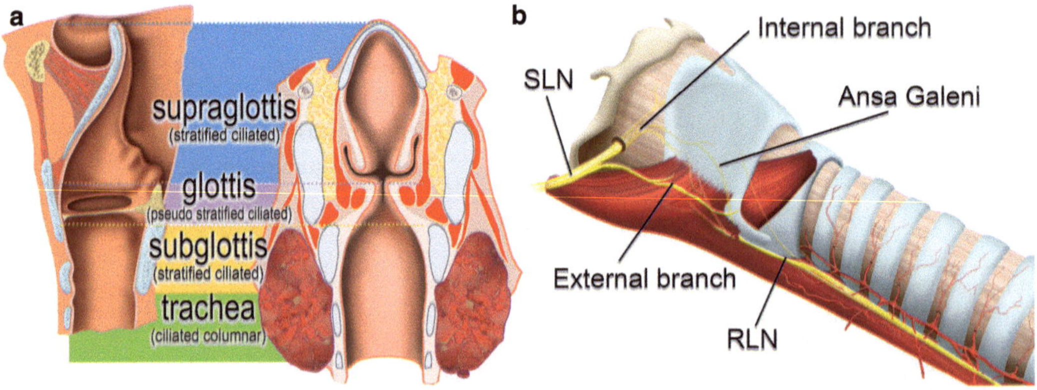

Fig. 17.1 Laryngotracheal anatomy. (**a**) In children, the supra- and the subglottic mucosa is lax and therefore more prone to edema, inflammation, and trauma. (**b**) The trachea is supplied via a rich segmental microcirculation coming from its posterolateral aspect leaving the anterior portion precarious to ischemic trauma. Note that the superior and recurrent laryngeal nerves are critical for sensory and protective functions of the vocal larynx

and this makes the LTS management more challenging in the smaller airways.

The percentage of trachea affected by a stenosis should be estimated using the number of rings as compared to the total number of rings which is normally between 16 and 20, but can be as little as 12 in some patients [3]. In managing tracheal stenoses, one should bear in mind the segmental nature of the blood supply to the trachea and the importance of preserving the lateral arterial supply by minimal dissection, though this is more of an issue in adults than children [4].

The superior laryngeal nerve (SLN) branches off from the vagus nerve approximately 2.5 cm below the base of the skull; its internal branch is responsible for sensory innervation to the superior portion of the larynx and the epiglottis and must be preserved to avoid the risk of postoperative dysphagia and aspiration, especially after laryngeal release maneuvers [5]. Its external branch controls the cricothyroid muscle; if it cannot be spared, this results in lowered voice fundamental frequency and projection, fatigue, and inability to achieve high-pitched voice [6].

The left RLN branches off from the vagus nerve inferior to the aortic arch and posterior to ligamentum arteriosum, while the right RLN branches off the vagus around the right subclavian artery. Both nerves continue superiorly behind the thyroid gland in the tracheoesophageal groove and enter the larynx posterior to the cricothyroid joints through the pharyngeal constrictor muscle. They innervate all intrinsic muscles of the larynx and are responsible for the subglottic sensitivity. Careful dissection and preserving both RLNs are of utmost importance when performing open airway surgery.

17.3 Etiologies

Airway stenosis can arise anywhere from the nasal cavity to the bronchial tree. This chapter will focus on laryngotracheal stenosis (LTS), more specifically at the subglottic and tracheal levels.

17.3.1 Children

17.3.1.1 Subglottis

Congenital SGS (Fig. 17.2)

Congenital SGS is the third most common (10–15%) of all congenital airway anomalies (after laryngomalacia and vocal fold palsy VFP) and the first cause for performing a tracheostomy in newborns [7]. It is due to the incomplete canalization of the laryngeal lumen in the tenth week of gestation. It is more likely to be part of a syndrome such as trisomy 21, CHARGE, and 22q11 deletion syndromes [8], and half of the cases have associated cardiovascular, tracheobronchial, or esophageal anomalies [9].

The diameter of the lumen at the level of the cricoid cartilage in a normal newborn is 5–6 mm. A subglottic lumen diameter less than 4 mm in newborns and less than 3 mm in premature children is pathological.

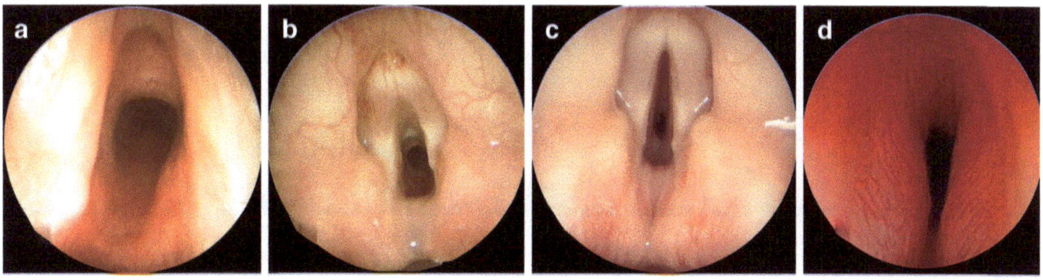

Fig. 17.2 Congenital subglottic stenosis. (**a**) Thick anterior cricoid lamina. (**b**) Generalized cricoid thickening. (**c**) Elliptic-shaped cricoid. (**d**) Prominent V-shape posterior cricoid plate

Holinger classified the histopathological etiologies of SGS as (1) cartilaginous, which are mainly congenital, and (2) soft tissue, which are mainly acquired [10]. Cartilaginous deformities include small size with normal-shaped cricoid, elliptical shape, generalized thickening, prominent V-shape posterior cricoid plate, flattened shape, thick anterior or posterior laminae, as well as clefts. An entrapped first tracheal ring can sometimes be found and further reduces the cricoid lumen.

Soft tissue stenoses include submucosal cysts, mucous gland hyperplasia, submucosal fibrosis, and granulation tissue, as well as hemangiomas.

Subglottic stenosis (SGS) becomes symptomatic when 50% or more of the lumen is obstructed, leading to biphasic stridor, recurrent or long-lasting croup, OSA with retractions, and barking cough. Severe croup before 1 year of age is rare and should prompt early endoscopic exploration [11].

Mild congenital SGS can be managed conservatively until the child outgrows the problem, while more severe cases require prompt surgical airway management and reconstruction.

Glottic Webs and Atresia (Fig. 17.3)

Webs and atresia cause varying degrees of obstruction at the glottic level. In Cohen types III and IV, laryngeal webs and laryngeal atresia, dilation, and endoscopic incision/resection are not a viable option as they will lead to granulation tissue formation with subsequent development of mixed acquired stenoses.

Congenital high airway obstruction syndrome (CHAOS) is a very rare entity in which the upper airway is intrinsically obstructed, most often the larynx and sometimes the trachea [12]. It encompasses atresia, webs, cysts, stenoses, or agenesis at various levels. Prenatal diagnosis using ultrasonography and magnetic resonance imaging enables proper antenatal and perinatal

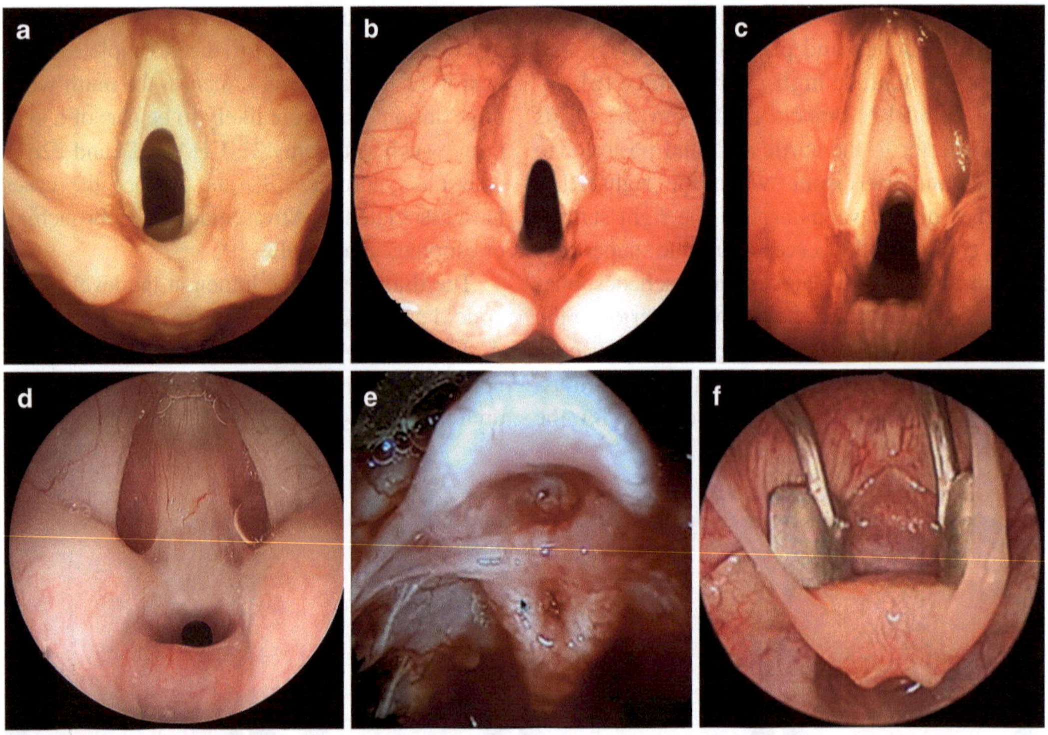

Fig. 17.3 Glottic webs and atresia. (**a–d**) Cohen type I, II, III, and IV webs are obstruction of <35% of the glottis length (GL), 35–50% of GL and minimal subglottic extension (SGE), 51–75% of GL with significant SGE possibly with cartilaginous component, and 71–90% of GL, severe SGE with cartilaginous component. (**e, f**) Transglottic and glottic atresia with complete lumen obliteration

management by determining the precise obstructive site and the associated anomalies. Ex utero intrapartum treatment (EXIT) procedure and tracheostomy are the procedures of choice to rescue the baby and initiate ventilatory support [13].

Acquired Glotto-SGS (Fig. 17.4)

Most pediatric G-SGS are acquired. Ninety percent of all acquired laryngotracheal stenoses result from intubation injuries (Fig. 17.5) and can already be seen 2–3 days after intubation due to pressure necrosis with subsequent mucosal ulcerations, edema, and submucosal cysts.

Other causes include iatrogenic complications (dilations, laser, and heat dissipation through the fragile infantile mucosa), trauma, benign tumors, chronic inflammatory disorders, and an idiopathic etiology.

Duration of intubation is an important factor, but other factors such as oversized or an inadequate tube, repeated intubations, poor nursing, infection, as well as patient factors (critical illness, underlying conditions such as diabetes, gastrointestinal reflux (GER), cardiopulmonary conditions) all contribute to the pathogenesis of soft tissue scarring and stenosis.

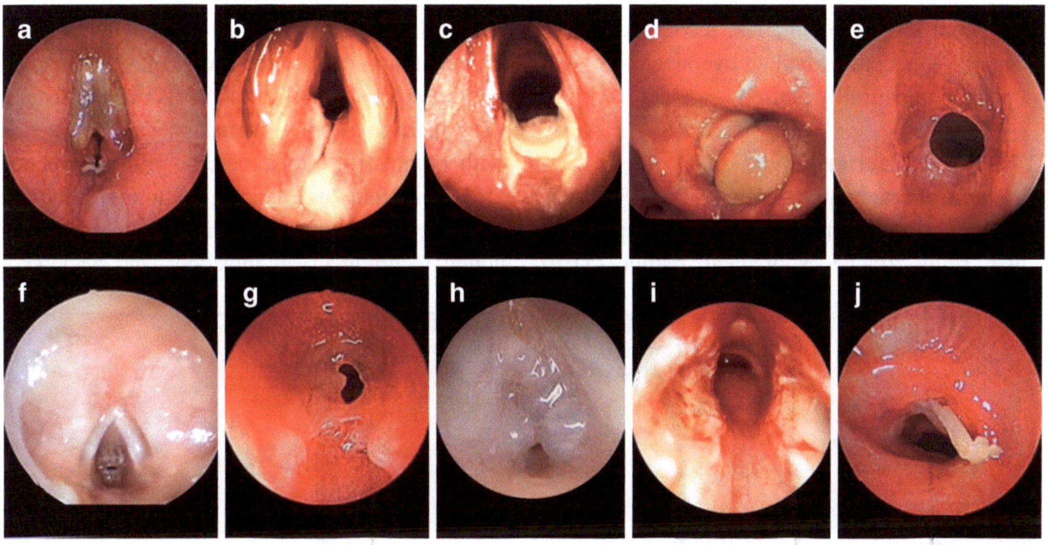

Fig. 17.4 Laryngotracheal lesions of intubation. (**a**) Severe vocal cords edema with posterior commissure ulceration. (**b**) Posterior commissure granulations. (**c**) Posterior cricoid cartilage denuded of mucosa. (**d**) Multiple intubation granulomas. (**e**) Grade I subglottic stenosis SGS. (**f**) Severe SGS. (**g**) Severe SGS with posterior glottic cicatricial band. (**h**) Severe bilateral subglottic retention cysts. (**i**) Arytenoid cicatricial furrows. (**j**) Tracheal cartilage trauma

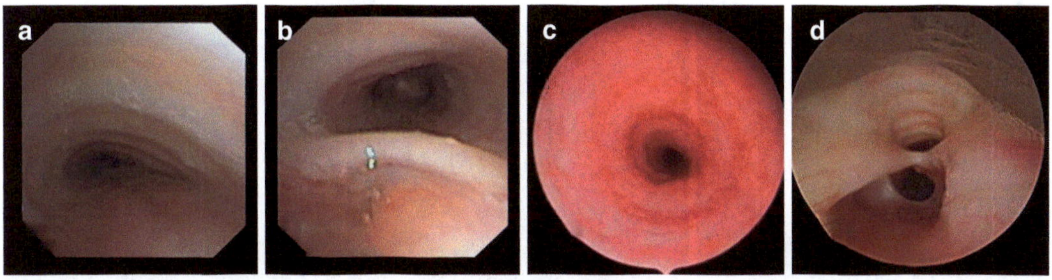

Fig. 17.5 Congenital tracheal stenosis. (**a**, **b**) Severe tracheomalacia with tracheoesophageal fistula. (**c**) Complete tracheal rings. (**d**) Type IV (Benjamin) laryngotracheoesophageal cleft

Prevention is of paramount importance and includes using age-appropriate endotracheal tubes made of polyvinyl chloride, maintaining correct cuff pressures between 10 and 30 cm H_2O, minimizing tube mobilizations, and optimal nursing.

In the mid-twentieth century, the advent of neonatal ICUs and ventilator support of premature infants with endotracheal intubation led to an increase of acquired SGS; but in the last decades, further developments, notably optimization of endotracheal tubes and cuffs as well as ventilator management, have decreased the rate of acquired LTS from 12% to approximately 1% [8, 14].

Acquired lesions may worsen pre-existing congenital cricoid anomalies, leading to mixed stenoses, especially when an oversized tube with poor biocompatibility is used.

17.3.1.2 Trachea

Congenital tracheal stenosis (CTS) (Fig. 17.6) is secondary due to tracheomalacia, complete circular rings, tracheoesophageal fistula (TEF), laryngotracheoesophageal clefts (LTOC), and tracheal webs [7]. Cardiac comorbidities are frequent and should be explored and addressed. Symptoms depend on location, severity (more than 50%), length, and type of the obstruction. They include recurrent pulmonary infections, barking cough, biphasic stridor, expiratory wheeze, *washing machine* type breathing, respiratory distress, cyanotic or apneic spells, failure to thrive, and life-threatening episodes. Children adopt a classic position with hyperextension of the neck to render the airway patent.

Tracheomalacia (TM) is a deficient support of the cartilaginous rings to keep a patent airway lumen open by more than 50% during expiration. It can be diffuse and congenital in premature or syndromic infants or acquired and localized associated with vascular anomalies, tracheoesophageal fistulas (TEFs), tracheostomy, trauma, failed reconstruction with progressive dehiscence, or graft destruction [15]. Symptoms are variable in time and include prolonged expiratory phase with wheezing, barking cough, recurrent airway infections, and cyanotic or

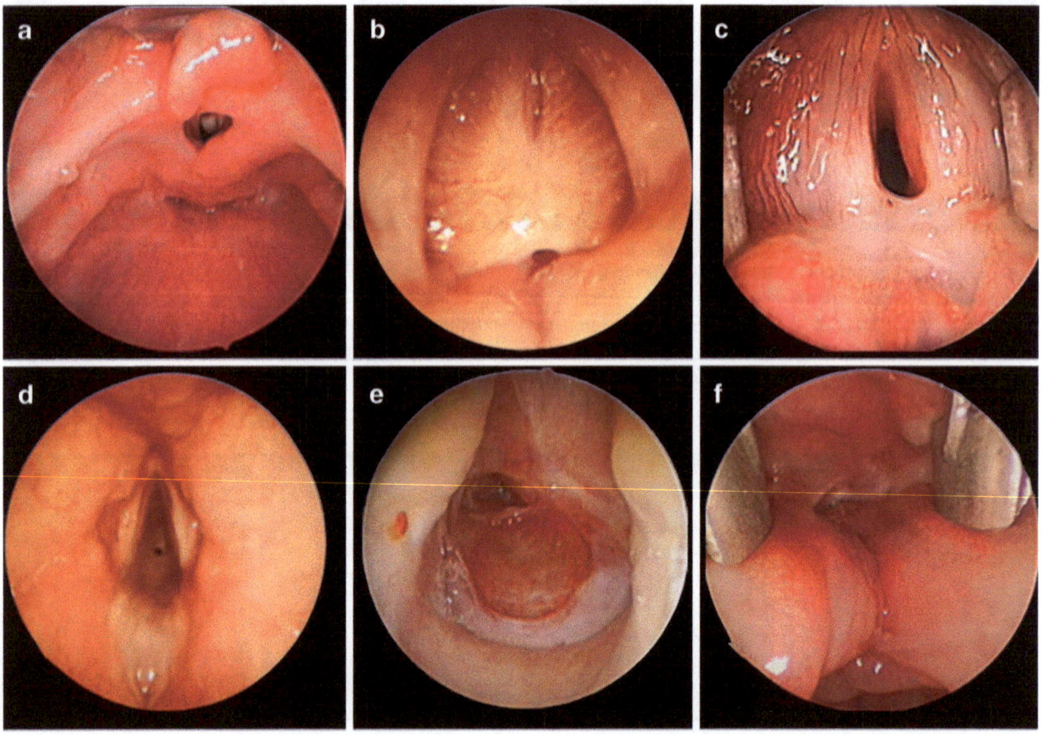

Fig. 17.6 Acquired laryngotracheal stenosis. (**a**) Supraglottic stenosis. (**b**) Vocal fold synechia. (**c**) Posterior glottic stenosis. (**d**) Grade III subglottic stenosis (SGS). (**e**) Grade IV SGS. (**f**) Complex glotto-subglottic stenosis

apneic spells during feeding, coughing, and crying. Neck hyperextension position helps with keeping the airway patent.

Tracheomalacia (TM) usually only requires supportive care in congenital cases with physiotherapy and GERD treatment, but depending on severity and exacerbations, BiPAP (bi-level positive airway pressure) can be used. In severe cases, aortopexy is the gold standard procedure for tracheomalacia and can be combined with other cardiovascular procedures when required, though it is not as effective in the presence of bronchial involvement [16]. Low-placed tracheostomy is the last alternative in severe cases until outgrowth of this usually self-limiting pathology.

Acquired TS is mainly due to tracheostomy (Fig. 17.7) or can be secondary to intubation lesions, airway injuries, or factors mentioned in the introduction of Sect. 17.2 [17].

17.3.2 Adults

17.3.2.1 Subglottis

Acute lesions of intubation (Fig. 17.5) may mature into cicatricial sequelae of the subglottic region, similar as in children [18]. Other causes include trauma, inhalation injuries, and stenosis after a high tracheostomy or cricothyroidotomy.

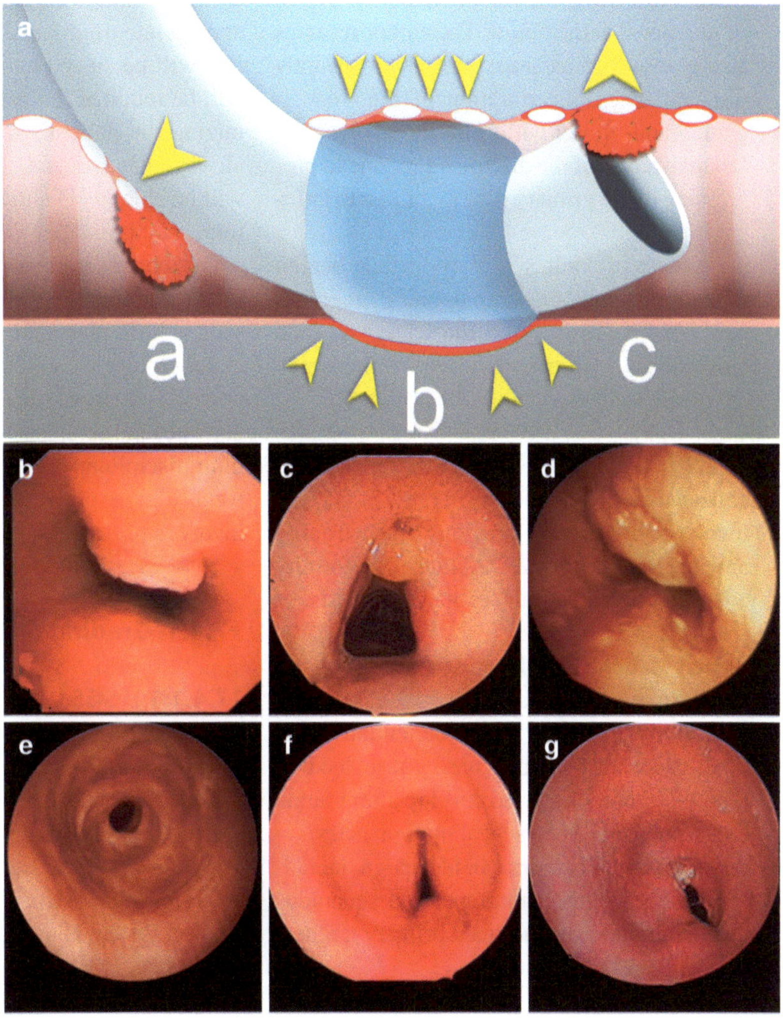

Fig. 17.7 Tracheostomy-induced stenosis. (**a**) Schema showing tracheostomy cannula-induced stenosis. a, suprastomal collapse and granuloma; b, cuff-induced trauma; c, cannula tip granuloma. (**b**) Suprastomal collapse. (**c**) A-shape deformity with granuloma. (**d**) Cannula tip granulations. (**e**) Cannula tip stenosis. (**f**, **g**) Severe A-shape tracheal stenosis

Idiopathic subglottic stenosis (I-SGS) is a rare cause of SGS that can extend to the trachea with the maximum point of stenosis being at the cricoid and the first tracheal ring [19]. It mostly affects Caucasian adult women. Being a mucosal disease, endoscopic ablation and balloon dilation are the treatments of choice, but may cause recurrence or disease extension to the glottis (iatrogenic causes included) that might require a tracheostomy. Therefore, a single-stage cricotracheal resection and anastomosis are favored as definitive treatments with excellent results [20].

Wegener's granulomatosis is a multisystemic granulomatous disease with necrotizing vasculitis that may be the cause of subglottic stenosis in approximately 10–20% of cases [21]. Similar to I-SGS, endoscopic treatments must be attempted at the outset. The author reserves airway resection and anastomosis for severely resistant cases, deterioration of the stenosis grade, and those with glottic involvement (cranialization of the disease either due to progression of the primary disease or due to iatrogenic causes).

Other causes of adult SGS may include benign or malignant tumors, pemphigoid, Langerhans cell histiocytosis of the larynx, and amyloidosis. Gastroesophageal reflux may aggravate lesions and alter the healing.

17.3.2.2 Trachea

Localized tracheal stenosis (Fig. 17.7) is commonly secondary to previous tracheostomy and leads to a typical "A-shape" deformity after anterior tracheal cartilage necrosis or stomal infection.

Acquired tracheoesophageal fistulas result from prolonged intubation in 75% cases [18], due to the pressure from the endotracheal tube, especially when a nasogastric feeding tube is present. It can also develop after trauma and esophageal and tracheal malignancies.

Primary tracheal tumors can be benign, including endobronchial hamartoma and squamous cell papilloma, but malignant primary tracheal tumors are more common, including squamous cell carcinomas and adenoid cystic carcinomas [22]. Smoking is a known risk factor for tracheal squamous cell carcinomas. Direct tumoral invasion arising from nearby structures, such as the thyroid gland, the lung, the larynx, or the esophagus, is also possible.

17.4 Preoperative Evaluation

Decision-making and successful outcome for patients suffering from laryngotracheal stenosis heavily depend on a thorough and systematic multidisciplinary evaluation of the disease and its context with respect to the existing comorbidities. Once a comprehensive evaluation is done, the multidisciplinary team will choose the appropriate timing and type of surgery, deciding if it will be staged and if postoperative stenting will be required. Efforts will be directed at optimizing the patient's medical status prior to the airway management. By doing this, the team will be able to (1) anticipate risks and complications, (2) have a fair idea of the expected results, (3) provide proper information to the patient and/or the family, (4) obtain an appropriate consent, and (5) plan an optimal strategy with all the collaborators (e.g., intensivists, cardiac surgeons, infectious disease specialists, swallow and speech therapists, etc.). At our institution, a multidisciplinary airway meeting is planned weekly to assess each patient together with the involved professionals.

17.4.1 Grading Systems

17.4.1.1 SGS

The severity of SGS is determined by comparing the appropriate endotracheal tube size with age-matched norms as per the Cotton-Myer grading system [23].

When vocal cord immobility is present from posterior glottic stenosis, the Bogdasarian classification system is used [24]:

- Type I: inter-arytenoid adhesion with normal residual mucosal bridge between the arytenoids.
- Type II: inter-arytenoid and posterior commissure scarring with no residual normal mucosa between the arytenoids.
- Type III: posterior commissure scarring with fixation of one cricoarytenoid joint.
- Type IV: posterior commissure scarring with fixation of both cricoarytenoid joints.

A recent consensus paper of the European Laryngological Society (ELS) [25] (Fig. 17.8 Table I) proposes a **five-step endoscopic airway assessment method as well as a standardized scoring system** to help surgeons tailor their surgery to offer the best surgical option to their specific patient and the stenosis for optimal outcomes. This system integrates not only the severity of the stenosis but also patient comorbidities, maturity of a cicatricial stenosis, as well as other levels of obstruction. For both adults and pediatric populations, this revised system enables precise classification and accurately predicts success in procedures, thereby helping caregivers to correctly counsel their patients. **Its use in common practice and future research is strongly recommended** [26, 27].

A **checklist of patient assessment for LTS** (Fig. 17.9 Table II) should be used as an everyday tool during the workup stage and endoscopic evaluation.

17.4.2 Basic Assessment

17.4.2.1 History

Birth history, prematurity, prior intubations, associated syndromes, and congenital anomalies must be systematically obtained.

Respiratory status will orient toward the stenotic site: SGS usually is associated with biphasic stridor; supraglottic stenosis is responsible for inspiratory stridor; and intrathoracic tracheal stenosis is associated with an expiratory stridor. Tracheostomy and eventual oxygen dependence are noted, and the impact of the breathing function on the child's quality of life is assessed.

Nutritional habits, reflux symptoms, and thriving difficulties are evaluated. A perioperative swallowing assessment, with tools such as the fiberoptic endoscopic evaluation of swallowing (FEES), should be used in a multidisciplinary fashion, as LTS patients have a higher incidence of underlying dysphagia but swallowing tends to

The ELS Classification system for benign laryngotracheal stenosis

ELS classification score, Myer-Cotton grade		No. of affected airway subsites (supraglottis, glottis, subglottis or trachea)		Comorbidities	
I	> 50%	a	1	+	Yes
II	51% - 70%	b	2		
II	71% - 99%	c	3	/	No
IV	100%	d	4		

ELS = European Laryngological Society

Fig. 17.8 Table I. The ELS classification system for benign laryngotracheal stenosis. (Reprinted by permission from John Wiley and Sons: The Laryngoscope, Multicentric study applying the European Laryngological Society classification of benign laryngotracheal stenosis in adults treated by tracheal or cricotracheal resection and anastomosis, C. Sittel et al.(C) 2019)

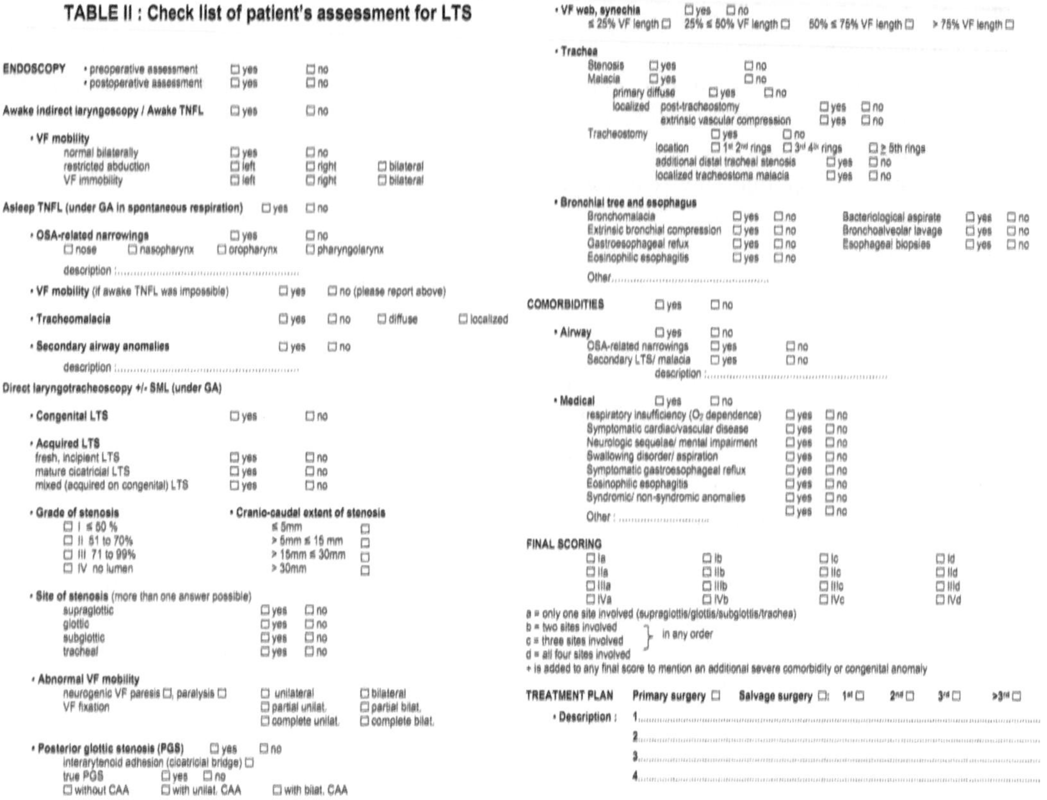

TABLE II : Check list of patient's assessment for LTS

ENDOSCOPY • preoperative assessment ☐ yes ☐ no
• postoperative assessment ☐ yes ☐ no

Awake indirect laryngoscopy / Awake TNFL ☐ yes ☐ no

• **VF mobility**
normal bilaterally ☐ yes ☐ no
restricted abduction ☐ left ☐ right ☐ bilateral
VF immobility ☐ left ☐ right ☐ bilateral

Asleep TNFL (under GA in spontaneous respiration) ☐ yes ☐ no

• **OSA-related narrowings** ☐ yes ☐ no
☐ nose ☐ nasopharynx ☐ oropharynx ☐ pharyngolarynx
description :……………………………

• **VF mobility** (if awake TNFL was impossible) ☐ yes ☐ no (please report above)

• **Tracheomalacia** ☐ yes ☐ no ☐ diffuse ☐ localized

• **Secondary airway anomalies** ☐ yes ☐ no
description :……………………………

Direct laryngotracheoscopy +/- SML (under GA)

• **Congenital LTS** ☐ yes ☐ no

• **Acquired LTS**
fresh, incipient LTS ☐ yes ☐ no
mature cicatricial LTS ☐ yes ☐ no
mixed (acquired on congenital) LTS ☐ yes ☐ no

• **Grade of stenosis**
☐ I ≤ 50 %
☐ II 51 to 70%
☐ III 71 to 99%
☐ IV no lumen

• **Cranio-caudal extent of stenosis**
≤ 5mm ☐
> 5mm ≤ 15 mm ☐
> 15mm ≤ 30mm ☐
> 30mm ☐

• **Site of stenosis** (more than one answer possible)
supraglottic ☐ yes ☐ no
glottic ☐ yes ☐ no
subglottic ☐ yes ☐ no
tracheal ☐ yes ☐ no

• **Abnormal VF mobility**
neurogenic VF paresis ☐, paralysis ☐ ☐ unilateral ☐ bilateral
VF fixation ☐ partial unilat. ☐ partial bilat.
☐ complete unilat. ☐ complete bilat.

• **Posterior glottic stenosis (PGS)** ☐ yes ☐ no
interarytenoid adhesion (cicatricial bridge) ☐
true PGS ☐ yes ☐ no
☐ without CAA ☐ with unilat. CAA ☐ with bilat. CAA

• **VF web, synechia** ☐ yes ☐ no
≤ 25% VF length ☐ 25% ≤ 50% VF length ☐ 50% ≤ 75% VF length ☐ > 75% VF length ☐

• **Trachea**
Stenosis ☐ yes ☐ no
Malacia ☐ yes ☐ no
primary diffuse ☐ yes ☐ no
localized post-tracheostomy ☐ yes ☐ no
extrinsic vascular compression ☐ yes ☐ no
Tracheostomy ☐ yes ☐ no
location ☐ 1st 2nd rings ☐ 3rd 4th rings ☐ ≥ 5th rings
additional distal tracheal stenosis ☐ yes ☐ no
localized tracheostoma malacia ☐ yes ☐ no

• **Bronchial tree and esophagus**
Bronchomalacia ☐ yes ☐ no
Extrinsic bronchial compression ☐ yes ☐ no
Gastroesophageal reflux ☐ yes ☐ no
Eosinophilic esophagitis ☐ yes ☐ no
Bacteriological aspirate ☐ yes ☐ no
Bronchoalveolar lavage ☐ yes ☐ no
Esophageal biopsies ☐ yes ☐ no
Other……………………………

COMORBIDITIES ☐ yes ☐ no

• **Airway** ☐ yes ☐ no
OSA-related narrowings ☐ yes ☐ no
Secondary LTS/ malacia ☐ yes ☐ no
description :……………………………

• **Medical** ☐ yes ☐ no
respiratory insufficiency (O_2 dependence) ☐ yes ☐ no
Symptomatic cardiac/vascular disease ☐ yes ☐ no
Neurologic sequelae/ mental impairment ☐ yes ☐ no
Swallowing disorder/ aspiration ☐ yes ☐ no
Symptomatic gastroesophageal reflux ☐ yes ☐ no
Eosinophilic esophagitis ☐ yes ☐ no
Syndromic/ non-syndromic anomalies ☐ yes ☐ no
Other : …………………… ☐ yes ☐ no

FINAL SCORING

☐ Ia	☐ Ib	☐ Ic	☐ Id
☐ IIa	☐ IIb	☐ IIc	☐ IId
☐ IIIa	☐ IIIb	☐ IIIc	☐ IIId
☐ IVa	☐ IVb	☐ IVc	☐ IVd

a = only one site involved (supraglottis/glottis/subglottis/trachea)
b = two sites involved
c = three sites involved } in any order
d = all four sites involved
+ is added to any final score to mention an additional severe comorbidity or congenital anomaly

TREATMENT PLAN **Primary surgery** ☐ **Salvage surgery** ☐: 1st ☐ 2nd ☐ 3rd ☐ >3rd ☐

• **Description :** 1……………………………
2……………………………
3……………………………
4……………………………

Fig. 17.9 Table II. Checklist for assessment of LTS. (Reprinted by permission from Springer Nature: European Archives of Oto-Rhino-Laryngology, Preoperative assessment, and classification of benign laryngotracheal stenosis: a consensus paper of the European Laryngological Society, Ph. Monnier et al. (C) 2015)

return to baseline with appropriate postoperative rehabilitation [28].

Though dyspnea and dysphagia have the greatest impact on quality of life (QoL) [29], voice evaluation preoperatively using tools, such as the GRBAS scale [30] and QoL questionnaires, is important as significant dysphonia is frequent in LTS patients [31], especially when the glottis is involved [32, 33], warranting proper counseling by establishing priorities and clarifying expectations prior to the surgical management.

Assessment of QoL in airway disease patients is emerging as a key outcome to consider when counseling families and helping them in defining their expectations. Significant gain in terms of QoL may accurately define success for the patients and their families, and airway management has shown substantial success even for neurologically impaired children [34].

17.4.2.2 Assessment of General Condition and Preoperative Preparation

Preparation for the surgical procedure includes definitive weaning from mechanical ventilation, treatment of respiratory infection, physiotherapy, and correction of malnutrition through enteral feeding [35].

- **Antibiotic Prophylaxis**: Graft loss and dehiscence can result from surgical site infection with considerable morbidity; and pulmonary superinfection secondary to perioperative atelectasis and mediastinitis can complicate the postoperative course [36]. Ninety-five percent of tracheostomized patients have lower airway colonization, frequently with *Pseudomonas aeruginosa* and methicillin-resistant *Staphylococcus aureus* (MRSA)

Timing	MRSA protocol	Pseudomonas aeruginosa protocol
Preoperative	TMP and SMX[ab] 6-12mg TMP/kg/d orally divided twice daily for 72 hours before surgery or	▲ tracheostomy tube. Topical or nebulized antipseudomonal (tobramycin or Ciprodex)
Perioperative	Intravenous vancomycin 1 hour before incision	Intravenous piperacillin and tazobactam 1 hour before incision
Postoperative	Intravenous vancomycin every 6 to 8 hours for 24 to 48 hours; then change to oral TMP/SMX for total of 14 days' treatment	Intravenous piperacillin and tazobactam every 6 hours for 24 to 48 hours

Abbreviations. MRSA, methicillin-resistant *Staphylococcus aureus*; SMX, sulfamethoxazole, TMP, trimethoprim

a Children who have MRSA-positive cultures from the nares are treated with mupirocin ointment twice daily for 72 hours before surgery.

b MRSA resistant to TMP is treated with en alternate oral antibiotic based on sensitivities.

Fig. 17.10 Table III. Antibiotic prophylaxis protocol for airway surgery. (Reprinted from Otolaryngologic Clinics of North America, Volume 41, Issue 5, A. de Alarcon et al., Revision Pediatric Laryngotracheal Reconstruction, Pages 959–980, (C) 2008, with permission from Elsevier)

which can be responsible for such complications [37]. Thus, a perioperative antibiotic screening protocol and prophylaxis are reasonable measures to reduce this risk, usually pursued during the first postoperative week [38]. We routinely perform a preoperative identification of tracheal colonization based on pulmonary aspirate cultures taken from preoperative endoscopic assessments and base our choice of perioperative antibiotic prophylaxis accordingly [39] (Fig. 17.10 Table III).

- GER can contribute to the development or exacerbation of airway conditions, and patients with uncontrolled GER have a higher rate of failure following laryngotracheal reconstructions. Patients undergoing treatment for SGS are best managed when GER treatment is optimized [40].
- "Active larynx" is a chronic inflammation of the larynx thought to be due to GER, eosinophilic esophagitis (EE), or idiopathic causes. It creates technical difficulty during surgery due to edema, erythema, and poorer healing and can lead to surgical failure. It should be treated prior to undertaking any complex reconstructions. Azithromycin can be used in idiopathic active larynx for its anti-inflammatory and immunomodulatory properties, after an electrocardiogram evaluation [39, 41].
- A special attention is given to associated comorbidities:
  - Vocal fold immobility can lead to chronic aspiration and lung infection that may worsen after surgery.
  - Neurological impairment may compromise or severely delay successful decannulation.
  - Cardiac or pulmonary conditions: adequate pulmonary function, minimal oxygen supplementation, and resolution of mechanical ventilation needs should be ensured before airway reconstruction. Cardiovascular conditions should be optimized, and surgical correction should be combined with open airway surgery for complete tracheal rings. A laryngeal stenosis correction must be

done only after the pre-existing cardiopulmonary condition has been adequately repaired.

17.4.2.3 Radiological Evaluation

Conventional radiographs give limited information on laryngotracheal stenosis, but are critical in evaluating pulmonary parenchymal disorders and in postoperative follow-up period [8]. Tracheobronchography with iso-osmolar contrast is a simple tool which may provide useful information regarding the stenosis [3]. Cross-sectional imaging using computed tomography (CT) is used for imaging the trachea and bronchi [42], though they will exaggerate the stenosis in the presence of secretions and do not give any information on the airway mucosal quality. Contrast 3D CT and MRI scans are important in the assessment of cardiopulmonary anomalies.

In our opinion, CT scans will be of significant value in the following conditions:

1. LTS following neck trauma to document cartilage fractures.
2. Low neck tracheostomy with severe neck scarring that might need a sternotomy. This will document the mediastinal vessels, and care can be taken while opening the thoracic cage.
3. Previous sternotomy.
4. In cases with history of mediastinitis.

Virtual bronchoscopy accurately assesses the stenosis width and length in severely obstructed airway lesions (advanced grades of glottic webs and atresia, long-segment congenital tracheal stenosis with complete rings) and should be used as a complimentary tool to endoscopic evaluation [43].

Modified barium swallow study provides useful information in patients with coexisting dysphagia or aspiration.

17.4.3 Endoscopic Workup

Systematic photo and video documentation of endoscopic explorations is critical for team preparation, treatment planning, and educational purposes. **In addition to the checklist for LTS** mentioned earlier, *a* ***schematic endoscopy report*** *is useful in this task and for patient counseling* (Fig. 17.11).

17.4.3.1 Awake Trans-nasal Flexible Laryngoscopy (TNFL)

Using a flexible nasofibroscope and topical nasal anesthetic, an awake TNFL can be performed at

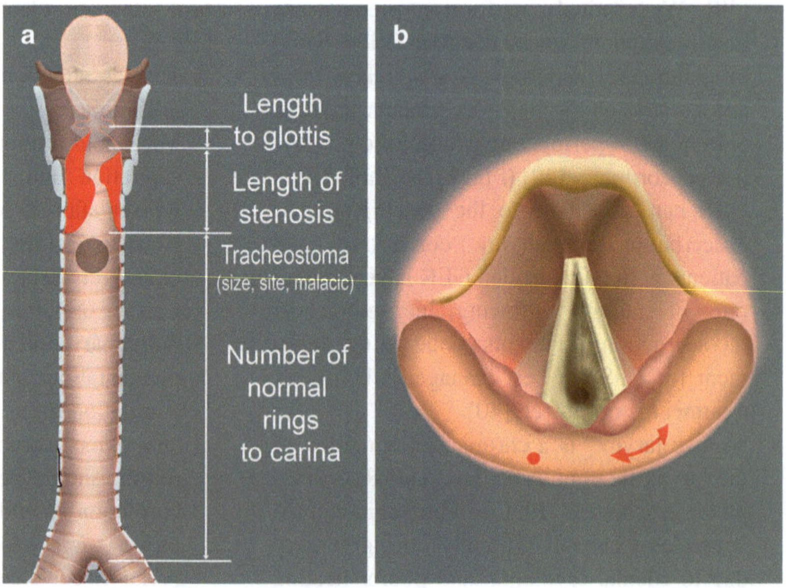

Fig. 17.11 Endoscopy report. Schema showing dynamic examination documenting upper airway extra-laryngeal sites of obstruction, vocal cord mobility, and tracheobronchomalacia. A rigid endoscopy gives details of the airway pathology, the remaining normal tracheal rings, tracheostomy site, and the airway mucosa quality

the bedside in collaborative patients and enables evaluation of the upper aerodigestive tract down to the vocal folds, giving valuable information regarding nasal cavities, nasopharynx, oro- and hypopharynx, dynamic function of the larynx, vocal fold mobility, presence of obstructive lesions and occasional laryngomalacia, as well as signs of GERD [8]. Functional evaluation of swallowing study (FEES) will efficiently assess swallowing function [44].

17.4.3.2 Asleep TNFL (Fig. 17.12)

In addition to the previously explored sites, a flexible bronchoscope is passed trans-nasally through the ventilation mask, under general anesthesia, spontaneous ventilation, and topical laryngeal anesthesia. The presence of associated laryngomalacia, vocal fold immobility, and tracheobronchomalacia are carefully noted, as they are potential causes of surgical failure when not identified and addressed [39].

17.4.3.3 Direct Laryngotracheoscopy with a Bare 0° Rod-Lens Telescope

Direct visualization of the larynx is made with a Macintosh laryngoscope tip in the vallecula, using a 0° 2.7 mm sinusoscopy telescope for children and 0° Hopkins 4 mm telescope for adults to examine the glottis and the posterior glottis. Using the telescope gently to lateralize the vocal fold, the subglottis and the trachea up to the carina can be explored. The anterior commissure can be visualized using a 30°/70° endoscope placed in the subglottis. A blunt probe is used to palpate the posterior commissure and exclude immobility of the arytenoids from posterior glottic stenosis (Fig. 17.13).

A rigid bronchoscope, starting with a 3 mm diameter for the newborn, can be gently used to palpate a cartilaginous stenosis to confirm its nature and objectively measure it. The numbers of tracheal rings proximal, distal to, and within a stenosis are carefully counted; when the mucosa is swollen, the visualization can be aided using narrow-band imaging (NBI) when available. No attempt is made to pass a severe grade III or IV LTS. A very fine telescope (1.9 mm 0° Hopkins telescope or 1 mm sialendoscopy optical fiber) can be used to assess a narrow concentric ring tracheal stenosis. Rough manipulations during endoscopy can induce dangerous airway edema in these very narrow airways, leading to a potential "cannot intubate and cannot ventilate" critical situation.

17.4.3.4 Broncho-Esophagoscopy

The trachea is evaluated for complete tracheal rings; external tracheal compression from adjacent vascular structures, such as in the setting of a vascular ring or aberrant subclavian artery; anatomical variants such as a pig bronchus; and the presence of tracheoesophageal fistula.

Flexible esophagoscopy helps in the evaluation of the esophagus and stomach for signs of GERD, and biopsies can be taken to search for *H. pylori* infection. It is our routine at the beginning of open airway surgery to place a naso-jejunal feeding tube and a nasogastric aspiration tube. This allows transpyloric feeding in the

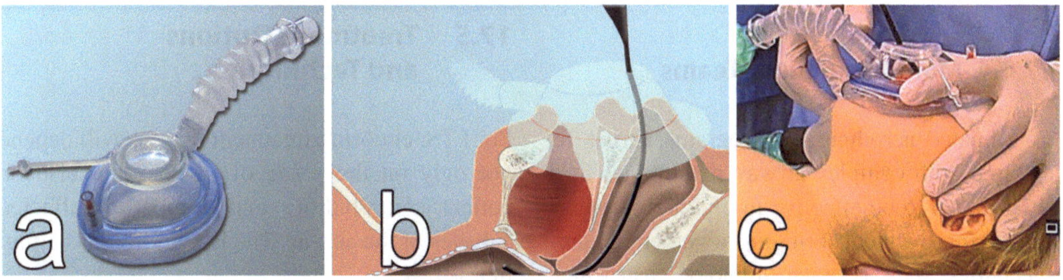

Fig. 17.12 Dynamic airway examination. (**a**–**c**) With the child in spontaneous respiration, an age-appropriate flexible bronchoscope is passed through a ventilation mask (VBM Medizintechnik GmbH, Germany), and dynamic inspiratory-expiratory responses are noted

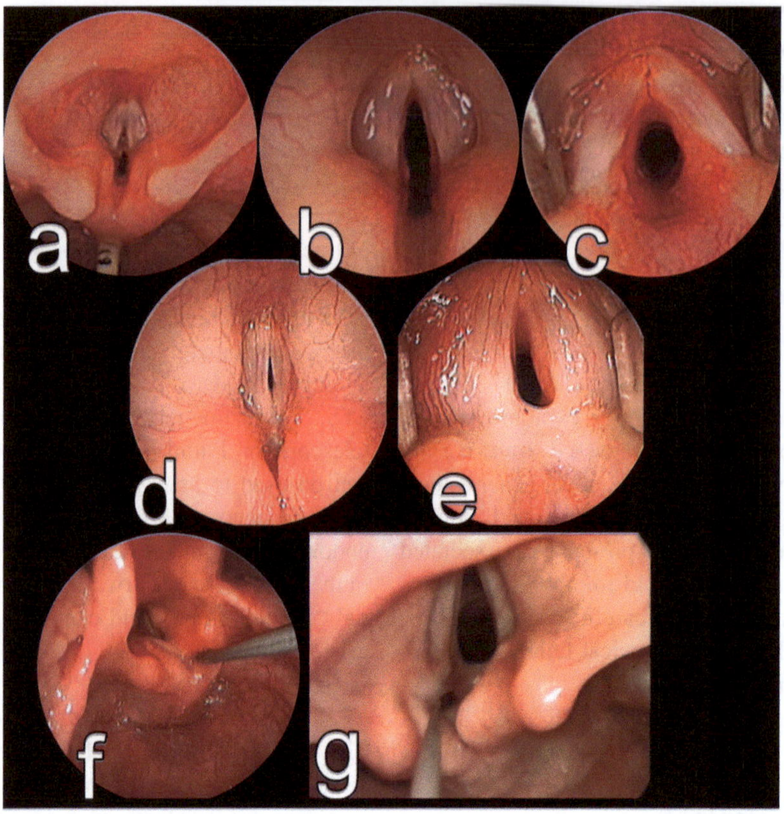

Fig. 17.13 Differentiating between bilateral vocal cord palsy (BVCP) and posterior glottic stenosis (PGS) and passive arytenoid palpation. (**a**) BVCP. Note the infraglottic edema secondary to severe negative subglottic pressure. (**b**, **c**) Posterior commissure mucosa is normal, and this is confirmed by placing a vocal fold spreader. (**d**) PGS with scarred posterior glottic mucosa—confirmed after spreading the vocal folds (**e**). (**f**) Arytenoid palpation under suspension laryngoscopy. A blunt probe is used to passively palpate the arytenoid cartilages. In the presence of an inter-arytenoid cicatricial tissue, the contralateral arytenoid will follow the palpated arytenoid in a lateral and outward direction. (**g**) In this case, palpation of both arytenoid cartilages revealed bilateral cricoarytenoid joint fixation

postoperative period while limiting both reflux and gastric hyperinflation due to non-invasive ventilation after extubation.

17.4.4 Multidisciplinary Teams

Coordinated aerodigestive programs caring for children with complex airway pathologies have been shown to be effective in optimizing preoperative management, bringing together required specialties, such as otolaryngology, gastroenterology, pulmonology, and speech-language pathology (SLP), and when required cardiologists, geneticists, neurologists, and radiologists [45]. This has a significant impact on the management and optimizes the success rates [46].

17.5 Treatment Options and Techniques

For LTS, choosing treatment options will depend not only on the grade of stenosis but also on patient comorbidities and number of affected subsites of the airway. The ELS system is helpful in this task.

A treatment algorithm for LTS (Fig. 17.14) is helpful in decision-making and choosing the appropriate treatment—keeping in mind that

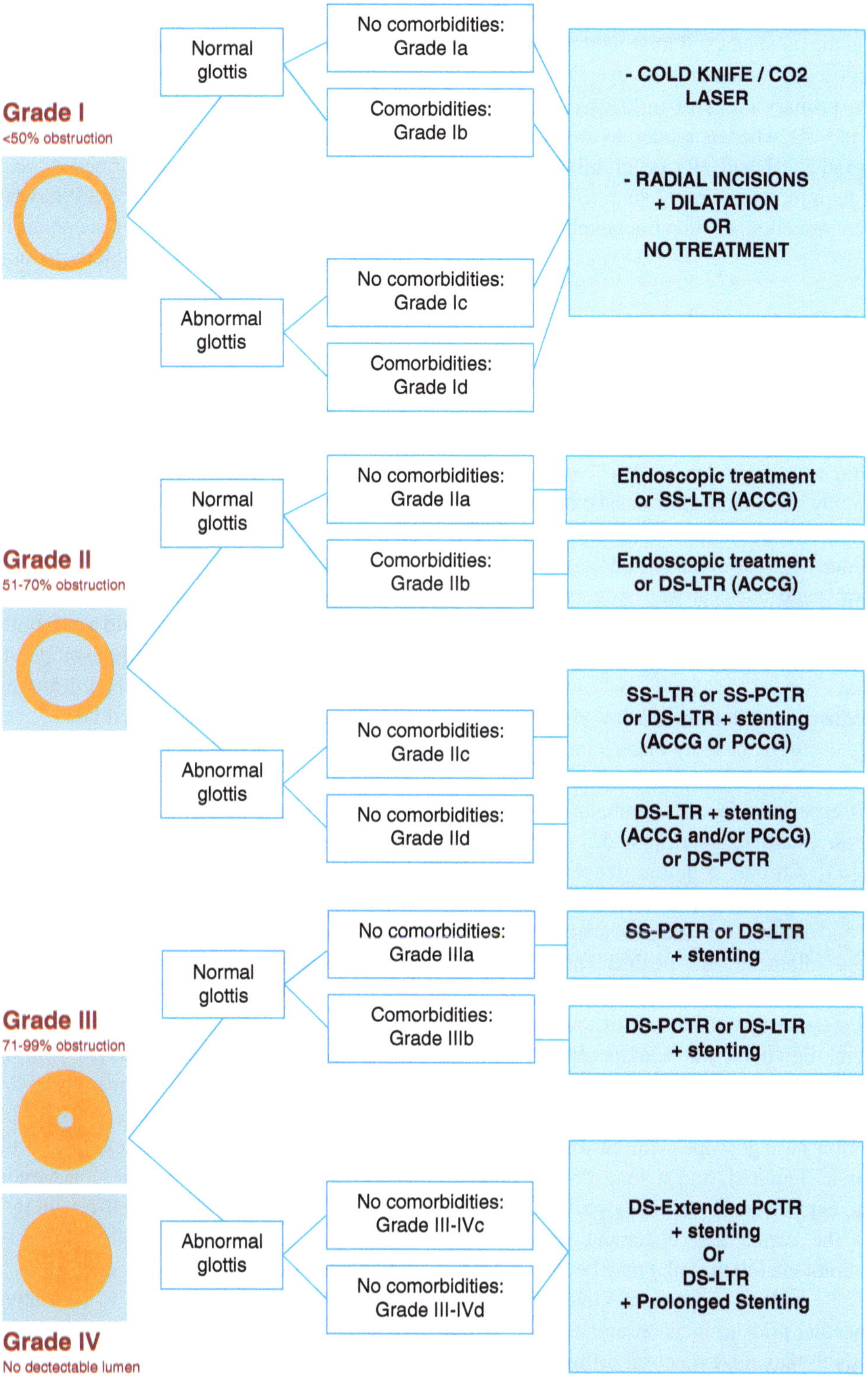

Fig. 17.14 Treatment algorithm for LTS

each situation must be individually assessed to choose the most adapted treatment and timing.

Endoscopic treatments are usually most effective in primary cases of mild cases of isolated SGS and TS, whereas moderate to severe stenoses (grades III and IV) or multilevel stenoses often require open surgery such as LTR, PCTR, tracheal resection, or slide tracheoplasty [47, 48].

17.5.1 Primary Endoscopic

Various anesthesia techniques exist for endoscopic procedures. Spontaneous breathing anesthesia, intermittent apnea, continuous endotracheal intubation, and jet ventilation are commonly used. High-flow nasal oxygen therapy under apneic conditions is a promising novel technique to safely extend apneic intervals and perform endoscopic airway surgery in selected adult and pediatric patients [49, 50]. Each technique has its own specific advantages and pitfalls.

Endoscopic dilation is a low-risk procedure mostly useful in the early management of mild to moderate acquired stenosis, with excellent outcomes especially for soft, immature, gossamer-like thin cicatricial scars [51, 52] or idiopathic SGS [53]. Chronic acquired dense stenoses are less likely to benefit from this technique due to firm consistency of mature scar tissue and reduced diameter of healthy mucosa [54]. Modern dilation balloons allow application of a radial pressure up to 20 atm with a predetermined diameter based on the age-appropriate airway size.

The patient is exposed using a Benjamin-Lindholm laryngoscope with customized dental guards as required, and a long 0° telescope is used to explore the larynx, subglottis, and trachea up to the carina and document the stenosis. Triamcinolone (40 mg/mL) may be injected submucosally with an endoscopic Kleinsasser injection needle, prior to incision and dilation of the stenosis to maximize mucosal diffusion. Using a Kleinsasser sickle knife or the CO_2 laser (*125 mJ/cm², 50 Hz UltraPulse with 250 μm microspot at 400 mm focal distance*), radial incisions of the stenosis following Shapshay's technique are performed for circular stenoses [55], and wedge excisions are considered in asymmetrical LT stenoses affecting less than 50% of the circumference. Preoxygenation is performed with a short intubation. Dilatation is performed either with CRE/Cordis balloons or Savary-Gilliard tapered bougies under vision with 0° telescope or though the working channel of a flexible bronchoscope for distal lesions [56]. We favor ballooning as bougies exert mucosal shearing and cause further airway injury. Noncompliant rectilinear designs of balloons are preferred as they allow for a uniform pressure application on the stenosis. The balloon size is chosen based on the outer diameter of an age-appropriate endotracheal tube; and then adding 1 mm for the larynx and 2 mm for the trachea. The balloon is kept inflated for 2 min after inflation or until the oxygen saturation decreases, and occasionally, this can be repeated.

Endoscopic anterior cricoid split with balloon dilation can be used in mild to moderate stenosis, after repeated failed extubation attempts or after failed endoscopic balloon dilation.

Endoscopic posterior cricoid split with cartilage graft (EPCS or Inglis procedure) (Fig. 17.15) is an effective alternative to open laryngotracheal reconstruction (LTR) or to ablative endoscopic procedures such as vocal cordotomy or arytenoidectomy. Described in 2003 by Inglis [57, 58], the technique allows for a high decannulation rate and is mostly effective in posterior glottic stenosis, but can be indicated in posteriorly based mature subglottic stenosis and bilateral vocal cord paralysis [59].

Under general anesthesia through the former or a new tracheostomy, using a laser-compatible tube, the posterior glottis is exposed with the largest possible vallecular laryngoscope (Lindholm) and Lindholm self-retaining false vocal fold retractor. A rib cartilage graft is harvested and designed as described in Fig. 17.15, adapting the width and length to the native cricoid without overexpansion of the posterior glottis. Using the operative microscope combined with the CO_2 laser (same parameters as mentioned above) and a micromanipulator, the interarytenoid musculature and scar are divided on the

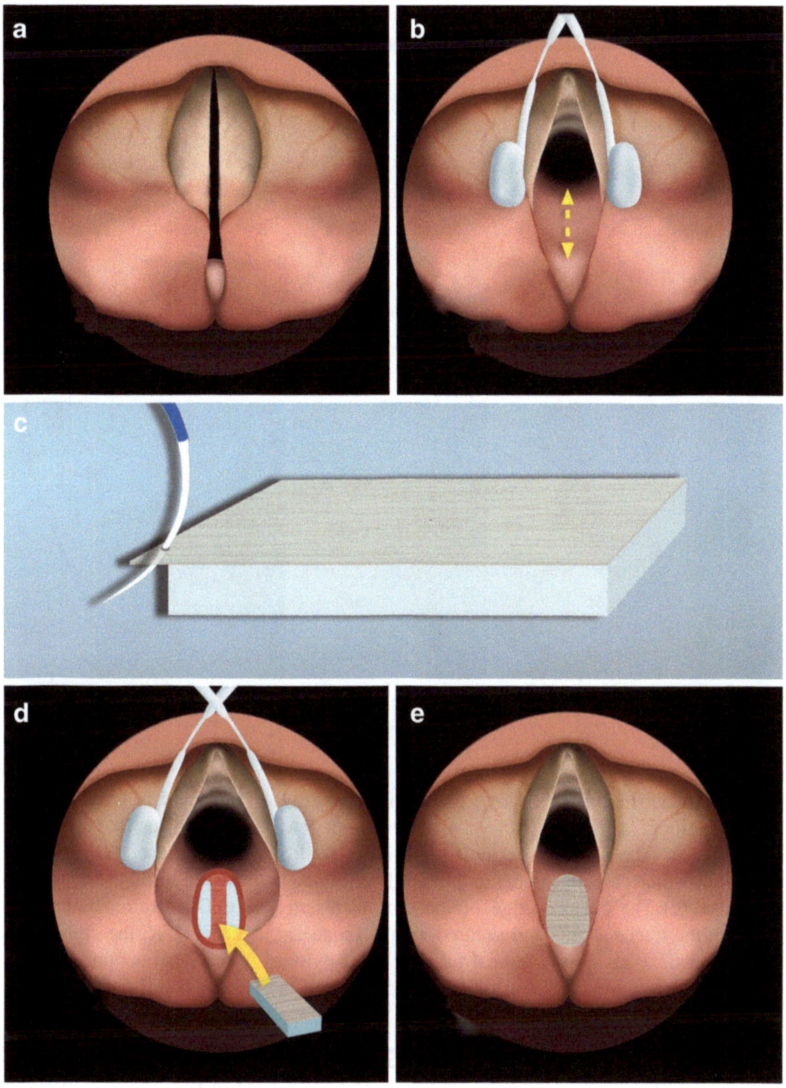

Fig. 17.15 Endoscopic posterior cricoid split and rib cartilage grafting for posterior glottic stenosis (PGS). (**a, b**) Under suspension microlaryngoscopy and after spreading the vocal folds, the CO_2 laser is used to divide the inter-arytenoid muscles and the posterior cricoid plate avoiding trauma to the posterior cricoid and tracheal mucosae. (**c–e**) A rib cartilage is harvested keeping a cranial perichondrial extension that is sutured with the posterior glottic mucosa

midline to prevent postoperative arytenoid prolapse, followed by a posterior cricoid split, preserving as much as possible the posterior perichondrium and avoiding injury of the pharyngeal mucosa. No extra undermining is attempted to enhance the stability of the graft. The graft is then snapped in the cricoid split, thus achieving posterior expansion. The cranial perichondrium extension of the graft is sutured with the posterior glottic mucosa to reduce salivary contact with the graft. No graft-to-cricoid cartilage sutures are placed, and in tracheostomized patients, an LT-Mold™ is placed endoscopically to further stabilize the graft [7].

Subglottic cysts are endoscopically managed by marsupialization, using either cold instruments or CO_2/diode laser. Microdebrider and Bugbee fulguration electrode device can also be used for this purpose [60]. Balloon dilation can be used as an adjunct after marsupialization.

Mitomycin C (MMC), an anti-fibroblastic agent, is sometimes used topically to avoid or at least delay recurrence of SGS after endoscopic treatment, though its efficacy still lacks scientific proof [51, 61]. It may cause delayed healing with subsequent fibrinous debris causing obstruction [62]. Direct application of MMC on exposed cartilage must be avoided.

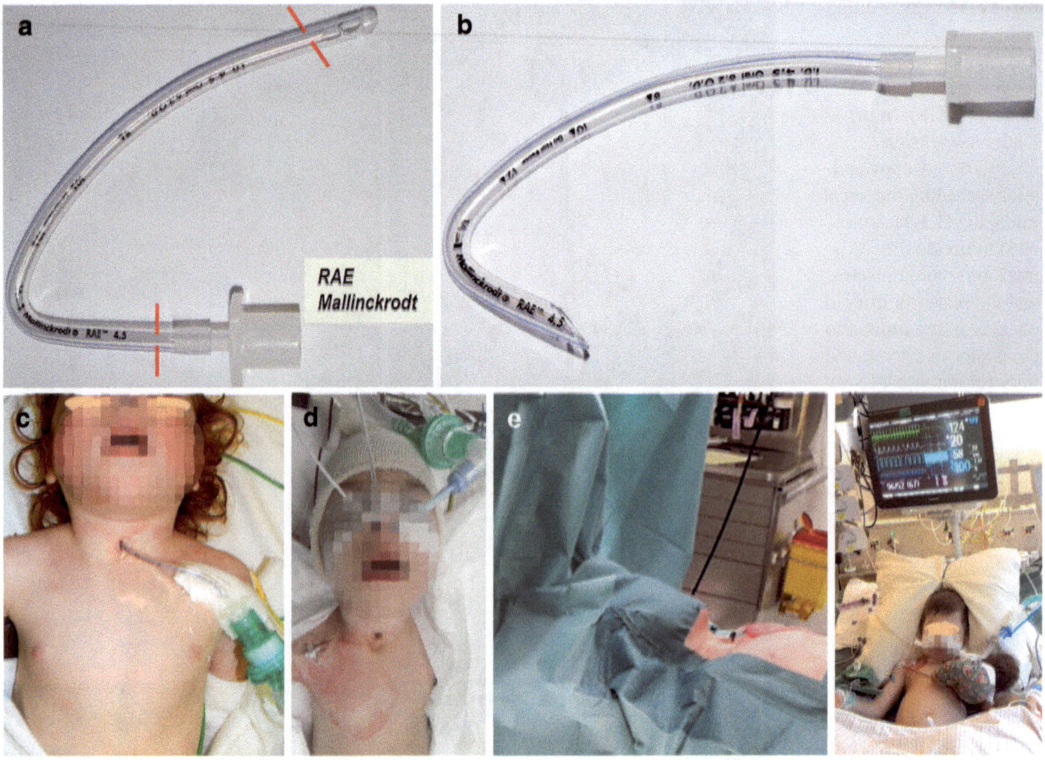

Fig. 17.16 Open airway surgery: general intraoperative considerations. (**a**, **b**) The ends of a Mallinckrodt RAE endotracheal tube are cut (interrupted red lines), and the side of the connector attachment to the ventilator tubing is reversed. (**c**) The beveled edge of the tube is inserted through the tracheostoma and secured with a Tegaderm. (**d**) The patient has a naso-jejunal tube for trans-pyloric alimentation and a nasogastric tube for gastric exsufflation, and in case of a single-stage PCTR/LTR, a nasal Portex Blue line endotracheal tube is placed in the glottis and retrieved during surgery. The modified RAE tube is passed through the tracheostoma and is not shown here. (**e**) Disinfection and draping of the patient. (**f**) Post PCTR or EPCTR, the child is placed in a semi-sitting position with head supports. [Note that **d**, **e**, and **f** represent the same child]

17.5.2 Open Airway Surgery: General Intraoperative Considerations (See Fig. 17.16)

Anesthesia is carried out through the tracheostoma with in-field ventilation system in tracheostomized patients using a modified Mallinckrodt tube or a flexible armored cuffed tube on a sterile circuit in the operating field. In non-tracheostomized patients, inhalation induction is performed under mask ventilation using sevoflurane, followed by propofol, fentanyl, and vecuronium maintenance [63]. This allows dilation of the stenosis (balloon or bougies) and naso-/orotracheal intubation using the smallest tube with adequate ventilation; the dilation-induced trauma is acceptable as the stenosis will anyways be resected. Once the airway is open, the patient is ventilated through the opened tracheal stump, using a second set of sterile flexo-metallic tube passed via the open trachea [64]. At the end of the procedure, the naso-/orotracheal tube is placed distal to the anastomosis. For long-segment congenital tracheal stenosis with severe stenosis, a tube may be placed in the glottis just above the obstruction. Alternately, a laryngeal mask could be used until ECMO is in place. Any attempt to intubate through the stenosis may compromise the airway.

Feeding tubes In small children, a flexible nasogastroscope is used to place a naso-jejunal feeding tube for postoperative transpyloric feeding, as well as a nasogastric tube for gastric aspiration to prevent any reflux.

Positioning For all open procedures, the patient is placed supine with a shoulder pad to enhance exposure. In procedures including airway resections, this will be removed when performing the anastomosis to relieve tension.

Patient is prepped, and the sterile surgical drapes are placed from the chin to the umbilicus. A 3M™ loban antimicrobial incision film (or equivalent) can be applied to the chest to reduce the risk for thoracic wound infection. A vertical frame holds the sterile drapes cranially and allows for a proper working space for both surgeons and the anesthesiologist at the head end of the patient. A sterile ventilation circuit is passed through this field and tested prior to incision.

Rib cartilage grafts Rib cartilage is the best option for cartilage graft augmentation after the first year of life, before which an autologous thyroid cartilage may be used [65]. When required and if possible, the procedure should be carried out prior to airway incision to avoid contamination from oral secretions that may be encountered during open neck surgery. An incision is performed over the chosen rib after local anesthesia injection, in the inframammary crease in females or adapted to the patient's muscle mass. The choice can vary from the fifth to sixth rib allowing for a straight graft to the ninth or tenth rib synchondrosis for a simple and safe harvest [66, 67]. A self-retaining retractor is placed, and the muscular attachments are sharply removed up the bony-cartilaginous junction using monopolar cautery, preserving the anterior perichondrium, and ensuring proper hemostasis. Blunt dissection at the deep portion of the cartilage is carefully performed with a raspatory in a sub-perichondrial plane to avoid perforation of the pleura, and lateral attachment of the cartilage is incised using a scalpel over the raspatory as a safeguard, followed by the medial incision in the same fashion after checking that adequate length is available. The assistant irrigates the wound with saline during a Valsalva maneuver to check for pleural effraction. An aspiration drain is placed in the wound which is closed in layers with muscle approximation. A postoperative chest X-ray is done systematically to rule out pneumothorax.

The surgeon carves the cartilage as required, designing flanges on the denuded side of the cartilage so as to keep the graft steady when inserted in the airway and keeping the perichondrium on the lumen side to avoid chondritis and granulations. For posterior costal cartilage graft (PCCG), the shape is rectangular, and for anterior costal cartilage graft (ACCG), it is diamond-shaped to accommodate the vertical incision on the trachea, cricoid, and thyroid cartilage. The ideal size of a posterior graft is unknown, but recommendations are about 5 mm for a 2-year-old and 8–10 mm in a teenager according to Rutter [39] so as to prevent overcorrection and subsequent persistent dysphonia and aspiration.

Surgical approach A horizontal collar incision is made 2 cm above the sternal notch or an ellipse at the level of the tracheostoma if it is to be excised. Subplatysmal flaps are elevated, strap muscles are divided in the midline, the thyroid gland is exposed, and an isthmotomy with lateral retraction of the lobes is performed. Elastic stay hooks are useful to moor the tissues to a Denys-Brown Lone Star® retractor and enhance exposure. As required, sternotomy is performed by the thoracic surgeon.

During open surgeries including airway resections, tracheal mobilization is always performed taking great care to limit the dissection laterally and preserve the vascular supply in the tracheo-esophageal groove to avoid anastomosis ischemia. In addition, staying close to the trachea will avoid damage to the recurrent laryngeal nerves, which are not identified. Further mobilization is achieved by detaching the anterior attachments from the mediastinal structures.

The integrity of the anastomosis is tested by filling the surgical field with saline and asking the anesthetist to perform a Valsalva maneuver after cuff deflation. Any air leaks are corrected with extra sutures, and fibrin glue is applied to the suture line. Thyroid lobes are sutured at the midline over the anastomosis to enhance its vascularity by contact. Additional tension-reducing sutures can be placed between the inferolateral cricoid and/or thyroid cartilage and the trachea. The thymus can be mobilized and interposed to protect the innominate artery from being exposed to the anastomosis as described by Grillo [68].

A Penrose silicone drain is left in the thoracic inlet to drain serous secretions and emphysema—should a dehiscence occur. Strap muscles are sutured at the midline, and the skin is closed in two layers.

17.5.3 Laryngotracheal Reconstruction (LTR) with Cartilage Expansion

Cotton described the technique in the 1970s [69], after which it became the gold standard in the treatment of SGS before the advent of PCTR.

Nowadays, severe grade I to minor grade III SGSs with/without comorbidities are theoretically best candidates amenable to single-stage LTR with A +/– PCCG. Staging and stenting are best for LTR with comorbidities and glottic involvement.

LTR with PCCG is the procedure of choice for all cases involving the vocal fold level such as higher-grade posterior glottic stenoses, cricoarytenoid joint fixation, and bilateral vocal cord immobility to restore the inter-arytenoid distance, in cases not amenable to endoscopic treatment [39, 70]. Care is taken to split the posterior cricoid exactly in the midline to avoid injuring the posterior cricoarytenoid ligament and the joint itself, as this might later result in arytenoid prolapse and surgical failure [37].

LTR is technically less demanding, does not risk the recurrent laryngeal nerves or an anastomotic dehiscence, and is not a surgeon-dependent operation.

17.5.3.1 Procedure (Figs. 17.17 and 17.18)

For simple LTR with ACCG, a partial laryngofissure is performed through the lower third of the thyroid cartilage just below the anterior commissure, the cricothyroid membrane, the cricoid, and the first two tracheal rings. The costal cartilage is harvested as previously described, is shaped, and placed with the perichondrium facing the airway lumen. The lateral flanges of the graft are tied to the thyroid, cricoid, and tracheal rings with Vicryl sutures to avoid graft displacement into the airway. The tracheostoma can be included in the reconstruction and requires transient intubation to manage postoperative subglottic edema in pediatric cases.

If a PCCG is required, a partial or full laryngofissure is required. The full laryngofissure consists of the anterior thyro-tracheal incision that is extended through the anterior commissure staying exactly in the midline to minimize the risk of vocal fold injury and passing through the anterior cricoid lamina and two tracheal rings. The posterior cricoid plate is incised in the midline, and the scar tissue is sharply resected from the subglottic and inter-arytenoid regions. Vicryl stitches are placed on the graft and cricoid plate and the rectangular graft is snapped in the posterior cricoid plate with the perichondrium facing toward the lumen side and the sutures are tied intraluminally. An ACCG is added if required, a tracheostomy is performed, and the reconstruction stented with an LT-Mold™.

Single- vs. Double-Stage LTR A double-stage LTR is performed for grade I, grade II, and minor grade III SGS in the presence of comorbidities or glottic involvement or both. The LT-Mold stent can be removed under suspension microlaryngoscopy, and a duration of 4 weeks to 3 months might be sufficient for satisfactory cartilage healing and epithelization [71, 72].

17.5.4 Partial Cricotracheal Resection (PCTR)

PCTR is the treatment of choice for severe grade III and IV SGS, even in infants and small children.

Single-stage PCTR (SS-PCTR) is adapted to treat isolated SGS without glottic involvement nor comorbidities (severe grade IIIa or IVa in the ELS classification).

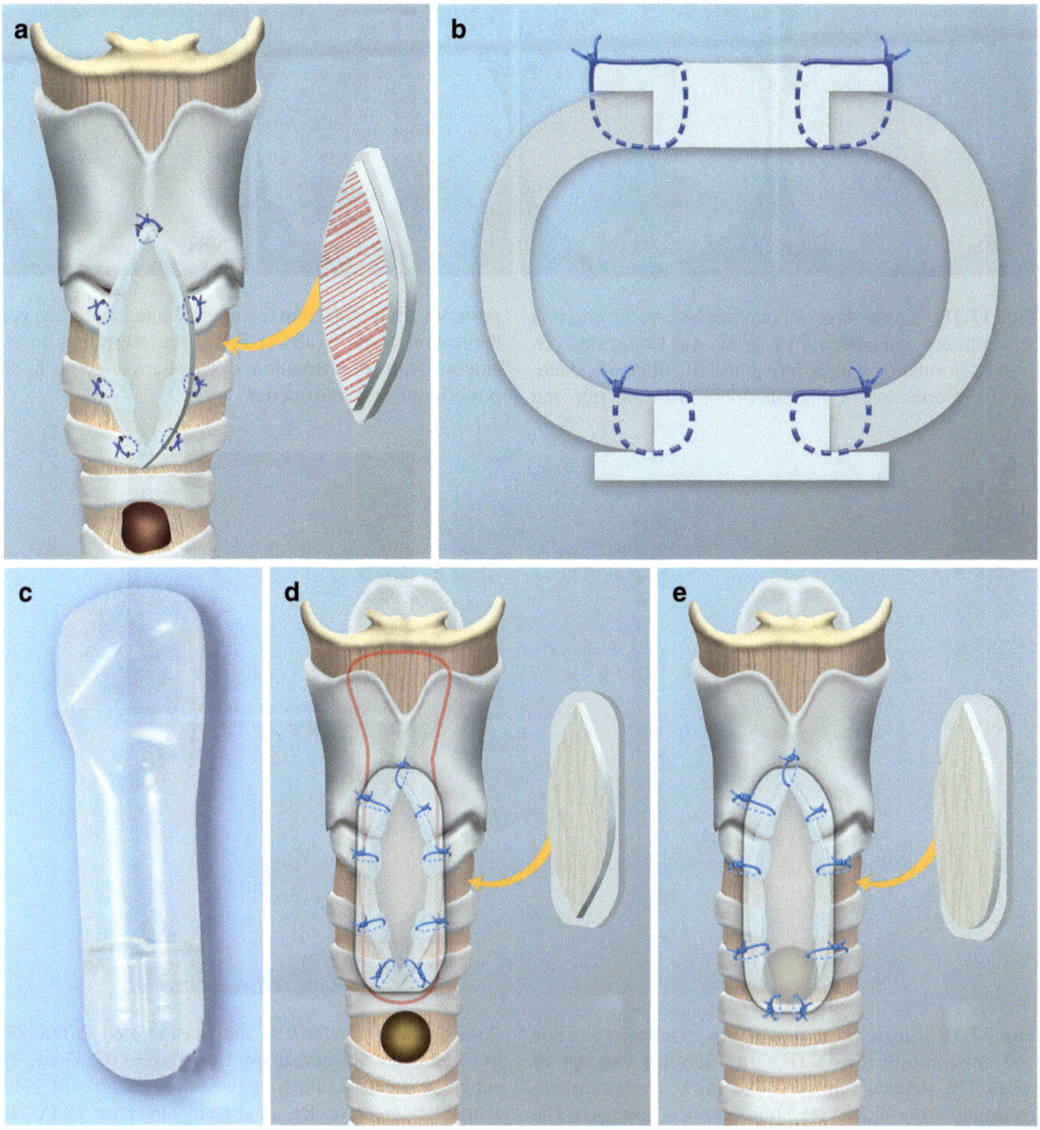

Fig. 17.17 Laryngotracheal reconstruction-operative steps. (**a**) Sub-commissural partial laryngofissure with anterior cricoid split. A diamond-shaped rib cartilage graft is used for anterior subglottic expansion. (**b**) Anterior and posterior cricoid splits with cartilage graft expansion. (**c**) Monniers' laryngotracheal mold. (**d**) An LT-Mold is used to stent the reconstruction in a two-stage procedure. (**e**) A rib cartilage graft is used to expand the subglottis and close the tracheostomy in a single-stage operation. A soft nasogastric endotracheal tube is used for temporary stenting

Double-stage PCTR (DS-PCTR) is preferred in case of glottic involvement and severe comorbidities or when the length of resection exceeds five tracheal rings causing excessive anastomotic tension.

First described by Pearson in 1975 and perfected by Grillo in 1982 for adult patients [68, 73], the procedure was introduced to the pediatric population by Savary in 1978 and established as a reference treatment for severe SGS in children by Monnier.

The technique (Fig. 17.19) consists of completely removing the anterolateral cricoid arch with the subglottic stenotic tissue, tracheostoma

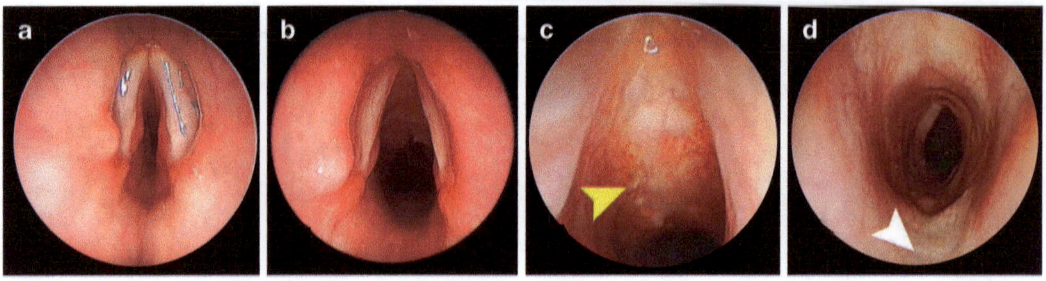

Fig. 17.18 Single-stage laryngotracheal reconstruction with anterior and posterior rib grafts. (**a**) Congenital cricoid malformation with severe grade III subglottic stenosis. (**b**) Correction of the subglottis with anterior and posterior rib grafts. Note the optimal integration and epithelization of the grafts (**c**, yellow arrow points to the anterior graft reconstruction; **d**, white arrow points to the posterior graft reconstruction)

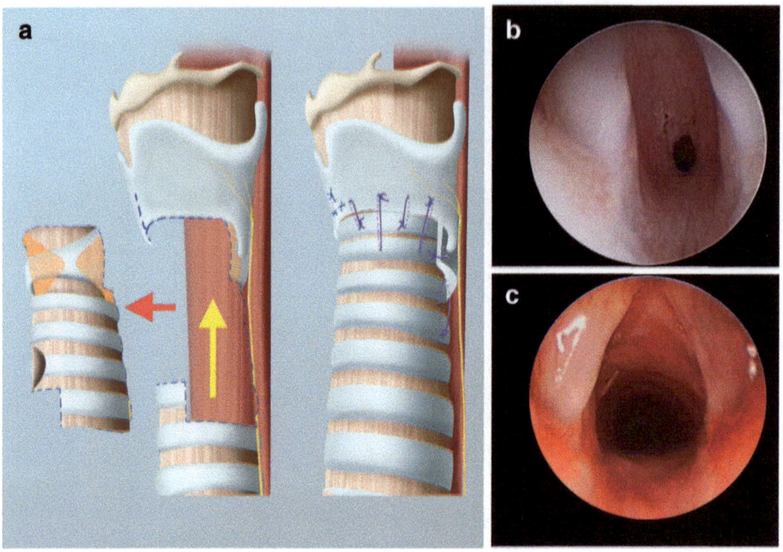

Fig. 17.19 Single-stage partial cricotracheal resection and anastomosis (SS-PCTR). (**a**) Surgical concept of SS-PCTR: stenotic subglottis and the tracheostomy are concomitantly removed via a trans-cervical approach. The distal trachea is mobilized and anastomosed to the posterolateral cricoid and thyroid cartilages. (**b**) Grade III subglottic stenosis following two failed attempts of endoscopic treatment. (**c**) Result at 12 months after SS-PCTR

if present, preserve the recurrent laryngeal nerves, and finally obtain a fully mucosalized airway reconstruction [74, 75].

17.5.4.1 Procedure (Fig. 17.20)

Adequate exposure and tracheal mobilization are achieved as previously described. Infrahyoid release is performed in long resections including more than five tracheal rings or revision cases with short tracheas. The medial insertions of the cricothyroid muscles are sharply incised, dissected off the anterior cricoid arch, and reflected laterally as a protective landmark anterior to the RLNs. Stay sutures are placed on the distal tracheal to help with mobilization. The airway is opened horizontally at the lower end of the stenosis, and distal intubation is performed with the in-field circuit. In a single-stage procedure, the incision is carried out directly above the tracheostoma, and a lower cut will be performed shortly after with subsequent reintubation of the distal stump. The second incision is placed at the lateral aspects of the anterior cricoid arch, anterior to the cricoarytenoid joints to preserve the RLNs. The cranial extent of the stenosis is assessed under direct vision, and the distal tracheal stump is

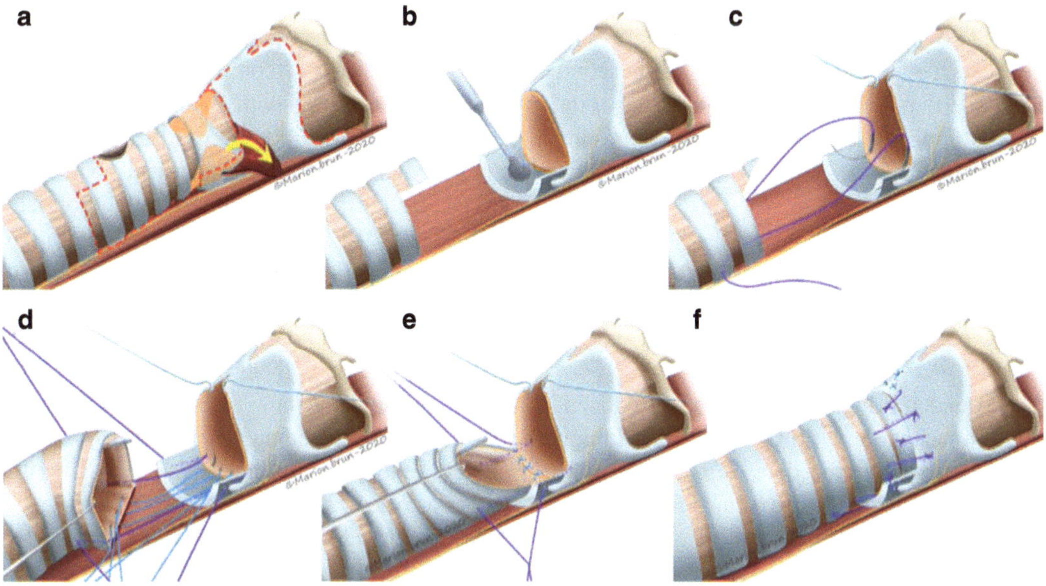

Fig. 17.20 Surgical steps of single-staged partial cricotracheal resection and anastomosis. (**a**) After exposing the laryngotracheal cartilage framework, the dissection is carried out medial to the cricothyroid muscle (curved yellow arrow) and joint, without identifying the recurrent laryngeal nerve(s). Please note the incision of the stenosis (dotted lines). (**b**) The anterior cricoid arch with the stenotic block is removed, but posterior cricoid plate is preserved. Using a diamond burr, the plate is thinned and cicatricial tissue removed. (**c**) Passing the posterolateral anastomotic sutures. These are passed submucosally through the trachea, then through the posterolateral glottic mucosa, and finally through the posterior cricoid plate in the subperiosteal plane. (**d**) Posterior anastomosis between the membranous trachea and posterior glottic mucosa. (**e**) Completion of the posterior and posterolateral anastomosis. (**f**) Completion of the lateral and anterior thyro-tracheal anastomotic sutures. Note the tension-reducing stitch between the inferior lateral edge of the cricoid and the trachea

carefully dissected off the esophagus for a limited distance equal to the height of the posterior cricoid plate. This prepares the future resurfacing of the cricoid with a posterior tracheal membranous pedicled flap. This usually requires resecting the lateral aspects of the first healthy tracheal ring, but care is taken to preserve its anterior portion to serve as a triangular cartilaginous wedge. The latter will accommodate into an inferior midline thyrotomy carried out up to the anterior commissure without transecting it, thus enlarging the reconstructed subglottis. It is important to match the tracheal lumen with that of the thyroid cartilage whose diameters differ.

The integrity of the posterior cricoid is respected except in cases where it is abnormal and must then be thinned with a diamond burr.

Anastomosis ensues, using interrupted resorbable sutures to reduce the risk of dehiscence in case a suture comes loose. The first two stitches are critical, as they are kept under tension on clamps to perform the posterior anastomosis. 3.0 Vicryl is used; each stitch is passed submucosally through the posterolateral aspect of the first one-and-half normal tracheal ring and through the cricoid plate laterally in a sub-perichondrial plane emerging on the outer surface of the cricoid plate in front of the cricoarytenoid joint to avoid harming the RLNs. The posterior anastomosis between the membranous trachea and the inter-arytenoid mucosa is carried out using full-thickness 4.0 or 5.0 Vicryl sutures tied on the lumen side. At this stage, the shoulder pad is removed to reduce anastomotic tension, and the two cricotracheal posterolateral stitches are tied. Secretions are aspirated from the distal trachea, and the ET tube is passed distal to the anastomosis. Lateral and anterior thyro-tracheal anastomosis are placed using 3.0 or 4.0 Vicryl, knotted on the outside, alternating between the first and the second tracheal rings of the distal stump to distribute tension. Two tension-releasing sutures are added between the inferolateral border of the cricoid plate and the second distal tracheal rings. Fibrin glue is applied to the anastomosis to ensure a watertight closure.

17.5.5 EPCTR for SGS Combined with Glottic Pathology (Figs. 17.21 and 17.22)

The extended PCTR (EPCTR) was introduced in 1999 in cases where a PCTR and an additional airway expansion procedure were combined [76, 77]. Usually, a PCTR is performed in conjunction with a PCCG augmentation to treat severe grade III or IV SGS with concomitant severe glottic involvement (posterior glottic stenosis PGS, vocal cord fusion, and transglottic stenosis).

The surgical steps are comparable to PCTR, and a full laryngofissure and a posterior cricoid split are added. The glotto-subglottic cicatricial tissue is excised, and maximum normal posterior glottic mucosa is spared. The transverse inter-arytenoid muscle is fully transected. PCCG is performed as previously described to enlarge the inter-arytenoid space. The anastomosis is comparable to PCTR, but the inter-arytenoid space and PCCG are resurfaced with a pedicled flap of membranous trachea sutured to the mucosa of the posterior laryngeal commissure. The thyro-tracheal anastomosis with a small pedicled anterior tracheal cartilaginous wedge to accommodate the laryngofissure is performed as in a PCTR. Before tying the sutures, an appropriate-size LT-Mold™ is placed and secured with two transfixing 3.0 Prolene stitches to stent the reconstruction. Stenting is necessary as the cartilaginous framework is destabilized by the posterior cricoid split and will allow cicatrization in an abducted glottis. A new tracheostoma is placed three to four rings below the reconstruction. The stent is removed endoscopically after 3–6 months as per the case.

Monnier and Sandu modified the technique to address the risk of covert progressive anastomotic dehiscence around the stent, which when undetected leads to stenosis recurrence [78]. Thinning and preserving the split anterior cricoid arch allows intussusception of the thyro-tracheal anastomosis and enhances its security. Furthermore, this allows better preservation of the lateral cricothyroid muscles and maintains arytenoid stability. This approach allows mobilization of fixed cricoarytenoid joints as an attempt to relieve them from ankylosis, without extra risk.

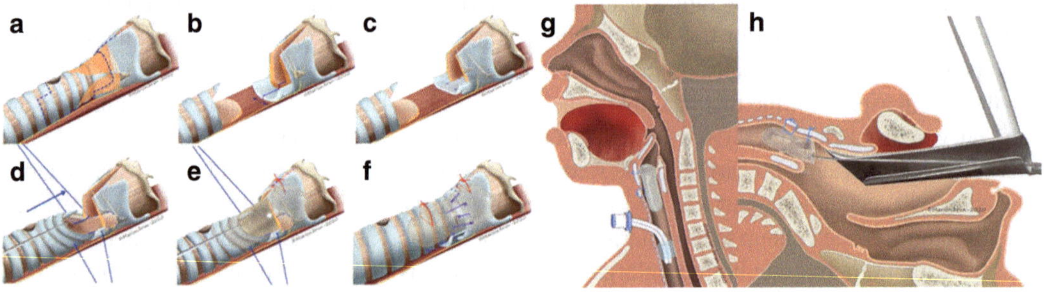

Fig. 17.21 Surgical steps for extended PCTR. (**a**) Early dissection is similar to PCTR (steps a–c). Additionally, a full laryngofissure and posterior cricoid split are performed. Please note the incision (dotted lines). (**b**) Posterior cricoid split. (**c**) Expansion with posterior costal cartilage graft. (**d**) Mobilization of the distal trachea (blue arrow) and mucosal anastomosis between posterior tracheal membranous flap and posterior glottis mucosa. Tracheostomy is performed three rings distally. (**e**) Insertion of an LT-Mold that is fixed with two 3.0 Prolene sutures (in the supraglottis and trachea). (**f**) Laryngofissure is closed and completion of the thyro-tracheal anastomosis (similar to PCTR). (**g**) Lateral view showing LT-Mold in place, implying a double-staged procedure. (**h**) Endoscopic removal of the LT-Mold. Under suspension microlaryngoscopy, a hole is made in the superior portion of the prosthesis with endoscopic scissors. Then, the Prolene anchoring sutures are cut and the prosthesis is removed

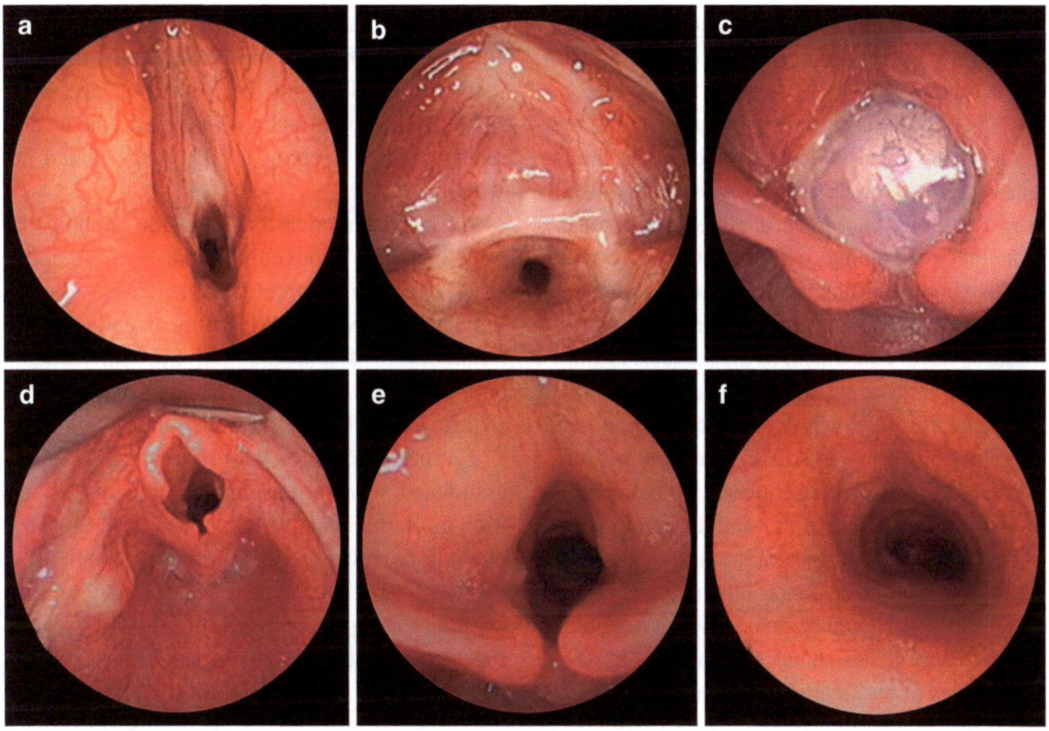

Fig. 17.22 Extended partial cricotracheal resection and anastomosis (EPCTR). (**a**, **b**) Severe grade III mixed (acquired on congenital) glotto-subglottic stenosis. (**c**) EPCTR with LT-Mold in situ. (**d**–**f**) Postoperative results after 15 months. Decannulation was done on postoperative day 92

17.5.6 Tracheal Resection with End-to-End Anastomosis

Tracheal resection with end-to-end anastomosis (TRA) is a common indication for adults and children presenting with acquired tracheal stenosis (TS) such as suprastomal collapse and stenosis, stomal malacia, and A-shape deformity following tracheostomy, stenosis from intubation lesions, and tracheal tumors. TEFs can also be treated with this technique, though slide tracheoplasties have recently been shown to bear significant success in these indications [39]. For the repair of TEFs, a cervical approach, with or without a median sternotomy, enables tracheal resection and anastomosis with or without muscle interposition, yielding a high success rate of 90–95% fistula closure.

TRA implies resecting the stenotic segment and ensuring a tension-free anastomosis, therefore limiting the length of trachea that can be resected safely and rendering the use of *tension-releasing maneuvers* mandatory when long resections are necessary. A maximum of half of the pediatric trachea can be resected due to its elasticity, but the risk of dehiscence is high if resection exceeds above 30%. Resecting more than a third of the adult trachea is usually not possible nor is safe.

Immediate postoperative extubation is possible in cooperative adults, while short-term intubation is preferred in children.

17.5.6.1 Procedure

The trachea is dissected anterolaterally close to the tracheal rings, taking care to preserve the vascular supply in the tracheoesophageal groove and leaving the RLNs laterally without identifying them. If the stenosis is high and if anterolateral tracheal dissection sufficiently mobilizes the distal trachea, sternotomy can be avoided. Laryngeal release procedures are performed if required.

The stenotic segment is defined by an intraoperative flexible endoscopy done via the endotracheal tube.

A horizontal incision is performed at the midpoint of the stenosis. From this incision, the trachea is further incised anteriorly vertically distally down to the normal tracheal rings, and confirmation that proceeding with resection is possible without undue tension is established. Cranial anterior vertical incision is not immediately performed because the cranial extent of the stenosis is known from the endoscopic preoperative evaluation. At this stage, if resection is deemed too risky, it is still possible to opt for an ACCG tracheoplasty or in some cases a slide tracheoplasty if quality of the mucosa permits it. Bear in mind that acquired stenoses are made of cicatricial tissue; therefore, anastomosis in these conditions may not be optimal, and TRA should be favored when possible. If RA is chosen, horizontal cuts are made at the extremities of the stenosis "in sano," without traumatizing the anterior esophageal wall. We dissect the tracheal stenotic segment off the esophagus, limiting the posterior dissection to a few millimeters and thus preserving the vascularization of the proximal and distal trachea.

After securing it with a stay suture, the ET tube is withdrawn by the anesthetist up to the subglottis, and the ventilation is switched to the in-field sterile circuit through the distal stump. Under intermittent apneas or spontaneous ventilation [79], the posterior anastomosis is carried out using either inverted and interrupted Vicryl stitches or a running PDS suture. The lateral and anterior anastomoses are performed with interrupted Vicryl sutures placed prior to being tied, alternating between one and two tracheal rings on each side of the anastomosis to optimally distribute tension. After aspirating blood and mucus from the distal airway, the naso-/orotracheal ET tube is positioned distal to the anastomosis, and the lateral and anterior anastomotic sutures are tied.

17.5.7 Slide Tracheoplasty

Slide tracheoplasty (ST), first described by Tsang in 1989, involves transverse division of the trachea at the midpoint of the stenosis and "sliding" spatulated proximal and distal ends together, therefore quadrupling the lumen surface while reducing the total tracheal length and the airflow resistance and keeping a fully mucosalized airway [80, 81].

ST has emerged as the technique of choice for long-segment congenital tracheal stenosis (LSCTS) with complete tracheal rings, but its indications have recently been extended to the treatment of TEFs, acquired tracheal stenosis, and combined subglotto-tracheal stenoses that require longer lengths of resection [39, 47, 82].

Former procedures used to treat LSCTS were associated with largely unfavorable results and high morbidity and mortality rates [83]. Slide tracheoplasty revolutionized the management of this malformation, bearing the advantage of both keeping a completely mucosalized airway, avoiding a tracheostomy, and the doubling operative success while reducing mortality by more than 50% [39]. Approximately two-thirds of the intrathoracic trachea can undergo a ST before tension-relieving maneuvers are required [84]. The long and oblique suture line decreases risk of anastomotic dehiscence or stenosis [37, 39]. The tracheal bronchus is an abnormal tracheal insertion of the right upper lobe bronchus, present in one in ten to four CTS patients. The usual posterior-anterior slide tracheoplasty technique described below can usually be performed regardless, as the RULB usually arises from the posterolateral aspect of the trachea [85].

Cardiopulmonary bypass or extracorporeal membrane oxygenation (ECMO) is usually required during the procedure as in most cases the stenosis is close to the carina, and up to 70% of the patients have associated cardiopulmonary malformations such as pulmonary artery sling, which warrant concomitant correction [39, 86, 87]. These should be performed prior to entering the trachea so as to avoid contamination from tracheal secretions [88].

The available data suggests that 10% of cases with mild symptoms and no respiratory decompensations may not require immediate or any surgical management, warranting for an observation period when possible [83, 89]. As a matter of fact, circular rings are sometimes discovered at an adult age without having been previously symptomatic or misdiagnosed as asthma [90–92]. Tracheal growth after ST is normal, similar to unrepaired tracheal rings [87, 93, 94]. Occasional follow-up endoscopies may be necessary to optimize results, namely, to treat "figure of 8" deformities or granulations.

Tracheal slide tracheoplasty (TST) is performed via a sternotomy allowing cardiovascular corrections. Cervical slide tracheoplasty (CST) is performed via a cervical incision only and without ECMO, with intermittent in-field intubation and ventilation. The choice depends on the size and extent of the stenosis.

CST is also successful in treating acquired high TS and revision cases, as well as TEFs [47].

17.5.7.1 **Procedure** (Fig. 17.23)

The trachea is mobilized and transected horizontally at the midpoint of the stenosis. This point can be confirmed prior to incision using an intraoperative flexible bronchoscopy and insertion of fine needles through to the tracheal lumen to mark the distal and proximal ends of the stenosis.

Vertical incisions are made from that point on the midline, on the anterior aspect of the distal tracheal stump with a posterior bevel, and on the posterior aspect of the proximal stump with an anterior bevel, until normal trachea is reached. This opens the complete tracheal rings. The proximal and distal ends are "slid" on top of one another. The anastomosis is performed starting distally, with a double arm running polydioxanone suture.

A final bronchoscopy through the endotracheal tube confirms the immediate result and enables aspiration of distal airway blood and secretions. The ET tube is secured with the tip at the midportion of the slid segment.

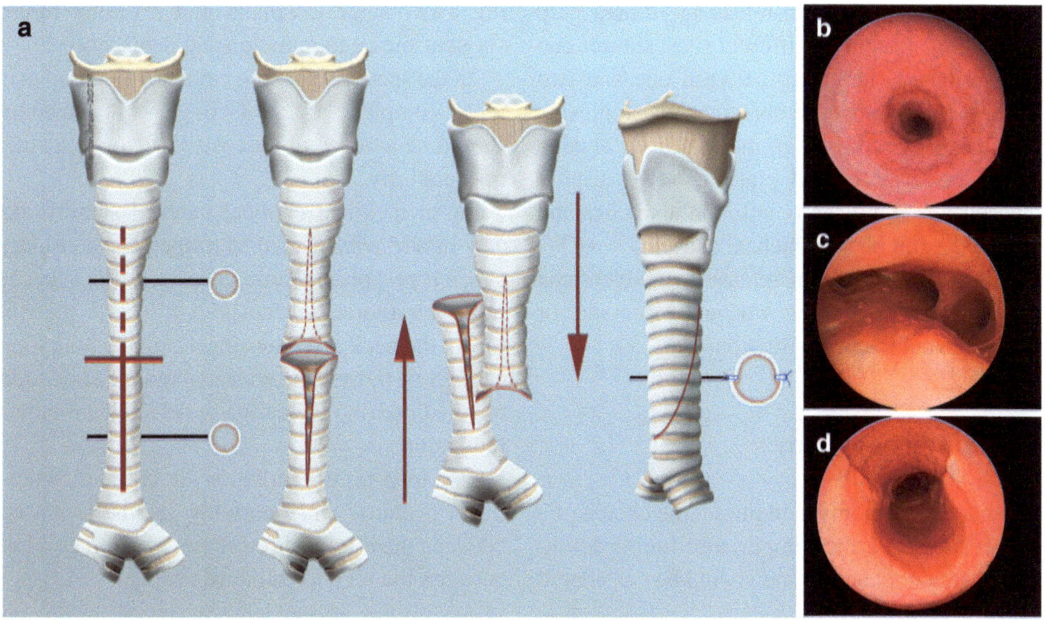

Fig. 17.23 Long-segment congenital tracheal stenosis (LSCTS) and slide tracheoplasty (ST). (**a**) Surgical concept of ST: tracheal stenotic segment is fully transected at its midpoint. All the complete rings in the proximal segment are incised at the back up to the normal rings. The distal segment rings are incised in front, and then the two tracheal segments are slid on top of each other. This will shorten the stenotic segment by half, increase the diameter two times, and by Poiseuille's law reduce airway resistance four times. (**b**) LSCTS due to complete tracheal rings. (**c**) Right upper lobe bronchus arising from the trachea (*pig bronchus or bronchus suis*). (**d**) Postoperative result after slide tracheoplasty

17.5.8 Tension-Releasing Maneuvers in Extensive Airway Resection

Commitment to totally resecting a stenotic segment of the airway ensures an optimal anastomosis with healthy mucosa. This is a key factor in reducing the risk of dehiscence and favoring optimal cicatrization. A second important factor in airway resection surgeries is reducing as much as possible the anastomotic tension using different maneuvers [39].

Infrahyoid laryngeal release consists of sectioning the thyroid insertion of the thyrohyoid muscles and dividing the thyrohyoid membrane along the upper rim of the thyroid cartilage up to its superior cornu which can also be sectioned bilaterally. This ensures a 1.5-cm-long release sparing the superior laryngeal nerves [7]. In small children, laryngeal release procedures seldom induce dysphagia nor aspiration due to the high position of the thyroid cartilage in the neck, whereas in adults, this should be considered.

Intraoperative tension-releasing sutures help in reducing tension on different sites; sutures can be distributed alternating between one and two tracheal rings below and above the anastomosis.

Sutures passed through the inferolateral edge of the posterior cricoid plate and two distally placed rings significantly pull up the trachea and reduce tension in cricotracheal anastomoses.

Hilar and pericardial release maneuvers can be beneficial in thoracic tracheal resections or long-segment tracheal resections [95].

17.5.9 Tracheostomy

When a tracheostomy is required, the choice of a proper site is of critical importance for the definitive treatment planning and should be considered individually for each situation. The objectives of airway management in an incipient airway stenosis are:

- Creating a safe airway, by bypassing the stenotic site: the tip of the cannula should always be placed in the lumen, distal to the stenotic site.
- Sparing as much healthy tracheal length as possible so as to avoid a more complex reconstruction and a potential second stenotic site in the future.
- Avoid iatrogenic lesions to the glottis and the cricoid, the recurrent laryngeal nerves, the thyroid gland, and the esophagus.

17.5.9.1 Recommended Sites of Performing the Tracheostomy (Fig. 17.24)

In an LTS, it is best placed either close to the stenosis (first ring) allowing concomitant resection of stenosis and stoma or distal (sixth ring) allowing a two-stage treatment and avoiding future surgical site contamination and dehiscence.

In the specific of a congenital tracheal stenosis with complete tracheal rings, tracheostomy should be avoided at all costs in favor of a slide tracheoplasty.

In an incipient cervical tracheal stenosis or/and in the presence of a former tracheostomy site, it is best placed through the stenosis, whereas in an intrathoracic stenosis, it is best to place it low in the neck and choosing a cannula both long enough to bypass the stenosis and short enough to avoid injuring the carina or selective bronchus intubation.

For long-term ventilation or chronic aspiration, pediatric tracheostomy is best placed between the third and fourth rings and in an adult between the second and third rings.

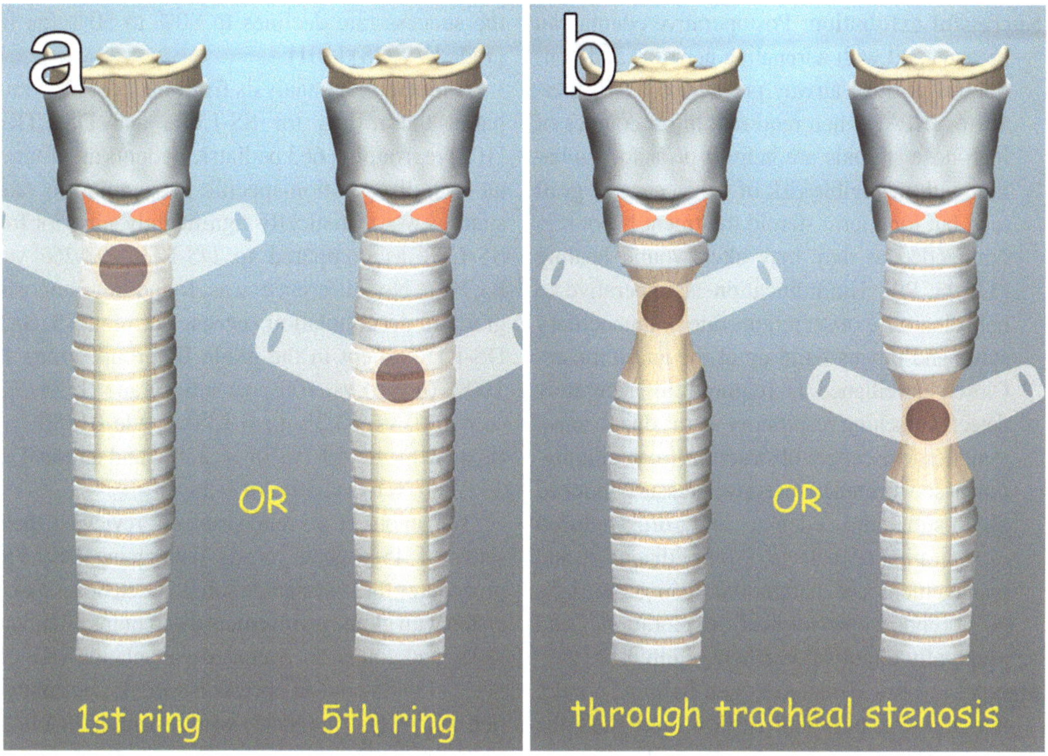

Fig. 17.24 Tracheostomy placement site: (**a**)* In incipient subglottic stenosis, tracheostomy is performed either between the cricoid, first, and second tracheal rings or between the fifth and sixth rings. (**b**) In existing tracheal stenosis, the tracheostomy is placed directly through the stenotic site. *This strategy will allow a single- or double-stage procedure in the future. The decision of tracheostomy site allows maximum preservation of the normal trachea for future airway corrective surgery. (Reprinted/adapted by permission from Springer Nature: Pediatric Airway Surgery by P. Monnier © 2011)

17.6 Postoperative Care and Follow-Up in Open Airway Surgery

Stable position: Keeping neck at a 30° flexion and limiting movements are important aspects of postoperative management after airway resection procedures. To achieve this analgesia, sedation +/− neuromuscular blockade are key in avoiding a dehiscence and achieving good results. Form-retaining pillows are helpful (see Fig. 17.16f). Chin-to-chest sutures are not recommended as they have been reported to induce ischemic myelopathy and irreversible paraplegia or tetraplegia [96].

Antibiotics are given as per the preoperative tracheobronchial aspirate and always after consulting the infectious disease specialist. Off-label use of nebulized Ciprodex (ciprofloxacin-dexamethasone suspension) appears to be helpful in controlling granulation tissue [88].

Limited intubation: Children remain electively intubated for 5–7 days to bypass postoperative vocal cord edema and facilitate wound healing without neck extension and movements. For tracheal resection and anastomosis, 24–48 h are sufficient due to limited glottic edema. Generally, nasotracheal intubation using soft Portex Blue Line® tubes is well tolerated with less gag reflex. When no airway resection is involved such as in LTRs, older children could stay awake while maintaining the nasotracheal tube, and this dramatically decreases the incidence of postoperative adverse events secondary to sedatives and effectively reduces length of PICU stay [97]. Adults undergo the same procedure with cuffed soft naso-/orotracheal tubes, but maintaining patients awake intubated is rarely tolerated.

Successful extubation: Postoperative edema can be managed with adrenaline aerosols and continuous positive airway pressure (CPAP) therapy or BiPAP when required. Short courses of high-dose steroids are helpful prior to extubation with negligible risk of dehiscence or graft loss, but long-term steroid treatment is not recommended as they may alter wound healing [37, 98, 99]. Humidification is imperative to help clearance of secretions due to mucociliary stasis and mucus build-up at the anastomoses. Close surveillance is required to accurately detect worsening respiratory status due to anastomotic dehiscence, obstruction from granulation tissue formation, negative pressure-induced glotto-subglottic edema, and drug-induced exaggeration of malacia. Prompt diagnosis and management are paramount, using aerosols, NIV, endoscopic/surgical exploration, and eventually reintubation when required.

Heliox® is a low-density oxygen-helium mixture that reduces turbulent airflow and thus the work of breathing; it is exceptionally used as a temporizing measure in acute airway situations not responding to non-invasive ventilation, before appropriate definitive management can be achieved [100].

Postoperative nutrition is administered using a transpyloric naso-jejunal feeding tube, while a nasogastric feeding tube allows for gastric exsufflation.

Follow-up endoscopy is performed before extubation in the PICU and then usually at 3 weeks and 3 months. If required, additional endoscopic procedures to treat granulations or if a dehiscence is suspected are performed. A fresh reconstruction should ideally not undergo dilation before 6 weeks to avoid iatrogenic dehiscence.

17.7 Results

17.7.1 Pediatric LTR and PCTR and Slide Tracheoplasty

17.7.1.1 LTR

A decannulation rate of just under 90% for grade I and II SGS following LTR is common in experienced centers. For advanced grades of stenosis, the success rate declines to 80% to 50% (as in grade IV SGS) [101].

A recent meta-analysis from Padia et al. compared the results for SS-LTRs and DS-LTRs [102] regrouping 663 pediatric patients and found an overall operation-specific decannulation rate success was statistically significantly superior for SS-LTR as compared to DS-LTR (93.2% vs. 83.7%). No difference was found for stenosis grade in decannulation success between SS- and DS-LTR except in the grade III group: grade I, 100% ($n = 6$) vs. 100% ($n = 6$); grade II, 84.9% ($n = 106$) vs. 83.3% ($n = 138$); grade III, 80.2% ($n = 101$) vs. 69.7% ($n = 238$); and grade IV, 33.3% ($n = 6$) vs. 50% ($n = 58$).

Yamamoto et al. retrospectively reviewed their series of 45 patients mostly undergoing DS-LTR procedures for lower-grade subglottic stenoses associated with glottic involvement that required stenting [103] and found an overall decannulation rate of 86.7% (39/45) and an operation-specific decannulation rate of 66.7% (30/45) with restenosis in 11/45 (24%) patients that were endoscopically or surgically treated. Revision surgery was required in ten patients, and two children died of mucus cannula obstruction. The respiratory, voice, and swallowing functions were excellent or good in 86%, 75%, and 84% of patients, respectively.

For grade IV stenoses, the Great Ormond Street team confirmed a higher decannulation rate with CTR than with laryngotracheal reconstruction (LTR) with ACCG + PCCG (92% versus 81%), and patients were less likely to need additional open procedures to achieve decannulation (18% versus 46%) [104]. The same team published their experience on 199 patients with overall good results for LTRs [105], with post-LTR success in 100% with grade I stenosis, 92.3% with grade II stenosis, 88.1% in grade III stenosis, and 83.3% in grade IV stenosis. Restenosis remained a problem, and children with grade IV stenosis treated with LTR were more likely to require subsequent open procedure(s) to achieve decannulation than those treated with CTR [106].

17.7.1.2 PCTR and TR

Over the years, the technique of PCTR for SGS has been well described and accepted, with an overall decannulation rate of more than 90% in primary and salvage PCTRs [75, 107–110]. In the previous edition of this book, Monnier showed this figure was higher in the two centers with the largest experience with better results for primary PCTRs (98–100%), salvage PCTRs (93–95%), and extended PCTR cases (94–95%) though this last group required more than one open surgery to achieve decannulation [111].

The recent ELS classification was shown to reliably predict surgical outcomes in the pediatric population undergoing segmental airway resection. The authors retrospectively applied the new classification to restage a group of 191 pediatric LTS patients accordingly in 2018 [27]. They found a mean decannulation rate of 88%, consistent with the available literature. A higher rate was statistically significant for patients without comorbidities (95.7% vs. 78.1%), when the stenosis involved two or fewer subsites involved (89% vs. 72%), and in patients classified with an ELS score of IIIa+ or less (96% vs. 82%). Surgical complications depended on the number of affected subsites and on the presence of associated comorbidities, but interestingly they were not dependent on the degree of stenosis, which reinforces our opinion that CTR is best adapted to grade IV stenoses as opposed to LTRs. The need for re-treatment depended on the length of resection, ELS stage, and presence of surgical complications.

Overall, LTR is a less extensive procedure and favored for grade II and selected grade III stenosis, while CTR is the preferred option for severe grade III and grade IV.

Slide tracheoplasty Grillo showed excellent results for ST with 100% success in a small series and normal tracheal growth [112]. Wertz et al. also reported an overall success of 87% in children and 85% cases not requiring no additional intervention. The Cincinnati team confirmed an operation-specific success of 79% for CST [47] and found similar success rates between primary TST and revision TST. The same team of Manning et al. published that a series of 80 pediatric patients who received TST [113] had a mortality rate of 5% associated with the duration of cardiopulmonary bypass and mechanical ventilation. 42.5% patients required re-intervention, and 62.5% patients were extubated within 48 h, mainly those undergoing isolated airway reconstruction alone. Zhang et al. reported an overall mortality rate of 9.9% in a series of 81 patients [114] with clear reduction over time in relation to their learning curve. They found a higher mortality in patients <10 months old and >24 months due to airway obstruction from obstructive granulation tissue at the anastomotic site. The Great Ormond Street team studied their series of 101 patients undergoing TST and found an overall mortality rate of 11.8% with preoperative ECMO, severe distal airway malacia, and bronchial stenosis being significant predictors of mortality [87]. This relates to the high prevalence of cardiopulmonary-associated conditions in this population.

17.7.2 Adult PCTR, LT, and TR

17.7.2.1 PCTR

Monnier described in the previous edition of this book the overall results in the international literature published from 1972 to 2000 on 249 adult patients with a 95% success rate and a 1% (2/249 cases) mortality rate, comparable to the pediatric population [111].

As for the pediatric population, the recent ELS classification was recently shown to reliably predict surgical outcomes in the adult population undergoing segmental airway resection [26]. The authors retrospectively applied the new classification to restage a group of 166 adult LTS patients undergoing TRA and CTRA procedures. They found an impressive ODR of 99% of patients without and in 88% of patients with surgical complications in patients with an ELS score < IIIb bearing a lower complication rate (32.8% vs. 57.7%). Additional treatment was required in 44% of patients. ELS score ≥ IIIb, length of resection, and occurrence of surgical complications were predictive of additional treatment. Surgical complications were related to increased ELS score.

17.7.2.2 LTR

Data for LTR in the adult population is heterogeneous due to varied etiologies. The Cincinnati team published their results for 95 adult patients undergoing LTR over a 10-year period [115]. 14.7% patients failed to decannulate by one postoperative year. The patients with diabetes, gastroesophageal reflux disease, and grade IV stenosis were at higher risk for decannulation failure; and requirement of endoscopic dilation with T-tube placement and were predictive of decannulation failure. At UCLA, Ching et al. evaluated their series of 81 adult patients, of which 61 underwent LTR [116], and found 80.3% ODR for LTR and an 90.0% ODR for CTR, respectively, with a significant association between stenosis grade and decannulation in the LTR group as in children. Also as in children, ODR was not associated with stenosis grade for CTR.

Lewis et al. performed a systematic review of the surgical treatment of LTS in adults and adolescents in 2017 [117] with 834 pooled patients to compare open versus endoscopic outcomes. Patients undergoing open procedures (CTR and LTR) underwent less additional surgery (32% versus 38%) and had a higher ODR (89% versus 83%), as compared to endoscopically managed cases, of which 44% required additional surgery and 63% were decannulated. Patients with LTS acquired after intubation/tracheostomy had better decannulation rates (88%), compared to traumatic etiologies (78%) and idiopathic stenosis (63%).

17.7.2.3 TR

Grillo published a large series of 503 patients who underwent segmental tracheal resection for postintubation stenosis with a 94% good (no exertional dyspnea) to satisfactory (no normal activity dyspnea) postoperative result [118]. Other studies reported similar results [119].

17.8 LTS and COVID-19 Pandemic (Fig. 17.25)

Following the first wave of COVID-19 pandemic, the Laryngotracheal Stenosis Committee of the European Laryngological Society (ELS) alerted the medical and scientific communities of the possibility of a surge in the number of airway injuries [120] secondary to prolonged intubation and tracheostomy and suggested that specialists in this field should see these patients at the earliest.

Several mechanisms [121] specifically related to COVID-19 treatment that increase the suscep-

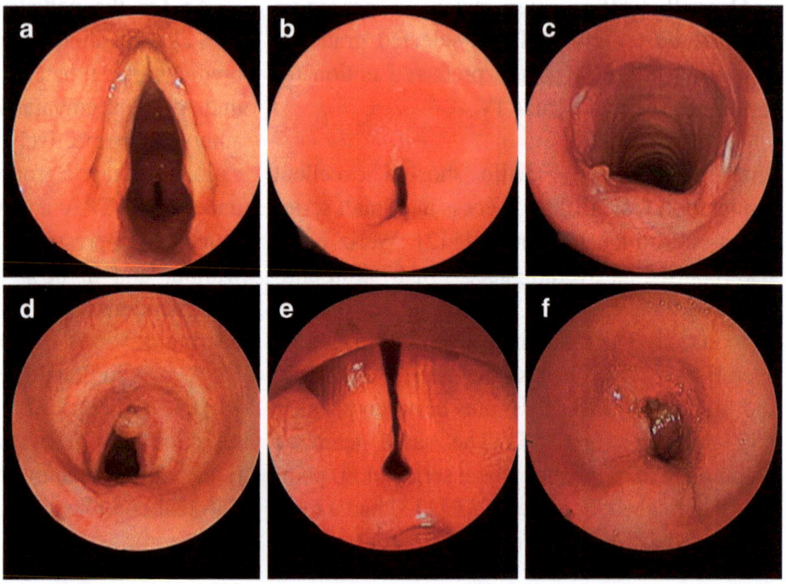

Fig. 17.25 Intubation- and tracheostomy-related LT stenosis in adult patients during the SARS-CoV-2 pandemic. (**a–c**) Severe tracheal stenosis following a single-stage five tracheal ring resection and anastomosis. (**d**) A-shape deformity with granuloma. (**e**) Severe posterior glottic stenosis. (**f**) Distal tracheal stenosis

tibility of the larynx and the trachea to intubation and tracheostomy complications are

1. Pronation maneuvers.
2. Prothrombotic and antifibrinolytic state of the patients affecting the laryngotracheal and esophageal microcirculation, thus predisposing the mucosa to more ischemia and necrosis.
3. High viral replication in the tracheal epithelium could weaken the mucosa.
4. Chronic high-dose corticosteroid use thins down the tracheal mucosa.
5. Lower PaO_2/FiO_2 ratio causes increased hypoxia of the laryngotracheal mucosa.
6. Emotional and physical exhaustion of the caregivers can add to the iatrogenic trauma.
7. Existing comorbidities.

In our early experience while treating LTS in these patients, we observed that the treatment is challenging because of their pre-existing comorbidities and the sequelae secondary to long and complicated ICU stays. Surgeons must be well trained to choose the appropriate treatment option that best suits their patient. Management strategies during the current and future months of the pandemic must aim at reducing laryngotracheal injuries.

17.9 Tips and Pearls to Avoid Complications

It cannot be emphasized enough that **optimizing patient status before surgery is crucial to achieve success**. Airway surgery should never be undertaken without a thorough global evaluation of the patient and without performing an in-depth evaluation of the airway problem(s) [36, 37].

Careful selection of timing and type of surgical procedure are key, because the highest chance of success lies in the first operation [7].

Perfect execution of the surgical technique and ensuring a quality anastomosis without tension are also of utmost importance in avoiding dehiscence. When performing resection and anastomosis, always place stitches in a submucosal plane to avoid devascularization of the mucosa at the site of anastomosis. When dissecting the trachea, always avoid unrequired circumferential mobilization to avoid ischemia and anastomotic failure.

Choosing a two-stage procedure instead of a single-stage procedure is appropriate in patients having SGS with glottic involvement, comorbidities, or both.

Performing a preoperative bacterial screening protocol and antibiotic prophylaxis such as previously described is important in reducing the postoperative infection risk.

Airway surgeons should be well trained and master a complete armamentarium of skills and techniques to ensure optimal management of these challenging cases and adapt to incurrent events or difficulties [39].

These measures will help in avoiding most complications such as dehiscence or graft loss.

Airway patients are challenging, and success is the fruit of multidisciplinary collaboration. Airway surgeons should invest time in sensitizing fellow pediatricians and anesthesiologists to the specificities of the pediatric airway and work in close collaboration with intensivists to ensure best possible care when using endotracheal tubes and cannulas.

A simple but invaluable tool in the everyday practice is an institutional airway pocket card, in the form of either a physical plastic card or a mobile phone application [122], detailing airway dimensions and their matching endotracheal tubes, tracheostomy cannulas, and endoscopes. It is readily available and may buy precious time in the management of airway emergencies.

17.10 Future Developments

Future advances in endoscopic airway techniques and instrumentation might allow more precise treatment and further avoid the need to perform open surgical airway procedures.

Further research is needed to address the complex challenge of tracheal replacement, which is still facing important setbacks.

Improvement in materials with the use of custom-made 3D-printed bioresorbable prostheses such as internal or external stents are promising solutions and will need further validation [123].

The growing use of platelet-derived concentrated growth factors may become an option to enhance results after cartilage grafting or airway resection to promote healing and vascularization of grafts and anastomoses [124–127].

The use of apneic oxygenation with high-flow nasal oxygen for laryngeal surgery is gaining attention in both adults and children during endoscopic procedures and may be a paradigm change in the way certain shared airway procedures are managed in the future.

Data regarding swallowing outcome is still lacking [31]; swallowing assessment perioperatively needs to be systematized to avoid the complications, costs, and morbidity of prolonged nutritional support.

Developing and integrating QoL measurement tools in routine practice should help to better define success for individual airway patients in the future.

References

1. Isaiah A, Moyer K, Pereira KD. Current trends in neonatal tracheostomy. JAMA Otolaryngol Head Neck Surg. 2016;142:738–42.
2. Adly A, Youssef TA, El-Begermy MM, Younis HM. Timing of tracheostomy in patients with prolonged endotracheal intubation: a systematic review. Eur Arch Otorhinolaryngol. 2018;275:679–90.
3. Torre M, Varela P, Romero D, Leopold E. Complex tracheal resection in children: myths, reality and lessons learned. Semin Pediatr Surg. 2021;2021:151059.
4. Grillo HC. Slide tracheoplasty for long-segment congenital tracheal stenosis. Ann Thorac Surg. 1994;58:613–20.
5. Allen E, Minutello K, Murcek BW. Anatomy, head and neck, larynx recurrent laryngeal nerve. Treasure Island, FL: StatPearls; 2021.
6. Potenza AS, Araujo Filho VJF, Cernea CR. Injury of the external branch of the superior laryngeal nerve in thyroid surgery. Gland Surg. 2017;6:552–62.
7. Monnier P, editor. Pediatric airway surgery: management of laryngotracheal stenosis in infants and children. New York: Springer; 2011. https://doi.org/10.1007/978-3-642-13535-4.
8. Marston AP, White DR. Subglottic stenosis. Clin Perinatol. 2018;45:787–804.
9. Morimitsu T, Matsumoto I, Okada S, Takahashi M, Kosugi T. Congenital cricoid stenosis. Laryngoscope. 1981;91:1356–64.
10. Holinger LD, Oppenheimer RW. Congenital subglottic stenosis: the elliptical cricoid cartilage. Ann Otol Rhinol Laryngol. 1989;98:702–6.
11. Hiebert JC, Zhao YD, Willis EB. Bronchoscopy findings in recurrent croup: a systematic review and meta-analysis. Int J Pediatr Otorhinolaryngol. 2016;90:86–90.
12. D'Eufemia MD, Cianci S, Di Meglio F, et al. Congenital high airway obstruction syndrome (CHAOS): discussing the role and limits of prenatal diagnosis starting from a single-center case series. J Prenat Med. 2016;10:4–7.
13. Kumar M, Gupta A, Kumar V, Handa A, Balliyan M, Meena J, Roychoudhary S. Management of CHAOS by intact cord resuscitation: case report and literature review. J Matern Fetal Neonatal Med. 2019;32:4181–7.
14. Walner DL, Loewen MS, Kimura RE. Neonatal subglottic stenosis—incidence and trends. Laryngoscope. 2001;111:48–51.
15. Stramiello JA, Mohammadzadeh A, Ryan J, Brigger MT. The role of bioresorbable intraluminal airway stents in pediatric tracheobronchial obstruction: a systematic review. Int J Pediatr Otorhinolaryngol. 2020;139:110405.
16. Rijnberg FM, Butler CR, Bieli C, et al. Aortopexy for the treatment of tracheobronchomalacia in 100 children: a 10-year single-centre experience. Eur J Cardiothorac Surg. 2018;54:585–92.
17. Smith MM, Cotton RT. Diagnosis and management of laryngotracheal stenosis. Expert Rev Respir Med. 2018;12:709–17.
18. Benjamin B. Prolonged intubation injuries of the larynx: endoscopic diagnosis, classification, and treatment. Ann Otol Rhinol Laryngol Suppl. 1993;160:1–15.
19. Axtell AL, Mathisen DJ. Idiopathic subglottic stenosis: techniques and results. Ann Cardiothorac Surg. 2018;7:299–305.
20. Donahoe L, Keshavjee S. Contemporary management of idiopathic laryngotracheal stenosis. Thorac Surg Clin. 2018;28:167–75.
21. Alaani A, Hogg RP, Drake Lee AB. Wegener's granulomatosis and subglottic stenosis: management of the airway. J Laryngol Otol. 2004;118:786–90.
22. Harris C, Cao C, Croce B, Cao C. Tracheal tumors. Ann Cardiothorac Surg. 2018;7:317.
23. Myer CM, O'Connor DM, Cotton RT. Proposed grading system for subglottic stenosis based on endotracheal tube sizes. Ann Otol Rhinol Laryngol. 1994;103:319–23.
24. Bogdasarian RS, Olson NR. Posterior glottic laryngeal stenosis. Otolaryngol Head Neck Surg. 1980;88:765–72.
25. Monnier P, Dikkers FG, Eckel H, Sittel C, Piazza C, Campos G, Remacle M, Peretti G. Preoperative assessment and classification of benign laryngotracheal stenosis: a consensus paper of the European Laryngological Society. Eur Arch Otorhinolaryngol. 2015;272:2885–96.
26. Fiz I, Monnier P, Koelmel JC, Di Dio D, Fiz F, Missale F, Piazza C, Peretti G, Sittel C. Multicentric

study applying the European Laryngological Society classification of benign laryngotracheal stenosis in adults treated by tracheal or cricotracheal resection and anastomosis. Laryngoscope. 2020;130:1640–5.
27. Fiz I, Monnier P, Koelmel JC, Di Dio D, Torre M, Fiz F, Missale F, Piazza C, Peretti G, Sittel C. Implementation of the European Laryngological Society classification for pediatric benign laryngotracheal stenosis: a multicentric study. Eur Arch Otorhinolaryngol. 2019;276:785–92.
28. Haywood M, Lovell L, Roe J, Clunie G, Sandhu G, Al Yaghchi C. Perioperative instrumental swallowing evaluation in adult airway reconstruction: a retrospective observational cohort study. Clin Otolaryngol. 2021; https://doi.org/10.1111/coa.13820.
29. Nouraei SAR, Makmur E, Dias A, Butler CR, Nandi R, Elliott MJ, Hewitt R. Validation of the Airway-Dyspnoea-Voice-Swallow (ADVS) scale and Patient-Reported Outcome Measure (PROM) as disease-specific instruments in paediatric laryngotracheal stenosis. Clin Otolaryngol. 2017;42:283–94.
30. Webb AL, Carding PN, Deary IJ, MacKenzie K, Steen N, Wilson JA. The reliability of three perceptual evaluation scales for dysphonia. Eur Arch Otorhinolaryngol. 2004;261:429–34.
31. Clunie GM, Roe JWG, Alexander C, Sandhu G, McGregor A. Voice and swallowing outcomes following airway reconstruction in adults: a systematic review. Laryngoscope. 2021;131:146–57.
32. Pullens B, Hakkesteegt M, Hoeve H, Timmerman M, Joosten K. Voice outcome and voice-related quality of life after surgery for pediatric laryngotracheal stenosis. Laryngoscope. 2017;127:1707–11.
33. Cohen W, Lloyd S, Wynne DM, Townsley RB. Perceptual evaluation of voice disorder in children who have had laryngotracheal reconstruction surgery and the relationship between clinician perceptual rating of voice quality and parent proxy/child self-report of voice-related quality of life. J Voice. 2019;33:945.e27–35.
34. Kokje VBC, Mermod M, Bertinazzi M, Sandu K. A new dimension of success in the management of airway disease in children with neurological deficit. Int J Pediatr Otorhinolaryngol. 2020;139:110483.
35. Bibas BJ, Cardoso PFG, Minamoto H, Pêgo-Fernandes PM. Surgery for intrathoracic tracheoesophageal and bronchoesophageal fistula. Ann Transl Med. 2018;6:210.
36. Ludemann JP, Hughes CA, Noah Z, Holinger LD. Complications of pediatric laryngotracheal reconstruction: prevention strategies. Ann Otol Rhinol Laryngol. 1999;108:1019–26.
37. de Alarcon A, Rutter MJ. Revision pediatric laryngotracheal reconstruction. Otolaryngol Clin N Am. 2008;41:959–80.
38. Polubothu S, Harrison S, Clement A, Kubba H. An audit of prophylactic antibiotic use in laryngeal reconstruction surgery. Int J Pediatr Otorhinolaryngol. 2009;73:1157–9.
39. Kou Y-F, Rutter MJ, Sandu K, Guilcher P. Pediatric open airway reconstruction. Curr Otorhinolaryngol Rep. 2021; https://doi.org/10.1007/s40136-020-00317-3.
40. Gray S, Myer CM, Miller R, Cotton RT. Adjunctive measures for successful laryngotracheal reconstruction. Ann Otol Rhinol Laryngol. 1987;96:509–13.
41. Themes UFO. 47 endoscopic airway surgery. Ento Key;2021.
42. Shepard J-AO, Flores EJ, Abbott GF. Imaging of the trachea. Ann Cardiothorac Surg. 2018;7:197–209.
43. Burke AJ, Vining DJ, McGuirt WF, Postma G, Browne JD. Evaluation of airway obstruction using virtual endoscopy. Laryngoscope. 2000;110:23–9.
44. Willging JP, Thompson DM. Pediatric FEESST: fiberoptic endoscopic evaluation of swallowing with sensory testing. Curr Gastroenterol Rep. 2005;7:240–3.
45. Boesch RP, Balakrishnan K, Acra S, et al. Structure and functions of pediatric aerodigestive programs: a consensus statement. Pediatrics. 2018; https://doi.org/10.1542/peds.2017-1701.
46. Wertz A, Ryan M, Jacobs I, Piccione J. Impact of pre-operative multidisciplinary evaluation on laryngotracheal reconstruction outcomes. Laryngoscope. https://doi.org/10.1002/lary.29338.
47. de Alarcon A, Rutter MJ. Cervical slide tracheoplasty. Arch Otolaryngol Head Neck Surg. 2012;138:812–6.
48. White DR, Bravo M, Vijayasekaran S, Rutter MJ, Cotton RT, Elluru RG. Laryngotracheoplasty as an alternative to tracheotomy in infants younger than 6 months. Arch Otolaryngol Head Neck Surg. 2009;135:445–7.
49. Riva T, Theiler L, Jaquet Y, Giger R, Nisa L. Early experience with high-flow nasal oxygen therapy (HFNOT) in pediatric endoscopic airway surgery. Int J Pediatr Otorhinolaryngol. 2018;108:151–4.
50. Lyons C, Callaghan M. Apnoeic oxygenation with high-flow nasal oxygen for laryngeal surgery: a case series. Anaesthesia. 2017;72:1379–87.
51. Warner D, Brietzke SE. Mitomycin C and airway surgery: how well does it work? Otolaryngol Head Neck Surg. 2008;138:700–9.
52. Durden F, Sobol SE. Balloon laryngoplasty as a primary treatment for subglottic stenosis. Arch Otolaryngol Head Neck Surg. 2007;133:772–5.
53. Rutter MJ, Cohen AP, de Alarcon A. Endoscopic airway management in children. Curr Opin Otolaryngol Head Neck Surg. 2008;16:525–9.
54. Lang M, Brietzke SE. A systematic review and meta-analysis of endoscopic balloon dilation of pediatric subglottic stenosis. Otolaryngol Head Neck Surg. 2014;150:174–9.
55. Shapshay SM, Beamis JF, Hybels RL, Bohigian RK. Endoscopic treatment of subglottic and tracheal stenosis by radial laser incision and dilation. Ann Otol Rhinol Laryngol. 1987;96:661–4.
56. Management of the difficult airway: a handbook for surgeons. Routledge & CRC Press. https://

www.routledge.com/Management-of-the-Difficult-Airway-A-Handbook-for-Surgeons/Thompson-Vieira-Rutter/p/book/9781909836051. Accessed 29 May 2021.
57. Inglis AF, Perkins JA, Manning SC, Mouzakes J. Endoscopic posterior cricoid split and rib grafting in 10 children. Laryngoscope. 2003;113:2004–9.
58. Thakkar K, Gerber ME. Endoscopic posterior costal cartilage graft placement for acute management of pediatric bilateral vocal fold paralysis without tracheostomy. Int J Pediatr Otorhinolaryngol. 2008;72:1555–8.
59. Dahl JP, Purcell PL, Parikh SR, Inglis AF. Endoscopic posterior cricoid split with costal cartilage graft: a fifteen-year experience. Laryngoscope. 2017;127:252–7.
60. Soloperto D, Spinnato F, Di Gioia S, Di Maro F, Pinter P, Bisceglia A, Marchioni D. Acquired subglottic cysts in children: a rare and challenging clinical entity. A systematic review. Int J Pediatr Otorhinolaryngol. 2021;140:110523.
61. Smith ME, Elstad M. Mitomycin C and the endoscopic treatment of laryngotracheal stenosis: are two applications better than one? Laryngoscope. 2009;119:272–83.
62. Hueman EM, Simpson CB. Airway complications from topical mitomycin C. Otolaryngol Head Neck Surg. 2005;133:831–5.
63. McRae K. Anesthesia for airway surgery. Anesthesiol Clin North Am. 2001;19:497–541.
64. Daumerie G, Su S, Ochroch EA. Anesthesia for the patient with tracheal stenosis. Anesthesiol Clin. 2010;28:157–74.
65. Klemm E, Nowak A, editors. Tracheotomy and airway: a practical guide. Cham: Springer; 2020. https://doi.org/10.1007/978-3-030-44314-6.
66. Gallagher TQ, Hartnick CJ. Costal cartilage harvest. Adv Otorhinolaryngol. 2012;73:39–41.
67. Kearns DB, Olson TS, Pransky SM, Seid AB. Technique for costal cartilage harvest for use in laryngotracheal reconstruction. Int J Pediatr Otorhinolaryngol. 1989;18:73–5.
68. Grillo HC. Primary reconstruction of airway after resection of subglottic laryngeal and upper tracheal stenosis. Ann Thorac Surg. 1982;33:3–18.
69. Cotton RT, Evans JN. Laryngotracheal reconstruction in children. Five-year follow-up. Ann Otol Rhinol Laryngol. 1981;90:516–20.
70. Rutter MJ, Cotton RT. The use of posterior cricoid grafting in managing isolated posterior glottic stenosis in children. Arch Otolaryngol Head Neck Surg. 2004;130:737–9.
71. Zalzal GH, Cotton RT, McAdams AJ. The survival of costal cartilage graft in laryngotracheal reconstruction. Otolaryngol Head Neck Surg. 1986;94:204–11.
72. Pashley NR, Jaskunas JM, Waldstein G. Laryngotracheoplasty with costochondral grafts—a clinical correlate of graft survival. Laryngoscope. 1984;94:1493–6.
73. Pearson FG, Brito-Filomeno L, Cooper JD. Experience with partial cricoid resection and thyrotracheal anastomosis. Ann Otol Rhinol Laryngol. 1986;95:582–5.
74. Ikonomidis C, George M, Jaquet Y, Monnier P. Partial cricotracheal resection in children weighing less than 10 kilograms. Otolaryngol Head Neck Surg. 2010;142:41–7.
75. Yamamoto K, Jaquet Y, Ikonomidis C, Monnier P. Partial cricotracheal resection for paediatric subglottic stenosis: update of the Lausanne experience with 129 cases. Eur J Cardiothorac Surg. 2015;47:876–82.
76. Rutter MJ, Hartley BEJ, Cotton RT. Cricotracheal resection in children. Arch Otolaryngol Head Neck Surg. 2001;127:289–92.
77. Monnier P, Lang F, Savary M. Cricotracheal resection for pediatric subglottic stenosis. Int J Pediatr Otorhinolaryngol. 1999;49(Suppl 1):S283–6.
78. Sandu K, Monnier P. Partial cricotracheal resection with tracheal intussusception and cricoarytenoid joint mobilization: early experience in a new technical variant. Laryngoscope. 2011;121:2150–4.
79. Sivakumar RK, Panneerselvam S, Uthaman D, Rudingwa P, Ravi R. Spontaneous ventilation as a key ventilation technique during open airway phase in tracheal resection and reconstruction: a case series. Indian J Anaesth. 2019;63:1029–32.
80. Tsang V, Murday A, Gillbe C, Goldstraw P. Slide tracheoplasty for congenital funnel-shaped tracheal stenosis. Ann Thorac Surg. 1989;48:632–5.
81. Yong MS, Konstantinov IE. Understanding the impact of slide tracheoplasty in congenital tracheal stenosis. Transl Pediatr. 2019;8:462–4.
82. Provenzano MJ, Rutter MJ, von Allmen D, Manning PB, Paul Boesch R, Putnam PE, Black AP, de Alarcon A. Slide tracheoplasty for the treatment of tracheoesophogeal fistulas. J Pediatr Surg. 2014;49:910–4.
83. Ywakim R, El-Hakim H. Congenital tracheal stenosis managed conservatively: systematic review of the literature. J Otolaryngol Head Neck Surg. 2012;41:288–302.
84. Chen S-J, Wu E-T, Wang C-C, Chou H-W, Chen Y-S, Huang S-C. Excessive tracheal length in patients with congenital tracheal stenosis. Ann Thorac Surg. 2019;108:138–45.
85. Morita K, Yokoi A, Fukuzawa H, Hisamatsu C, Endo K, Okata Y, Tamaki A, Mishima Y, Oshima Y, Maeda K. Surgical intervention strategies for congenital tracheal stenosis associated with a tracheal bronchus based on the location of stenosis. Pediatr Surg Int. 2016;32:915–9.
86. Hofferberth SC, Watters K, Rahbar R, Fynn-Thompson F. Evolution of surgical approaches in the management of congenital tracheal stenosis: single-center experience. World J Pediatr Congenit Heart Surg. 2016;7:16–24.
87. Butler CR, Speggiorin S, Rijnberg FM, Roebuck DJ, Muthialu N, Hewitt RJ, Elliott MJ. Outcomes

of slide tracheoplasty in 101 children: a 17-year single-center experience. J Thorac Cardiovasc Surg. 2014;147:1783–9.
88. Stephens EH, Wiedermann JP, Dearani JA, Backer CL. Expert technique: pediatric tracheal surgery. World J Pediatr Congenit Heart Surg. 2021;12:414–7.
89. Nonoperative management of complete tracheal rings. Congenital defects. JAMA Otolaryngol Head Neck Surg. JAMA Network. https://jamanetwork.com/journals/jamaotolaryngology/fullarticle/647378. Accessed 23 May 2021.
90. Esener Z, Tür A, Diren B. Difficulty in endotracheal intubation due to congenital tracheal stenosis: a case report. Anesthesiology. 1988;69:279–81.
91. Donnelly J. Congenital tracheal stenosis in an adult, complicated by asphyxial pulmonary oedema. Anaesth Intensive Care. 1988;16:212–5.
92. Lee JC, Kim GS, Lee SJ, Yoo CG, Kim YW, Han SK, Shim YS. An adult case of pulmonary sling with complete tracheal ring. Korean J Intern Med. 1996;11:175–7.
93. Speggiorin S, Gilbert TW, Broadhead M, Roebuck DJ, McLaren CA, Elliott MJ. Do tracheas grow after slide tracheoplasty? Ann Thorac Surg. 2012;93:1083–6.
94. Wilcox LJ, Schweiger C, Hart CK, de Alarcon A, Peddireddy NS, Rutter MJ. Growth and management of repaired complete tracheal rings after slide tracheoplasty. Otolaryngol Head Neck Surg. 2019;161:164–70.
95. Broussard B, Mathisen DJ. Tracheal release maneuvers. Ann Cardiothorac Surg. 2018;7:293–8.
96. Noh KB, Mohamad I, Maruthamuthu T, Nadarajah S, Hassan NFHN. Paraplegia as a rare complication of tracheal resection anastomosis. Int J Otorhinolaryngol Head Neck Surg. 2018;4:823–5.
97. Jacobs BR, Salman BA, Cotton RT, Lyons K, Brilli RJ. Postoperative management of children after single-stage laryngotracheal reconstruction. Crit Care Med. 2001;29:164–8.
98. Lee C-H, Peng M-J, Wu C-L. Dexamethasone to prevent postextubation airway obstruction in adults: a prospective, randomized, double-blind, placebo-controlled study. Crit Care. 2007;11:R72.
99. Veyckemans F. Tracheal extubation in children: planning, technique, and complications. Pediatr Anesth. 2020;30:331–8.
100. McGarvey JM, Pollack CV. Heliox in airway management. Emerg Med Clin North Am. 2008;26: 905–20.
101. Cotton RT, Gray SD, Miller RP. Update of the Cincinnati experience in pediatric laryngotracheal reconstruction. Laryngoscope. 1989;99:1111–6.
102. Padia R, Sjogren P, Smith M, Muntz H, Stoddard G, Meier J. Systematic review/meta-analysis comparing successful outcomes after single vs. double-stage laryngotracheal reconstruction. Int J Pediatr Otorhinolaryngol. 2018;108:168–74.
103. Yamamoto K, Monnier P, Holtz F, Jaquet Y. Laryngotracheal reconstruction for pediatric glotto-subglottic stenosis. Int J Pediatr Otorhinolaryngol. 2014;78:1476–9.
104. Gustafson LM, Hartley BE, Cotton RT. Acquired total (grade 4) subglottic stenosis in children. Ann Otol Rhinol Laryngol. 2001;110:16–9.
105. Bajaj Y, Cochrane LA, Jephson CG, Wyatt ME, Bailey CM, Albert DM, Hartley BEJ. Laryngotracheal reconstruction and cricotracheal resection in children: recent experience at Great Ormond Street Hospital. Int J Pediatr Otorhinolaryngol. 2012;76:507–11.
106. Hartley BE, Cotton RT. Paediatric airway stenosis: laryngotracheal reconstruction or cricotracheal resection? Clin Otolaryngol Allied Sci. 2000;25:342–9.
107. Sandu K, Monnier P. Cricotracheal resection. Otolaryngol Clin N Am. 2008;41:981–998, x.
108. Ranne RD, Lindley S, Holder TM, Ashcraft KW, Sharp RJ, Amoury RA. Relief of subglottic stenosis by anterior cricoid resection: an operation for the difficult case. J Pediatr Surg. 1991;26:255–258; discussion 258–9.
109. Triglia JM, Nicollas R, Roman S. Primary cricotracheal resection in children: indications, technique and outcome. Int J Pediatr Otorhinolaryngol. 2001;58:17–25.
110. White DR, Cotton RT, Bean JA, Rutter MJ. Pediatric cricotracheal resection: surgical outcomes and risk factor analysis. Arch Otolaryngol Head Neck Surg. 2005;131:896–9.
111. Monnier P. Subglottic and tracheal stenosis. In: Remacle M, Eckel HE, editors. Surgery of larynx and trachea. Berlin: Springer; 2010. p. 137–58.
112. Grillo HC, Wright CD, Vlahakes GJ, MacGillivray TE. Management of congenital tracheal stenosis by means of slide tracheoplasty or resection and reconstruction, with long-term follow-up of growth after slide tracheoplasty. J Thorac Cardiovasc Surg. 2002;123:145–52.
113. Manning PB, Rutter MJ, Lisec A, Gupta R, Marino BS. One slide fits all: the versatility of slide tracheoplasty with cardiopulmonary bypass support for airway reconstruction in children. J Thorac Cardiovasc Surg. 2011;141:155–61.
114. Zhang H, Wang S, Lu Z, Zhu L, Du X, Wang H, Xu Z. Slide tracheoplasty in 81 children: improved outcomes with modified surgical technique and optimal surgical age. Medicine (Baltimore). 2017; 96:e8013.
115. Tawfik KO, Houlton JJ, Compton W, Ying J, Khosla SM. Laryngotracheal reconstruction: a ten-year review of risk factors for decannulation failure. Laryngoscope. 2015;125:674–9.
116. Ching HH, Mendelsohn AH, Liu IY, Long J, Chhetri DK, Berke GS. A comparative study of cricotracheal resection and staged laryngotracheoplasty for adult subglottic stenosis. Ann Otol Rhinol Laryngol. 2015;124:326–33.
117. Lewis S, Earley M, Rosenfeld R, Silverman J. Systematic review for surgical treatment of

adult and adolescent laryngotracheal stenosis. Laryngoscope. 2017;127:191–8.

118. Grillo HC, Donahue DM, Mathisen DJ, Wain JC, Wright CD. Postintubation tracheal stenosis. Treatment and results. J Thorac Cardiovasc Surg. 1995;109:486–492; discussion 492–3.
119. Kanlikama M, Celenk F, Gonuldas B, Gulsen S. Cervical tracheal resection and anastomosis for postintubation tracheal stenosis. J Craniofac Surg. 2018;29:e578–82.
120. Piazza C, Filauro M, Dikkers FG, Nouraei SAR, Sandu K, Sittel C, Amin MR, Campos G, Eckel HE, Peretti G. Long-term intubation and high rate of tracheostomy in COVID-19 patients might determine an unprecedented increase of airway stenoses: a call to action from the European Laryngological Society. Eur Arch Otorhinolaryngol. 2021;278:1–7.
121. Fiacchini G, Tricò D, Ribechini A, Forfori F, Brogi E, Lucchi M, Berrettini S, Bertini P, Guarracino F, Bruschini L. Evaluation of the incidence and potential mechanisms of tracheal complications in patients with COVID-19. JAMA Otolaryngol Head Neck Surg. 2021;147:70.
122. Free Mobile Airway Card app is a great tool for ENT physicians. iMedicalApps; 2016.
123. Morrison RJ, Hollister SJ, Niedner MF, Mahani MG, Park AH, Mehta DK, Ohye RG, Green GE. Mitigation of tracheobronchomalacia with 3D-printed personalized medical devices in pediatric patients. Sci Transl Med. 2015;7:285ra64.
124. Gürsoy K, Teymur H, Göktaş Demircan FB, Tanas Işikçi Ö, Gümüş M, Koçer U. Effect of platelet-derived concentrated growth factor on single-layer, multi-layer, and crushed onlay cartilage grafts. Aesthet Surg J. 2021;41:537–47.
125. Gómez-Caro A, Ausin P, Boada M. Platelet rich plasma improves the healing process after airway anastomosis. Interact Cardiovasc Thorac Surg. 2011;13:552–6.
126. Sahin Onder S, Sahin Yilmaz A, Erkmen B, Topal CS, Gergin O, Canpolat MS. Platelet-rich plasma for laryngotracheal reconstruction: an experimental study. Eur Arch Otorhinolaryngol. 2020;277:3103–9.
127. Topkara A, Özkan A, Özcan RH, Öksüz M, Akbulut M. Effect of concentrated growth factor on survival of diced cartilage graft. Aesthet Surg J. 2016;36:1176–87.

Tracheotomy

18

Georges Lawson, Marius Claude Flatin,
and Sébastien Van der Vorst

18.1 Introduction

Tracheostomy is one of the oldest surgical procedures in the history of head and neck surgery. The evolution of tracheotomy stretches back over many centuries. It has been performed for more than 3500 years, but the first successful well-documented tracheotomy is attributed to Antonio Musa Brasavolo in 1546. In 1932, Chevalier Jackson [1, 2] standardized the technique and taught the medical community about a well-performed tracheotomy and routine surgical care; more specifically, he pointed out the side effects of "high tracheotomy." The procedure is described as a potential lifesaving surgery performed sometimes in emergency situations but more often as a planned surgery in the operating room or intensive care unit.

Tracheotomy is a surgical opening into the trachea. It is performed for the purpose of ventilation and/or pulmonary toilet. Today, in the English-language literature, the terms tracheotomy and tracheostomy are used interchangeably. To clarify, *tracheotomy* is used here for the procedure of opening the trachea and *tracheostomy* is a permanent opening and exteriorizing the trachea to the cervical skin until the opening has become epithelialized. Performed under ideal circumstances (in an operating room, as an elective procedure, on a patient with a slender neck without airway obstruction), tracheotomy is a simple, safe, and easy procedure.

Successful management of the airway requires a complete understanding of the structure and function of the upper aerodigestive tract. The goal is to apply the appropriate solution for each specific case to avoid complications and a life-threatening situation.

This chapter is designed to provide information about the following:

- Indications for tracheotomy
- Decision making for open neck tracheotomy versus percutaneous tracheotomy
- Surgical technique
- Management of the tracheostomy

18.2 Indications for Tracheotomy

Tracheotomy means "making a stoma into the trachea." This temporary or permanent opening of the trachea may be necessary when circumstances exist that compromise adequate respira-

G. Lawson (✉) · S. Van der Vorst
Otolaryngology, Head and Neck Surgery Department, CHU UCL Namur - site Godinne, Yvoir, Belgium
e-mail: georges.lawson@chuuclnamur.uclouvain.be; sebastien.vandervorst@chuuclnamur.uclouvain.be

M. C. Flatin
Chirurgien Cervico-Facial et ORL, Maître de Conférences Agrégé, ENT & Head and Neck Surgery Medical School, University of Parakou, Parakou, Benin

M. Remacle, H. E. Eckel (eds.), *Textbook of Surgery of Larynx and Trachea*,
https://doi.org/10.1007/978-3-031-09621-1_18

tion. There are several situations in which tracheotomy is needed:

- Upper airway obstruction
  - Inflammatory disease
  - Benign laryngeal pathology
  - Malignant laryngeal tumors
  - Benign and malignant tracheal tumors
  - Laryngeal trauma or stenosis
  - Tracheal stenosis
- Need for assisted ventilation over a prolonged period of time
- Deficit of lower airway protection against aspiration of oral or gastric secretions
- Clearance of lower respiratory tract secretions

There is no fixed list of circumstances and morphological or pathological situation for tracheotomy. However, there are a variety of alternatives to tracheotomy:

- Noninvasive positive-pressure ventilation with a face mask or a laryngeal mask
- Endotracheal intubation
- Endoscopic procedure to remove some foreign bodies

An appropriate decision should be made for each patient, taking into account the following facts:

- The laryngeal mask airway is not suitable for all patients, particularly for patients at risk for aspiration, and it requires close intensive care monitoring.
- Endotracheal intubation is not always possible, depending on the patient's anatomy or pathological situation. In case of difficult airway management, tracheotomy should be considered according to the "Practice Guidelines for Management of the Difficult Airway" [3].
- Prolonged intubation for more than a week can induce laryngeal and tracheal damage [4].

18.3 Decision Making for Open Neck Tracheotomy Versus Percutaneous Tracheotomy

Conventional surgical tracheotomy reported as open neck tracheotomy is a safe, less easy procedure when performed under ideal circumstances. However, many complications following the operation have been reported [5]. Since the report by Ciaglia et al. [6] in 1985 on percutaneous dilatation tracheostomy (PCDT), several studies demonstrated that this technique is safe and easy with a low complication rate; furthermore, it is superior to the conventional surgical tracheostomy as immediate complications as well as complications with the tracheostomy tube in situ are fewer and less severe [7].

It must be stressed that PCDT is suitable only in adult patients without a midline neck mass and if cricoid cartilage can be palpated above the sternal notch. All patients below the age of 18 years or with a neck deformity and/or unidentifiable anatomy of the neck represent a group for whom PCDT is contraindicated.

During PCDT, the surgeon is sharing the airway with the anesthetist from the start of the procedure. The endotracheal tube is deflated and withdrawn above the vocal cord. In emergency cases or in patients with difficult airway management, this maneuver can result in a nonfunctional airway. In such a situation, conventional tracheostomy is more advisable.

18.4 Tracheotomy Techniques

18.4.1 Conventional or Open Neck Tracheotomy

Conventional or open neck tracheotomy can be performed in various situations: in an emergency or as an elective operation, under general or local anesthesia, in the operating room or by the bedside.

Elective tracheotomy is best carried out in the operating room under general anesthesia, where efficient assistance is available with adequate equipment (light, suction, electrocautery, tracheostomy tubes of different sizes and shapes). The patient is placed on supine position, with the head extended using a shoulder roll (Fig. 18.1a). A horizontal incision is made midway between the sternal notch and the cricoid cartilage. A sharp dissection is carried down through the subcutaneous tissue and platysma. The strap muscles are identified, and then the dissection is changed to the vertical plane (Fig. 18.2a). The strap muscles are separated in the midline with a retractor until the thyroid isthmus is encountered and the anterior wall of the trachea is identified (Fig. 18.2b). Inferior and median thyroid blood vessels are ligated; the thyroid isthmus is transected, and each side is suture-ligated to prevent bleeding (Fig. 18.2c). The anterior wall of the trachea is incised between the second and third tracheal incision to determine the correct level at which to enter the trachea. To secure the opening of the stoma, an inferiorly based flap consisting of the anterior portion of a single tracheal ring is sutured to the inferior skin margin (Fig. 18.2d).

During surgery, a special curved endotracheal tube (Montandon endotracheal tube) is introduced in the stoma and replaced by a tracheotomy tube at the end of the surgery. The placement begins with the tracheotomy tube at right angles to the trachea (Fig. 18.3a, b); then as the tube is inserted, it is rotated so its axis is parallel to that of the trachea. The tracheotomy tube is sutured to the skin as an added precaution to prevent accidental dislodgement of the tube (Fig. 18.3c). To avoid subcutaneous emphysema, pneumothorax, and infection, a tracheotomy wound is never closed tightly around the tube.

18.4.2 Percutaneous Dilatation Tracheotomy

Percutaneous dilatation tracheotomy (PDT) is a safe, simple, accepted alternative to conventional tracheotomy. Some studies [8–10] have demonstrated advantages of less cost, infection,

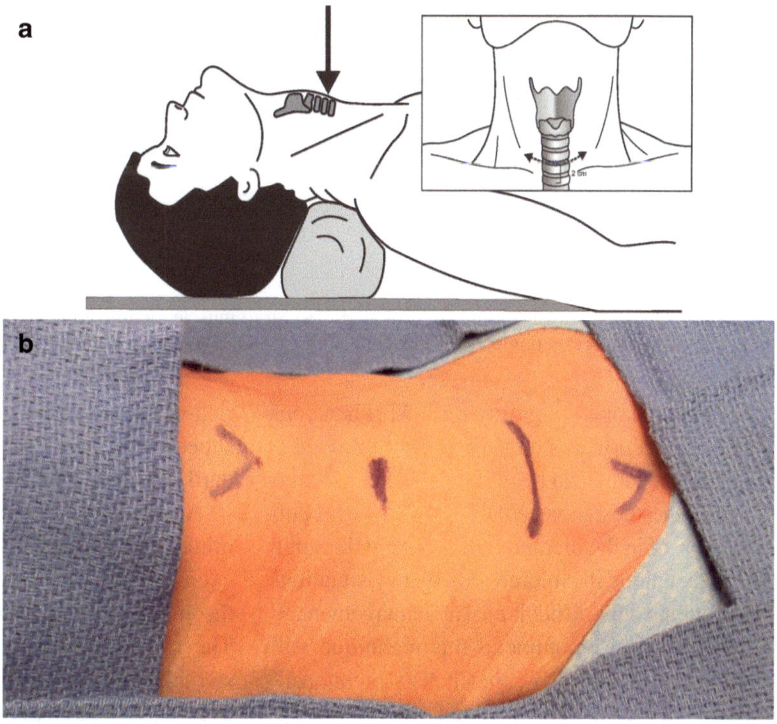

Fig. 18.1 (**a**) Patient's position: supine with the head extended. (**b**) Landmark for tracheotomy

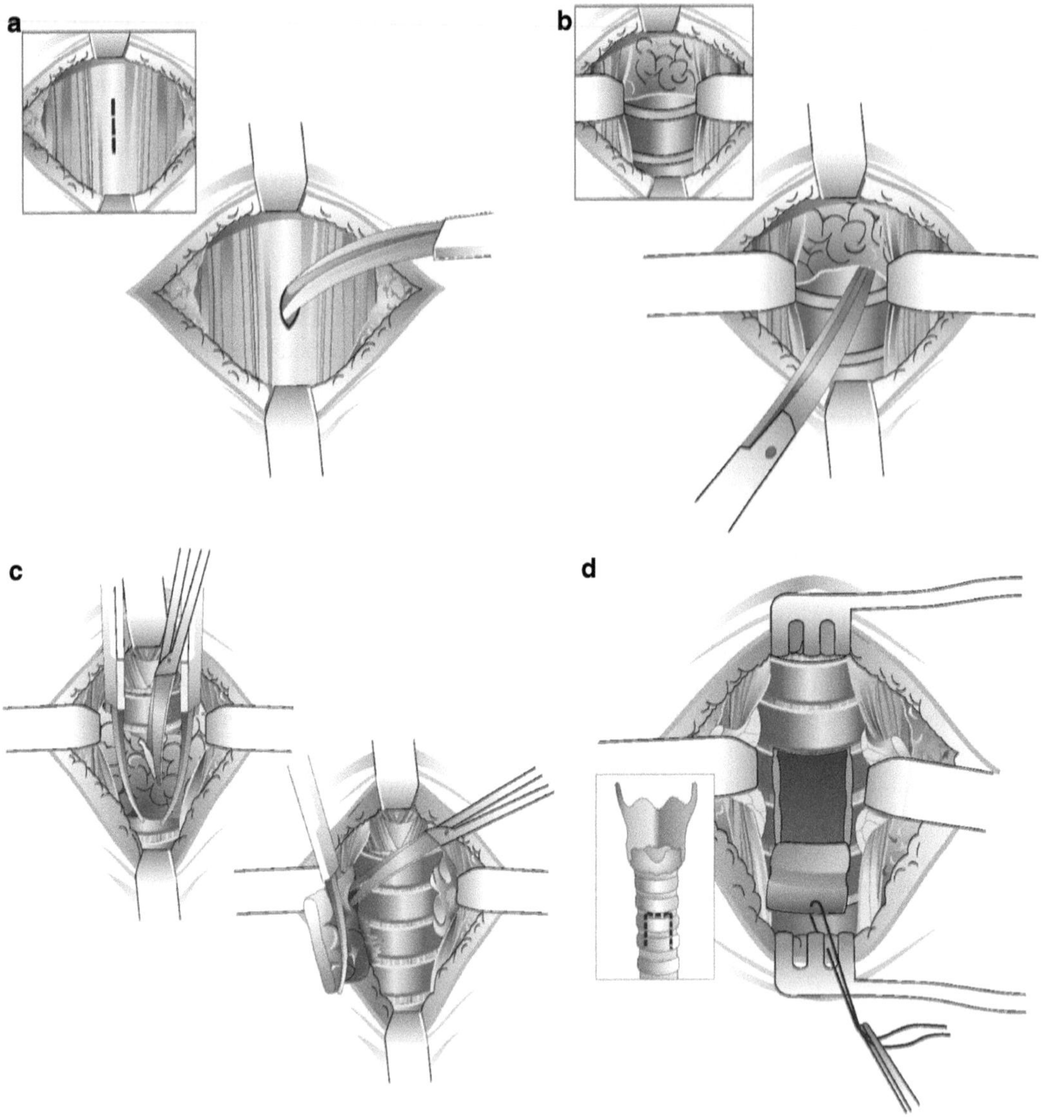

Fig. 18.2 Open neck tracheotomy surgical steps: (**a**) Strap muscle identification and dissection, (**b**) tracheal anterior wall identification, (**c**) sectioning of the thyroid isthmus, and (**d**) opening of the tracheal with an inferiorly based flap

bleeding, and operating time for PDT when compared to traditional open neck tracheotomy.

The procedure can be performed under local or general anesthesia. Nevertheless, there is no published proof in the literature to guarantee the safety of the technique in children, emergency situations, and patients with difficult airway management.

We strongly recommend this technique with good airway control by anesthetists or intensivists, ideally under direct vision with fiberscopy during the procedure. The surgery should be carried out by a skilled surgeon (or under his or her supervision), with the ability to perform a standard tracheotomy.

Anatomical suitability for PDT must be determined preoperatively with the patient's neck extended. A contraindication to the procedure is the inability to palpate the laryngeal landmark. The cricoid cartilage should be felt above the sternal notch. Similarly, the patient with a midline neck mass, a large thyroid gland, should be a candidate for conventional tracheotomy.

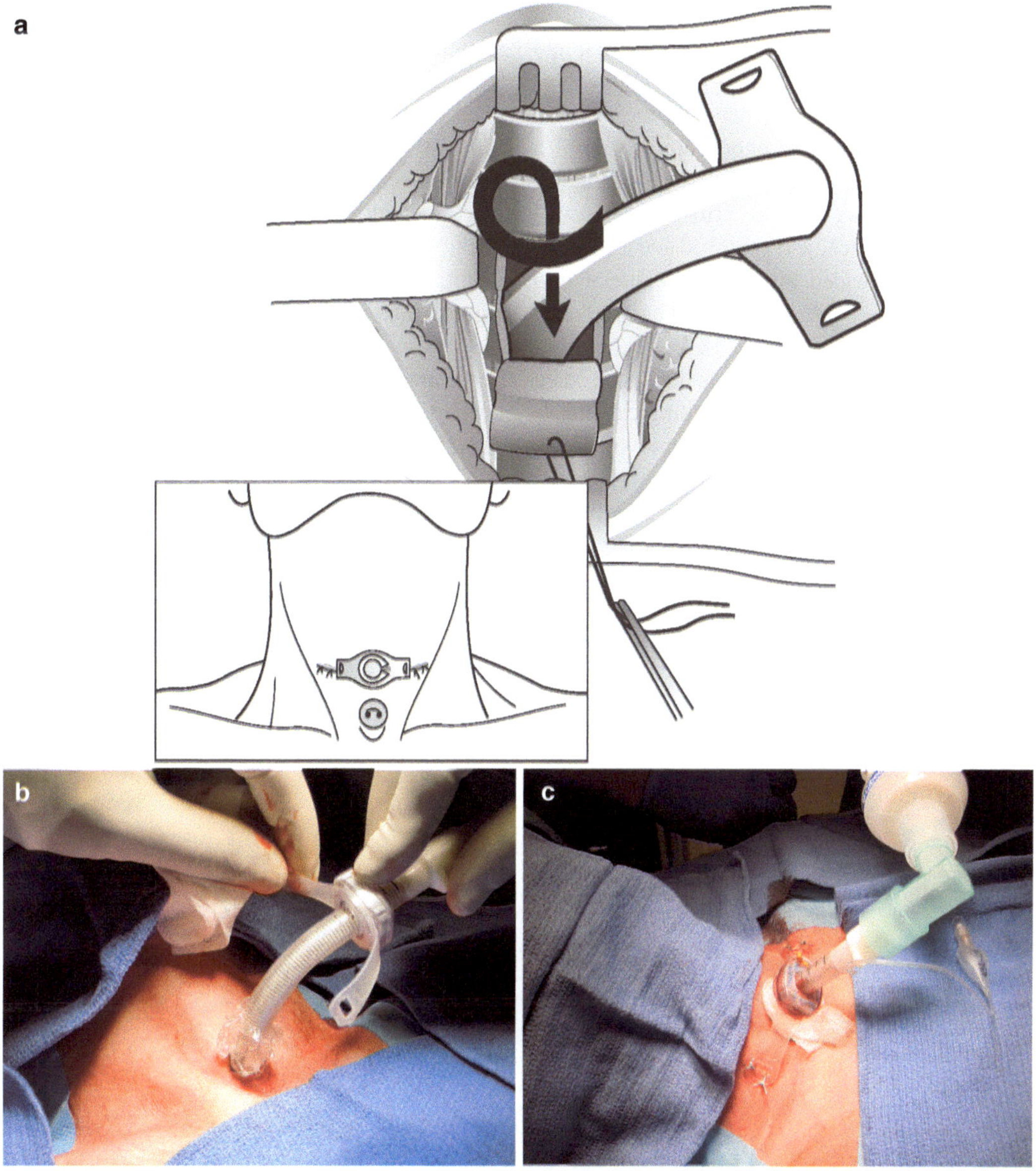

Fig. 18.3 Rotation movement for introduction of the tracheotomy tube (**a**) direction of tracheostomy tube rotation (**b**) Initial position of the tracheostomy tube before introduction (**c**) Tracheostomy tube in place and secure

The patient receives appropriate sedation and is then positioned in supine with the neck extended by using a shoulder roll. The patient's neck and upper chest are prepped and draped as for open neck tracheotomy (Fig. 18.1).

Fiber-optic tracheobronchoscopy is carried out through the endotracheal tube. If needed, 2 mL of 4% lidocaine is injected into the trachea through the bronchoscope, and pulmonary toilet is performed. The distal extremity of the fiber-scope is placed at the tip of the endotracheal tube, and the cuff is deflated.

Under fiber-optic vision, the endotracheal tube is slowly withdrawn from the trachea just below the level of the glottic opening and held securely to prevent accidental extubation. Laryngeal and tracheal landmarks are palpated. The light is visualized through the skin, and the tracheal rings are palpated to confirm the proper position of the tip of the tube.

A Teflon catheter introducer needle with a syringe attached is inserted between the first and second tracheal rings. Aspiration of air bubbles confirms entry into the trachea, and the location of the needle is verified endoscopically until a midline position is achieved inside of the trachea without puncturing the posterior tracheal wall (Fig. 18.4a). The needle is removed and a J-tipped guidewire is threaded through the catheter into the trachea. The catheter is removed and replaced by the introducer dilator (Fig. 18.4b). A horizontal skin incision of 1.0–1.5 cm is then performed at the level of the puncture; a guiding catheter is placed over the guidewire after removal of the introducer dilator.

A hydrophilically coated Ciaglia Blue Rhino dilator is now introduced over the guiding catheter into the trachea until the 38-F marking is identified endoscopically (Fig. 18.4d). A tracheotomy tube with the inner cannula replaced by a corresponding loading dilator from the Ciaglia set is introduced over the guiding catheter into the trachea (Fig. 18.4c). The correct intratracheal position of the tracheotomy tube is confirmed endoscopically, the guidewire and guiding catheter are removed, and the inner cannula is put back. The respirator is disconnected from the endotracheal tube and is connected to the tracheostomy tube. The latter is fixed and adjusted, and the cuff is inflated. Final endoscopy control is performed through the tracheostomy tube, and if needed, excess secretions and/or blood are aspirated to prevent airway obstruction.

Postoperative chest radiography should be performed to ensure the absence of pneumothorax and pneumomediastinum.

The tracheotomy tube is first changed 7 days postoperatively.

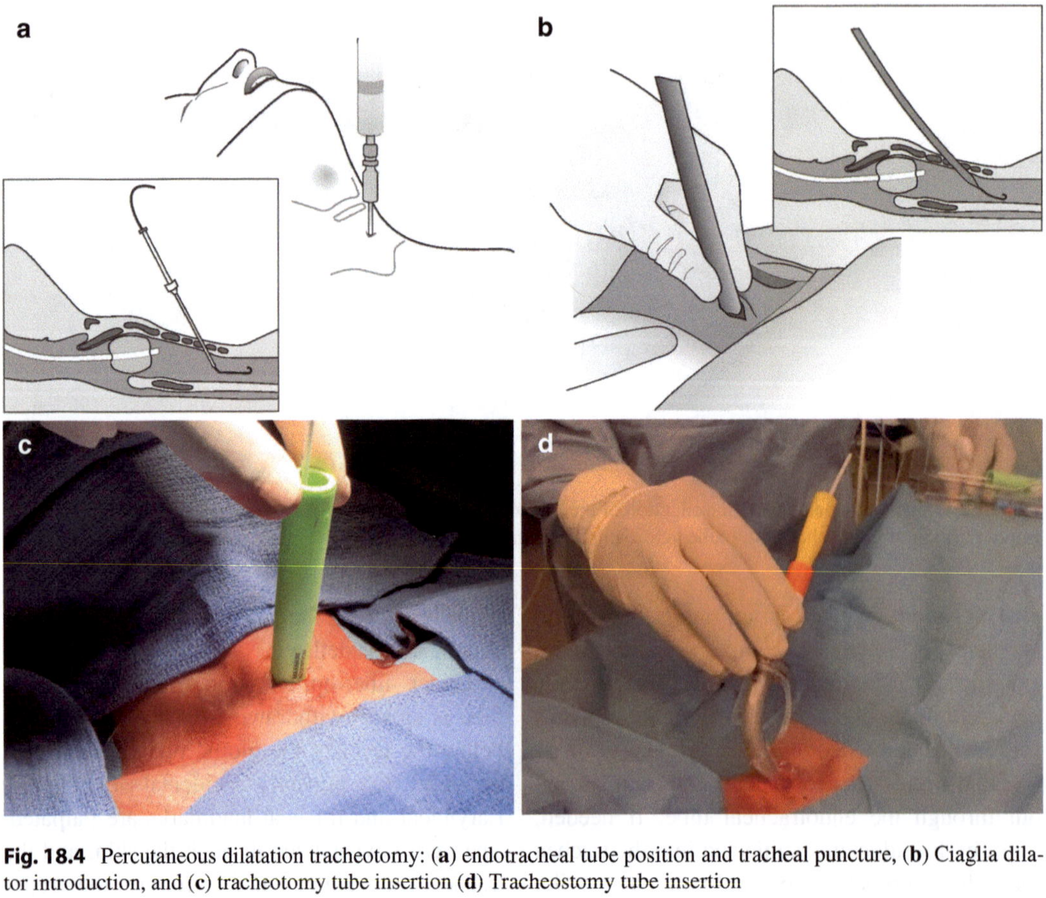

Fig. 18.4 Percutaneous dilatation tracheotomy: (**a**) endotracheal tube position and tracheal puncture, (**b**) Ciaglia dilator introduction, and (**c**) tracheotomy tube insertion (**d**) Tracheostomy tube insertion

18.4.3 Tracheotomy in the Pediatric Age Group

To prevent complications, preoperative planning is the first step to successful tracheotomy in a child. All patients should be examined and the airway secured before surgery. The surgical procedure is carried out in a manner similar to that in adults, in the operating room when possible.

More than in adults, care must be taken to avoid excessive dissection lateral to the trachea to prevent the possibility of recurrent nerve injury and dissection of air into the tissues. The thyroid isthmus is divided only if it cannot be retracted superiorly. The tracheal opening is a simple vertical incision made in the second and third tracheal rings. Nylon traction sutures are placed on either side of the incision line before the incision is performed and then after a second pair of traction sutures is placed along the lateral edge of the trachea (Fig. 18.5a). Those sutures will be helpful for the stoma opening and tracheostomy tube reinsertion (Fig. 18.5b). Excision of any anterior trachea wall during tracheotomy should be avoided in this age group.

Pediatric tracheostomy tubes generally have no cuff. The size of the tracheostomy tube is determined according to the age of the child with respect to the carina.

18.4.4 Bedside Open Tracheotomy

Intensive care unit patients are at higher risk for complications than other groups of patients due to frequent multisystem diseases. When tracheotomy is required for these patients, they are taken to the operating room for conventional tracheotomy. Operating room time is expensive, in high demand, and often in short supply. On the other hand, moving critically ill patients is associated with a number of risks (e.g., accidental extubation, changes in the vital signs).

Open tracheotomy can also be performed at the bedside in the intensive care unit setting [11]. In such a situation, surgeons must ensure that proper lighting, some assistance, and proper equipment are available. Patients with unfavorable anatomy (morbid obesity, short and fat neck, cervical mass lesions, enlarged thyroid gland) should proceed to the operating room for a standard tracheotomy under ideal circumstances.

The surgical technique is the same as describe above for conventional open neck tracheotomy. The advantages of performing a tracheotomy at the bedside is that operating room coasts are defrayed, the procedure is generally less expensive than a PDT, and the procedure can be performed as soon as the surgeons are available. As for main dis-

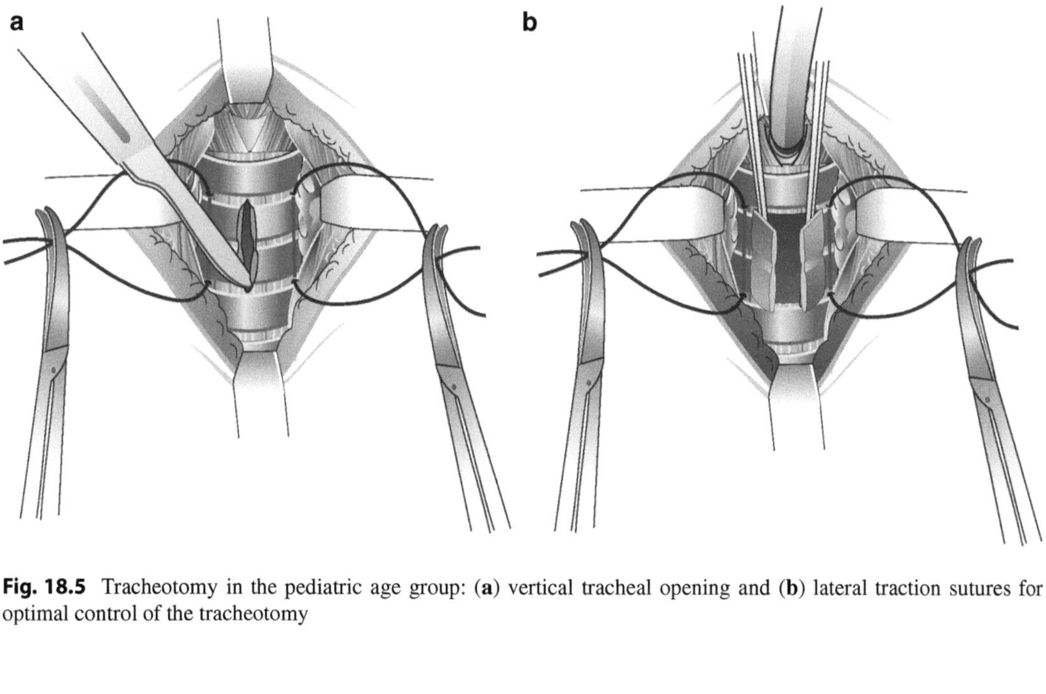

Fig. 18.5 Tracheotomy in the pediatric age group: (**a**) vertical tracheal opening and (**b**) lateral traction sutures for optimal control of the tracheotomy

advantages, the procedure is longer compare to PDT, it requires transporting electrocautery, instrument trays, and extra lighting from operating room to intensive care unit. Often there are no available trained operating room nurses and assistants.

18.4.5 Emergency Tracheotomy

18.4.5.1 Open Tracheotomy

It is widely accepted by head and neck surgeons that emergent tracheotomy is a procedure to be avoided. Nevertheless, in an acute airway emergency that cannot be handled by other options, tracheotomy should be considered.

Patients are positioned in supine with the neck extended using a shoulder roll. The patient's neck and upper chest are prepared and draped as for open neck tracheotomy. A median vertical incision of 3–4 cm is performed starting at the level of the cricoid and extended to the sternal notch. The incision is continued through the skin, platysma, and subcutaneous tissues. The strap muscles are divided with retractors, and the thyroid isthmus is pushed inferiorly (or superiorly) with the index finger. The trachea is palpated and incised at about the second or third tracheal ring. The endotracheal tube or tracheostomy tube is introduced inside the trachea; sometimes a tracheal dilator is helpful during the introduction and so must be prepared as a part of the equipment for emergent tracheotomy.

The tracheostomy is securely fixed. As soon as the patient's situation allows, the tracheotomy is carefully assessed to control hemostasis to determine the exact location of the tracheal incision and, if needed, to perform appropriate revisions.

18.4.5.2 Cricothyroidotomy

Cricothyroidotomy is a rapid technique to create an opening in the cricothyroid membrane followed by placement of a stenting tube. The procedure is a good alternative to emergent tracheotomy. Its main advantage is that the cricothyroid membrane is near the skin surface and much less dissection is necessary. The major disadvantage is possible damage to the subglottis area, often because the cricothyroidotomy tube is too large and/or is left in place for a long time.

The surgical technique is simple: the cricothyroid space is palpated, and a short, transverse incision is performed directly over the cricothyroid membrane. The scalpel is inserted into the cricothyroid membrane and twisted vertically to open it (Fig. 18.6a). An endotracheal tube is inserted and secured (Fig. 18.6b).

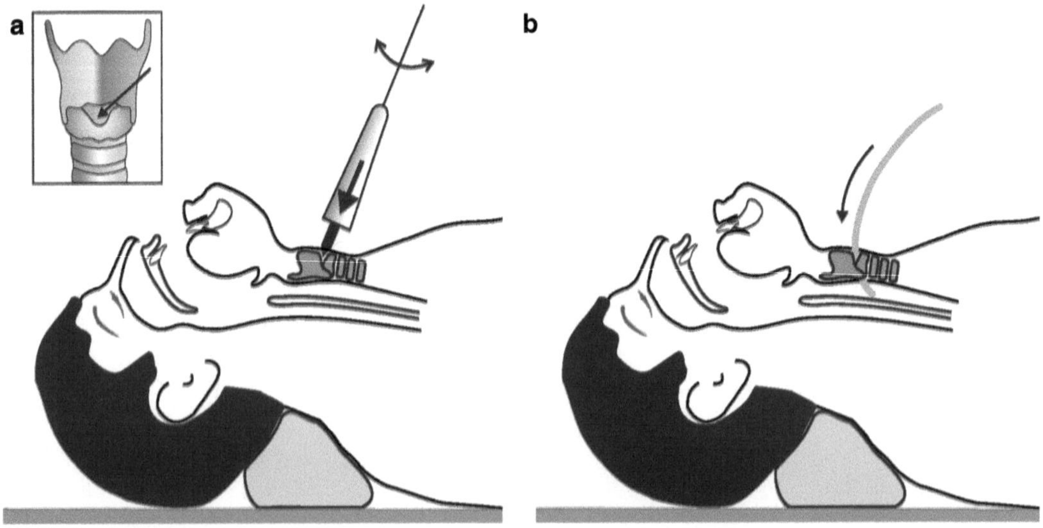

Fig. 18.6 Cricothyroidotomy: (**a**) cricothyroid membrane opening and (**b**) endotracheal tube insertion through the cricothyroidotomy

When the patient's condition has stabilized, if respiratory support through the surgical airway is needed for more than 2–4 days, the cricothyroidotomy should be converted to a conventional tracheotomy.

18.4.6 Mediastinal Tracheostomy (MT)

Mediastinal tracheostomy (MT) is a very rare and specific procedure with the final stoma located in the lower position in the middle of the chest. Its indications are as follows:

1. Extensive laryngotracheal resection where the residual trachea is too short to accommodate a cervical tracheostomy.
2. Radical surgery to cure or obtain long-term control of advanced or recurrent carcinoma of the lower neck necessitating relocation of the trachea to the anterior chest wall.

MT is a complex and risky surgical technique requiring close collaboration with the thoracic surgeon or personal experience in head neck and thoracic surgery.

18.4.6.1 The Procedure

Skin incision combining horizontal neck incision, as for open neck tracheostomy, or thyroidectomy with a midline upper sternal incision starts at the sternal notch and is carried down past the sterno-manubrium junction and onto the middle of the sternum (Fig. 18.7a).

Skin flaps are gently dissected on each side of the incision and the soft tissues in the midline are divided down to the bony sternum and manubrium. Sternum and manubrium are prepared for sternotomy by dividing the premanubrium and sternal musculature. A longitudinal sternal split is then performed for optimal visual access onto the anterior mediastinum. With caution, excision of the two halves of the manubrium as well as proximal portions of the first two ribs and medial clavicular heads is performed. A wide and safe access to the superior mediastinum is then created (Fig. 18.7b). All major vessels are visualized and easily accessible throughout the procedure.

To avoid devascularization, the distal trachea is mobilized only as much as necessary for connection to the chest. It is obliquely transected at the appropriate level, leaving a longer flap posteriorly (Fig. 18.7c). The distal tracheal portion is then intubated with a sterile (cuffed and curved) endotracheal tube that is passed under the drapes to the anesthetist (Fig. 18.8).

To secure the tracheal stoma and protect the great vessels, a reconstruction is done with a large pectoralis major musculocutaneous flap. A skin paddle is designed and preserved to fit onto the new mediastinal window, and the muscular part of the flap is large, enough to close the entire defect without tension and still allows a tracheostomy deep within the mediastinum (Fig. 18.9). A site for the proposed tracheal stoma is chosen somewhere in the middle of the flap. A circular defect is created by excision of the skin, fat, and muscle, avoiding the major vessels on the deep surface of the muscle. There is, in optimal condition, no need to displace the trachea inferior to the innominate artery because the flap will reach down to the trachea even if it is beneath that vessel (Fig. 18.8).

The pectoralis major musculocutaneous flap is our preferred closure material in this indication because its pedicle is safe and robust, and the musculature is large enough to adapt to any defect size with a lowest risk of necrosis. Finally, the donor site can be closed primarily without tension.

All of the interrupted sutures are first placed through the full thickness of the tracheal rim and then brought through the opening of the flap for an additional bite of the flap skin edges [12]. After all sutures are in place, the endotracheal tube is repositioned through the opening of the flap, and the flap is lowered with the sutures tied sequentially.

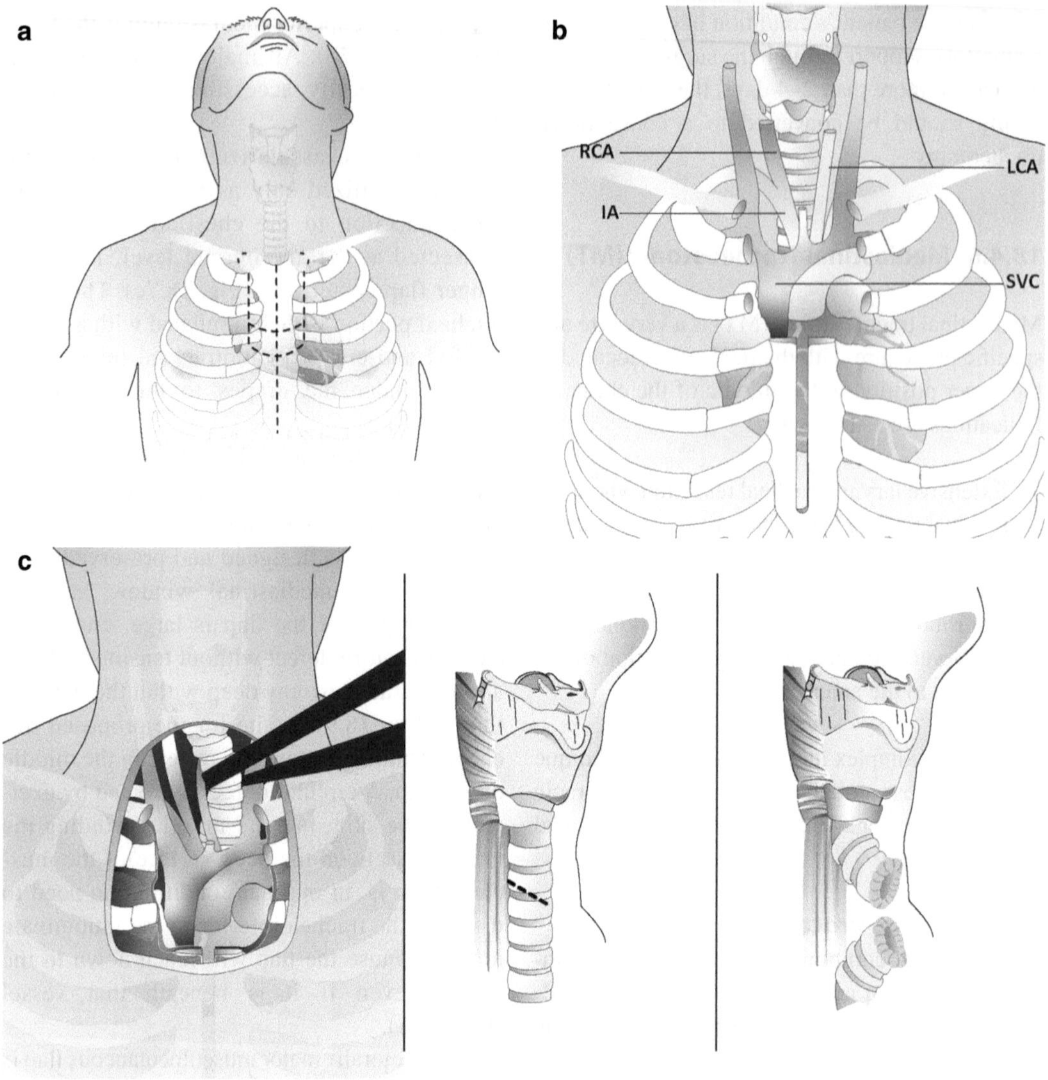

Fig. 18.7 Mediastinal tracheostomy: (**a**) surgical landmark, (**b**) intraoperative mediastinal exposure after sternal split and manubrium excision (*IA* the innominate artery, *RCA* right carotid artery, *LCA* left carotid artery, *SVC* superior vena cava), and (**c**) opening of the trachea

Precise apposition of the skin and the tracheal mucosa is imperative (Figs. 18.9 and 18.10). The tracheal stoma remains as the most superior structure in the mediastinum, and the great vessels and mediastinum are protected by a two-layer (skin and muscle) seal around the tracheal stoma.

18.4.6.2 Technical Comments

- En bloc removal of the manubrium and medial segments of the adjacent ribs and clavicles without a preliminary sternotomy is considered to be hazardous due to a failure to gain control of the great vessels. A longitudinal sternal split in standard fashion is recommended.

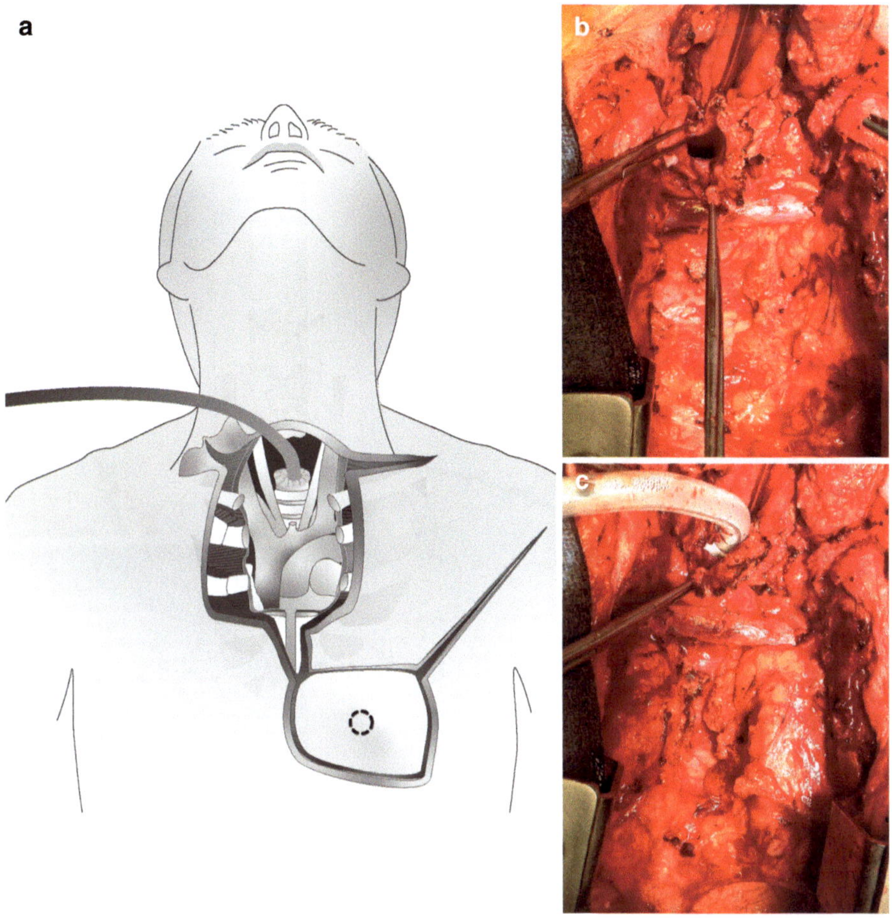

Fig. 18.8 Mediastinal tracheostomy—pectoralis major musculocutaneous flap for reconstruction of the anterior and superior portions of the chest. (**a**) Pectoralis major musculocutaneous flap dissection. (**b** and **c**) The final mediastinal tracheotomy site before the flap position

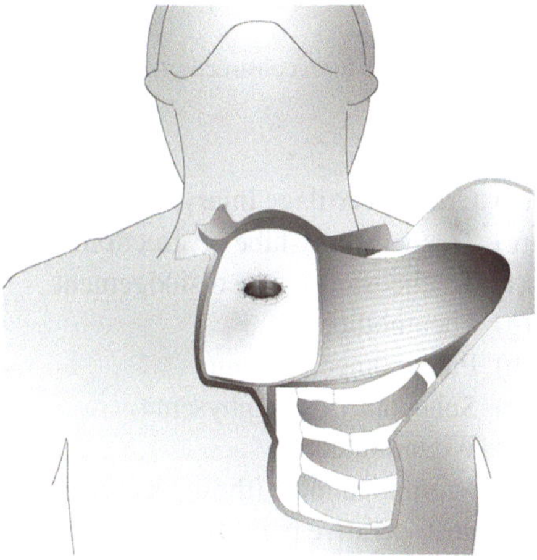

Fig. 18.9 Mediastinal tracheostomy—pectoralis major musculocutaneous flap for reconstruction with tracheostomy passing through the flap

- In case of hypertrophic thymus, a limited thymectomy allows for increased visualization of the innominate vessels.
- The patient ventilation to 100% oxygen saturation is a key security attitude before tracheal opening.
- After transection of the anterior half of the trachea, stay sutures are placed on each side at 9 and 3 o'clock positions. The tracheal transection is completed while pulling forward on the stay sutures and an over-the-field ringed endotracheal tube is placed into the distal trachea and the balloon reinflated.
- When the trachea is short, the innominate vessels are elevated, and the trachea is passed underneath using the stay sutures, allowing a more direct route to the anterior chest wall.

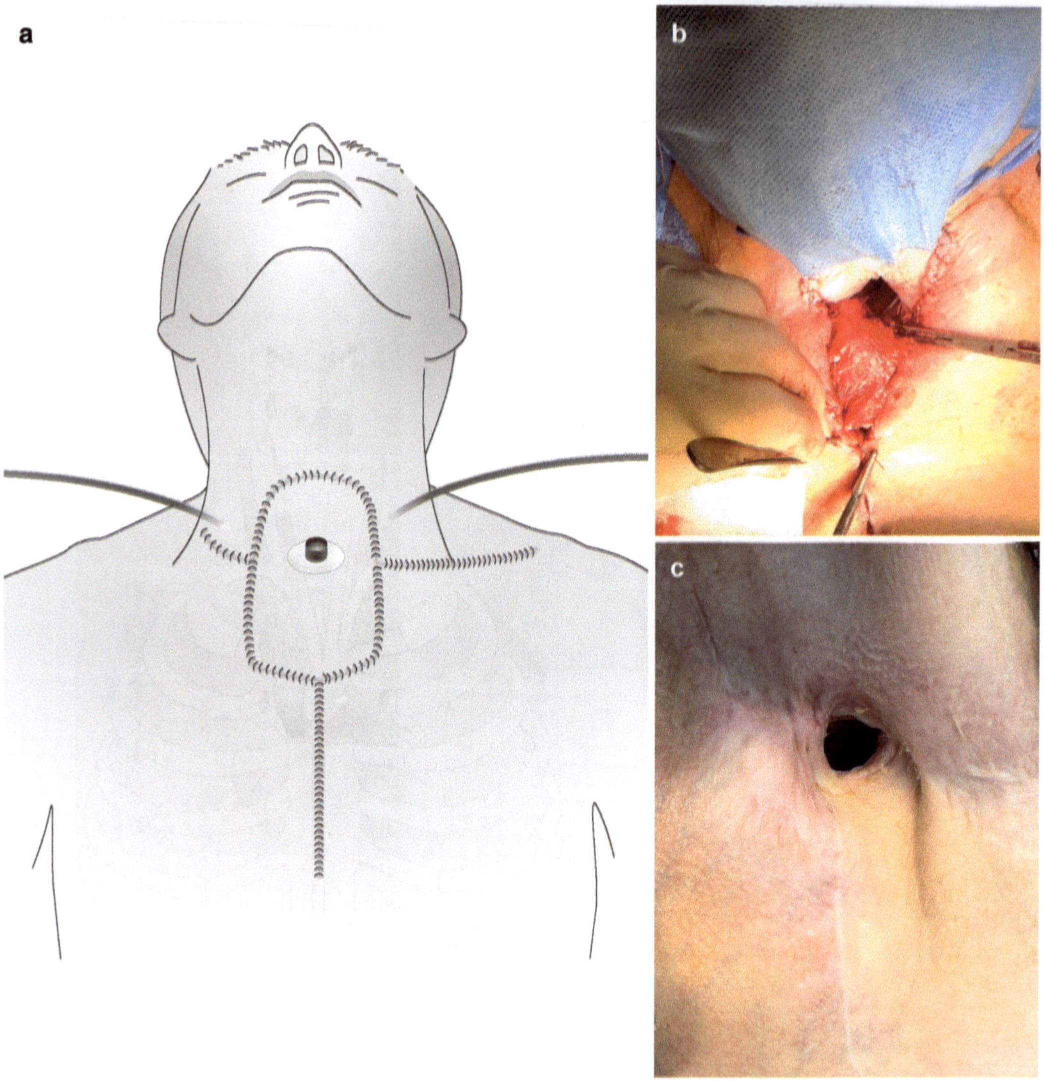

Fig. 18.10 Mediastinal tracheostomy—pectoralis major musculocutaneous flap for reconstruction: (**a**, **b**) final closure and (**c**) late healing aspect

18.5 Complications of Tracheotomy

As for any surgical procedure, complications of tracheotomy may occur even with the use of optimal surgical techniques. Those complications can be generally divided into two categories: early and late.

1. Early complications (those occurring intraoperatively and early in the postoperative period)
   (a) Hemorrhage
   (b) Tracheoesophageal perforation
   (c) Recurrent nerve injury
   (d) Cricoid cartilage injury
   (e) Tracheostomy tube obstruction
   (f) Tracheostomy tube dislodgement
   (g) Pneumothorax
   (h) Pneumomediastinum
   (i) Subcutaneous emphysema
   (j) Wound infection
2. Late complications (those occurring in the late postoperative period)
   (a) Infection
   (b) Hemorrhage
   (c) Granuloma
   (d) Aspiration

(e) Laryngotracheal stenosis
(f) Subglottic stenosis
(g) Tracheoesophageal fistula
(h) Tracheomalacia

The best way to prevent complications during tracheotomy and in tracheotomized patients is a good knowledge of the following:

- Potential complications of tracheotomy
- Variety of strategies available for airway management
- Various surgical techniques for tracheotomy and their application
- Proper cannula selection based on the patient's anatomy and pathology
- Appropriate postoperative care for each specific situation

As soon as the complication is recognized, it must be managed efficiently to achieve the expected positive outcome.

18.6 Pearls and Tips

18.6.1 Pearls

- Tracheotomy stands out as one of the most helpful therapies in the management of compromised airway. In decision making for tracheotomy, appropriate solutions must be taken for each specific case, in order to avoid complications and life-threatening situations.
- The key features in preventing complications are good knowledge of:
  - The potential complications of tracheotomy
  - The variety of strategies available for airway management
  - The different surgical techniques for tracheotomy and their applications

18.6.2 Practical Tips

- *Conventional or open neck tracheotomy*
  - Secure the airway first before performing the surgical procedure.
  - Be sure that efficient assistance and adequate equipment are available.
  - Dissecting in the midline to prevent:
    - Bleeding from the jugular vein, carotid artery, thyroid isthmus, or aberrant innominate arteries
    - Injury to recurrent laryngeal nerves
    - Pneumothorax or pneumomediastinum
- Secure the opening of the stoma, by suturing the anterior portion of a single tracheal ring to the inferior skin margin, and insert the tracheotomy tube into the trachea under direct vision to prevent false passage between the trachea and the sternum.
- Prevent tracheotomy tube displacement by:
  - Appropriate selection of the tube according to the patient's anatomy
  - Sewing the tracheotomy tube to the peristomal skin
  - Setting the low-pressure cuff pressure under 25 mmHg
- *Percutaneous dilatation tracheotomy (PDT)*
  - The principal contraindication to the PDT procedure is the inability to palpate the laryngeal landmarks.
  - Flexible bronchoscopy for endoscopic guidance is mandatory to:
    - Visualize the trachea
    - Confirm the proper position of the tip of the endotracheal tube
    - Transilluminate for palpation of anatomic landmarks and visualize needle placement through the anterior tracheal wall
    - Confirm safe tracheal dilation and proper tube placement
  - Have a standard tracheotomy tray available
  - The tracheotomy tube should be securely fixed to avoid accidental decannulation
  - Never perform unnecessary change of the tracheotomy tube during the first postoperative 3 days
  - If the tube replacement is inevitable, be prepared with:
    - Endotracheal tube for patient reintubation if needed
    - A good preoxygenation of the patient
    - Tracheotomy dilatation forceps
    - Fiberscope for tracheal assessment

- When long-term tracheotomy is planned, it is preferable to perform conventional tracheotomy.
- *Emergency tracheotomy*
  - Depending on the severity and primary cause of the airway impairment
    Other airway management options should be considered
  - All information related to the patient must be shared with the operating team and anesthesiologist prior to the procedure
- Avoid the following:
  Percutaneous dilatation tracheotomy
  A high tracheotomy through or near the cricoid cartilage
- Cricothyroidotomy should be converted to conventional tracheotomy
- *Tracheotomy in the pediatric age group*
  - The tracheal opening must have a simple vertical incision
  - Place nylon traction sutures on either side of the incision line before tracheal opening
  - Avoid any anterior trachea wall excision
  - The tracheostomy tube size is determined according to the child's age
- *Mediastinal tracheostomy (MT)*
  - En bloc removal of the manubrium and medial segments of the adjacent ribs and clavicles without a preliminary sternotomy is considered to be hazardous due to a failure to gain control of the great vessels. A longitudinal sternal split in standard fashion is recommended.
  - In case of hypertrophic thymus, a limited thymectomy allows for increased visualization of the innominate vessels.
  - Patient ventilation to 100% oxygen saturation is a key security attitude before tracheal opening.
  - After transection of the anterior half of the trachea, stay sutures are placed on each side at 9 and 3 o'clock positions. The tracheal transection is completed while pulling forward on the stay sutures and an over-the-field ringed endotracheal tube is placed into the distal trachea and the balloon reinflated.
  - When the trachea is short, the innominate vessels are elevated, and the trachea is passed underneath using the stay sutures, allowing a more direct route to the anterior chest wall.

References

1. Jackson C. High tracheotomy and other errors: the chief causes of chronic laryngeal stenosis. Surg Gynecol Obstet. 1923;32:392.
2. Jackson C, Jackson CL. The larynx and its diseases. Philadelphia, PA: W.B. Saunders; 1937.
3. Practice guidelines for management of the difficult airway. A report by the American Society of Anaesthesiologists task force on management of the difficult airways. Anaesthesiology. 1993;78:597–602.
4. Benjamin B. Prolonged intubation injuries of the larynx: endoscopic diagnosis, classification, and treatment. Ann Otol Rhinol Laryngol. 1993;102(Suppl. 160):1–15.
5. Stauffer JL, Oison DE, Petty TL. Complications and consequences of endotracheal intubation and tracheostomy. Am J Med. 1981;70:65–75.
6. Ciaglia P, Firsching R, Syniec C. Elective percutaneous dilatation tracheostomy. A new simple bedside procedure: preliminary report. Chest. 1985;87:715–9.
7. Holdgaard HO, Pedersen J, Jensen RH, Outzen KE, Midtgaard T, Johansen LV, Mailer J, Paaske PB. Percutaneous dilatational tracheostomy versus conventional surgical tracheostomy. Acta Anaesthesiol Scand. 1998;42:545–50.
8. Ciaglia P, Graniero KD. Percutaneous dilatation tracheostomy. Results and long-term follow-up. Chest. 1992;101:464–7.
9. Griggs WM, Myburgh JA, Worthley LI. A prospective comparison of a percutaneous tracheostomy technique with standard surgical tracheostomy. Intensive Care Med. 1991;17:261–3.
10. Hazard P, Jones C, Benitone J. Comparative clinical trial of standard operative tracheostomy with percutaneous tracheostomy. Crit Care Med. 1991;19:1018–24.
11. Wang SJ, Sercaz JA, Blackwell KE, et al. Open bedside tracheotomy in intensive care unit. Laryngoscope. 1999;109:891–3.
12. Grant C, Marshall MB. Mediastinal tracheostomy with vessel transposition and minimally invasive transhiatal esophagectomy. Oper Tech Thor Cardiovasc Surg. 2016;21(1):47–64.

Neurolaryngology

19

Orlando Guntinas-Lichius, Andreas H. Müller,
and Christian Sittel

Key points

- Neurolaryngology: important definitions and applications are presented.
- Laryngeal electromyography: when and how—described in detail.
- Beyond electromyography: more electrodiagnostic tests are described.
- Neurolaryngological disorders: systematic overview is given.
- Laryngeal dystonia: clinical classification is introduced.
- Botulinum toxin: a practical guide is presented.
- Neurostimulation: proven technique with new innovative diagnostic role for laryngeal pacing.

O. Guntinas-Lichius (✉)
Department of Otorhinolaryngology, Jena University Hospital, Friedrich-Schiller-University Jena, Jena, Germany
e-mail: orlando.guntinas@med.uni-jena.de

A. H. Müller
Klinik für HNO-Heilkunde/Plastische Operationen, SRH Wald-Klinikum Gera, Gera, Germany
e-mail: andreas.mueller@wkg.srh.de

C. Sittel
Department of Otolaryngology, Klinikum der Landeshauptstadt Stuttgart gKAöR, Stuttgart, Germany
e-mail: c.sittel@klinikum-stuttgart.de

19.1 Introduction

Although the term neurolaryngology has come into use more than 30 years now, this important field of laryngology still is often neglected. In the last years, neurolaryngology has developed rapidly in response to the advances in diagnosis and treatment of laryngeal disorders (for a detailed description of the various possibilities of neurolaryngology, see a recent textbook exclusively on neurolaryngology: [1]). Diagnostic procedures include many technical innovations that have expanded the armamentarium for treatment of benign and malignant diseases. Nevertheless, neurolaryngology is a challenge for many otolaryngologists. Laryngeal neurophysiology depends on neuromuscular forces acting on the framework of the cartilage, soft tissue and vocal cords. Understanding its pathophysiology requires knowledge of specific neurological processes that affect voice and airway regulation. It is essential that the practitioner becomes familiar with the basics of electromyography. Laryngeal electromyography (LEMG) is the most important tool for diagnostics in neurolaryngology. Therefore, this chapter is opened by practical guidelines on how to use this essential method. The technical approach is explained in detail. The clinical significance and the limits of the method are pinpointed. Thereafter, a review is given on the most frequent neurolaryngological disorders. The most important diseases in daily

M. Remacle, H. E. Eckel (eds.), *Textbook of Surgery of Larynx and Trachea*,
https://doi.org/10.1007/978-3-031-09621-1_19

practice, vocal cord paralysis and laryngeal dystonia, are described in detail. Many practitioners are not aware that many central nervous disorders may cause laryngeal diseases. Hence, explaining the relationship between central nervous system diseases and laryngeal pathology is of great importance. Finally, the important role of botulinum toxin therapy in neurolaryngeal disorders is revealed through practical guidelines on how to use this medicament in neurolaryngology.

19.2 Electromyography

19.2.1 Definition

Laryngeal electromyography (LEMG) comprises a set of electrophysiological procedures for the diagnosis, prognosis and treatment of laryngeal movement disorders including laryngeal dystonias, vocal fold paralysis and other neurolaryngological disorders. It is performed by otolaryngologists, often in collaboration with a neurologist. LEMG requires special skills and equipment as well as considerable experience, although no formal education exists so far for the laryngeal electromyographer. LEMG may provide useful information that cannot be obtained by other techniques, but it is still not considered a routine examination available at every ENT department in Europe. Although LEMG has been the subject of much investigation over the past decades for the management of various laryngological disorders, until today there is much variability in the opinions on and use of LEMG among otolaryngologists for the management of unilateral vocal fold immobility [2, 3]. Trained neurolaryngologists show a high inter-rater agreement interpreting LEMG results [4].

19.2.2 Technique

Electromyography evaluates the integrity of the motor system by recording action potentials generated in the muscle fibres. Several consensus statements or clinical guidelines are now available, for instance, the European Laryngological Society (ELS), American Association of Neuromuscular & Electrodiagnostic Medicine (AANEM) or the American Academy of Otolaryngology Head and Neck Surgery Neurolaryngology Subcommittee/Neurolaryngology Study Group [5–7]. These guidelines give detailed recommendations on technical prerequisites and the examination procedures.

Principally all five major laryngeal muscles (thyroarytenoid muscle [TA], lateral cricoarytenoid muscle [LCA], posterior cricoarytenoid muscle [PCA], interarytenoid muscle, cricothyroid muscle [CT]) lend themselves for electrophysiological examination, with the TA being investigated most frequently. However, more and more studies are performed including other important extrinsic and intrinsic laryngeal muscles, first of all the PCA and CT. These muscles may be approached in the awake patient either transcutaneously or transorally. For the transcutaneous approach, bipolar concentric needle electrodes are passed through the cricothyroid membrane, and then the tip of the needle is angled to the affected side laterally and superiorly at 30°–45°. If the patient coughs, which indicates penetration of the airway space, the needle is withdrawn and repositioned. Increase of LEMG activity while the patient is phonating validates correct electrode position within the TA. If there is no muscle activity detectable at all, electrode displacement cannot be discriminated from complete vocal fold paralysis using the transcutaneous technique.

For transoral LEMG, bipolar hooked-wire electrodes are available. The hooks at the end of these thin flexible wires act as barbs, keeping the electrode in place once positioned in the muscle. Electrodes are positioned using a special device for application, which is inserted into the endolarynx under endoscopic guidance with the needle tip being secured in the applicator. Surface anaesthesia of the oropharynx and endolarynx prior to the procedure is mandatory. When the applicator is positioned correctly above the medio-dorsal aspect of the vocal fold, the tip of the needle is pushed into the thyroarytenoid muscle. Due to the hooks at the distal end of the wire, the electrode remains in position when the applicator is withdrawn. While this technique allows better control over electrode position, it is more time-consuming, significantly more expensive and technically more difficult. LEMG recordings are made visible on a monitor and made audible through a loudspeaker.

Interestingly, not much is known yet about the prevalence of abnormal LEMG findings in healthy asymptomatic adults across a large age spectrum. Recently, it has been confirmed that abnormal qualitative and quantitative LEMG findings were uncommon and minor in severity in our group of asymptomatic healthy adults. The likelihood of abnormal LEMG results in asymptomatic adults was reported to be 2.2% for qualitative findings, 9.3% for synkinesis and 5.4% for turns/s [8].

19.2.3 Other Techniques

Spontaneous needle LEMG provides useful information regarding the innervation status of a muscle, but cannot yield quantitative data for several reasons. Sampled recordings from a single site in a muscle may not reflect the overall status of innervation of the muscle. Recordings from a single site may be influenced by many variables, like size and shape of electrodes, slight changes in electrode position relative to each motor unit within a muscle or variation in voluntary effort between trials and between participants.

In theory, these shortcomings can be overcome by employing nerve stimulation instead of voluntary effort to evoke a muscular response. In so doing, consistent responses in repeated trials would be warranted and maximal stimulation could ensure that all motor units composing the muscle would be activated and potentially contribute to the recorded response. This should give a far more representative picture of the innervation status of a large portion of the muscle during the initial phase of degeneration or the subsequent phase of reinnervation, allowing for a more accurate diagnosis and prognosis. Recent animal investigations could show the potential value of the technique [9]. There have been attempts to establish transcutaneously evoked LEMG as a routine tool in humans [10–12]; however, these techniques are lacking reliability and reproducibility. Applying a sufficient electrical stimulus to the recurrent laryngeal nerve in a way acceptable for patients is still an unsolved problem. Invasive direct stimulation is not an option for diagnostic use for obvious reasons. Transcutaneous stimulation requires considerably high voltage to elicit a response from the deeply hidden recurrent laryngeal or vagal nerve, making the procedure inaccurate and uncomfortable for the patient. Magnetic stimulation is not sufficiently focalized to activate a target nerve with certainty.

Besides these technical considerations, an alleged superiority of evoked LEMG over spontaneous LEMG is far from self-evident. Both techniques are well comparable to facial nerve electroneurography (evoked) and needle electromyography of facial muscles (spontaneous). Among the abundance of investigations over the last decades, yielding often confusing results, there are strong arguments casting some shadow on the reliability and accuracy of evoked electromyography techniques in the facial nerve [13, 14].

19.2.4 New Techniques and Tools

Needle LEMG is the standard LEMG technique. The needle records electrical potentials named motor unit action potentials (MUPs) generated by muscle fibres close to the needle. The use of single-fibre electromyography (SFEMG) has not yet been established as part of clinical routine. Single-fibre LEMG allows recording of potentials from single muscle fibres [15]. Transcutaneous SF-ELMG using bipolar microelectrodes with a diameter of 25 μm with repeated insertions is well tolerated and is able to analyse the muscle fibre density in the TA. Thereby, it can be used to study abnormalities of neuromuscular transition and the MUP architecture. This can be helpful in diagnosing a myopathy, for instance, in a case of dysphonia due to myasthenia gravis, or to detect a motor neuron disease like amyotrophic lateral sclerosis in the TA [15]. Limitations of needle LEMG include patient discomfort and limited duration of recording. The potential of surface LEMG (sLEMG) is not much investigated yet. High-density sEMG may be used to identify differences in anterior neck muscle activity between rest, low- and high-pitch phonation. This might allow to include also these muscles into the analysis of laryngeal muscle activity in the future [16].

Verification of the correct needle position for LEMG recording is crucial for the validity of the results. For this reason, laryngeal ultrasound and, more recently, ultrasound-guided needle tracking have been introduced to place EMG needles [17, 18].

LEMG is primarily a qualitative examination. There are first approaches to establish quantitative norms for motor unit recruitment in healthy controls and in patients with unilateral vocal fold paralysis. Interference pattern analysis in the TA and LCA in healthy adults and patients with unilateral VFP seems to indicate that motor unit recruitment is different between controls and patients with unilateral VFP [19].

19.2.5 Electrostimulation to Select Cases for Laryngeal Pacing

The future introduction of selective laryngeal stimulation systems (laryngeal pacing) will create new indications for LEMG [20]. Laryngeal pacing in case of bilateral VFP will only work if the intramuscular neurostimulation of the PCA evokes a selective abductor movement without co-stimulating the adductor muscles. Therefore, before indicating a laryngeal pacing system, screening with electrical stimulation of the terminal abductor fibre in the PCA has to be performed to identify suitable patients. Continuous electric needle stimulation with 1.5 mA at 3 Hz can be used to localize a so-called hot spot in the PCA that if electrically stimulated induces vocal fold abduction [21].

19.3 Clinical Significance

19.3.1 Diagnosis

When reduced or absent abductor or adductor movement of the true vocal fold is observed on laryngeal examination, a diagnosis of laryngeal paresis is suspected, and EMG becomes an important diagnostic tool, especially if performed within 6 months of onset of the voice problem. Normal electrical activity patterns on LEMG suggests arytenoid fixation [22], whereas abnormal electrical activity, including patterns of denervation or reinnervation, suggests unilateral vocal fold paresis/paralysis [23].

Abnormal activity can include the presence of fibrillation potentials, insertional fibrillations (insertional activity), complex repetitive discharges, sharp positive waves and nascent and polyphasic motor unit potentials. Specifically, fibrillation potentials are defined as low-amplitude, short-duration units, and insertional activity is defined as mechanical discharge associated with repeated needle movement within a muscle. Polyphasic units are large-amplitude units with five or more baseline crossings with increased duration compared with normal units, whereas nascent units are defined as low-amplitude units with an increased number of baseline crossings and do not meet the amplitude or duration criteria of polyphasic units. Abnormal activity can also be manifested as decrements in the number of normal motor unit potentials and a reduction in recruitment during volitional activity. Recruitment is defined as activation of motor units with increasing strength of voluntary muscle contraction and reflects the number of motor unit potentials identifiable during increasing activation during voicing tasks in the TA or sniffing in the PCA.

Interpretation of electrophysiological findings is based on the following criteria: LEMG allows for distinction between normal silent resting potential, voluntary motor unit potential, spontaneous fibrillation potential and polyphasic reinnervation potential. The absence of any electrical activity either on electrode insertion or on attempted voluntary motion is called electrical silence. Normal voluntary action potentials are diphasic or triphasic and are extremely variable in amplitude (Figs. 19.1 and 19.2). Spontaneous fibrillation activity is defined as involuntary potential generated by a single muscle fibre, indicating axonal degeneration (Fig. 19.3). However, this symptom of degeneration does not appear earlier than 10–14 days after injury. Polyphasic motor units have four or more phases and are heralding nerve regeneration (Fig. 19.4).

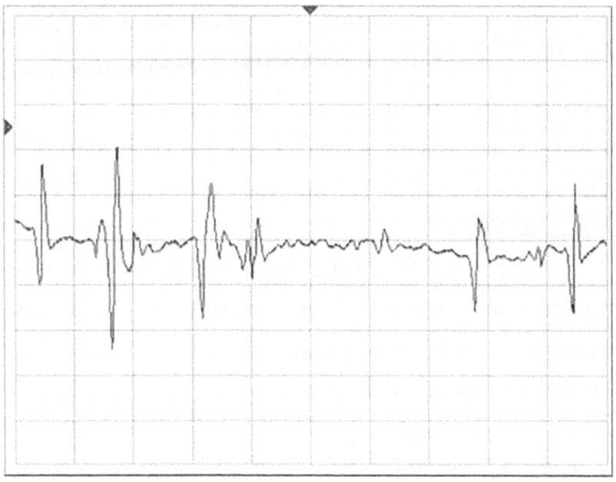

Fig. 19.1 Extremely rarefied firing pattern on phonation, but no spontaneous activity at rest: neurapraxia

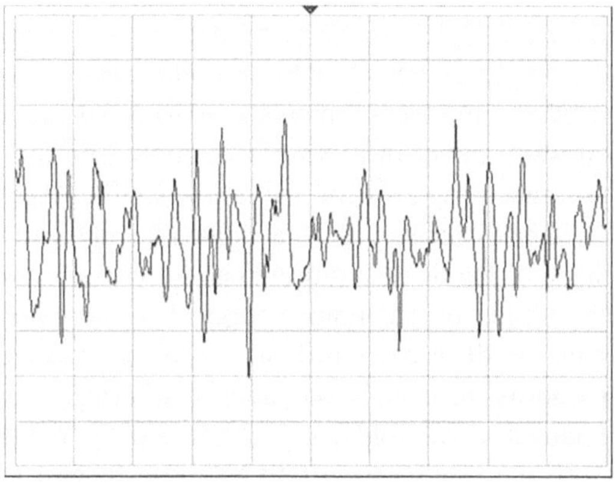

Fig. 19.2 Slightly reduced recruitment on phonation, no spontaneous activity at rest: neurapraxia

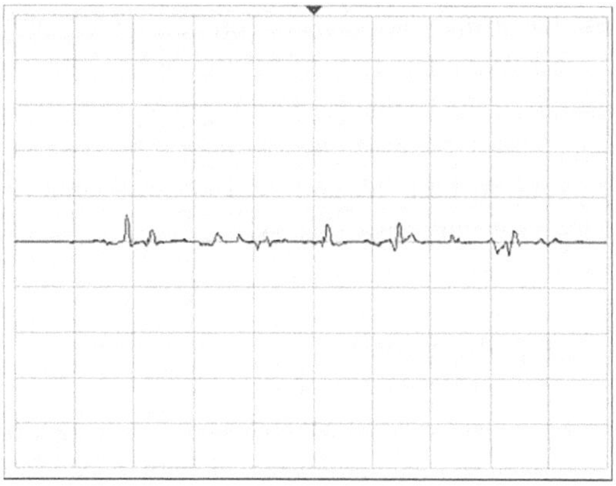

Fig. 19.3 Spontaneous fibrillation activity at rest, minimal recruitment on voluntary action: axonotmesis

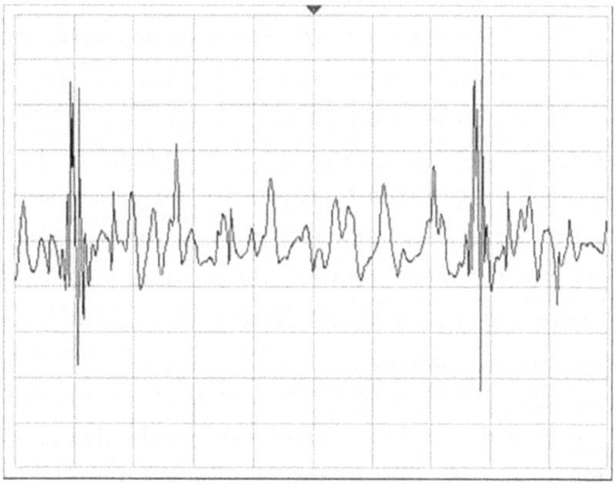

Fig. 19.4 Polyphasic, prolonged action potentials with giant amplitudes: reinnervation 4 months after nerve injury

For clinical routine use, it is convenient to classify electrophysiological findings according to Seddon [24] into neurapraxia, axonotmesis or neurotmesis. For neurapraxia the diagnostic criteria in LEMG are detection of a rarefied recruitment pattern or single action potentials on voluntary action without fibrillation activity and without spontaneous positive sharp waves. Axonotmesis is suspected when spontaneous activity, indicating neural degeneration, can be detected. Usually this is the case not earlier than 10–14 days after onset of paralysis. There is an inherent statement on prognosis in this classification [25], since a patient with neurapraxia is most likely to recover completely within 8–12 weeks, while a patient with axonotmesis is thought to have only a poor chance of recovery to a functional level. If reinnervation occurs following axonotmesis, usually it is associated with sequelae like synkinesis due to neuronal misdirection [26–28]. The presence of electrical synkinesis seems to decrease the likelihood of motor recovery, but only few data are available [7, 29]. The result is simultaneous activation of adducting and abducting intrinsic laryngeal muscles defined by Roger L. Crumley as laryngeal synkinesis [30]. For the same situation in facial nerve disorder, the term "autoparalytic syndrome" has been coined [31]. Neurotmesis, representing complete destruction of the whole nerve structure over its full diameter, apparently cannot be expected to recover at all. Finally, one should be aware that Crumley's synkinesis classification is helpful in describing and understanding synkinesis but it does not always correlate predictably with LEMG data [32]. If LEMG only addresses the TA, it can be that laryngeal synkinesis is overseen. The PCA might be the more reliable target muscle. At best, TA and PCA are evaluated for laryngeal synkinesis [33, 34].

19.3.2 Prognosis

The clinical use of LEMG has been advocated for the diagnosis and prognostication of vocal fold palsy for over two decades [10, 28, 35–37]. Surprisingly, until today there are only very few reports on the usefulness of this technique in terms of reliability and prognostic accuracy. Min et al. [38] reported a prognostic accuracy of impressive 89% in patients with unilateral vocal fold palsy. This study is seriously flawed for at least two reasons: first, the study population comprised 14 individuals only. Second, criteria for prognostication were defined very generously: A positive prognosis for laryngeal recovery was assumed when motor unit waveform morphology was normal and significant persistent overall electromyography activity as well as no electrical silence during voluntary tasks could be found. Obviously, this combination of favourable findings should be considered more an indication of a very discrete lesion than an actual prognosis. Another study investigating 18 patients [39] was not truly focused on the prognostic accuracy of LEMG. The authors of this study concluded cautiously that LEMG may be of prognostic value. Newer data showed that LEMG can be used to predict recurrent nerve recovery, but timing is important and LEMG results earlier than 3 months may overestimate a negative prognosis [40].

The Pittsburgh working group around Rosen and Munin see for quantitative LEMG and turns analysis the potential of a near 100% positive prediction of vocal fold movement return [41]. However, as in the aforementioned studies, the concern of a too small number of cases (4 out of 23 had a positive prognosis) also applies here. Only when this can be confirmed in larger multicentre studies will the predictive power of the LEMG improve in this respect. The group published new quantitative LEMG data recently showing that long-term VFP is infrequently associated with absent motor unit recruitment, indicating at least some degree of preserved innervation and/or reinnervation in most of these patients [42].

Another study suggests that detection of neural degeneration in LEMG allows for the prediction of poor functional outcome with high reliability in an early phase of the disease process [43]: LEMG had been used in 98 patients on 111 paralyzed vocal folds. Thirty-nine patients had been diagnosed with neurapraxia, while 72 laryngeal palsies had been characterized as axonotmesis. Neurotmesis was found in no case. Based on these data, a positive predictive value of 94% for the event "defective recovery," defined as absence of completely free vocal fold mobility, was calculated. For the event "complete recovery," prognosis was accurate in 12.8% of cases only. The quite accurate prognosis of the unfavourable event "defective recovery" at a comparatively early stage of the disease process can be valuable for the timing of a definitive surgical intervention, most of all in cases of bilateral recurrent nerve paralysis. In a study on patients suffering from bilateral vocal fold palsy conducted by Eckel [44], the routine use of LEMG was helpful to decide on posterior cordectomy (for widening of the glottic chink) at a comparatively early stage. Consequently, tracheotomy was required in 21% of the study population only. On the other hand, the absence of degeneration signs may not lead to the assumption that complete recovery is to be expected automatically. Based on data available today it seems safe to say that in patients suffering from vocal fold palsy of the lower motoneuron type, the detection of well-defined signs of neural degeneration in LEMG allows for the prediction of poor functional outcome with high reliability in an early phase of the disease process. In the presence of signs of neural degeneration detected by LEMG, the decision for definitive surgical interventions like thyroplasty or vocal fold augmentation in unilateral or partial cordectomy in bilateral vocal fold paralysis can be made safely at an earlier stage of the disease process. Thus, LEMG can be helpful to significantly shorten the process of voice rehabilitation. However, the absence of degenerative alterations in LEMG is not necessarily indicating recovery to a normal or near-normal functional level. Hypothetically, these findings may reflect secondary fibrosis of the cricoarytenoid joint following prolonged vocal fold immobility of primarily neurogenic aetiology. On the other hand, histological examinations in patients with vocal fold paralysis many years after onset have not confirmed a fibrosis [45].

In summary, LEMG is a valuable tool in the workup of patients suffering from vocal fold palsy. Since prognostic accuracy for favourable results is comparatively low LEMG cannot replace clinical monitoring over at least 6 months or until complete recovery has been reached.

19.3.3 LEMG-Guided Injections

LEMG guidance of botulinum toxin injections into the TA in patients with adductor spasmodic dysphonia is an establish method since many years. To be effective in the much rarer cases of paradoxical motion of the vocal fold (postneuroleptic laryngeal dyskinesia, laryngeal dyspnoea), the LEMG guidance of the botulinum toxin injection into the TA, PCA, or CA is essential [46]. Now, it has been shown that LEMG guidance could also be used for vocal fold injection laryngoplasties. In a prospective study of 60 patients observed for at least 6 months, an office-based awake LEMG-guided hyaluronic acid vocal fold injection for unilateral VFP was performed without using any anaesthesia [47]. A 26-G monopolar injectable needle electrode was used. The procedure led to satisfactory phonatory results and the majority needed only a single injection during the 6-month follow-up period.

19.3.4 Laryngeal Pacing

The editors invited us to include a section on laryngeal pacing in this neurolaryngology chapter. Like selective reinnervation as the most complex form of nerve reconstruction described in Chap. 20, the principle of laryngeal pacing aims to regain vocal fold abduction in bilateral recurrent laryngeal nerve paralysis (BRLNP). The first acute and chronic attempts of laryngeal neurostimulation, mostly in dogs, were carried out in the 1970s and 1980s of the last century [48, 49]. These early studies showed that artificially induced paralysis could be treated with neurostimulation even for over a longer period of time [50]. More denervated muscles require a high current intake, which leads to side effects of the neurostimulation and allows their long-term use only when reinnervation occurs [51]. Zealear et al. achieved the first application of laryngeal pacing in human in 1995 [52]. A standard pain therapy implant (Itrel II, Medtronic, USA) with spinal cord electrodes was applied as no implant adapted to the requirements of laryngeal neurostimulation was available. This pioneering work showed proof of principle but could not be continued with the available technology due to technical problems such as electrode corrosion.

Over the last decade, the concept of laryngeal pacing has been revived in Europe [20]. Based on preclinical research, it has been shown to be beneficial to avoid direct electrical muscle stimulation towards neuromuscular stimulation, which requires 10–100 times lower current intensity. In this way, while at the same time further developing the surgical method towards a minimally invasive procedure of injecting the stimulation electrode into the target muscle, the risk of tissue damage due to surgery and current intake can be significantly minimized [53]. The therapeutic approach of neuromuscular stimulation requires an at least partial, misdirected or dysfunctional, e.g. synkinetic reinnervation of the PCA in eligible patients, which in our experience is present in the vast majority of patients with persistent BRLNP after 4–6 months [54].

Research teams in Gera, Würzburg and Innsbruck in cooperation with the Austrian company MED-EL have advanced the development of a clinically applicable laryngeal neurostimulation solution in BRLNP, known by its project title "Laryngeal Pacemaker (LP) System" (Figs. 19.5 and 19.6), to the point where a feasibility study on nine symptomatic BRLNP

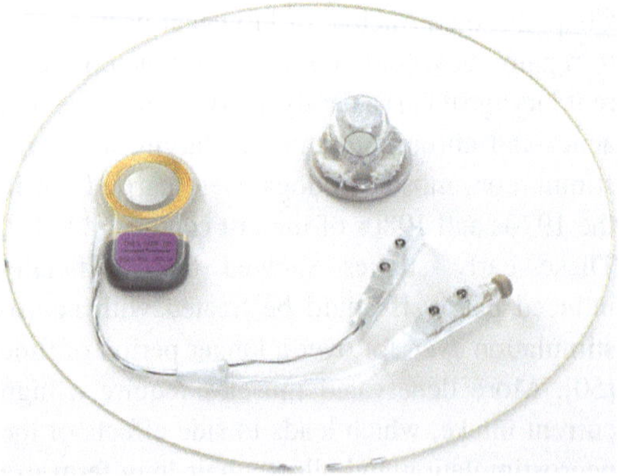

Fig. 19.5 Laryngeal pacemaker system (LP system) consisting of the LP processor (control unit with battery and a coil for inductive transmission), the LP implant (internal electronics in a titanium housing, the receiver inductive coil and connectors) and the active LP electrode for minimal invasive placement in the PCA muscle

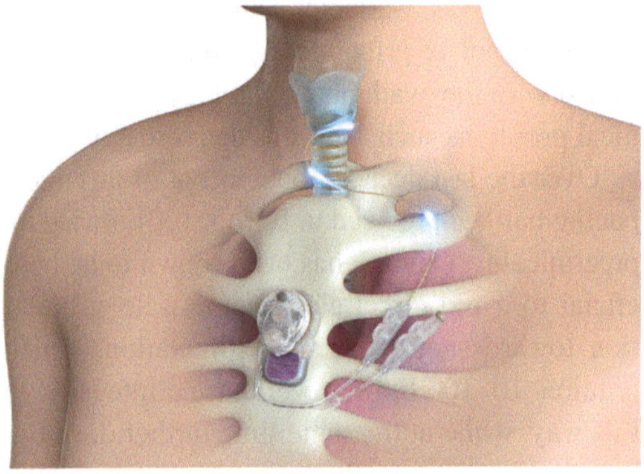

Fig. 19.6 Laryngeal pacing system in situ. One of the two possible LP electrodes is inserted into the left PCA muscle; LP implant is placed in a subcutaneous pocket in front of the sternum; LP processor is kept in place over the LP implant by magnetic pull

patients could be initiated [21]. This study demonstrated the safety of the surgical procedure and the implanted LP system. For safety reasons, in this first study of its kind, vocal fold abduction was only stimulated on one side. This new dynamic therapy resulted in an immediate improvement of the respiratory function, physical activity and quality of life to the extent of the established laser surgical glottis enlargement without compromising the patient's voice as it is the case with the standard therapy [55, 56].

Laryngeal pacing is still in the stadium of clinical trials. At present, a major research focus is on the development of even more durable electrodes and the synchronization of vocal fold abduction stimulation with the patient's breathing cycle. In the future, the suitability of this laryngeal neurostimulation principle for the stimulation of vocal fold adduction in unilateral paralysis with high voice demands will be investigated.

Due to its neurophysiological requirements, the laryngeal pacemaker is not suitable for all patients with permanent BRLNP. This future therapeutic option should be considered if no pronounced atrophy of the internal laryngeal muscles is expected and the LEMG shows any kind of pathological reinnervation. Furthermore, the cricoarytenoid joint should be mobile and intraoperative electrical test stimulation in the context of a routine panendoscopy should have shown visible vocal fold abduction. Candidates who meet these requirements and do not require immediate intervention may be included in future laryngeal pacemaker studies.

19.4 Neurolaryngological Disorders

Laryngeal physiology depends on dynamic neuromuscular forces acting on a basic framework of cartilage and specialized soft tissues, the vocal folds. Specific neurological processes may affect voice, swallowing or airway regulation. Neuromuscular impairment continues to be a dominant topic in the study of neurolaryngological disorders [57]. Table 19.1 gives an overview about the most common neurolaryngological disorders and their characteristics. Perhaps the most common neuromuscular impairment of the larynx is the vocal cord paralysis. In the majority of cases, this paralysis is caused by a lesion of recurrent or vagal nerve. In these cases, the typical signs of a lower motor neuron disease are found in the larynx: peripheral neuropathy, isolated flaccid paralysis, decreased agility, muscle atrophy but normal coordination of the laryngeal muscles.

Table 19.1 Characteristics of the most common neurolaryngological disorders

Disease	Laryngoscopic features	Electrodiagnostic features
Lower motor neuron vocal cord paralysis (recurrent or vagal nerve lesion)	Vocal fold immobility with reduced tension	Spontaneous activity in thyroarytenoid muscle starts 10–14 days after lesion for about 2–3 months. Reduced or no voluntary activity. In vagal nerve lesions: In addition features of superior laryngeal nerve lesion.
Vocal cord synkinesis	Vocal fold immobility with near normal tension	Polyphasic reinnervation potentials in thyroarytenoid muscle during phonation. No spontaneous activity.
Isolated lesion of the superior laryngeal nerve	Normal vocal fold movement, but bowing during phonation	Spontaneous activity in cricothyroid muscle starts 10–14 days after lesion for about 2–3 months. Reduced or no voluntary activity.
Upper motor neuron vocal cord paralysis	Vocal fold immobility	No spontaneous activity.
Adductor spasmodic dysphonia	Symmetrical glottic compression during phonation. Normal vocal fold mobility	Abnormal bursts of activity in the thyroarytenoid muscle during phonation. Some patients show enlarged or polyphasic potentials.
Abductor spasmodic dysphonia	Incomplete glottic opening during phonation. Normal vocal fold mobility	Abnormal bursts of activity in the posterior cricoarytenoid muscle during phonation. Some patients show enlarged or polyphasic potentials.
Essential voice tremor	No action-induced spasms. Rhythmic, periodic glottic spasms	Spontaneous activity in thyroarytenoid and/or lateral cricoarytenoid muscle. Tremor bursts in thyroarytenoid and/or lateral cricoarytenoid muscle.
Parkinson's disease	Vocal fold bowing during phonation. Delayed movements	Decreased voluntary activity in thyroarytenoid muscle. Single-fibre MEG may show increased variability of the inter-spike interval of single motor units.
Stroke	Different degrees of vocal fold immobility	Signs of lower and/or upper motor neuron vocal cord paralysis.

In the seldom case of the disorder of the neuromuscular junction, fatigability and fluctuating abnormalities are common signs of laryngeal movements. However, vocal cord paralysis or other vocal manifestations are frequently primary modes of presentation for neurological disease. The typical signs of an upper motor neuron disease could be found as in other central nervous diseases, of course, also in the larynx: spastic paralysis of muscles groups and decreased agility are symptoms of cerebral diseases. Disorders affecting the basal ganglia present a resting tremor, dystonia or rigidity of the laryngeal muscles. In cerebellar diseases, intention tremor and dysdiadokokinesis are seen during laryngoscopy. Myoclonus and choreatic movement in the larynx are unspecific signs of an upper motor neuron disease. The most important movement disorders affecting the larynx are presented. The major components of the neurolaryngological examination of all patients are a detailed history, evaluation of the voice, stroboscopy and electromyography of the larynx [58].

19.4.1 Vocal Cord Paralysis of the Lower Motor Neuron Type: Recurrent and Vagal Nerve Lesions

The potential causes of a vocal cord paralysis are manifold [59, 60]. Surgical trauma has long been recognized as the most common cause of unilateral and bilateral vocal cord paralysis. Thyroid surgery still is the major risk factor. Carotid endarterectomy or neck dissection is seen as another underlying cause. Other causes are neoplasms in the neck and mediastinum and traumatic and idiopathic conditions. Various neurologic disorders, including poliomyelitis, Guillain-Barre syndrome and multiple sclerosis, could lead to direct damage of the vagal nerve [61]. Lower motor neuron lesions could also be affected by diseases in the brainstem leading to direct damage of the motor neurons in the vagal nuclei. Typical examples are Wallenberg syndrome, bulbar polio, amyotrophic lateral sclerosis, syringomyelia, multiple sclerosis and encephalitis. When the reasons for unilateral and bilateral vocal cord paralysis are compared, there are no significant differences [59].

The major symptom indicating a lower motor neuron lesion of the recurrent or vagal nerve is a unilateral or bilateral vocal cord paralysis. The lesions are caused by injuries directly affecting the recurrent nerve or the vagal nerve. Localized lesions of the myelin sheath (neurapraxia) will regenerate without functional deficits. Axonal lesions (axonotmesis) or combined damage of axons and myelin sheaths (neurotmesis) induces the Wallerian degeneration of the distal nerve stump to the peripheral target muscle. Axon sprouting starts at the first Ranvier node proximal to the lesion site of the axon. In consequence, the regeneration time depends mainly on the site of the lesion. The first clinical signs of nerve regeneration after peripheral damage of the vagal nerve or the recurrent nerve are typically seen not before 3 months after the trauma. The axonal sprouting and the anatomical variety of Galen's anastomosis between recurrent und superior laryngeal nerve branches lead to misdirected reinnervation of the laryngeal muscles. Therefore, a retrieval of the muscle tone, for instance, in the vocal cords, is observed on some other months. But movement do not come back due to simultaneous movements of antagonistic laryngeal muscles caused by the misdirected reinnervation. Severe lesions within the brainstem and some forms of peripheral toxic lesions lead to a degeneration of the related motor neurons at the nuclear level in the brainstem. The reduction of the driving motor neuron pool results in a decreased muscle strength and limited movements. The therapeutic possibilities for transient and permanent vocal cord paralysis are described in Chaps. 4, 7, 12 and 21.

Information of the integrity of the recurrent nerve can be obtained by laryngeal EMG of the thyroarytenoid muscle [23, 62]. The superior laryngeal nerve is analysed by EMG of the cricothyroid muscle. The posterior cricoarytenoid muscle has to be analysed in individual cases, as this muscle can be preferentially damaged, especially in iatrogenic genesis [63]. Reduced insertion potentials indicate muscle wasting and atrophy. A loss of nerve function demonstrates a decrease or absence in frequency of firing in muscle action potential. If some fibres remain intact, the amplitude of the muscle action potential is normal. Axonal damage leads to Wallerian degeneration of the distal nerve fibres. In consequence, fibrillation potentials are seen about 10–14 days later that can persist for some weeks. The detection of neural degeneration by laryngeal EMG allows the prediction of poor functional outcome [43]. Polyphasic reinnervation potentials indicate an old lesion with definitive misdirected reinnervation. The laryngeal synkinesis is distinguishable from physiological antagonistic TA activity by LEMG [64]. Depending on the site of the lesion, polyphasic reinnervation potentials are not seen before 2–3 months after axonal lesion. Increase of polyphasic reinnervation potentials is typically seen up to 6–12 months after lesion.

LEMG is also an important tool to monitor the reinnervation and to determine the outcome after surgical reconstruction of the recurrent nerve by direct nerve anastomosis, cross-anastomosis with the ansa cervicalis or use of a nerve-muscle pedicle. Through LEMG, reinnervation and maturation of the voluntary action potential are typically seen over the first 1½ years [64].

If the site of the lesion is lying proximal to the recurrent or vagal nerve, i.e. the lesion is affecting the first motor neuron or complex cortical structures, spontaneous activity will be absent during LEMG recording despite clinically evident vocal cord paralysis. If the vocal cord immobility was caused by a cricoarytenoid joint fixation or by interarytenoid scar formation, the laryngeal EMG shows completely normal activity of the laryngeal muscles.

19.4.2 Vocal Cord Paralysis of the Upper Motor Neuron Type

In infants and children, bilateral vocal cord paralysis s most often congenital [65]. About half of the congenital cases are associated with other anomalies. Even many acquired cases are secondary to underlying congenital anomalies, particularly associated to meningomyeloceles, midbrain or brainstem dysgenesis, Arnold-Chiari malformation and hydrocephalus [61]. Patients with comorbid factors, especially severe neurological abnormalities, often require tracheotomy to manage the children's airway [66]. After laryngomalacia, vocal cord paralysis is the second most common cause of stridor in children. Onset of paralysis in children may not be immediate. Age of onset or its diagnosis may range from birth to 6–8 weeks of age. Unilateral paralysis is more common than bilateral paralysis. Recovery can be expected in only approximately 20–30% of the congenital cases. Other seldom reasons for vocal cord paralysis in children are birth trauma, surgical trauma or congenital infections. The acquired cases show a higher recovery rate up to 50–60% [67]. If an older child does not present other symptoms, the vocal cord dysfunction could be confused with exercise-induced asthma, because the disease tends to be triggered by exercise [68]. Management of vocal cord paralysis in children should be directed towards the establishment of a secure airway and treatment of the underlying disease. Whereas tracheotomy is normally not required in unilateral paralysis, the rate of tracheotomies is high for bilateral disease. The different techniques for airway management are described in detail in Chap. 7. The same is valid for upper motor type vocal cord paralysis in adults. The different diseases are described below in more detail. As explained above, LEMG is an important tool to differentiate an upper motor neuron-type lesion from a lower motor neuron lesion as the latter shows typical LEMG alterations.

19.4.3 Laryngeal Dystonia: Adductor and Abductor Spasmodic Dysphonia

Laryngeal dystonia, or spasmodic dysphonia, is a form of dystonia, a chronic neurologic disorder of central motor processing characterized by task-specific action-induced muscle spasms. Dystonia may be generalized or limited to one functional group of muscles. Laryngeal dystonia is usually focal. A strained and strangled quality to the voice with effortful voicing and voice fatigue is typical. Approximately four of five affected individuals have adductor spasmodic dysphonia, which causes inappropriate glottal closure and, consequently, strangled breaks in connected speech. A subentity is termed adductor breathing dystonia (or breathing dystonia) if the patients develop adductor spasms during breathing, producing paradoxical vocal cord motion [69]. LEMG is demonstrating burst of glottic compression in the TA during phonation at unpredictable intervals. Abductor spasmodic dysphonia, in contrast, causes inappropriate glottal opening in one of five patients that produces hypophonia and breathy breaks. Hence, the LEMG shows bursts of muscle activity in the PCA. Because of compensatory manoeuvres or mixed dystonic features, voice patterns encountered clinically may not always be typical or easy to discern [57]. LEMG is important for treatment planning [70]. It shows the major muscular source of the dystonia. Only LEMG detects the rare cases, where the lateral cricoarytenoid muscle, the interarytenoid muscle or the CA is the major focus of the dystonia [71, 72]. Spasms typically do not occur during singing. The most important forms of differential diagnosis that can cause voice breaks are essential voice tremor, muscle tension dysphonia and a functional disorder. As spasmodic dystonia is a disorder of the central nervous system rather than of the larynx, interventions at the end organ do not offer a definitive cure. Botulinum toxin (BTX) therapy is the treatment of first choice. After BTX injection, the typical laryngeal nerve evoked potentials are weakened or even disappear in the injected muscles [73]. There is report of a 90%

overall improvement after BTX therapy for adductor spasmodic dysphonia. Nevertheless, the results of BT for abductor spasmodic dysphonia have been less successful. Only 20–40% of patients improve after BTX treatment [74]. The BTX application technique is described in detail below. Voice therapy may be useful in addition to BTX therapy. In patients with contraindications for BTX, or if BTX fails, surgical treatment should be discussed with the patient: Lateralization thyroplasty is an easy but very mechanical approach to help patients with refractory adductor spasmodic dysphonia [75]. Long-term results are often disappointing. Alternatively, a selective section of the distal branches of the recurrent nerve leading to the thyroarytenoid and sometimes the lateral cricoarytenoid muscle, with immediate reinnervation using a non-laryngeal nerve, generally the sternohyoid branch of the ansa cervicalis, is proposed. In this way, they sought to prevent reestablishment of abnormal central motor control by connecting the laryngeal musculature to a nerve supply not affected by the disorder [57, 76]. In patients with refractory abductor spasmodic dysphonia, a bilateral medialization thyroplasty could be helpful [77, 78]. Recently, it was shown that a unilateral posterior cricothyroid myoplasty, i.e. a unilateral desertion of the muscle, could improve the effect of the medialization thyroplasty [79].

19.4.4 Stroke

Stroke is a highly prevalent disease that has significant potential to adversely affect the voice and swallowing. Expressive aphasia due to stroke in the frontal cortex (Broca area) and receptive aphasia due to stroke in the temporal cortex (Wernicke area) are well-known clinical signs of a stroke. But the corticobulbar tract and cranial nerves themselves could also be affected directly by the cerebrovascular accident. An isolated vocal paralysis is an uncommon manifestation of stroke. Most often, multiple cranial nerves are involved. Clinically, voice quality and speech production is affected. Of course, perhaps more common than these direct effects of the stroke on voice production are the multitude of indirect effects on the voice from the general neurological characteristics of stroke patients. Hoarseness and chronic laryngitis can go along with a vocal cord paralysis. The chronic laryngitis is the result of laryngopharyngeal reflux and/or prolonged nasogastric feeding. Therefore, the otolaryngological management of the stroke patient in most stroke patients is orientated by the urgent problems of protection of the airway, control of the respiration and last phonation. The need for prolonged ventilation should be recognized early. The patient may be converted appropriately to tracheotomy. Downsizing the tracheotomy tube when appropriate facilitates speech therapy for voice and communication.

19.4.5 Essential Voice Tremor

Essential tremor is an idiopathic disorder of involuntary movement. But the classification of voice tremor is controversial. The tremor has also been characterized as a separate subtype of laryngeal dystonia [80]. The tremor is believed to originate from a disordered cerebellar control of vocal cord length and tension. Patients generally will report slowly worsening symptoms over months to years. Voicing worsens with anxiety or stress and is especially troublesome under more demanding acoustic conditions, such as speaking against background noise. Laryngeal tremor is often not restricted to the intrinsic muscles of the larynx. The other muscles of the phonatory apparatus are often and variably involved. Tremor in the larynx characteristically is seen as bilateral, symmetrical, involuntary, rhythmic, periodic spasms of the laryngeal, supraglottic or pharyngeal muscles. The reliable periodicity of the spasms, similar to the ticking of a clock, is the key feature of a tremor. The tremor frequency has been documented between 3 and 6 Hz. Tremors can occur at rest or with intention, which in the larynx is seen during sustained phonation. Action-induced spasms as typical for spasmodic dysphonia are not seen. The larynx may be normal at rest. Myoclonus is differentiated from tremor in that the spasms seen during myoclonic activity are jerky and arrhythmic. LEMG is showing spontaneous activity at rest. Typically, LEMG exhibits tremor sign in all laryngeal muscles during phonation. The thyroarytenoid and the lateral crico-arytenoid muscle are most often involved [80]. Propranolol (a β-adrenergic blocker) and primidone (a neuroleptic) are mainstays of treatment. BTX treatment will not improve the essential tremor in any case. Generally, BTX only decreases the amplitude of the tremor. The result is a severe breathiness of the patient, but many patients are content with BTX treatment [58]. BTX injections are most effective if the dominating tremor muscles (shown by LEMG) are treated [80].

19.4.6 Parkinson's Disease

The majority of patients with Parkinson's disease complain of voice problems characterized by vocal tremor, decreased volume and hoarseness [81]. Vocal fold bowing is a common finding during laryngoscopy. The source of this bowing has not been fully elucidated but some patients show a dyskinesia of the intrinsic laryngeal muscles that might be the result of defective basal ganglia control. Often vocal cord closure is slowed or delayed. Tremor associated with Parkinson's disease will be evident at rest. Most importantly, the speech, although often breathy and of low intensity, does not demonstrate the characteristics in a rhythmic fashion like in patients with essential tremor. Rather, the characteristic hypophonia is relatively constant. The extrinsic laryngeal muscles (strap muscles) could also be affected. The result is a significant slowing of vertical laryngeal excursion during deglutition [82]. Additionally, poor breath support could be present as a result of chest wall rigidity. The disease is often exacerbated by articulatory difficulties and sometimes by cognitive and articulatory problems. Other findings are pooled hypopharyngeal secretions, decreased sensation and diminished cough reflex and aspiration. Laryngeal EMG demonstrates decreased firing rate and in older male Parkinson's patients increased variability of the inter-spike interval of single motor units [83]. Efficient therapy of the dysphonia in patients with Parkinson's disease is difficult. Vocal fold augmentation is often not effective in severe cases [84]. Standard Parkinson's disease treatment with L-dopa, deep brain stimulation or neurosurgical interventions have shown only limited results in dysphonia. Only behavioural therapy has shown sustained beneficial effect on the voice and speech functions of patients with Parkinson's disease [85].

19.4.7 Other Central Nervous System Diseases

Patients with amyotrophic lateral sclerosis could display several laryngological symptoms. Adductor-type spasmodic dysphonia has been described as a feature of the central motor neuron degeneration [86]. Multiple system atrophy encompasses three neurodegenerative syndromes (striatonigral degeneration, olivopontocerebellar atrophy and Shy-Drager syndrome). Besides the typical symptoms of autonomic, cerebellar and pyramidal dysfunction, stridor occurs in multiple system atrophy at different stages. Severe respiratory insufficiency sometimes requires tracheotomy. The cause of stridor in multiple system atrophy is a dystonia of the vocal cords. In most cases, laryngoscopy reveals normal bilateral movements of the vocal cords. LEMG during quiet breathing is showing persistent tonic activity in both abductor and adductor vocal cord muscles [87]. Botulinum toxin injection into the adductor muscles could be offered to the patients to reduce the tonic LEMG activity.

19.5 Botulinum Toxin Treatment in the Larynx

Botulinum toxin (BTX) has been used successfully in otolaryngology since over twenty years for the treatment of a still increasing number of diseases [88]. BTX blocks the release of acetylcholine from nerve terminals. Thereby, BTX causes flaccid paralysis of the muscle starting about 48 h after injection. Its effect is transient and non-destructive. Recovery starts after about 28 days. Recovery is complete after about 90 days, a length of time that correlates with the clinically observed duration of effect. Two serotypes of BTX, serotype A and B, are available for clinical use. Three compounds of BTX type A (Botox®, Dysport® and Xeomin®) and type B compound (NeuroBloc®)

Table 19.2 Comparison of four licensed botulinum toxin formulations[a]

	Botox®	Dysport®	Xeomin®	NeuroBloc®[b]
Company	Allergan, Inc., Irvine, CA 92612, USA	Ipsen Biopharm Ltd., UK-Wrexham LL13 9UF, United Kingdom	Merz Pharmaceuticals GmbH, 60048 Frankfurt, Germany	Solstice Neuroscience Inc., South San Francisco, CA 94080, USA
Neurotoxin type	A	A	A	B
Mouse units per vial	100	500	100	2500/5000/10,000
2–8 °C	2–8 °C or <–5 °C	2–8 °C	2–8 °C	2–8 °C
Durability	36 months	24 months	36 months	24 months
Solvent	0.9% saline	0.9% saline	0.9% saline	Pre-manufactured solution
Labelled therapeutic indications	Blepharospasm and strabismus in adults, cervical dystonia in adults, hemifacial spasm in adults, dynamic equinus foot deformity due to spasticity in children >2 years of age, focal hand spasticity of adults after stroke, chronic migraine, overactive bladder, leakage of urine (incontinence) due to overactive bladder caused by a neurologic condition, spasticity, severe underarm sweating (axillary hyperhidrosis) and wrinkles[c]	Blepharospasm in adults, cervical dystonia in adults, hemifacial spasm in adults, dynamic equinus foot deformity due to spasticity in children older than 2 years of age, axillar hyperhidrosis, moderate to severe glabellar lines associated with procerus and corrugator muscle activity in adult patients <65 years of age	Chronic sialorrhoea, upper limb spasticity, cervical dystonia, blepharospasm with onabotulinumtoxin A (Botox®) prior treatment, temporary improvement in the appearance of moderate to severe glabellar lines with corrugator and/or procerus muscle activity	Cervical dystonia in adults

[a]There are now other preparations from China (Prosigne®, Lantox®) and Korea (Neuronox®) not licenced in Europe or in the United States
[b]Named MyoBloc® in USA
[c]The commercial name for treatment of wrinkles is Botox Cosmetic® in the USA and Vistabel® in Switzerland

are commercially available (Table 19.2; a comparison of currently available neurotoxins is given in: [89]). To date, BTX treatment in the larynx still is of "off-label" use. But due to the large experience with the drug in the larynx, the AAO-HNS considers the laryngeal treatment safe and effective. The dosage is measured in mouse units (MU). A unit is defined by the median lethal intraperitoneal dose (LD50) in Swiss Webster mice. It is important to be aware that a unit of Botox® is not equivalent to a unit of Dysport®, Xeomin® or NeuroBloc®. Botox®, Dysport® and Xeomin® require rehydration with normal saline prior to usage. NeuroBloc® is directly delivered by the company as a solution. We recommend using the BTX type A formulation for first-line treatment. BTX type B should be reserved for patients with secondary treatment failure of BTX type A [90]. The concentration may be varied depending on the physician's need, the involved muscles and the prior experience in the individual patient. Treating the small muscles of the larynx, a concentration of 5 MU/0.1 mL Botox®, 20 MU/0.1 mL Dysport®, 5 MU/0.1 mL Xeomin® or 500 MU/0.1 mL NeuroBloc® is most useful. But a higher concentration may be useful in some patients, if side effects are seen as the result of diffusion of the toxin from the target muscle to adjacent muscles.

In general, multiple small-volume injections may contain the effect better with less risk of side effects. The clinical effect is dose-related, but the range of effective doses among patients with the same disease may vary extremely [91]. The physician will find the correct dose only through experience with each individual case. BTX should not be used in pregnancy, because teratogenicity and safety have not been established yet. It has been used for a long time in children suggesting that efficacy and side effects are the same as in adult patients. In general, BTX should be used very careful in patients with neuromuscular disease, due to the higher risk of systemic muscle weakness. Aminoglycoside antibiotics interfere with BTX and may potential its effect. Therefore, BTX therapy should be avoided during such an antibiotic treatment. The amount of toxin used in the larynx is very low. Hence, an overdose has never been described. Second, the risk of acquired resistance to BTX by patient's production of antibodies against the drug is very low. To our knowledge, immunoresistance in patients with laryngeal treatment have not been described yet. The development of immunoresistance seems to occur more often in patients treated with large doses and short treatment intervals. We recommend starting treatment with the smallest effective dose, to avoid booster injections and to maximize inter-treatment intervals.

If possible, we prefer endoscopic-assisted transoral injections of BTX into the intrinsic laryngeal muscles. If the transcutaneous way is used, LEMG is recommended to prove precisely the placing of BTX. Either the target muscle is identified by the EMG needle first as described above and the BTX syringe needle is injected parallel to the EMG needle to deliver the toxin into the muscle, or, alternatively, the BTX is delivered directly through a Teflon-coated needle attached to the electromyography machine. If both ways, the transoral and the transcutaneous way, fail to reach an effect, we recommend re-evaluating the indication. If the indication remains proven true, we recommend repeating the transoral injection in general anaesthesia. Guidelines for BTX dosages and injections sites for most the frequent indications in patients with neurolaryngological disorders are presented in Table 19.3.

Table 19.3 Recommended botulinum toxin injection technique for neurolaryngological disorders[a]

Disorder	Injection site and doses	Comment
Adductor spasmodic dysphonia	Thyroarytenoid muscle bilateral: 1–5 MU Botox®/1–5 MU Xeomin®/10–40 MU Dysport® per side	In some patients unilateral treatment is sufficient.
Abductor spasmodic dysphonia	Posterior cricoarytenoid muscle unilateral or bilateral: 2.5–5 MU Botox®/2.5–5 MU Xeomin®/20–40 MU Dysport® per side	The risk of dyspnoea is less after unilateral treatment of the most active side (as shown by LEMG).
Essential voice tremor	Thyroarytenoid muscle or lateral cricothyroid muscle unilateral or bilateral: 2.5 MU Botox®/2.5 MU Xeomin®/20 MU Dysport® per side	Selection of the target muscles by LEMG is very important.
Bilateral vocal fold paralysis	Thyroarytenoid muscle bilateral: 2.5–5 MU Botox®/2.5–5 MU Xeomin®/20–40 MU Dysport® per side	Only in selected cases as an adjuvant treatment to surgery.

[a] Only examples for formulations of Table 19.2 are shown. Of course, other formulations can be used. Be aware that botulinum toxin treatment in neurolaryngology is mainly off-label use

Take-Home Messages

- Differential diagnosis between vocal fold paralysis and arytenoid fixation using laryngeal electromyography is reliable.
- Laryngeal electromyography is the method of choice for the assessment of neural damage.
- Prognosis of a vocal fold paralysis can be assessed reliably within 2 weeks after onset.
- A proven electrical simulated vocal fold abduction demonstrates a viable condition for future larynx pacing strategies.
- Botulinum toxin therapy is the treatment of choice for laryngeal dystonia.

References

1. Sittel C, Guntinas-Lichius O. Neurolaryngology. Stuttgart: Thieme; 2018.
2. Halum SL, Patel N, Smith TL, Jaradeh S, Toohill RJ, Merati AL. Laryngeal electromyography for adult unilateral vocal fold immobility: a survey of the American Broncho-Esophagological Association. Ann Otol Rhinol Laryngol. 2005;114(6):425–8.
3. Ingle JW, Young VN, Smith LJ, Munin MC, Rosen CA. Prospective evaluation of the clinical utility of laryngeal electromyography. Laryngoscope. 2014;124(12):2745–9.
4. Ho GY, Leonhard M, Volk GF, Foerster G, Pototschnig C, Klinge K, Granitzka T, Zienau AK, Schneider-Stickler B. Inter-rater reliability of seven neurolaryngologists in laryngeal EMG signal interpretation. Eur Arch Otorhinolaryngol. 2019;276(10):2849–56.
5. Blitzer A, Crumley RL, Dailey SH, Ford CN, Floeter MK, Hillel AD, Hoffmann HT, Ludlow CL, Merati A, Munin MC, Robinson LR, Rosen C, Saxon KG, Sulica L, Thibeault SL, Titze I, Woo P, Woodson GE. Recommendations of the Neurolaryngology Study Group on laryngeal electromyography. Otolaryngol Head Neck Surg. 2009;140(6):782–93.
6. Volk GF, Hagen R, Pototschnig C, Friedrich G, Nawka T, Arens C, Mueller A, Foerster G, Finkensieper M, Lang-Roth R, Sittel C, Storck C, Grosheva M, Kotby MN, Klingner CM, Guntinas-Lichius O. Laryngeal electromyography: a proposal for guidelines of the European Laryngological Society. Eur Arch Otorhinolaryngol. 2012;269(10):2227–45.
7. Munin MC, Heman-Ackah YD, Rosen CA, Sulica L, Maronian N, Mandel S, Carey BT, Craig E, Gronseth G. Consensus statement: using laryngeal electromyography for the diagnosis and treatment of vocal cord paralysis. Muscle Nerve. 2016;53(6):850–5.
8. Leclerc AA, Munin MC, Smith LJ, Rosen CA. Abnormal laryngeal electromyography findings in asymptomatic adults across the age spectrum. Laryngoscope. 2020; https://doi.org/10.1002/lary.29213.
9. Zealear DL, Swelstad MR, Fortune S, Rodriguez RJ, Chung SM, Valyi-Nagy K, Billante MJ, Billante CR, Garren K. Evoked electromyographic technique for quantitative assessment of the innervation status of laryngeal muscles. Ann Otol Rhinol Laryngol. 2005;114(7):563–72.
10. Thumfart WF. Elektrodiagnostik bei Läsionen des N. recurrens. Arch Otorhinolaryngol. 1981;231:483–505.
11. Thumfart WF, Pototschnig C, Zorowka P, Eckel HE. Electrophysiologic investigation of lower cranial nerve diseases by means of magnetically stimulated neuromyography of the larynx. Ann Otol Rhinol Laryngol. 1992;101(8):629–34.
12. Thumfart WF. Endoscopic electromyography and neuromyography. In: Samii M, Jannetta PJ, editors. The cranial nerves. Heidelberg: Springer; 1998. p. 597–606.
13. Sittel C, Guntinas-Lichius O, Streppel M, Stennert E. Variability of repeated facial nerve electroneurography in healthy subjects. Laryngoscope. 1998;108(8 Pt 1):1177–80.
14. Sittel C, Stennert E. Prognostic value of electromyography in acute peripheral facial nerve palsy. Otol Neurotol. 2001;22(1):100–4.
15. Bertorini TE, Sharaf AG. An overview of laryngeal muscle single fiber electromyography. J Clin Neurophysiol. 2015;32(4):304–8.
16. Bracken DJ, Ornelas G, Coleman TP, Weissbrod PA. High-density surface electromyography: a visualization method of laryngeal muscle activity. Laryngoscope. 2019;129(10):2347–53.
17. Seo HG, Jang HJ, Oh BM, Kim W, Han TR. Use of ultrasonography to locate laryngeal structures for laryngeal electromyography. PM R. 2014;6(6):522–7.
18. Klinge K, Guntinas-Lichius O, Naumann A, Mueller AH. Ultrasonography-guided electromagnetic needle tracking in laryngeal electromyography. Eur Arch Otorhinolaryngol. 2019;276(4):1109–15.
19. Statham MM, Rosen CA, Nandedkar SD, Munin MC. Quantitative laryngeal electromyography: turns and amplitude analysis. Laryngoscope. 2010;120(10):2036–41. https://doi.org/10.1002/lary.21046.
20. Mueller AH. Laryngeal pacing for bilateral vocal fold immobility. Curr Opin Otolaryngol Head Neck Surg. 2011;19(6):439–43.
21. Mueller AH, Hagen R, Foerster G, Grossmann W, Baumbusch K, Pototschnig C. Laryngeal pacing via an implantable stimulator for the rehabilitation of subjects suffering from bilateral vocal fold paralysis: a prospective first-in-human study. Laryngoscope. 2016;126(8):1810–6.
22. Rontal E, Rontal M, Silverman B, Kileny PR. The clinical differentiation between vocal cord paralysis and vocal cord fixation using electromyography. Laryngoscope. 1993;103(2):133–7.
23. Koufman JA, Postma GN, Whang CS, Rees CJ, Amin MR, Belafsky PC, Johnson PE, Connolly KM, Walker FO. Diagnostic laryngeal electromyography: the Wake Forest experience 1995–1999. Otolaryngol Head Neck Surg. 2001;124(6):603–6.
24. Seddon H. Three types of nerve injury. Brain. 1943;66:237–88.
25. Pototschnig C, Thumfart WF. Electromyographic evaluation of vocal cord disorders. Acta Otorhinolaryngol Belg. 1997;51(2):99–104.
26. Blitzer A, Jahn AF, Keidar A. Semon's law revisited: an electromyographic analysis of laryngeal synkinesis. Ann Otol Rhinol Laryngol. 1996;105(10):764–9.
27. Kirchner JA. Semon's law a century later. J Laryngol Otol. 1982;96:645–57.

28. Sasaki CT, Horiuchi M, Ikari T, Kirchner JA. Vocal cord positioning by selective denervation. Old territory revisited. Ann Otol Rhinol Laryngol. 1980;89(6 Pt 1):541–6.
29. Statham MM, Rosen CA, Smith LJ, Munin MC. Electromyographic laryngeal synkinesis alters prognosis in vocal fold paralysis. Laryngoscope. 2010;120(2):285–90. https://doi.org/10.1002/lary.20629.
30. Crumley RL. Laryngeal synkinesis: its significance to the laryngologist. Ann Otol Rhinol Laryngol. 1989;98(2):87–92.
31. Stennert E. Why does the frontalis muscle "never come back"? Functional organization of the mimic musculature. Eur Arch Otorhinolaryngol. 1994;1994:S91–5.
32. Foerster G, Podema R, Guntinas-Lichius O, Crumley RL, Mueller AH. Crumley's classification of laryngeal synkinesis: a comparison of laryngoscopy and electromyography. Laryngoscope. 2020; https://doi.org/10.1002/lary.29275.
33. Paniello RC. Synkinesis following recurrent laryngeal nerve injury: a computer simulation. Laryngoscope. 2016;126(7):1600–5. https://doi.org/10.1002/lary.25730.
34. Foerster G, Mueller AH. PCA atrophy and synkinesis as the main factors for persistent vocal fold immobility in RLN paralysis. Laryngoscope. 2020; https://doi.org/10.1002/lary.29195.
35. Crumley RL. Unilateral recurrent laryngeal nerve paralysis. J Voice. 1994;8(1):79–83.
36. Ford CN. Laryngeal EMG in clinical neurolaryngology. Arch Otolaryngol Head Neck Surg. 1998;124(4):476–7.
37. Simpson DM, Sternman D, Graves-Wright J, Sanders I. Vocal cord paralysis: clinical and electrophysiologic features. Muscle Nerve. 1993;16(9):952–7.
38. Min YB, Finnegan EM, Hoffman HT, Luschei ES, McCulloch TM. A preliminary study of the prognostic role of electromyography in laryngeal paralysis. Otolaryngol Head Neck Surg. 1994;111(6):770–5.
39. Rodriquez AA, Myers BR, Ford CN. Laryngeal electromyography in the diagnosis of laryngeal nerve injuries. Arch Phys Med Rehabil. 1990;71(8):587–90.
40. Paniello RC, Park AM, Bhatt NK, Al-Lozi M. Recurrent laryngeal nerve recovery patterns assessed by serial electromyography. Laryngoscope. 2016;126(3):651–6. https://doi.org/10.1002/lary.25487.
41. Smith LJ, Rosen CA, Niyonkuru C, Munin MC. Quantitative electromyography improves prediction in vocal fold paralysis. Laryngoscope. 2012;122(4):854–9. https://doi.org/10.1002/lary.21884.
42. Lin RJ, Smith LJ, Munin MC, Sridharan S, Rosen CA. Innervation status in chronic vocal fold paralysis and implications for laryngeal reinnervation. Laryngoscope. 2018;128(7):1628–33. https://doi.org/10.1002/lary.27078.
43. Sittel C, Stennert E, Thumfart WF, Dapunt U, Eckel HE. Prognostic value of laryngeal electromyography in vocal fold paralysis. Arch Otolaryngol Head Neck Surg. 2001;127(2):155–60.
44. Eckel HE, Thumfart M, Wassermann K, Vossing M, Thumfart WF. Cordectomy versus arytenoidectomy in the management of bilateral vocal cord paralysis. Ann Otol Rhinol Laryngol. 1994;103(11):852–7.
45. Muller A, Paulsen FP. Impact of vocal cord paralysis on cricoarytenoid joint. Ann Otol Rhinol Laryngol. 2002;111(10):896–901.
46. Woisard V, Liu X, Bes MC, Simonetta-Moreau M. Botulinum toxin injection in laryngeal dyspnea. Eur Arch Otorhinolaryngol. 2017;274(2):909–17. https://doi.org/10.1007/s00405-016-4289-6.
47. Wang CC, Chang MH, Jiang RS, Lai HC, De Virgilio A, Wang CP, Wu SH, Liu SA, Liang KL. Laryngeal electromyography-guided hyaluronic acid vocal fold injection for unilateral vocal fold paralysis: a prospective long-term follow-up outcome report. JAMA Otolaryngol Head Neck Surg. 2015;141(3):264–71.
48. Zealear DL, Dedo HH. Control of paralysed axial muscles by electrical stimulation. Acta Otolaryngol. 1977;83(5–6):514–27.
49. Bergmann K, Warzel H, Eckhardt HU, Gerhardt HJ. Respiratory rhythmically regulated electrical stimulation of paralyzed laryngeal muscles. Laryngoscope. 1984;94(10):1376–80.
50. Bergmann K, Warzel H, Eckhardt HU, Hopstock U, Hermann V, Gerhardt HJ. Long-term implantation of a system of electrical stimulation of paralyzed laryngeal muscles in dogs. Laryngoscope. 1988;98(4):455–9.
51. Zrunek M, Carraro U, Catani C, Scabolcs M, Gruber H, Streinzer W, Mayr W, Thoma H (1986) [Functional electrostimulation of the denervated posticus muscle in an animal experiment: histo- and biochemical results]. Laryngorhinolotol. 65(11):621–7.
52. Zealear DL, Billante CR, Courey MS, Netterville JL, Paniello RC, Sanders I, Herzon GD, Goding GS, Mann W, Ejnell H, Habets AM, Testerman R, Van de HP. Reanimation of the paralyzed human larynx with an implantable electrical stimulation device. Laryngoscope. 2003;113(7):1149–56.
53. Foerster G, Arnold D, Bischoff S, Boltze K, Scholle HC, Schubert H, Mueller AH. Pre-clinical evaluation of a minimally invasive laryngeal pacemaker system in mini-pig. Eur Arch Otorhinolaryngol. 2016;273(1):151–8.
54. Muller AH. Laryngeal synkinesis: a viable condition for laryngeal pacing. Adv Otorhinolaryngol. 2020;85:112–9.
55. Mueller AH, Hagen R, Pototschnig C, Foerster G, Grossmann W, Baumbusch K, Gugatschka M, Nawka T. Laryngeal pacing for bilateral vocal fold paralysis: voice and respiratory aspects. Laryngoscope. 2017;127(8):1838–44. https://doi.org/10.1002/lary.26428.
56. Nawka T, Gugatschka M, Kolmel JC, Muller AH, Schneider-Stickler B, Yaremchuk S, Grosheva M, Hagen R, Maurer JT, Pototschnig C, Lehmann T, Volk GF, Guntinas-Lichius O. Therapy of bilateral vocal

fold paralysis: real world data of an international multicenter registry. PLoS One. 2019;14(4):e0216096.
57. Sulica L. Contemporary management of spasmodic dysphonia. Curr Opin Otolaryngol Head Neck Surg. 2004;12(6):543–8.
58. Merati AL, Heman-Ackah YD, Abaza M, Altman KW, Sulica L, Belamowicz S. Common movement disorders affecting the larynx: a report from the Neurolaryngology Committee of the AAO-HNS. Otolaryngol Head Neck Surg. 2005;133(5):654–65.
59. Hillel AD, Benninger M, Blitzer A, Crumley R, Flint P, Kashima HK, Sanders I, Schaefer S. Evaluation and management of bilateral vocal cord immobility. Otolaryngol Head Neck Surg. 1999;121(6):760–5.
60. Richardson BE, Bastian RW. Clinical evaluation of vocal fold paralysis. Otolaryngol Clin N Am. 2004;37(1):45–58.
61. Holinger LD, Holinger PC, Holinger PH. Etiology of bilateral abductor vocal cord paralysis: a review of 389 cases. Ann Otol Rhinol Laryngol. 1976;85(4 Pt 1):428–36.
62. Sulica L, Blitzer A. Electromyography and the immobile vocal fold. Otolaryngol Clin N Am. 2004;37(1):59–74.
63. Foerster G, Mueller AH. Laryngeal EMG: preferential damage of the posterior cricoarytenoid muscle branches especially in iatrogenic recurrent laryngeal nerve lesions. Laryngoscope. 2018;128(5):1152–6.
64. Maronian NC, Robinson L, Waugh P, Hillel AD. A new electromyographic definition of laryngeal synkinesis. Ann Otol Rhinol Laryngol. 2004;113(11):877–86.
65. Grundfast KM, Harley E. Vocal cord paralysis. Otolaryngol Clin N Am. 1989;22(3):569–97.
66. Miyamoto RC, Parikh SR, Gellad W, Licameli GR. Bilateral congenital vocal cord paralysis: a 16-year institutional review. Otolaryngol Head Neck Surg. 2005;133(2):241–5.
67. Emery PJ, Fearon B. Vocal cord palsy in pediatric practice: a review of 71 cases. Int J Pediatr Otorhinolaryngol. 1984;8(2):147–54.
68. Tilles SA. Vocal cord dysfunction in children and adolescents. Curr Allergy Asthma Rep. 2003;3(6):467–72.
69. Grillone GA, Blitzer A, Brin MF, Annino DJ Jr, Saint-Hilaire MH. Treatment of adductor laryngeal breathing dystonia with botulinum toxin type A. Laryngoscope. 1994;104(1 Pt 1):30–2.
70. Ludlow CL, Domangue R, Sharma D, Jinnah HA, Perlmutter JS, Berke G, Sapienza C, Smith ME, Blumin JH, Kalata CE, Blindauer K, Johns M, Hapner E, Harmon A, Paniello R, Adler CH, Crujido L, Lott DG, Bansberg SF, Barone N, Drulia T, Stebbins G. Consensus-based attributes for identifying patients with spasmodic dysphonia and other voice disorders. JAMA Otolaryngol Head Neck Surg. 2018;144(8):657–65.
71. Hillel AD, Maronian NC, Waugh PF, Robinson L, Klotz DA. Treatment of the interarytenoid muscle with botulinum toxin for laryngeal dystonia. Ann Otol Rhinol Laryngol. 2004;113(5):341–8.
72. Klotz DA, Maronian NC, Waugh PF, Shahinfar A, Robinson L, Hillel AD. Findings of multiple muscle involvement in a study of 214 patients with laryngeal dystonia using fine-wire electromyography. Ann Otol Rhinol Laryngol. 2004;113(8):602–12.
73. Yang Q, Xu W, Li Y, Cheng L. Value of laryngeal electromyography in spasmodic dysphonia diagnosis and therapy. Ann Otol Rhinol Laryngol. 2015;124(7):579–83.
74. Stong BC, DelGaudio JM, Hapner ER, Johns MM III. Safety of simultaneous bilateral botulinum toxin injections for abductor spasmodic dysphonia. Arch Otolaryngol Head Neck Surg. 2005;131(9):793–5.
75. Isshiki N, Haji T, Yamamoto Y, Mahieu HF. Thyroplasty for adductor spasmodic dysphonia: further experiences. Laryngoscope. 2001;111(4 Pt 1):615–21.
76. Berke GS, Blackwell KE, Gerratt BR, Verneil A, Jackson KS, Sercarz JA. Selective laryngeal adductor denervation-reinnervation: a new surgical treatment for adductor spasmodic dysphonia. Ann Otol Rhinol Laryngol. 1999;108(3):227–31.
77. Blitzer A, Brin MF, Stewart CF. Botulinum toxin management of spasmodic dysphonia (laryngeal dystonia): a 12-year experience in more than 900 patients. Laryngoscope. 1998;108(10):1435–41.
78. Postma GN, Blalock PD, Koufman JA. Bilateral medialization laryngoplasty. Laryngoscope. 1998;108(10):1429–34.
79. Shaw GY, Sechtem PR, Rideout B. Posterior cricoarytenoid myoplasty with medialization thyroplasty in the management of refractory abductor spasmodic dysphonia. Ann Otol Rhinol Laryngol. 2003;112(4):303–6.
80. Maronian NC, Waugh PF, Robinson L, Hillel AD. Tremor laryngeal dystonia: treatment of the lateral cricoarytenoid muscle. Ann Otol Rhinol Laryngol. 2004;113(5):349–55.
81. Blumin JH, Pcolinsky DE, Atkins JP. Laryngeal findings in advanced Parkinson's disease. Ann Otol Rhinol Laryngol. 2004;113(4):253–8.
82. Leopold NA, Kagel MC. Laryngeal deglutition movement in Parkinson's disease. Neurology. 1997;48(2):373–6.
83. Luschei ES, Ramig LO, Baker KL, Smith ME. Discharge characteristics of laryngeal single motor units during phonation in young and older adults and in persons with parkinson disease. J Neurophysiol. 1999;81(5):2131–9.
84. Kim SH, Kearney JJ, Atkins JP. Percutaneous laryngeal collagen augmentation for treatment of parkinsonian hypophonia. Otolaryngol Head Neck Surg. 2002;126(6):653–6.
85. Trail M, Fox C, Ramig LO, Sapir S, Howard J, Lai EC. Speech treatment for Parkinson's disease. Neuro Rehabil. 2005;20(3):205–21.
86. Roth CR, Glaze LE, Goding GS Jr, David WS. Spasmodic dysphonia symptoms as initial presentation of amyotrophic lateral sclerosis. J Voice. 1996;10(4):362–7.

87. Merlo IM, Occhini A, Pacchetti C, Alfonsi E. Not paralysis, but dystonia causes stridor in multiple system atrophy. Neurology. 2002;58(4):649–52.
88. Blitzer A, Sulica L. Botulinum toxin: basic science and clinical uses in otolaryngology. Laryngoscope. 2001;111(2):218–26.
89. Walker TJ, Dayan SH. Comparison and overview of currently available neurotoxins. J Clin Aesthet Dermatol. 2014;7(2):31–9.
90. Guntinas-Lichius O. Injection of botulinum toxin type B for the treatment of otolaryngology patients with secondary treatment failure of botulinum toxin type a. Laryngoscope. 2003;113(4):743–5.
91. Boutsen F, Cannito MP, Taylor M, Bender B. Botox treatment in adductor spasmodic dysphonia: a meta-analysis. J Speech Lang Hear Res. 2002;45(3):469–81.

20 Spasmodic Dysphonia

Juliëtta H. C. Schuering, Elisabeth V. Sjögren, and Antonius P. M. Langeveld

Key Points

- Two general types of spasmodic dysphonia are distinguished: adductor spasmodic dysphonia (AdSD) and abductor spasmodic dysphonia (AbSD). Of these, AdSD is the more common type.
- Botulinum toxin injection is the current gold standard of therapy. Temporarily, the voice quality can improve to an average of 80%–90% of normal vocal function after an injection.
- Surgical procedures could potentially offer a more stable and long-lasting beneficial effect than botulinum toxin treatment.
- The three most frequently used surgical techniques for AdSD over the past 10 years are selective laryngeal adductor denervation–reinnervation (SLAD-R), thyroplasty type II, and endoscopic laser thyroarytenoid myoneurectomy.

20.1 Introduction

- Definition
- Historical background (psychogenic versus organic approach)
- Etiology (fMRI, gamma-motor neurons)
- Adductor/abductor spasmodic dysphonia
- Symptomatology
- Diagnostic assessment

Spasmodic dysphonia is a rare voice disorder with unknown etiology that leads to severe problems in verbal communication. Historically, most clinicians viewed spasmodic dysphonia as a hysterical conversion reaction wherein some psychic conflict becomes somatized to the laryngeal sphincter. This theory prevailed for several decades, but nowadays spasmodic dysphonia is classified as a focal (laryngeal) dystonia. Dystonia is a neurological disorder of central motor processing with many different clinical manifestations. The neuroanatomical substrates for laryngeal dystonia are still only partly understood [1]. A potential etiology is an imbalance of sensory and motor signalling originating in the basal ganglia [2]. However, evidence from functional magnetic resonance imaging (fMRI) suggests a more heterogeneous localization in the brain, e.g., the somatosensory cortex [3]. More recently, authors have theorized that spasmodic dysphonia is a sensory disorder, induced by high activity of

J. H. C. Schuering (✉) · E. V. Sjögren
A. P. M. Langeveld
Department of Otorhinolaryngology, Head & Neck Surgery, Leiden University Medical Center, Leiden, Zuid-Holland, The Netherlands
e-mail: j.h.c.schuering@lumc.nl; E.V.sjogren@lumc.nl; A.P.M.Langeveld@lumc.nl

M. Remacle, H. E. Eckel (eds.), *Textbook of Surgery of Larynx and Trachea*,
https://doi.org/10.1007/978-3-031-09621-1_20

gamma-motor neurons [4]. Gamma-motor neurons regulate the innervation of the intrafusal fibers of the muscle spindle thereby increasing the firing rate and sensitivity of the afferent neuron [4]. Consensus on the precise etiology has not been reached yet.

Generally, two different types of spasmodic dysphonia are recognized: adductor spasmodic dysphonia (AdSD) and abductor spasmodic dysphonia (AbSD) [5]. AdSD and AbSD differ in their acoustic characteristics [6]. In AdSD, hyperactivity of the adductor muscles results in voice breaks and consequent alterations in phonation and pitch [6]. The most commonly involved laryngeal adductor muscles are the thyroarytenoid and the lateral cricoarytenoid [7]. The AdSD symptoms are a result of intermittent and involuntary contraction of these adductor muscles during phonation, which leads to tense vocal folds that are pressed against each other and to an increased glottic resistance [8]. In AbSD, the spasms occur in the posterior cricoarytenoid muscles resulting in breathy, segmented speech [6]. Patients with AdSD have greater difficulty with voiced sounds and AbSD with unvoiced sounds [6]. Mixed spasmodic dysphonia involves characteristics of both types [6]. Some authors believe that all of the patients are a mixed adductor/abductor with a predominance of one form [9]. The symptoms typically progress over 1–2 years and then remain chronic. A reduction or relief of symptoms is seen during uncontrolled voicing such as laughing, singing, coughing, whispering, humming, or with alcohol intake [10]. However, stress, fatigue, and communication through telephone often leads to an increase of complaints [11]. Spasmodic dysphonia patients often suffer from severe problems in communication, which has a huge impact on their quality of life [12, 13].

About one-third of the spasmodic dysphonia patients exhibit a co-occurring dystonic voice tremor, which often complicates the diagnosis and clinical management [14]. Therefore, the correct diagnosis is made by a team of experienced neurologists, otorhinolaryngologists, and speech therapists. This chapter focuses on the management of adductor spasmodic dysphonia (AdSD), the more common form of spasmodic dysphonia in approximately 90% of the cases. AbSD will be discussed briefly.

20.2 Treatment Options for AdSD

- Nonsurgical treatment
  - Botulinum toxin: gold standard therapy
  - Voice therapy
  - Oral medication
- Surgical treatment
  - Historical background
  - Selective laryngeal adductor denervation–reinnervation (SLAD-R)
  - Thyroplasty type II
  - Endoscopic laser thyroarytenoid myoneurectomy
  - Anecdotal/experimental procedures

There is no known cure for adductor spasmodic dysphonia. Various treatment modalities have been described over the past decades and they all focus on symptom management. Regardless of the treatment modality, the main challenge is to prevent the recurrence of symptoms.

20.2.1 Nonsurgical Treatment

20.2.1.1 Botulinum Toxin: The Current Gold Standard of Therapy

The concept of using "botulinum toxin" to treat patients with disorders of muscle function is credited to Dr. Alan B. Scott. He published the results of his first clinical trial with injection of botulinum toxin type A in patients with strabismus in 1980 [15]. Shortly after, in 1984, Blitzer was the first who injected botulinum toxin A into the vocal folds as treatment for AdSD [16]. Botulinum toxin A is a neurotoxin produced by *Clostridium botulinum*. Strains of *Clostridium botulinum* produce seven distinct neurotoxins (types A–G botulinum toxin) which act primarily on peripheral cholinergic synapses, but only botulinum toxin types A and B are currently available for clinical use [17, 18]. The mecha-

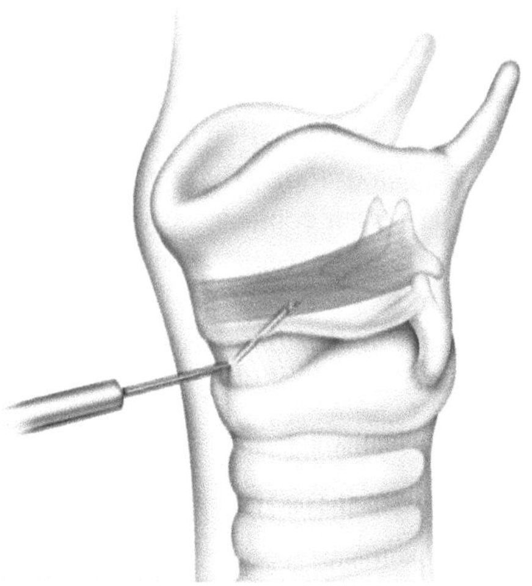

Fig. 20.1 EMG-guided injection of the thyroarytenoid muscle for adductor spasmodic dysphonia. Image from Sulica L, Blitzer A, Oper Tech Otolaryngol 15:76–80, 2004 © Elsevier, adapted and reprinted with permission [22]

nism of action of these potent neurotoxins is direct inhibition of the injected muscles by blocking the release of the neurotransmitter acetylcholine at the neuromuscular junction [17]. The result is a chemical denervation causing a dose-related muscle weakness, lasting several months. Recovery occurs by muscular reinnervation with smaller collateral nerve sprouts and an increase in the number of postsynaptic acetylcholine receptors [19]. The objective in AdSD patients is to inject botulinum toxin in the presumed main laryngeal adductor muscles affected in AdSD (the thyroarytenoid muscles) in the outpatient setting. This causes a temporary chemical denervation of these injected adductors. Currently, botulinum toxin A (BTX) injections in the adductor musculature are considered gold standard of care for AdSD patients.

Though widely accepted, BTX treatment for AdSD is not standardized; because no clear guidelines exist, protocols in BTX treatment vary among physicians [20]. There are different injection strategies. The most frequently used approach is the percutaneous route through the cricothyroid membrane under EMG control (Fig. 20.1), as described by Blitzer et al. [21].

In our center, the patient is placed in a supine position with the neck extended. A modified 1.5-inch hollow-bore 27-gauge Teflon-coated EMG needle is used both as a monopolar electrode to locate the thyroarytenoid muscle and as a port for injection of the botulinum toxin. The needle is placed through the skin and cricothyroid membrane and angled superiorly and slightly laterally into the thyroarytenoid muscles. Correct position of the needle tip is confirmed by the presence of crisp action potentials on phonation. The botulinum toxin is then injected in the muscles. Topical anesthesia is not necessary. The main disadvantage of this approach is that the needle tip can easily be placed more posteriorly or laterally than intended, injecting the lateral cricoarytenoid or cricothyroid muscles. Alternatively, botulinum toxin may also be injected percutaneously transcartilaginous through the thyroid cartilage, wherein the needle position is confirmed by flexible laryngoscopy [23]. Although less frequently used, an indirect laryngoscopic peroral approach or injection through an operative channel of a flexible laryngoscope have also been suggested [24, 25]. The duration of benefit of unilateral injections appear to be less than bilateral injections [26]. Therefore, most patients receive bilateral injections. However, if patients cannot tolerate the side effects of bilateral injections, a unilateral injection is offered [26]. Preference and/or prior experience of the patient/physician may influence that decision. Injection dosages range widely in literature. In a recent survey among 70 American laryngologists, a mode of 1.25 units (range 0.5–5.0 units) per injection side was described [20]. Decisions regarding dose of the injection are generally based on the experience and empirical judgement of the otolaryngologist and the patient. Good results can be accomplished with botulinum injections: voice quality can improve to an average of 80%–90% of normal vocal function [26, 27]. However, there are several drawbacks to BTX injection therapy. The main disadvantage is the need for repeated injections, since the BTX effect is temporary. The duration of improvement of symptoms varies by individual, but lasts about 3–4 months [28]. Thus, if patients want to maintain improved voice, they usually return 3–4 times a year for injections [28]. Second, an initial period of breathiness as a side effect of the injection usually leads to a decline in voice quality [27]. This breathiness typically starts immediately after the injection and lasts for 2–3 weeks before the optimal BTX voice quality is reached. As a result of either awaiting the full therapeutic effect or experiencing a therapeutic decline, optimal voicing is achieved during only 30% of the injection cycle [27]. Third, there is a lack of uniform responses to the injections among and within patients, causing wide cycle-to-cycle differences. This results in an unpredictable voice and emotional stress with high impact on quality of life [13]. Besides the breathy dysphonia, the most frequently reported side effects of botulinum toxin treatment are swallowing problems. Swallowing difficulties (i.e., mild choking on fluids) appear as early as the breathy voice and usually resolves within 2 weeks. Less common complications include hyperventilation, a "sore throat" feeling, and diplophonia. In the literature, there are no major complications reported [26].

20.2.1.2 Oral Medication

The utility of treatment of AdSD with oral medication (muscle relaxants, tranquilizers, etc.) is often limited by significant central nervous system side effects like sedation and memory loss [22]. It usually results in an incomplete response and is frequently unsuccessful. After a report showing that more than half of patients with SD experienced dramatically improved voice quality after ingestion of alcohol, Rumbach et al. have focused on the use of GABA receptor agonists, which produce effects through mechanisms similar to the action of alcohol, to improve symptoms [10]. A metabolite of sodium oxybate has been found to improve SD symptoms in 82% of patients who had improvement following alcohol ingestion [14].

20.2.1.3 Voice Therapy

Voice therapy has shown little therapeutic effect in AdSD patients, but can be useful in differentiating between the diagnosis of AdSD and voice disorders of other origins [29]. Additionally, behavioral treatment approaches may enhance the effectiveness of other AdSD treatment strategies, by reducing hyperfunctional vocal behaviors such as hard glottal attacks and excessive laryngeal tension [30]. These hyperfunctional behaviors are often compensatory in nature and are developed over time by individuals with AdSD as a means of countering vocal spasms and may persist even after the spasms are eliminated via injection [30, 31].

20.2.2 Surgical Treatment

Surgical procedures could potentially offer a more stable and long-lasting beneficial effect than botulinum toxin treatment. In 1976, Dedo introduced recurrent laryngeal nerve sectioning (RLNS) [32]. He hypothesized that "if a recurrent laryngeal nerve were paralyzed in a patient with spastic dysphonia, the other vocal cord might prove to be 'precompensated' so that its excessively strong adduction would carry it across the midline to the deliberately paralyzed cord, giving a relatively normal phonation" (p. 453) [32]. In the following years, several institutes reported their results after RLNS. Unfortunately, after initially promising outcomes, it showed disappointing long-term results with reoccurrence of symptoms [33–36]. This recurrence of spasmodic closure has been attributed to increased function of the opposite vocal fold and/or to regeneration of the resected laryngeal nerve [37, 38]. Due to the disappointing results, RLNS is nowadays abandoned. Currently, different surgical modalities are used. However, there is no consensus as to which procedure gives the best results. Therefore, the most commonly performed surgical modalities are highlighted below. The aim of every surgical treatment is to permanently reduce the endolaryngeal constriction activity during phonation.

20.2.2.1 Selective Laryngeal Adductor Denervation–Reinnervation (SLAD-R)

Berke presented the SLAD-R procedure in 1999 [39]. The concept is to produce thyroarytenoid and lateral cricoarytenoid muscle paralysis in patients with AdSD, by selectively denervating the recurrent laryngeal nerve (RLN) branches to these muscles [39]. In order to prevent unwanted reinnervation by RLN efferents and preserve muscle tone, a problem that limited the effectiveness of the previously described RLNS, the thyroarytenoid nerve branch is reinnervated with a branch of the ansa cervicalis [39]. The procedure does not affect the third adductor of the larynx, the interarytenoid muscle, which receives innervation from a nerve branch that divides more proximally from the RLN [40].

The steps of the SLAD-R procedure are shown in Figs. 20.2, 20.3, 20.4. After a low transverse incision in the neck, an inferiorly based window of approximately 14 × 18 mm is made in the thyroid lamina as a cartilaginous flap [39]. The distal portion of the anterior branch of the RLN is identified and followed distally [39]. The thyroarytenoid branch is located beneath the perichondrium and ligated 3 mm from its termination [39]. Generally, the sternohyoid branch of the ansa nerve is appropriately sized for thyroarytenoid reinnervation [39]. The ansa is sutured to the distal thyroarytenoid nerve stump to maintain muscle tone and bulk and also to presumably prevent regeneration of RLN axons to the neuromuscular endplates of the thyroarytenoid and lateral cricoarytenoid muscles [39, 40]. The proximal stump of the thyroarytenoid nerve branch is ligated with a 2–0 silk suture and sutured outside the cartilage window to the posterior lamina [39]. Initially, Berke added a lateral cricoarytenoid myotomy after several recurrences after thyroarytenoid SLAD-R in some patients, to provide maximal reduction of adductory force [39, 40]. Although lateral cricoarytenoid myotomy appeared to increase the potential for long-term success, it also increased the risk of severe breathiness because of incomplete posterior commissure closure [40]. Therefore, this additional step has been abandoned [40].

Berke achieved excellent preliminary results with the SLAD-R: he reported that 19 of 21 consecutive SLAD-R patients had moderate to severe dysphonia prior to the operation and mild voice symptoms postoperatively [39, 40]. From the same research group, Chettri et al. reported good long-term results of 86/136 patients in 2006 (50 lost to follow-up) [40]. They showed a high degree of patient satisfaction, with 91% agreeing that their voice is more fluent after the surgery [40]. Additionally, the group of Berke et al. compared the postoperative SLAD-R voice outcomes (i.e., VHI-10, voice questionnaire, and panel voice ratings) with the voice outcomes of a patient cohort 5–8 weeks after BTX treatment [42]. They described 77 participating SLAD-R patients (out of 157 patients who underwent a SLAD-R procedure between 1995 and 2007) and the prospectively collected results of 28 patients receiving BTX treatment [42]. A majority of the postoperative SLAD-R patients had a stable, long-lasting resolution of spasmodic voice breaks

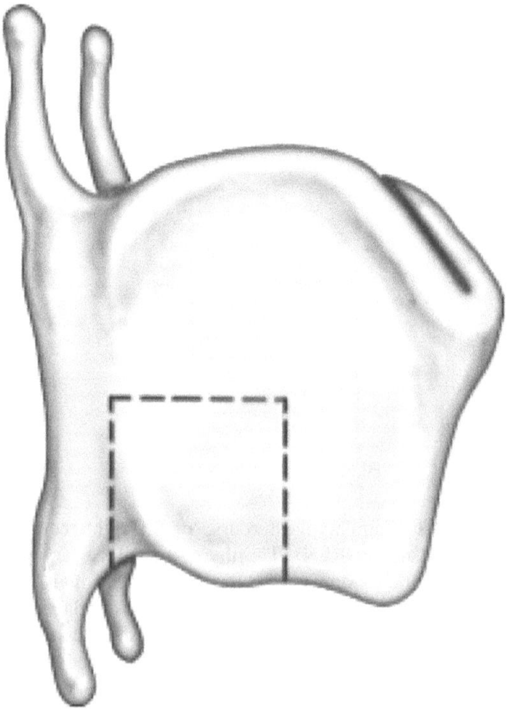

Fig. 20.2 "Lateral oblique view of right thyroid cartilage. The hashed lines show the trapdoor laryngotomy window, crossing the oblique line after removing inferior constrictor muscle attachments. The posterior limb is just anterior to the inferior cornu, the anterior limb passes through the inferior tubercle, and the superior limb is below the vertical midpoint of the cartilage." [41] Image from Long J, Berke G, Oper Tech Otolaryngol 23: 183–187, 2012 © Elsevier, adapted and reprinted with permission

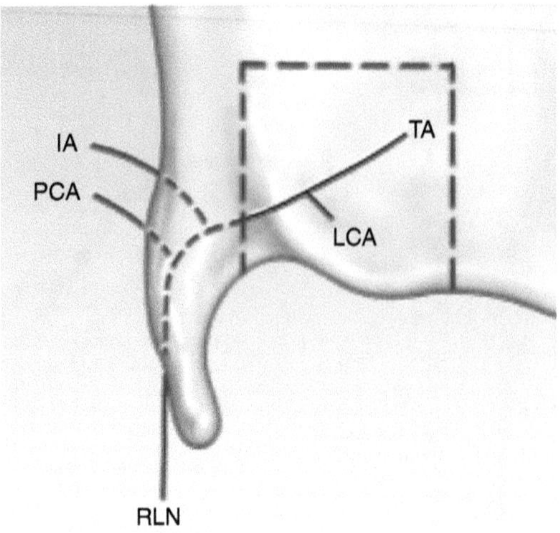

Fig. 20.3 "Intralaryngeal course of the right recurrent laryngeal nerve (RLN). The thyroid cartilage laryngotomy window is drawn with the long hashed lines. The short dashed lines represent nerves behind cartilage. The characteristic oblique anterosuperior course of the adductor nerve within the window is shown, destined for the thyroarytenoid muscle (TA) fibers. Other branches to the posterior cricoarytenoid (PCA) and interarytenoid (IA) muscles are not encountered during the dissection. Lateral cricoarytenoid (LCA) branch may be seen, although it is short and fine." [41] Image from Long J, Berke G, Oper Tech Otolaryngol 23: 183–187, 2012 © Elsevier, adapted and reprinted with permission

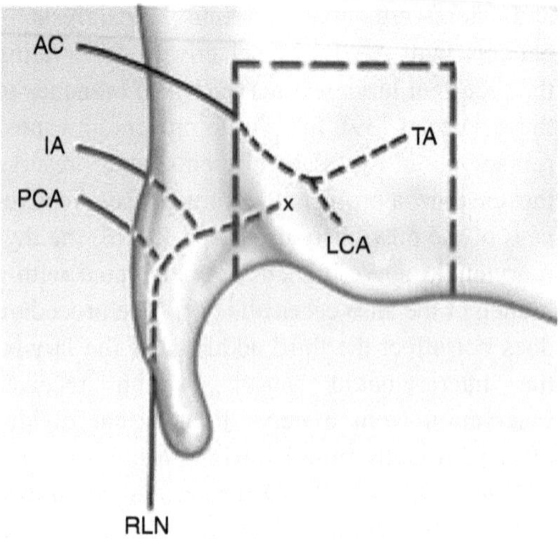

Fig. 20.4 "The postoperative arrangement of laryngeal nerves, after closure of laryngotomy trapdoor (outlined with long hashed lines). The ansa cervicalis (AC) enters through the cartilage window and anastomoses the distal stump of the adductor branch serving the thyroarytenoid muscle (TA) and the lateral cricoarytenoid (LCA) muscles. The proximal adductor branch from the recurrent laryngeal nerve (RLN) is divided and secured out of the larynx. The branches to the posterior cricoarytenoid (PCA) and the interarytenoid (IA) are unaltered." [41] Image from Long J, Berke G, Oper Tech Otolaryngol 23: 183–187, 2012 © Elsevier, adapted and reprinted with permission

and voice outcomes equal or superior to those after BTX treatment [40, 42]. Besides a case series, there no large studies on the SLAD-R procedure reported by other research groups other than Berke/Chettri et al. [43] Reported side effects are postoperative breathiness [40]. Aside from one aspiration pneumonia, no major surgical complications were noted [40, 44].

20.2.2.2 Thyroplasty Type II (TP II)

TP II as treatment for AdSD was initially suggested by Isshiki in 1998 [45]. His "basic idea behind this type of surgery is that any wide surgical intervention into the vocal folds should be avoided, and the vocal fold position and tension can be set optimally for the voice by reshaping the laryngeal framework" (p. 1761). The concept of the TP II in AdSD patients was to create "an imperfect closure of the glottis" to prevent their excessive glottic adduction [46]. It was thought that this would provide a longer-lasting result without the adverse effects of botulinum toxin injection [47]. The advantages of the surgery include the following: (1) optimal glottal closure for phonation can be adjusted, (2) no recurrence is likely to occur, (3) no damage is induced on the physiological function of phonation such as paralysis, (4) it is reversible if it were found ineffective intraoperatively, and (5) readjustment is possible when needed [46].

The procedure, as described initially by Isshiki and later modified by Sanuki, is performed under local anesthesia [47, 48]. A 4-cm horizontal skin incision is made at approximately the level of the vocal folds [47]. The anterior third of the thyroid cartilage is fully cut at the midline with a BP 11 scalpel [47]. The incised edges are pulled apart laterally by 3–4 mm, to test the effect of lateralization on the voice [47]. The required width of midline cartilage separation is determined and was initially maintained by a silicone shim [47]. The shim was fixed to the incised edges of the thyroid cartilage with mattress sutures [47]. However, the suture fixation of the silicone shim to a fragile cartilage edge was not easy, requiring considerable time and caution [48]. Therefore, nowadays a titanium bridge of different sizes, as described by Sanuki et al., is used to fix the position of the cartilage (Figs. 20.5 and 20.6) [48].

Reported results in literature vary. Isshiki and Sanuki described excellent results in relieving vocal stress–strain [48–51]. Nearly 70% of the patients judged their postoperative voice as normal [49]. In a more recent case series, roughly 30% of the patients who received thyroplasty type 2 reported that they were completely relieved of their AdSD voice symptoms (strangulation, interruption, and tremor) [51]. Concerning the symptom of strangulation, 25.8% of patients were completely relieved after surgery, 22.6% reported little strangulation, and 51.6% answered that they still sometimes experienced strangulation [51]. Only 1 of the 47 patients who underwent TP II with an titanium bridge had disease recurrence [51].

However, Chan et al. stated that only about 30% of patients had moderate to good improvements in their symptom severity and vocal effort 1 year after TP II [52]. No major complications were reported in literature. A total of 5.6% patients needed a revision surgery [49].

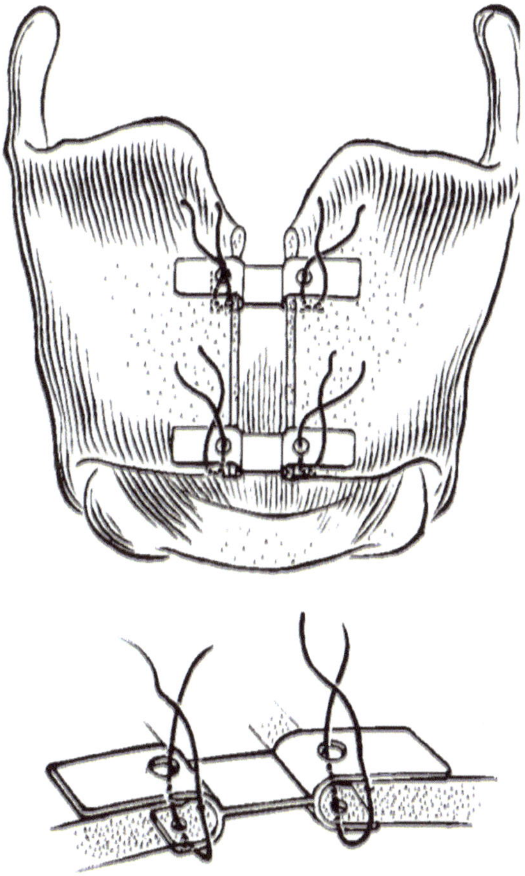

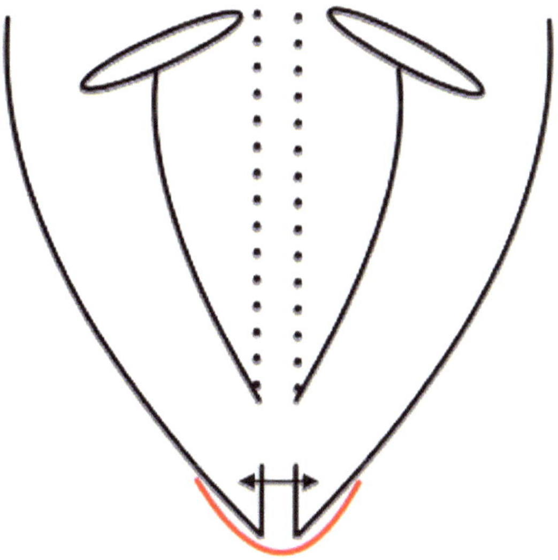

Figs. 20.5 and 20.6 Titanium bridges (various sizes are available) are put in place to fix the position of the cartilage. The device consists of bilateral receptors that grasp the cartilage edges and a connector between them to enable adjustment of the distance of separation. The optimal distance is usually +/−4 mm. Schematic image of the vocal cords and the 'imperfect close of the glottis' (dotted line) by reshaping the laryngeal framework [48]

20.2.2.3 Endoscopic Laser Thyroarytenoid Myoneurectomy (TA Myoneurectomy)

TA myoneurectomy, in which an endoscopic CO_2 laser myectomy of the thyroarytenoid muscle is combined with neurectomy of the thyroarytenoid branch of the recurrent laryngeal nerve, was defined by Su and Tsuji et al. [8, 53]. The concept of TA myoneurectomy is to mimic the effect of botulinum toxin injections on the thyroarytenoid muscle, by removing this muscle and its innervating nerves. By removal of the thyroarytenoid muscle, potential muscle reinnervation by regeneration of the resected laryngeal nerves is very unlikely (Figs. 20.7, 20.8, 20.9, 20.10) [31].

The TA myoneurectomy is performed under general anesthesia. In our center, we perform a modification of the procedure earlier described by Tsuij et al. [8]. And as in most studies, in general, we perform TA myoneurectomy bilaterally. A triangular piece of the thyroarytenoid muscle is resected with a CO2 laser through a transoral approach [54]. To get a clear view of the resection area, partial resection of the ventricular fold is performed, with preservation of the mucosal

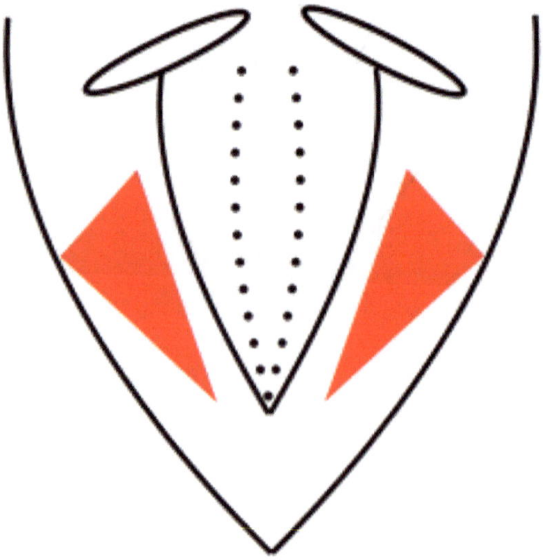

Fig. 20.7 The concept of thyroarytenoid (TA) myoneurectomy consists of a triangular resection of this muscle. The medial border of this triangle is just lateral of the vocal ligament. The lateral boundary of this triangle is the inner perichondrium of the thyroid lamina. The posterior border of the triangle is formed by the insertion of the thyroarytenoid muscle, lateral at the level of the vocal process. The deepest part of the resection is the fascia of the lateral cricoarytenoid (LCA). The neurovascular bundle, which enters the larynx inferolaterally, is coagulated. Schematic image of the vocal cords

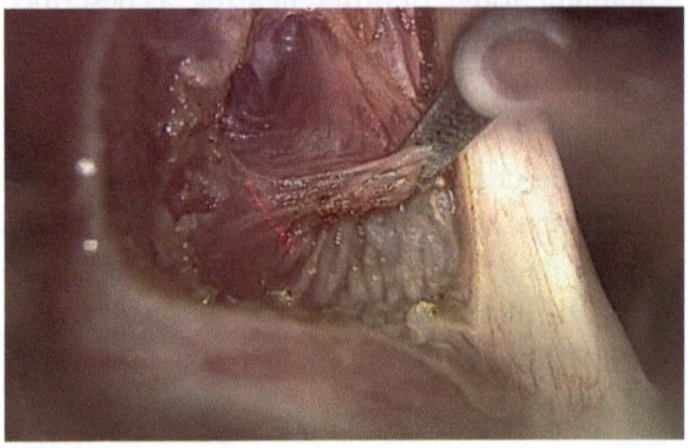

Fig. 20.8 Myotomy: laser resection of the thyroarytenoid muscle

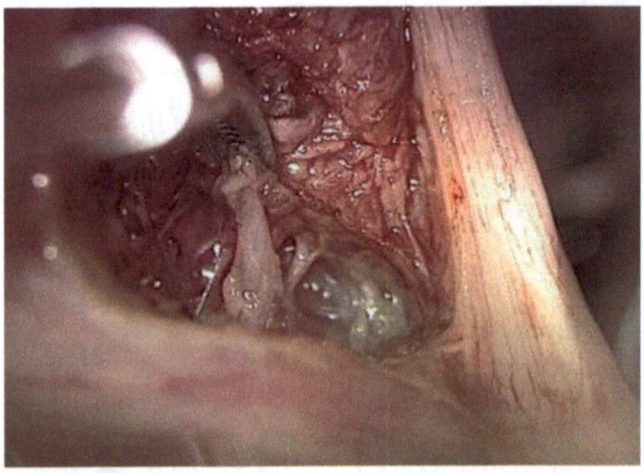

Fig. 20.9 Neurectomy: resection of the distal thyroarytenoid branch of the recurrent laryngeal nerve

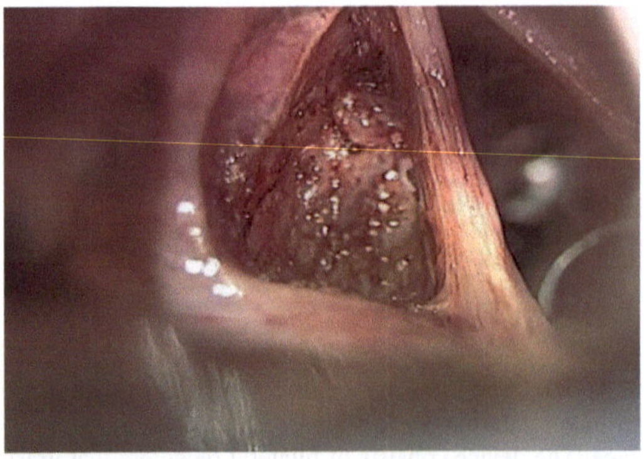

Fig. 20.10 Per-operative result after a TA myoneurectomy on the left side

strip in the apex of the ventricle. This is followed by a delineation of the triangular resection plane. The medial edge of the resection is located just lateral of the vocal ligament. The internal perichondrium of the thyroid cartilage is considered the lateral limit. The posterior/base edge of this triangular resection plane is formed by the insertion of the thyroarytenoid muscle, at the level just lateral of the vocal process. Guided by the inner perichondrium of the thyroid, the muscle fibers of the thyroarytenoid are resected, until the fascia of the lateral cricoarytenoid muscle is visible. Inferolaterally, the neurovascular thyroarytenoid bundle enters the endolarynx, which is coagulated. The inferior limit of the resection is defined by palpation of the free caudal edge of the thyroid, the fascia of the lateral cricoarytenoid muscles, and the edge of the elastic cone.

The results of different studies suggest that the long-term outcomes of TA myoneurectomy are encouraging. Several authors describe significant long-term improvement in voice quality in terms of reduced speech brakes, effort, and strain in voice [8, 55, 56]. Su et al. reported on 29/52 patients who were followed 12 months or more [55]. Approximately 90% (26/29) of these patients achieved moderate and marked vocal improvement [55]. This was confirmed by Tsuij et al., who prospectively analyzed 15 patients and described a postoperative median VHI-10 score improvement in 80%, after a median of 31 months follow-up postoperatively [8]. Schuering et al. were the first who conducted a comparative study, which compared the results after a TA myoneurectomy versus botulinum toxin in the same patient [54]. They found an initially improved stable voice quality after TA myoneurectomy in all 22 patients [54]. The postoperative voice quality was comparable to the best voice with botulinum toxin in the same patient [54]. However, after good results initially, voice deterioration was seen in 45% (10/22) of the patients during a follow-up of >12 months due to reoccurrence of symptoms. All these patients underwent a second procedure with varying success [54]. Nomoto et al. compared the outcomes of 35 TP II patients with 30 TA myoneurectomy patients [54, 57]. Voice quality improved in both procedures, but significant differences in severity outcomes favoring TA myoneurectomy were found in strangulation, interruption, tremor, and grade [57]. Postoperative VHI-10 scores did not differ significantly between the two procedures [57]. Given favorable improvement rates, both surgical procedures were considered effective [57].

Other than surgical removal of granuloma tissue in a few patients, there were no major complications or side effects reported in literature [54].

20.2.2.4 Anecdotal/Experimental Therapies

Anecdotal case reports on bipolar radiofrequency-induced thermotherapy (RFITT) with varying positive results have been described (Fig. 20.11). And again, "The goal is to weaken the force of laryngeal closure during spasms by creating fibrosis of the terminal branches of one recurrent nerve through coagulation" [58]. It consists of transoral coagulation of the terminal branches of the recurrent nerve using RFITT [4, 58, 59].

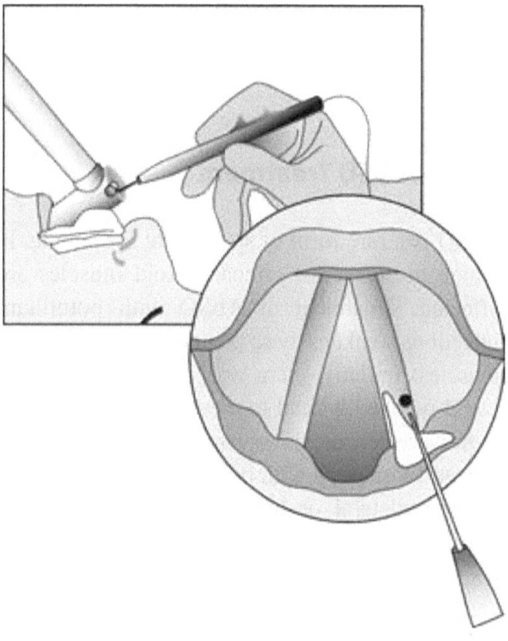

Fig. 20.11 Drawing of the transoral approach with insertion of the RFITT probe into the vocal fold externally and anteriorly to the vocal process. The location of the region of maximal stimulation is usually just lateral and anterior to the vocal process of the arytenoids [58]

Pitman et al. presented a report on the use of an implantable electrical stimulation device to treat spasmodic dysphonia via neuromodulation of the muscle spindle gamma loop [4]. This would modulate the afferent nerve signal, in contrast to all previously mentioned treatments where the efferent nerve signal is modulated. This is based on theory that SD is likely due to a sensory dysfunction, with the muscle spindle playing a central role [4]. Accordingly, the benefit of botulinum toxin injections may be in their modulation of the gamma loop of the muscle spindle via inhibition of the c-motor neuron and not via induction of muscle weakness [4]. They hypothesized that neuromodulation of the c-motor neuron and/or the 1a afferent neuron of the muscle spindle via electrical stimulation can inhibit these nerves, modulate the gamma loop, and mitigate the symptoms of spasmodic dysphonia [4]. In a small test case series, the left thyroarytenoid muscle of five human study participants was stimulated on 5 consecutive days below the level of alpha-motor neuron activation [4]. The spasmodic dysphonia symptoms were reduced in four out of five patients and no major complications were reported. However, no firm conclusions can be drawn from this concept study.

20.3 AbSD Treatment

AbSD is a rare form of spasmodic dysphonia, in which the posterior cricoarytenoid muscles are affected. Treatment of AbSD with botulinum injections weakens these posterior cricoarytenoid muscles. Initially, there was a concern that this could potentially lead to a compromised airway. However, there are now several studies describing successful therapy with botulinum injection with either unilateral or bilateral injection [60–62]. The injection can be applied through a transcricoid or retrocricoid approach (see Figs. 20.12 and 20.13). An average posttreatment voice function of 70% has been achieved [60].

For refractory AbSD cases, different surgical techniques have been mentioned in literature [63]. Case reports of posterior cricoarytenoid myoplasty with medialization thyroplasty and endoscopic partial posterior cricoarytenoid myectomy

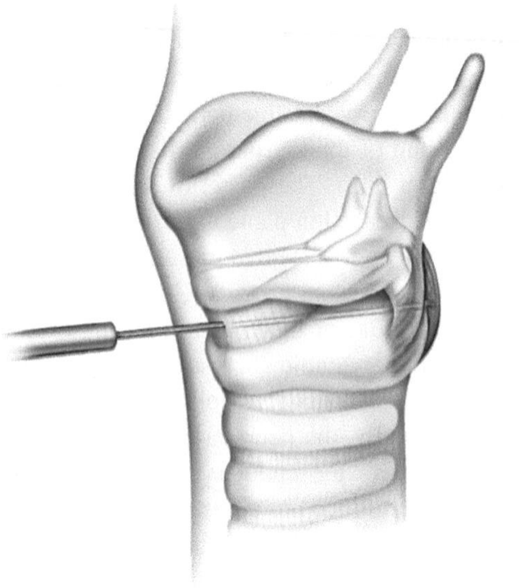

Fig. 20.12 Transcricoid EMG-guided injection of the posterior cricoarytenoid muscle for abductor spasmodic dysphonia. Image from Sulica L, Blitzer A, Oper Tech Otolaryngol 15:76–80, 2004 © Elsevier, adapted and reprinted with permission [22]

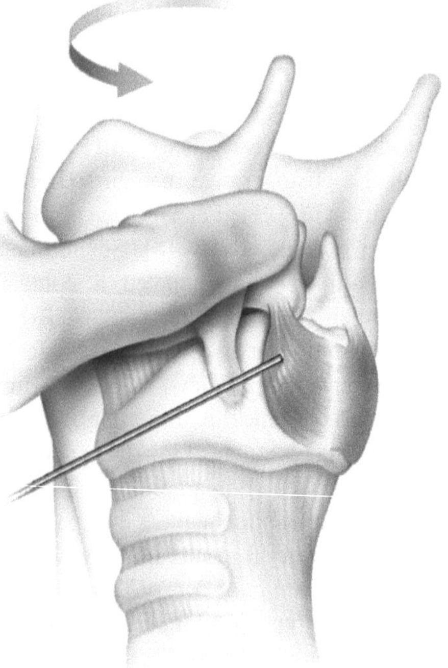

Fig. 20.13 Retrocricoid EMG-guided injection of the posterior cricoarytenoid muscle for abductor spasmodic dysphonia. Image from Sulica L, Blitzer A, Oper Tech Otolaryngol 15:76–80, 2004 © Elsevier, adapted and reprinted with permission [22]

have been described as treatment for AbSD [63, 64]. In some AbSD patients, decreased adductor muscle activity contributes to their symptoms and may be corrected by conventional medialization (type I) thyroplasty or bilateral medialization laryngoplasty [64, 65]. However, long-term outcomes in larger cohorts studies for these surgical procedures are rarely reported [63].

20.4 Concluding Remarks

Spasmodic dysphonia is a rare voice disorder with unknown etiology. The most common subtype is adductor spasmodic dysphonia, in which hyperactivity of the laryngeal adductor muscles occurs. Patients suffer from severe problems in communication, resulting in a significant decrease in quality of life. The current standard of therapy is injection with botulinum toxin in the main laryngeal adductor muscle: the thyroarytenoid muscle. Excellent voice quality can be achieved with an injection in the outpatient setting. However, the temporary effect and the unpredictable dose–response relationship between and within patients are serious disadvantages of botulinum injection treatment. A surgical procedure could potentially offer a more stable and long-lasting beneficial effect than botulinum toxin treatment. To achieve this, there are several surgical procedures described in literature. The three most frequently used techniques over the past 10 years are the SLAD-R, TP II, and TA myoneurectomy. Based on the current literature, no definitive conclusions can be drawn about what would be the best surgical procedure.

20.5 Recommendations for the Future

Botulinum toxin injections currently remain the gold standard for the treatment of AdSD as there is disagreement as to whether a surgical procedure is an equivalent alternative and, if this is the case, which procedure yields the best results. However, for some patients experiencing severe disadvantages of the temporal and unpredictable injection effect, a surgical procedure can offer the possibility of having more stable and long-lasting results. Currently, it is difficult to determine which surgical procedure is best. Most reported studies on postoperative results are based on small single-center case series, all using different outcome parameters. To be able to make a better assessment of the advantages and disadvantages of each surgical procedure, further research is needed. A single-center study comparing different surgical modalities in a randomized setting, or a multicenter study using standardizes diagnostic and outcome measurement protocols, is recommended.

References

1. Neychev VK, et al. The functional neuroanatomy of dystonia. Neurobiol Dis. 2011;42(2):185–201.
2. Izdebski K. Symptomatology of adductor spasmodic dysphonia: a physiologic model. J Voice. 1992;6(4):306–19.
3. Simonyan K, Ludlow CL. Abnormal activation of the primary somatosensory cortex in spasmodic dysphonia: an fMRI study. Cereb Cortex. 2010;20(11):2749–59.
4. Pitman MJ. Treatment of spasmodic dysphonia with a neuromodulating electrical implant. Laryngoscope. 2014;124(11):2537–43.
5. Cannito MP, Kahane JC, Chorna L. Vocal aging and adductor spasmodic dysphonia: response to botulinum toxin injection. Clin Interv Aging. 2008;3(1):131–51.
6. Whurr R, Lorch M. Review of differential diagnosis and management of spasmodic dysphonia. Curr Opin Otolaryngol Head Neck Surg. 2016;24(3):203–7.
7. Hillel AD. The study of laryngeal muscle activity in normal human subjects and in patients with laryngeal dystonia using multiple fine-wire electromyography. Laryngoscope. 2001;111(4 Pt 2 Suppl 97):1–47.
8. Tsuji DH, et al. Endoscopic laser thyroarytenoid myoneurectomy in patients with adductor spasmodic dysphonia: a pilot study on long-term outcome on voice quality. J Voice. 2012;26(5):666.e7–12.
9. Cannito MP, Johnson JP. Spastic dysphonia: a continuum disorder. J Commun Disord. 1981;14(3):215–33.
10. Kirke DN, Frucht SJ, Simonyan K. Alcohol responsiveness in laryngeal dystonia: a survey study. J Neurol. 2015;262(6):1548–56.
11. Barkmeier JM, Case JL, Ludlow CL. Identification of symptoms for spasmodic dysphonia and vocal tremor: a comparison of expert and nonexpert judges. J Commun Disord. 2001;34(1–2):21–37.
12. Hintze JM, et al. Spasmodic dysphonia: a review. Part 1: pathogenic factors. Otolaryngol Head Neck Surg. 2017;157(4):551–7.

13. Paniello RC, Barlow J, Serna JS. Longitudinal follow-up of adductor spasmodic dysphonia patients after botulinum toxin injection: quality of life results. Laryngoscope. 2008;118(3):564–8.
14. Rumbach AF, et al. An open-label study of sodium oxybate in Spasmodic dysphonia. Laryngoscope. 2017;127(6):1402–7.
15. Scott AB. Botulinum toxin injection into extraocular muscles as an alternative to strabismus surgery. Ophthalmology. 1980;87(10):1044–9.
16. Blitzer A, et al. Electromyographic findings in focal laryngeal dystonia (spastic dysphonia). Ann Otol Rhinol Laryngol. 1985;94(6 Pt 1):591–4.
17. Hambleton P. Clostridium botulinum toxins: a general review of involvement in disease, structure, mode of action and preparation for clinical use. J Neurol. 1992;239(1):16–20.
18. Cha W, et al. Liquid-type botulinum toxin type a in adductor spasmodic dysphonia: a prospective pilot study. J Voice. 2017;31(3):378 e19–24.
19. Wong DL, et al. Effect of neuromuscular activity on the response to botulinum toxin injections in spasmodic dysphonia. J Otolaryngol. 1995;24(4):209–16.
20. Shoffel-Havakuk H, et al. Common practices in botulinum toxin injection for spasmodic dysphonia treatment: a national survey. Laryngoscope. 2019;129(7):1650–6.
21. Blitzer A, Brin MF, Stewart CF. Botulinum toxin management of spasmodic dysphonia (laryngeal dystonia): a 12-year experience in more than 900 patients. Laryngoscope. 1998;108(10):1435–41.
22. Sulica L, Blitzer A. Botulinum toxin treatment of spasmodic dysphonia. Oper Tech Otolaryngol Head Neck Surg. 2004;15(2):76–80.
23. Green DC, et al. Point-touch technique of botulinum toxin injection for the treatment of spasmodic dysphonia. Ann Otol Rhinol Laryngol. 1992;101(11):883–7.
24. Ford CN, Bless DM, Lowery JD. Indirect laryngoscopic approach for injection of botulinum toxin in spasmodic dysphonia. Otolaryngol Head Neck Surg. 1990;103(5 (Pt 1)):752–8.
25. Rhew K, Fiedler DA, Ludlow CL. Technique for injection of botulinum toxin through the flexible nasolaryngoscope. Otolaryngol Head Neck Surg. 1994;111(6):787–94.
26. Blitzer A. Spasmodic dysphonia and botulinum toxin: experience from the largest treatment series. Eur J Neurol. 2010;17(Suppl 1):28–30.
27. Novakovic D, et al. Botulinum toxin treatment of adductor spasmodic dysphonia: longitudinal functional outcomes. Laryngoscope. 2011;121(3):606–12.
28. Zhao K, Guillaud M, Hu A. Factors associated with failure of botulinum toxin injection in adductor spasmodic dysphonia. Ann Otol Rhinol Laryngol. 2020;129(10):996–1002.
29. Silverman EP, et al. Combined modality treatment of adductor spasmodic dysphonia. J Voice. 2012;26(1):77–86.
30. Murry T, Woodson GE. Combined-modality treatment of adductor spasmodic dysphonia with botulinum toxin and voice therapy. J Voice. 1995;9(4):460–5.
31. Pearson EJ, Sapienza CM. Historical approaches to the treatment of Adductor-Type Spasmodic Dysphonia (ADSD): review and tutorial. NeuroRehabilitation. 2003;18(4):325–38.
32. Dedo HH. Recurrent laryngeal nerve section for spastic dysphonia. Ann Otol Rhinol Laryngol. 1976;85(4 Pt 1):451–9.
33. Aronson AE, De Santo LW. Adductor spastic dysphonia: three years after recurrent laryngeal nerve resection. Laryngoscope. 1983;93(1):1–8.
34. Biller HF, Som ML, Lawson W. Laryngeal nerve crush for spastic dysphonia. Ann Otol Rhinol Laryngol. 1983;92(5 Pt 1):469.
35. Fritzell B, et al. Long-term results of recurrent laryngeal nerve resection for adductor spasmodic dysphonia. J Voice. 1993;7(2):172–8.
36. Weed DT, et al. Long-term follow-up of recurrent laryngeal nerve avulsion for the treatment of spastic dysphonia. Ann Otol Rhinol Laryngol. 1996;105(8):592–601.
37. Blitzer A, Brin MF. Laryngeal dystonia: a series with botulinum toxin therapy. Ann Otol Rhinol Laryngol. 1991;100(2):85–9.
38. Ludlow CL, et al. Spasmodic dysphonia: botulinum toxin injection after recurrent nerve surgery. Otolaryngol Head Neck Surg. 1990;102(2):122–31.
39. Berke GS, et al. Selective laryngeal adductor denervation-reinnervation: a new surgical treatment for adductor spasmodic dysphonia. Ann Otol Rhinol Laryngol. 1999;108(3):227–31.
40. Chhetri DK, et al. Long-term follow-up results of selective laryngeal adductor denervation-reinnervation surgery for adductor spasmodic dysphonia. Laryngoscope. 2006;116(4):635–42.
41. Long JL, Berke GS. Selective laryngeal adductor denervation-reinnervation surgery for spasmodic dysphonia. Oper Tech Otolaryngol Head Neck Surg. 2012;23(3):183–7.
42. Mendelsohn AH, Berke GS. Surgery or botulinum toxin for adductor spasmodic dysphonia: a comparative study. Ann Otol Rhinol Laryngol. 2012;121(4):231–8.
43. Hussain A, Shakeel M. Selective lateral laser thyroarytenoid myotomy for adductor spasmodic dysphonia. J Laryngol Otol. 2010;124(8):886–91.
44. Allegretto M, et al. Selective denervation: reinnervation for the control of adductor spasmodic dysphonia. J Otolaryngol. 2003;32(3):185–9.
45. Isshiki N. Vocal mechanics as the basis for phonosurgery. Laryngoscope. 1998;108(12):1761–6.
46. Isshiki N, et al. Thyroplasty for adductor spasmodic dysphonia: further experiences. Laryngoscope. 2001;111(4 Pt 1):615–21.
47. Isshiki N, et al. Midline lateralization thyroplasty for adductor spasmodic dysphonia. Ann Otol Rhinol Laryngol. 2000;109(2):187–93.
48. Isshiki N, Yamamoto I, Fukagai S. Type 2 thyroplasty for spasmodic dysphonia: fixation using a titanium bridge. Acta Otolaryngol. 2004;124(3):309–12.

49. Sanuki T, Isshiki N. Overall evaluation of effectiveness of type II thyroplasty for adductor spasmodic dysphonia. Laryngoscope. 2007;117(12):2255–9.
50. Sanuki T, Isshiki N. Outcomes of type II thyroplasty for adductor spasmodic dysphonia: analysis of revision and unsatisfactory cases. Acta Otolaryngol. 2009;129(11):1287–93.
51. Sanuki T, Yumoto E. Long-term evaluation of type 2 Thyroplasty with titanium bridges for adductor spasmodic dysphonia. Otolaryngol Head Neck Surg. 2017;157(1):80–4.
52. Chan SW, et al. Long-term results of type II thyroplasty for adductor spasmodic dysphonia. Laryngoscope. 2004;114(9):1604–8.
53. Tsuji DH, et al. Impact in vocal quality in partial myectomy and neurectomy endoscopic of thyroarytenoid muscle in patients with adductor spasmodic dysphonia. Braz J Otorhinolaryngol. 2006;72(2):261–6.
54. Schuering JHC, et al. Adductor spasmodic dysphonia: botulinum toxin a injections or laser thyroarytenoid myoneurectomy? A comparison from the patient perspective. Laryngoscope. 2020;130(3):741–6.
55. Su CY, et al. Transoral laser ventricular fold resection and thyroarytenoid myoneurectomy for adductor spasmodic dysphonia: long-term outcome. Laryngoscope. 2010;120(2):313–8.
56. Nakamura K, et al. Surgical treatment for adductor spasmodic dysphonia—efficacy of bilateral thyroarytenoid myectomy under microlaryngoscopy. Acta Otolaryngol. 2008;128(12):1348–53.
57. Nomoto M, et al. The comparison of thyroarytenoid muscle myectomy and type II thyroplasty for spasmodic dysphonia. J Voice. 2015;29(4):501–6.
58. Remacle M, et al. Bipolar radiofrequency-induced thermotherapy (rfitt) for the treatment of spasmodic dysphonia. A report of three cases. Eur Arch Otorhinolaryngol. 2005;262(10):871–4.
59. Kim HS, et al. Radiofrequency thyroarytenoid myothermy for treatment of adductor spasmodic dysphonia: how we do it. Clin Otolaryngol. 2008;33(6):621–5.
60. Blitzer A, et al. Abductor laryngeal dystonia: a series treated with botulinum toxin. Laryngoscope. 1992;102(2):163–7.
61. Woodson G, Hochstetler H, Murry T. Botulinum toxin therapy for abductor spasmodic dysphonia. J Voice. 2006;20(1):137–43.
62. Klein AM, et al. Vocal outcome measures after bilateral posterior cricoarytenoid muscle botulinum toxin injections for abductor spasmodic dysphonia. Otolaryngol Head Neck Surg. 2008;139(3):421–3.
63. Benito DA, Ferster APO, Sataloff RT. Bilateral posterior cricoarytenoid myoneurectomy for abductor spasmodic dysphonia. J Voice. 2020;34(1):127–9.
64. Shaw GY, Sechtem PR, Rideout B. Posterior cricoarytenoid myoplasty with medialization thyroplasty in the management of refractory abductor spasmodic dysphonia. Ann Otol Rhinol Laryngol. 2003;112(4):303–6.
65. Postma GN, Blalock PD, Koufman JA. Bilateral medialization laryngoplasty. Laryngoscope. 1998;108(10):1429–34.

Nerve Reconstruction

21

Jean-Paul Marie, Kate Heathcote,
Frederic Crampon, and Sophie Deneuve

21.1 Introduction

Laryngeal nerve lesions are a common occurrence. They have medical or surgical etiologies. Depending on the level of the lesion, uni- or bilaterally, the presentation is different as well as the type of treatment. Moreover, the clinical outcome will evolve over time, depending of the degree of natural reinnervation.

In unilateral vocal cord paralysis, dysphonia is the major problem encountered. Aspiration may be present at the onset of the disease. It can increase pulmonary pathology, especially because coughing is not efficient. The main goal of treatments is to place the paralyzed vocal fold on the midline. Medialization techniques are described in previous chapters. A nonselective reinnervation can be performed, even in children. This procedure is more and more developed.

In bilateral paralysis, vocal cords are usually in a paramedian position. This may result in inspiratory dyspnea. However, phonation is satisfactorily preserved. Classical modes of treatment for bilateral paralysis are aimed at enlarging the

Core Messages

- Trunk to trunk anastomosis of a recurrent laryngeal nerve (RLN) does not allow recovery of vocal cord mobility.
- Vocal cord mobility is not necessary to achieve good voice results, but good muscular trophicity is required.
- Nonselective reinnervation is the optimal treatment of unilateral recurrent laryngeal nerve lesion. It can be performed at the time of the injury or delayed.
- Dissection of the distal portion of the RLN is always possible by the retrograde intralaryngeal approach.
- Ansa hypoglossi to RLN trunk anastomosis is the optimal technique in unilateral vocal cord paralysis, even in children.
- Nerve transfers have to be long enough to follow the laryngeal movements during swallowing.
- In bilateral RLN lesion, with the vocal cords in adductory position, treatments must respect the vocal cord integrity.
- New techniques of bilateral motor selective reinnervation of the larynx should be considered, only in cases when the arytenoids remain passively mobile.
- The phrenic nerve is the optimal nerve supply for posterior cricoarytenoid muscle reinnervation. Preservation of some

J.-P. Marie (✉) · F. Crampon · S. Deneuve
Otolaryngology, Head & Neck Surgery Department, University Hospital of Rouen, Rouen, Normandy, France
e-mail: jean-paul.marie@chu-rouen.fr; frederic.crampon@chu-rouen.fr

K. Heathcote
Otolaryngology, Poole Hospital NHS Trust, Longfleet Road, Poole, Dorset, UK

M. Remacle, H. E. Eckel (eds.), *Textbook of Surgery of Larynx and Trachea*,
https://doi.org/10.1007/978-3-031-09621-1_21

of its roots can spare some diaphragm innervation and function.

- Functional reinnervation is achieved after some delay: it is the time for axons to get the targeted muscles.

glottis (described in other chapters); unpredictable hoarseness and some lack of protective closure result with some of them. Selective laryngeal reinnervation can solve these problems.

There is a long history of reinnervation research in animal models but still limited experience in humans, but with growing interest. In this chapter, we present the current state of clinical applications and outcomes.

21.2 Anatomical Landmarks and Prerequisites

The intrinsic laryngeal muscles, with the exception of the cricothyroid muscle, are all innervated by the recurrent laryngeal nerve (RLN). The cricothyroid muscle is innervated by the external branch of the superior laryngeal nerve (SLN).

The RLN enters the larynx posteromedially to the cricothyroid joint which is an important landmark for its surgical identification. Intralaryngeally, it divides into several motor branches. Roughly, the posteromedial bundle runs to the posterior cricoarytenoid muscle (PCA) and the interarytenoid muscles. The anteromedial bundle (adductor branch) innervates the remaining intrinsic laryngeal muscles. One branch of the RLN, usually branching extralaryngeally, forms a junction with the SLN (the ansa galeni). The precise intralaryngeal anatomy is very variable and has been studied by different authors [1–4]. The intralaryngeal RLN branch for the PCA is sometimes unique, sometimes multiple, originating from the common branch of the adductor muscles. The main trunk of the RLN carries motor fibers to both the intrinsic laryngeal adductor and abductor muscles and contains 500–1000 myelinated nerve fibers. The ratio of adductor and abductor fibers is approximately 3:1.

The intraneural structure of the RLN forms no topographical separation of the adductor and abductor fibers. Sunderland and Swaney found a constantly changing pattern with frequent communication between fascicules [5] .This plexiform disposition of the axons inside the nerve trunk explains the failure of direct nerve anastomosis: misdirected regeneration of the axons to the antagonist muscles (synkinesis) and subsequent lack of recovery of the vocal cord mobility in case of trunk to trunk anastomosis or spontaneous recovery after a severe RLN lesion.

The motor units of the adductor muscles are small and have 2–20 muscle fibers per motor unit and muscle fibers have mainly fast contraction times. The abductor muscle (PCA) has much larger motor units with 200–250 muscle fibers per motor unit, mainly fibers with slower contraction time. Characteristics of a muscle fiber (fast or slow contraction time) are determined by the axonal supply and can change if a new nerve supply is provided.

Nerve lesions, if not too much severe, have a strong tendency to recover. It is particularly important for the RLN. Several experimental studies have shown nerve regrowth through an interrupted RLN [6, 7]. However, synkinesis explains that the vocal cord stays immobile.

Some additional concepts have to be understood for laryngeal reinnervation. Nerve lesion stimulates axonal sprouting in the vicinity of the injured muscle. On the contrary, axon-sprouting inhibitor factor is normally found in innervated muscle. Moreover, an innervated muscle will not accept some additional innervation, except if the original or the suppletive nerve is injured. For that reason, at the time of a reinnervation procedure, it is necessary to remove the spontaneous recovered innervation in order to improve the ability to receive a new one [8].

Biochemical properties of a reinnervated muscle are determined by the nerve transfer. For this reason, the phrenic nerve, with slow contraction fibers and firing in inspiration, is an ideal nerve graft for PCA reinnervation.

Denervation atrophy hinders reinnervation. But spontaneous reinnervation by nerves coming from the vicinity or regenerated laryngeal nerves prevents severe denervation atrophy for a long time. For these reasons, reinnervation can be proposed some years after laryngeal nerve lesions [9, 10].

In general terms, reinnervation can be categorized as selective or nonselective.

1. Selective reinnervation is the technique of reinnervating the abductors and adductors separately with the aim of restoring the vocal cord mobility. Thus, inspiratory glottic opening may be achieved, and laryngeal tonicity or closure is obtained. This is required in bilateral vocal cord paralysis.
2. Nonselective reinnervation involves anastomosis to the main stem of the RLN, leading to reinnervation of both the abductor and adductor muscles. It can be performed at the time of an acute nerve injury or in chronic vocal cord paralysis. The aim is to increase tonicity and stabilize the arytenoids as do the springs of a trampoline on the central surface.

Properties of the donor nerve have to be very similar to the original nerve, having the same function of the targeted muscles, mainly for selective functional reinnervation. The phrenic nerve and branches of the hypoglossal nerves have these properties.

But what are the consequences of removal of the donor nerve?

It has been shown that harvesting some of the several cervical roots of one phrenic nerve can be used in animals but also in humans with negligible consequences on diaphragm function [11–13].

21.3 Nonselective Reinnervation (in Unilateral Nerve Lesion)

21.3.1 Acute Lesion of the Laryngeal Nerves

A common question for the laryngologist is what to do in case of acute laryngeal nerve resection, when the neck is open. The answer is simple: always try to fix it, by nerve reconstruction, during the same operating time.

At the cervical level, injury of the recurrent nerve can be induced by laryngeal trauma (cricotracheal desinsertion) or thyroid surgery. Nerve resection is sometimes performed at the time of thyroid cancer resection. Optimal rehabilitation can be obtained by nerve anastomosis. A direct anastomosis can be carried out between two stumps of the RLN, using free nerve graft if it is necessary to bridge the gap between them [14–16]. If the proximal stump for the RLN cannot be found, a neighboring nerve can be used, mainly the ansa hypoglossi, as described by Crumley [17] and later on by Simo et al. [16, 18, 19].

No mobility recovery will be observed; nevertheless, the nonselective reinnervation will achieve optimal voice results after a 4- to 8-month delay. Temporary improvement can be obtained while waiting for the axonal growth, by endoscopic medialization, if possible with resorbable material (Gelfoam, fat).

When the RLN is injured at the thoracic level, immediate treatment can be done using immediate passive medialization and/or reinnervation. Medialization, associated to an adaptated nutrition, is very useful to prevent aspiration and to help cough efficacy, which are important in pulmonary healing.

Vagus nerve lesion at the cervical or thoracic level can benefit from the same approach.

Moreover, a vagus nerve lesion done at the skull base or intracranial level will induce vocal cord paralysis (often in a lateral position) and a sensitive denervation of the homolateral hemilarynx. The risk of aspiration is very high and justifies an early reconstructive method. Early endoscopic or external additional medialization is required, not always sufficient to avoid aspiration.

In case of unilateral RLN or vagus lesion, nonselective reinnervation is required, even if some authors have proposed unilateral selective reinnervation [20].

Sensitive rehabilitation can be done, in some favorable cases, by superior laryngeal nerve (SLN) anastomosis (directly or using a free nerve graft) [21]. In animal experiments, anastomosis to the superficial cervical plexus was successful [22].

21.3.2 Reinnervation of Chronic Unilateral Vocal Cord Paralysis

21.3.2.1 Inferior Laryngeal Nerve Lesion (Recurrent Nerve Paralysis)

General Indications

Nonselective reinnervation becomes more and more popular, even in children.

In the previous version of this textbook, we mentioned that reinnervation is indicated:

- When the nerve lesion is severe, either by known resection or when the time elapsed since vocal fold palsy has not demonstrated any functional and electrophysiologic recovery. By now, we think that some incomplete denervation or unfavorable synkinesis [23, 24] can be some good indication [10].
- When an optimal voice result is required (voice professionals).
- When the functional handicap is mainly dysphonia, with breathy voice or diplophonia induced by the lack of adduction of the vocal cords. We now think with K Zur that chronic aspiration can be a good indication [10, 25]. In some cases where the arytenoid is rotated inside the larynx, the Nonselective laryngeal reinnervation can improve dyspnea [10].
- Recent lesions (less than 3 years) are preferred to old lesions. However, poor residual innervation preserves trophicity and can allow successful reinnervation in adults and children, after long-term denervation [9, 10, 26, 27].

Recurrent nerve lesion at the entrance of the larynx is not a contraindication. An intralaryngeal retrograde dissection can easily be done.

Reinnervation can be completed by passive medialization while awaiting axonal regrowth (remember the axonal growth is a slow phenomenon: 1 mm per day).

No recovery of the mobility is expected. Only an improved trophicity of the ipsilateral larynx and a better tone are achieved, allowing better approximation of the contralateral healthy vocal cord in phonation. Passive mobility (lack of cricoarytenoid ankylosis) of the arytenoid is not required.

Previous medical history should be carefully assessed, specifically previous operative report with description of the recurrent nerve lesions (severity, level) and extent of the neck dissection (to anticipate the status of the potential donor nerve).

However, previous resection of the RLN close to the larynx does not preclude some intralaryngeal identification by retrograde dissection and neurotization [10].

Previous radiotherapy or severe neck fibrosis will add some difficulties.

Physical examination verifies the lack of vocal cord scars and the integrity of the other cranial nerves: a high-level lesion of the vagus nerve, in the brain stem or skull base, in addition to sensitive and pharyngeal contraction disease, with subsequent poor result.

Because the technique of reinnervation usually requires recurrent nerve resection, it is usually necessary to make sure, via laryngeal EMG, that only poor or no residual innervation remains into the intrinsic laryngeal muscles. Severe neurogenic pattern or fibrillation potentials are best suitable traces. On the contrary, fair enrichment in phonation means good residual innervation and will preclude a good functional result (reinnervation will not improve the result). Replacement of bad synkinesis remains to be discussed.

Usual preoperative voice assessments are required: questionnaires (VHI 100 or 10, or others), voice recordings for perceptual analysis and future comparisons (and medicolegal reasons), computerized analysis, and videoscopy imaging.

Surgical Technique (Including Specific Recommendations)

The Ansa Cervicalis to RLN Anastomosis ("Ansa Technique") Fig. 21.1

The ansa cervicalis to RLN anastomosis described by Crumley [17, 28, 29] is today the more frequently used technique.

A horizontal skin crease incision is performed at the level of the lower border of the cricoid cartilage, or in place of a previous thyroidectomy scar (which necessitates a more extended dissection). The plathysma is incised and then the superficial fascia, watching for the ansa cervicalis, on the jugular vein. The ansa can usually be found at the surface of the jugular vein; it can also be located by careful examination of the posterior aspect of the omohyoid or sternohyoid muscles. Once identified, the nerve is dissected proximally to the lateral edge of the jugular vein and distally into the strap muscles (electric stimulation of the nerve can be performed for confirmation: no curarization for this step). If possible, the descending branch of the hypoglossi is chosen, ensuring the anterograde direction of the axons to the future recipient nerve. A rubber sling is placed around the nerve. It is not transected at this stage.

The recurrent laryngeal nerve is identified next. In cases of intact cervical area (when the RLN lesion was produced by thoracic lesion, for instance), the RLN can be identified inferior to the thyroid gland and dissected superiorly (Fig. 21.1).

In more frequent cases of cervical injury, a retrograde dissection can be performed. The larynx must be rotated by applying upward traction by a skin hook placed on the posterior border of the thyroid cartilage. The constrictor muscles are dissected off the cartilage and the RLN is revealed lying just deep to them, behind the cricothyroid joint, entering the larynx.

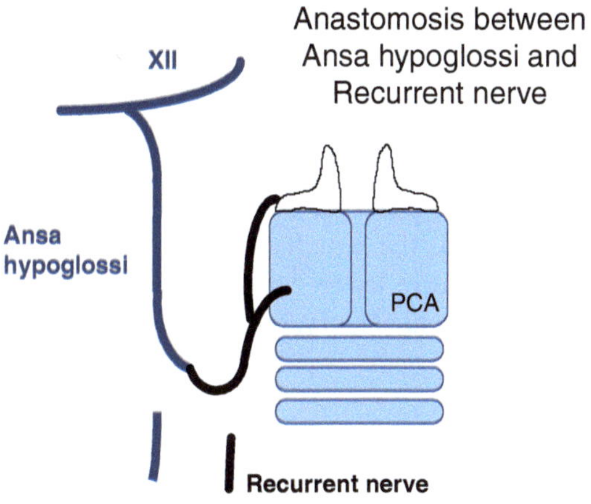

Fig. 21.1 Ansa-recurrent nerve anastomosis. Schematic posterior view of the procedure. Left side. XII, hypoglossal nerve; PCA, posterior cricoarytenoid muscle (courtesy of Jean-Paul Marie)

Once the nerves have been identified, it is possible to judge the lengths to form a tension-free anastomosis. Moreover, the ascending movement of the larynx on swallowing must be taken into account. The ansa will be cut at the place where the diameter is similar to that of the RLN.

End-to-end anastomosis is performed using standard microsurgical techniques, under magnification. After frank section of the nerves, extremities are prepared by resecting the axonal excess. The epineurium is preserved. Epi-perineural anastomosis is performed using 4–6 sutures of 9/0 spatulated needle. The anastomosis can be protected and stabilized either by biologic glue or by a surrounding vein or fat tissue. Hemostasis is secured and the wound closed in layers. It is usually not necessary to insert a drain. No antibioprophylaxis is required.

Even if a retrograde intralaryngeal dissection of the recurrent has been carried out, no hematoma or excessive laryngeal edema has been observed in our experience.

Usually, no postoperative aspiration is observed. No gastric feeding tube is required.

The procedure can be carried out as a day care.

Alteration of the voice can be observed for the next few weeks, which is a consequence of the removal of some remaining innervation of the hemilarynx, but more often, the resection of the RLN is performed in case of pretty severe larynx denervation.

Voice improvement is observed after 4 months, depending on the duration of denervation and the age of the patient. A temporary medialization can be performed at the time of surgery while awaiting efficacy of reinnervation, by Gelfoam (or fat injection in our experience).

Crumley has published very good phonatory results based on a large series [17, 28, 29].

Other authors have shown similar good longterm results [10, 27, 30, 31]. We have experienced this technique for 20 years.

Prospective randomized evaluation are lacking, even if a few comparative results with medialization are described [27, 32].

We have performed this technique as a salvage procedure with success [10].

It is now currently performed in **children**.

In the pediatric population, reinnervation offers several advantages over the alternative of injection medialization or framework surgery. It provides a permanent result without disruption of the growing larynx and can be performed under general anesthesia.

Smith et al. [26, 33, 34] and Zur et al. [25, 35] have developed this technique, followed by several authors [36–40]. A meta-analysis or prospective small series gave some advantage to nonselective reinnervation in comparison to medialization [41, 42].

Technical Variations

In order to solve the lack of ansa hypoglossi, the hypoglossal nerve trunk use was described by Paniello, as it is performed in facial nerve rehabilitation [43].

Contralateral ansa was used by Wang et al. [44].

Others have used the thyrohyoid branch of the hypoglossi (which can be found higher and in front of the ansa) [45].

Precious descriptions of the anatomical landmarks of hypoglossal branches have been reported [4, 46].

The Nerve-Muscle Pedicle Implantation of HM Tucker

Having introduced the nerve muscle pedicle (NMP) technique implantation for posterior cricoarytenoid reinnervation in bilateral vocal cord paralysis (see below), Tucker applied this technique for adductor muscle reinnervation [47–49]. Omohyoid muscle nerve supply was used, assuming that strap muscles are contracting in phonation during pitch control.

This technique can be performed in cases where RLN cannot be found.

The incision is performed horizontally in regard of the cricothyroid cartilage area. A block of omohyoid muscle is dissected and mobilized with the nerve supply (branch from the hypoglossal nerve). The strap muscles are then retracted and mobilized to expose the thyroid cartilage (as for thyroplasty). A posteriorly based perichondrial flap is created. A block of cartilage is removed with the Stryker saw (or the fissure burr) from the lower 50% of the thyroid ala so that an intact posterior and inferior strut of cartilage is left intact. Having incised the internal perichondrium, the fibers of the lateral thyroarytenoid muscle are exposed. The NMP pedicle is approximated to this muscle and sutured in place with two or three 5/0 nylon sutures. The wound is closed in a normal fashion.

Combinations

Reinnervation techniques can be performed in addition to medialization. It was proposed by HM Tucker who demonstrated that long-term results after thyroplasty are not so good, due to supposed muscular atrophy [48, 50].

The ansa recurrent technique can be combined to arytenoid adduction [51, 52].

21.3.2.2 Superior Laryngeal Nerve Lesions

The superior laryngeal nerve (SLN) is responsible for the sensitive innervation of the supraglottis area by the internal branch (iSLN). The external branch supplies the cricothyroid muscle. It can be injured at a high level, during skull base surgery, for instance, associating sensitive deficit and motor paralysis of all the intrinsic laryngeal muscles in the ipsilateral side, resulting in vocal cord paralysis often in an abductory position with breathy voice and aspiration (increased by lack of pharyngeal propulsion). More often, the external branch of the SLN laryngeal nerve lesion can result as a complication of thyroid surgery, or from a viral isolated disease.

External Branch (or Cricoid Branch) of the Superior Laryngeal Nerve Lesions

It is often misdiagnosed, if the patient presents with mild dysphonia that becomes worse with pitch control. EMG of the cricothyroid (CT) muscle confirms the diagnosis.

Spontaneous recovery or speech therapy effects must be achieved before performing surgery. In addition to the framework surgery technique (cricothyroid approximation, thyroplasty), some reinnervation can be proposed.

El-Kashlan has used with success the technique of muscle-nerve-muscle reinnervation [53] described in cats by Hogikyan [54]. The principle is to implant a free nerve graft in a donor muscle (here, the CT muscle) and to implant the other stamp in the receptor denervated muscle. Some reinnervation can be achieved and verified by electrical stimulation of the contralateral side.

Internal Branch of the SLN Lesions

They can produce some aspiration mainly if associated to a motor nerve as vagus nerve denervation. Sensory deficit can result also from stroke and induce some severe aspiration problems. Diagnosis can be confirmed by fibroscopic sensory tests, testing the ability of the patient to feel air pressure or fibroscope tip contact. In cases of failure in swallowing reeducation, this can be corrected by reinnervation.

Animal experiments in dogs [55], and rabbits by our research team [56], have demonstrated the feasibility of laryngeal sensory reinnervation either by direct iSLN anastomosis or by other nerve transfers, primarily by the great auricular nerve. This type of neurorraphy of the great auricular nerve was reported in two patients by Aviv et al. with success [21].

21.3.2.3 Vagus Nerve Lesion

It can be done at the time of schwannoma or vagus paraganglioma removal. Free nerve graft is usually required to bridge the gap between the two nerve stumps. Superficial cervical plexus (great auricular nerve) can be easily used, harvested even by the same wound, often by a separate incision placed below the external ear. A 5- to 7-cm portion can be harvested if the nerve is followed up in the parotid gland.

However, the longer the nerve graft is required, the longer time required for recovery. For that reason, we now perform a nonselective reinnervation with the ansa as described above. Some authors [20] have proposed selective unilateral reinnervation in one case of vagal paraganglioma resection.

If the vagus nerve lesion is at a very high level (skull base, or brain stem lesion), cricothyroid and sensory denervation is observed. The combination of RLN reinnervation and external and internal laryngeal nerve reinnervation can be proposed using the abovementioned techniques. In our limited experience, combination with passive medialization techniques or pharyngeal resection can also prevent severe aspiration while waiting for the nerve supply recovery.

21.4 Selective Motor Reinnervation (in Bilateral Nerve Lesion)

Selective reinnervation is defined as reinnervation of one or several groups of muscles dedicated to a function of adduction or abduction of the vocal cord. The ultimate goal of selective reinnervation is recovery of vocal cord mobility.

In cases of bilateral RLN paralysis, after some spontaneous reinnervation with subsequent synkinesis, the vocal cords are usually immobile in a paramedian position, with dyspnea but fairly good voice. The main problem is then to recover the abductory function.

A number of animal experiments have been done for decades with some success. The principle was to bring a motor supply, with an inspiratory trigger, to the abductor muscle (the posterior cricoarytenoid muscle [PCA]), often unilaterally, or sometimes on both sides. The motor nerve supply was either branches from the hypoglossal nerve or roots or the main trunk of the phrenic nerve.

Reinnervation was performed using three different techniques: nerve implantation into the muscle, nerve-muscle pedicle implantation, or selective nerve anastomosis. A combined method can be performed, and selective simultaneous reinnervation of both adductors and abductors can be done, on one or both sides [7].

We will consider only the techniques used in humans. Indications, techniques, follow-up, and results will be presented.

21.4.1 Surgical Techniques

21.4.1.1 Nerve-Muscle Pedicle with the Ansa Hypoglossi

The **nerve muscle pedicle technique described by Tucker et al.**, using an ansa hypoglossi nerve supply, was originally intended to be used as a means for reinnervating a transplanted larynx. It has since been modified and used in reinnervation of bilaterally paralyzed vocal cords in humans [47, 48]. The method was considered to be able to rapidly achieve some reinnervation. Adductor reinnervation was not performed because of the tendency of the vocal cords to return to the paramedian position when not actively abducted. Surgery was performed on one side alone.

Technique

Skin incision is made at the lower border of the thyroid cartilage. Incision of the plathysma and identification of the sternocleidomastoid muscle are performed. The anterior belly of the omohyoid muscle and the jugular vein are identified. The ansa hypoglossi can usually be seen lying on or crossing the internal jugular vein. The fascia overlying the ansa hypoglossi is carefully incised, and the nerve is traced proximally and distally to the first major branch, which is usually the one to the anterior belly of the omohyoid. A 2- to 3-mm square block of muscle, just large enough to include the point of entry and arborization of the nerve, is dissected from the omohyoid. The nerve-muscle pedicle is then isolated for a sufficient length to reach the larynx. The inferior constrictor muscle is then exposed. Blunt dissection and exposure of the PCA are carried out, whose fibers pass at a right angle to those of the inferior constrictor. Two or three 5-0 nylon sutures are placed in the posterior cricoarytenoid muscle and then sutured to the block of muscle that is part of the nerve-muscle pedicle.

Results

Tucker has reported a series of 214 patients with nerve-muscle pedicle in bilateral vocal cord paralysis of which 202 has at least 2 years of follow-up with 74% success. Deterioration was observed in 17% of these cases 2–5 years later (due to cricoarytenoid ankylosis for this author) [48]. Similar success was not confirmed by other authors and the technique is not often performed today. Main criticisms were the lack of active abduction of the arytenoid and the lack of EMG inspiratory activation. The procedure was thought to have some efficacy more by passive lateralization induced by the PCA scar than by efficient reinnervation. Moreover, the omohyoid and ansa activation during airway obstruction and hypoxia induces a self-limitation to its action [57].

Nevertheless, applying this technique, Fayoux et al. have recently published a series of 10 out of 16 abductions in children, with long-term outcome [58].

21.4.1.2 Selective Reinnervation Using the Phrenic Nerve

The phrenic nerve is able to produce an inspiratory firing to reinnervated muscles and was considered as an ideal nerve transfer for PCA reinnervation. Although unilateral phrenic nerve resection was considered to be well tolerated, some effort has been made to preserve nerve supply to the diaphragm.

Crumley et al. used a split phrenic nerve graft for PCA reinnervation [59] first in animals and then in humans [60] (Fig. 21.2).

The phrenic nerve was incised longitudinally on part of the circumference and a free nerve graft is then anastomosed to this harvested portion. The recurrent nerve trunk was sectioned to remove the residual innervation of the larynx and stimulate the ability of the muscle to accept a new innervation. The distal part of the nerve graft was anastomosed to the tiny abductor branch of the RLN inside the larynx.

Good results were achieved in animals, but the first human results, presented in 1983 [60], showed improvement in glottis diameter but no active arytenoid abduction.

Variations of this technique has been described in animals by Rice [61], Mahieu [62], and van Lith-Bijl et al. [62, 63]. They performed an extralaryngeal anastomosis of the phrenic nerve to the RLN main trunk and, sectioned inside the larynx, the adductor branch to implant it inside the PCA, guiding all the axons to that muscle.

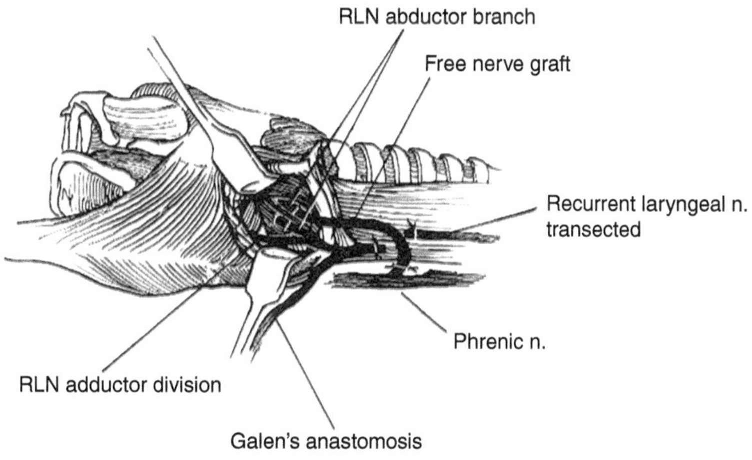

Fig. 21.2 Split-phrenic nerve graft procedure of RL Crumley (in bilateral vocal cord paralysis) [60]. Inspiratory phrenic nerve fibers are connected to the abductor branch of the RLN (for the PCA) through a free nerve graft

Crumley [64], Marie et al. [7, 65], and van Lith-Bijl et al. [66] refined this technique with selective simultaneous reinnervation of adductor (with the ansa) and abductor muscles (with the phrenic nerve graft), in animals, with some success.

Bilateral PCA reinnervation was performed in humans by Zheng at al. [67] on one side by phrenic nerve neurotization and on the contralateral side by the nerve muscle pedicle technique with the ansa. Arytenoid abduction was observed in five out of six patients, only on the phrenic nerve reinnervation side.

Li et al. [68] subsequently performed a series of bilateral PCA left phrenic nerve reinnervation in humans and reported some success.

Bilateral selective motor reinnervation of adductor and abductor laryngeal muscles (total motor reinnervation) by Marie et al. [7, 69] (Fig. 21.3a)

We have previously obtained successful results in dogs with unilateral selective reinnervation of both adductor and abductor muscles, using the ansa hypoglossi and the phrenic nerve, respectively [65]. In order to apply this technique in humans, we first studied the effects of partial phrenic nerve resection on respiration in rabbits and dogs and demonstrated that the resection of the upper phrenic nerve root had a slight effect on respiration [11, 70, 71]. Later on, we studied the possibilities of bilateral PCA reinnervation in dogs, in order to improve the glottis opening finally performing a total motor reinnervation of the larynx.

We showed that results were better with a few amount of axons for both PCA, provided by just one root from one phrenic nerve [57]. Contemporary reinnervation of adductors by the thyroid branch of both hypoglossal nerves can achieve optimal supply [72]. The technique can be used in a delayed manner, even in cases of synkinesis. Therefore, we were prompted to start a clinical prospective trial in humans. The first patient was operated on in 2003. Today, in our institution, more than 80 patients have undergone bilateral motor reinnervation with this technique.

Best indications are bilateral vocal cord paralysis in a paramedian position and dyspnea, without signs of recovery nor muscle atrophy (clinical and EMG diagnosis), without cricoarytenoid ankylosis. To check these conditions, a previous careful examination is performed, under awake and then general anesthesia with curarization [73, 74]. No previous laryngeal surgery must have been done, except tracheostomy or botulinum toxin (no scar on the vocal cord). Intact pulmonary function and diaphragm mobility must be verified. Transient tracheostomy at the time of surgery is required.

We have now extended indications to long-term denervation, in some bilateral vocal cord palsy in aperture (in rare cases of cricotracheal disruption) and in some cases of previous endolaryngeal treatments if passive mobility of the arycricoid joint is preserved. That is the subject of a prospective ethically approved trial.

Technique (Fig. 21.3a)

If not present, a tracheostomy is performed via a prior incision (usually, low neck horizontal scar after thyroidectomy). Horizontal cervicotomy at the level of the cricothyroid membrane, if possible, should be far from the unsterile tracheostomy.

Nerve Identification

A right phrenic nerve dissection ensues (convenient for right-handed surgeons; preserves the left diaphragm in case of aspiration and right lung atelectasis). Identification of the root distribution on the scalenus muscle is carefully assessed (Fig. 21.3c). A nerve stimulator is useful and lack of curarization is required. The upper phrenic nerve root will be used. Length is variable, sometimes no more than 2 cm, and necessitates the harvesting of a free nerve graft to elongate it. A 7- to 9-cm free nerve graft can be provided by the superficial cervical plexus (great auricular nerve [GAN]) (Fig. 21.3b). GAN can be harvested until the intraparotid branching: it will be used as a Y-shaped nerve graft for both PCA implantation. Alternatively, a sural nerve graft or some branches from the ansa can be used as interposition free nerve grafts.

Right and left dissection of the thyrohyoid branch of the hypoglossal nerves (THXII) is undertaken at the upper part of the anterior face of the thyrohyoid muscle (originating from the hypoglossal nerve, close to the hyoid bone, anterior from the ansa) (Fig. 21.3d).

Intralaryngeal dissection of the RLN branches proceeds: this necessitates hook positioning on the posterior border of the thyroid ala. The larynx is rotated and the cricothyroid joint identified. The inferior constrictor is sectioned just behind the joint. At this point, RLN distribution can be immediately found, even in scar situation which usually spares the retrocricoid area.

By now, we usually do not try to identify the RLN branch for the PCA which originates from a common branch for the interarytenoid muscle or from the adductor branch. The Y-shaped nerve graft will be inserted inside the PCA muscles.

A tunnel is created posterior to the cricoid cartilage, superficial to the PCA muscles.

The Y-shaped free nerve graft is passed left to right (single end first) through the retrocricoid tunnel such that the single end is ready to be attached to the previously identified root of the right phrenic nerve. The double ends of the Y graft then come to lie each one adjacent to its ipsilateral PCA. Each portion of the double-end Y graft is then implanted into each PCA. This is done by inserting the end of the graft in a small pocket, which is created in the muscle (vertical part). A 9/0 suture is used to secure the nerve in place and some tissue glue is applied.

The single end of the graft is anastomosed onto the root of the phrenic using a 9/0 epi-perineural suture. It is essential to ensure that there is no tension on these anastomoses and it may be prudent to pass the graft through a tunnel between the jugular vein and the carotid artery to shorten the distance.

The adductor muscles are reinnervated by transecting the main trunks of the RLNs. The distal stumps of the RLNs are swung upward and a free nerve graft is interposed between the stump and ipsilateral nerve to the thyrohyoid muscle on each side.

In the rare situation where the PCA branch has been identified, it is possible to make the anastomosis of the phrenic nerve root, via a lengthening graft, to the main trunk of the RLN. The adductor branch is then transected and the proximal stump anastomosed to another free cable graft (harvested from the ansa), which is passed through the retrocricoid tunnel to reach the contralateral side where it is anastomosed onto the PCA branch or implanted in the muscle. The distal stump of the adductor branch is then anastomosed via a free nerve graft to the thyrohyoid nerve on both sides.

Postoperatively, aspiration is present for a few days following surgery, necessitating a feeding tube, and tracheostomy can usually be removed within the fifth postoperative day. Resection of the RLN removes the paradoxical adduction during inspiration and usually decreases the laryngeal resistances. Voice recovery and improvement in ventilation should start within 6 to 9 months after the procedure.

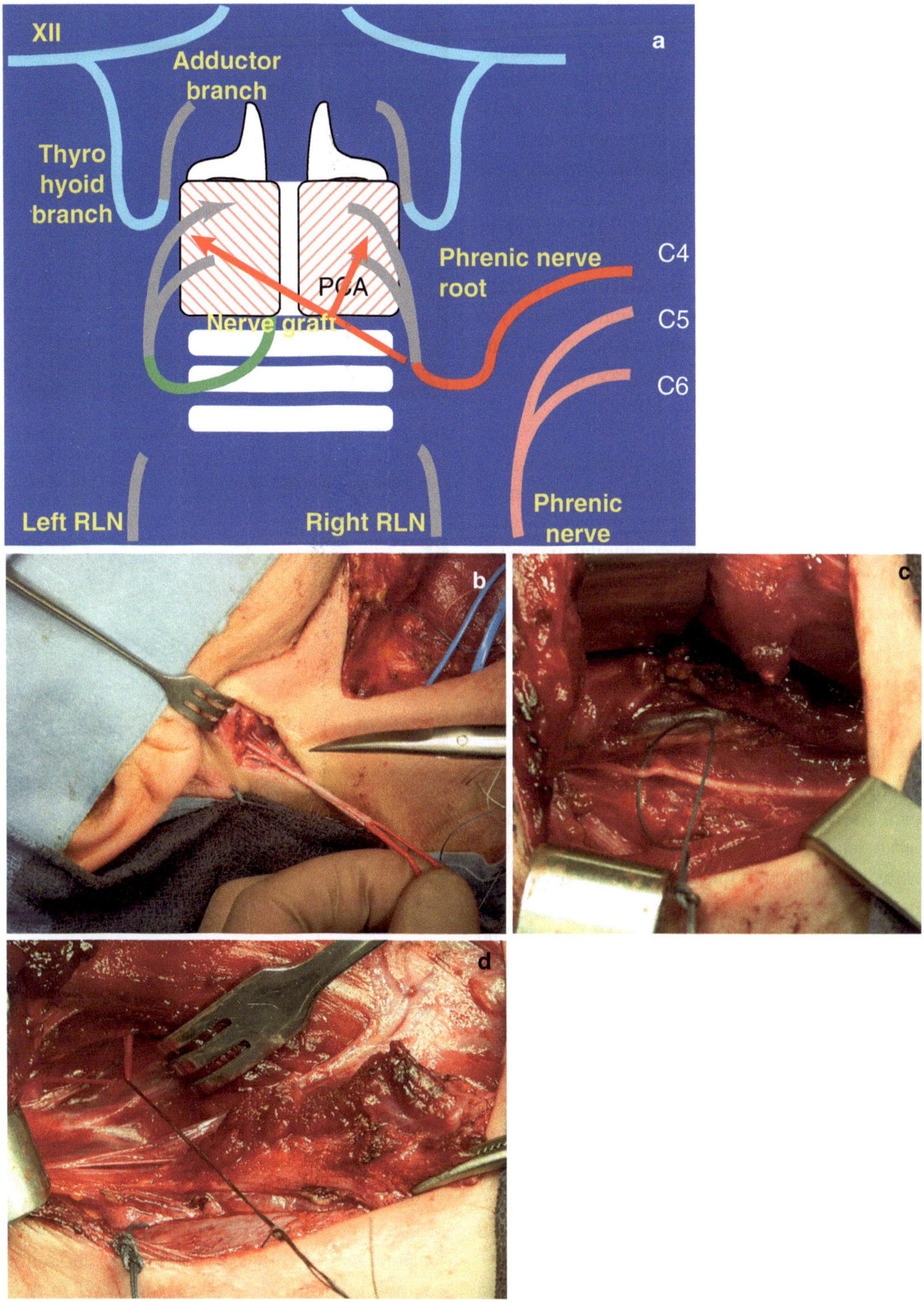

Fig. 21.3 (**a**) Total motor reinnervation of the larynx: both PCA reinnervation by the upper root of one phrenic nerve; reinnervation of both adductor muscles by thyrohyoid branches of both hypoglossal nerves. By now, the free interposition nerve graft is replaced by a Y-shaped lengthening nerve graft (in red) (courtesy of Jean-Paul Marie). (**b**) The greater auricular branch of the cervical plexus is dissected. (**c**) The phrenic nerve is carefully assessed and the upper branch identified. (**d**) The thyrohyoid branch of the hypoglossal nerve is identified

Results

To date, we have performed more than 80 cases. A recent retrospective analysis by questionnaire was done by a voice therapist regarding satisfaction and quality of life, some years after the procedure. A total of 83 questionnaires were sent to patients having received bilateral selective reinnervation (BSR) since 2003. Fifty-three patients with BSR for bilateral palsy in closure position answered. For the question, if it was necessary to have that surgery again, would you accept?, 96.4% of patients would accept, and 92.7% would advise this surgery to a family member or a friend. Publication is in preparation.

The evaluation of the first 40 patients with a follow-up of at least 1 year shows that the main etiology of bilateral palsy was thyroid surgery. There were children with congenital paralysis. And 10 patients had previous endoscopic enlargement.

Preservation or improvement of the voice was observed in almost all cases.

Thirty-five out of 40 cases showed improvement in ventilation parameters, although three required additional arytenoidectomy or posterior cricoid enlargement. Twenty-seven out of 40 patients had arytenoid abduction on inspiration on at least one side. Of these, 16 had bilateral abduction, although this figure is improved to 14 out of 30 patients if those with previous endolaryngeal scarring are excluded (Figs. 21.4 and 21.5). In one case with previous unsuccessful enlargement and scarring, the reinnervation result was good enough to allow secondary medialization of the scarred hemilarynx to improve voice.

The diaphragm function was recovered in most cases.

Selective reinnervation as a secondary procedure is the subject of a prospective trial in our center. The preliminary data show less good results in comparison to reinnervation performed as a first-line treatment.

The trend is now to perform this surgery in some cases of bilateral vocal fold palsy in aperture, for example, after laryngotracheal disruption. In some cases, we did it at the time of thyroid node recurrence resection, in esophageal reconstruction.

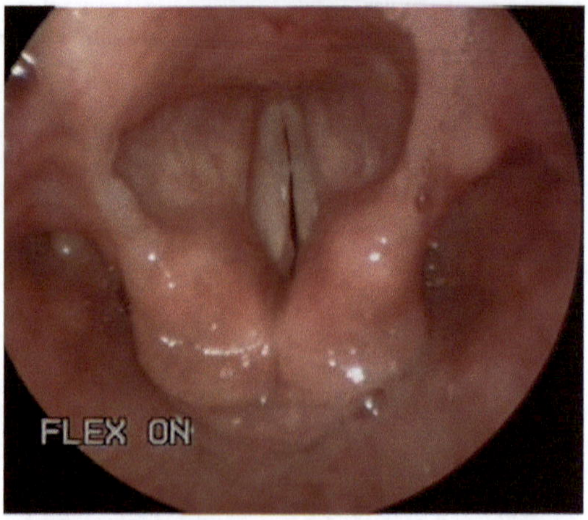

Fig. 21.4 Laryngoscopic view 7.5 months after bilateral selective reinnervation with the total selective reinnervation technique. Phonation (courtesy of Jean-Paul Marie)

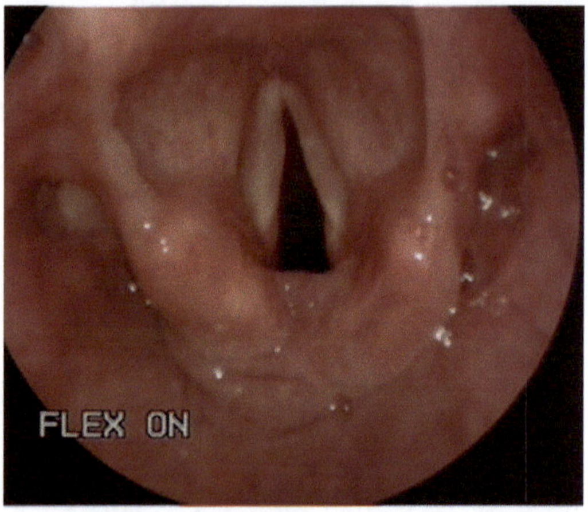

Fig. 21.5 Laryngoscopic view 7.5 months after bilateral selective reinnervation with the total selective reinnervation technique. Inspiration (courtesy of Jean-Paul Marie)

We have now published with Marshall Smith good results in eight children [75]. All were decannulated. A bilateral inspiratory abduction was observed in five of them, unilateral in two, and no movement in one.

21.5 Other Techniques or Indication of Nerve Reconstruction

21.5.1 Laryngeal Denervation-Reinnervation in Laryngeal Dystonia

Chhetri et al. have extensive experience on adductor muscle denervation/reinnervation in long-term, toxin-resistant, laryngeal dystonia [76]. Ansa hypoglossi is used to replace the adductor muscles by intralaryngeal bilateral anastomosis.

21.5.2 Laryngeal Pacing and Combination

Laryngeal pacing is the subject of more development in other chapters. It might be combined with laryngeal reinnervation in case of failure or synkinesis.

21.6 The Future of Nerve Reconstruction

In the future, the development of these different techniques, which may be in combination and contribution of nerve growth factors or stem cells, will help to improve reconstruction of sensation and motor function of the human larynx.

Functional recovery improvement and immunosuppressive and antimitotic drugs will allow to develop the concept of functional laryngeal transplantation.

Nimodipine can improve laryngeal nerve reconstruction in animals and humans [77–79].

We are currently investigating the use of olfactory stem cells to enhance regeneration of the RLN of the facial nerve in a rat model [69, 80–82].

Viral vector might increase the recovery potential of a RLN lesion.

Some drugs such as tacrolimus [83, 84] or antioxidant drugs [85] might have an effect on the targeting and recovery of the laryngeal nerve functions.

Refinement in nerve reconstruction techniques might allow to achieve functional laryngeal transplantation.

21.7 Conclusion

Laryngeal reinnervation gives good results for uni- or bilateral vocal cord paralysis even if it is not a "minute" treatment. It can be performed in children. In the future, it might replace some other techniques and might be used as a first-intention technique.

References

1. Damrose EJ, Huang RY, Ye M, Berke GS, Sercarz JA. Surgical anatomy of the recurrent laryngeal nerve: implications for laryngeal reinnervation. Ann Otol Rhinol Laryngol. 2003;112(5):434–8.
2. Maranillo E, León X, Ibañez M, Orús C, Quer M, Sañudo JR. Variability of the nerve supply patterns of the human posterior cricoarytenoid muscle. Laryngoscope. 2003;113(4):602–6. Epub 2003/04/03. eng.
3. Nguyen M, Junien-Lavillauroy C, Faure C. Anatomical intra-laryngeal anterior branch study of the recurrent (inferior) laryngeal nerve. Surg Radiol Anat. 1989;11(2):123–7.
4. Prades JM, Gavid M, Dubois MD, Dumollard JM, Timoshenko AT, Peoc'h M. Surgical anatomy of the ansa cervicalis nerve: which branch to use for laryngeal reinnervation in humans? Surg Radiol Anat. 2015;37(2):139–45. Epub 2014/08/29. eng.
5. Sunderland S, Swaney WE. The intraneural topography of the recurrent laryngeal nerve in man. Anat Rec. 1952;114:411–26.
6. Crumley RL, McCabe B. Regeneration of the recurrent laryngeal nerve. The Laryngoscope. 1982;90:442–7.
7. Marie J-P. (Contribution à l'étude de la réinnervation laryngée expérimentale. Intérêt du nerf phrénique). Laryngeal reinnervation: special interest with the phrenic nerve. [Thèse de Sciences]. Rouen: Rouen; 1999.
8. Obongo R, Bon-Mardion N, Duclos C, Strunski V, Guerout N, Marie JP. Dual innervation may occur in a partially denervated muscle. Muscle Nerve. 2019;59(1):108–15. Epub 2018/08/20. eng.
9. Li M, Chen S, Wang W, Chen D, Zhu M, Liu F, et al. Effect of duration of denervation on outcomes of ansa-recurrent laryngeal nerve reinner-

vation. Laryngoscope. 2014;124(8):1900–5. Epub 2014/01/30. eng.
10. Marie JP, Hansen K, Brami P, Marronnier A, Bon-Mardion N. Nonselective reinnervation as a primary or salvage treatment of unilateral vocal fold palsy. Laryngoscope. 2020;130(7):1756–63. Epub 2019/10/22. eng.
11. Marie JP, Lacoume Y, Laquerrière A, Tardif C, Fallu J, Bonmarchand G, et al. Diaphragmatic effects of selective resection of the upper phrenic nerve root in dogs. Respir Physiol Neurobiol. 2006;154(3):419–30. Epub 2006/06/10. eng.
12. Verin E, Marie JP, Tardif C, Denis P. Spontaneous recovery of diaphragmatic strength in unilateral diaphragmatic paralysis. Respir Med. 2006;100(11):1944–51. Epub 2006/04/19. eng.
13. Verin E, Marie JP, Similowski T. Cartography of human diaphragmatic innervation: preliminary data. Respir Physiol Neurobiol. 2011;176(1–2):68–71. Epub 2010/11/16. eng.
14. Sanuki T, Yumoto E, Minoda R, Kodama N. The role of immediate recurrent laryngeal nerve reconstruction for thyroid cancer surgery. J Oncol. 2010;2010:846235. Epub 2010/07/16. eng.
15. Hong JW, Roh TS, Yoo HS, Hong HJ, Choi HS, Chang HS, et al. Outcome with immediate direct anastomosis of recurrent laryngeal nerves injured during thyroidectomy. Laryngoscope. 2014;124(6):1402–8. Epub 2013/10/12. eng.
16. Simó R, Nixon IJ, Rovira A, Vander Poorten V, Sanabria A, Zafereo M, et al. Immediate intraoperative repair of the recurrent laryngeal nerve in thyroid surgery. Laryngoscope. 2020. Epub 2020/10/30. eng.
17. Crumley RL. Update: ansa cervicalis to recurrent laryngeal nerve anastomosis for unilateral laryngeal paralysis. Laryngoscope. 1991;101:384–8.
18. Mansor WNW, Azman M, Remli R, Yunus MRM, Baki MM. Primary nonselective laryngeal reinnervation in iatrogenic acute recurrent laryngeal nerve injury: case series and literature review. Ear Nose Throat J. 2021:145561321993605. Epub 2021/02/10. eng.
19. Wang W, Liu F, Zhang C, Li M, Chen S, Gao Y, et al. Immediate ansa cervicalis-to-recurrent laryngeal nerve anastomosis for the management of recurrent laryngeal nerve infiltration by a differentiated thyroid carcinoma. ORL J Oto-Rhino-Laryngol Relat Special. 2020;82(2):93–105. Epub 2020/02/10. eng.
20. Mat Baki M, Clarke P, Birchall MA. Immediate selective laryngeal reinnervation in vagal paraganglioma patients. J Laryngol Otol. 2018;132(9):846–51. Epub 2018/09/06. eng.
21. Aviv JE, Mohr JP, Blitzer A, Thomson JE, Close LG. Restoration of laryngopharyngeal sensation by neural anastomosis. Arch Otolaryngol Head Neck Surg. 1997;123(2):154–60. Epub 1997/02/01. eng.
22. Bouchetemblé P, Marcolla A, Lacoume Y, Verin E, Dehesdin D, Marie JP. Laryngeal sensation recovery by reinnervation in rabbits. Laryngoscope. 2007;117(5):897–902. Epub 2007/05/03. eng.
23. Crumley RL. Laryngeal synkinesis revisited. Ann Otol Rhinol Laryngol. 2000;109(4):365–71. Epub 2000/04/25. eng.
24. Foerster G, Podema R, Guntinas-Lichius O, Crumley RL, Mueller AH. Crumley's classification of laryngeal synkinesis: a comparison of laryngoscopy and electromyography. Laryngoscope. 2021;131(5):E1605–e10. Epub 2020/11/22. eng.
25. Zur KB, Carroll LM. Recurrent laryngeal nerve reinnervation for management of aspiration in a subset of children. Int J Pediatr Otorhinolaryngol. 2018;104:104–7. Epub 2017/12/31. eng
26. Smith ME, Houtz DR. Outcomes of laryngeal reinnervation for unilateral vocal fold paralysis in children: associations with age and time since injury. Ann Otol Rhinol Laryngol. 2016;125(5):433–8. Epub 2015/11/11. eng.
27. Lee SW, Park KN. A long-term comparative prospective study between reinnervation and injection laryngoplasty. Laryngoscope. 2018;128(8):1893–7. Epub 2018/02/17. eng.
28. Crumley RL, Izdebski K. Voice quality following laryngeal reinnervation by ansa hypoglossi transfer. Laryngoscope. 1986;96:611–6.
29. Crumley RL. Teflon versus thyroplasty versus nerve transfer : a comparison. Ann Otol Rhinol Laryngol. 1990;99:759–63.
30. Lorenz RR, Esclamado RM, Teker AM, Strome M, Scharpf J, Hicks D, et al. Ansa cervicalis-to-recurrent laryngeal nerve anastomosis for unilateral vocal fold paralysis: experience of a single institution. Ann Otol Rhinol Laryngol. 2008;117(1):40–5.
31. Wang W, Chen D, Chen S, Li D, Li M, Xia S, et al. Laryngeal reinnervation using ansa cervicalis for thyroid surgery-related unilateral vocal fold paralysis: a long-term outcome analysis of 237 cases. PLoS One. 2011;6(4):e19128. Epub 2011/05/12. eng.
32. Paniello RC, Edgar JD, Kallogjeri D, Piccirillo JF. Medialization versus reinnervation for unilateral vocal fold paralysis: a multicenter randomized clinical trial. Laryngoscope. 2011;121(10):2172–9. Epub 2011/09/08. eng.
33. Smith ME. Pediatric ansa cervicalis to recurrent laryngeal nerve anastomosis. Adv Oto-Rhino-Laryngol. 2012;73:80–5. Epub 2012/04/05. eng.
34. Smith ME, Roy N, Houtz D. Laryngeal reinnervation for paralytic dysphonia in children younger than 10 years. Arch Otolaryngol Head Neck Surg. 2012;138(12):1161–6. Epub 2012/12/19. eng.
35. Zur KB, Carroll LM. Recurrent laryngeal nerve reinnervation in children: acoustic and endoscopic characteristics pre-intervention and post-intervention. A comparison of treatment options. Laryngoscope. 2015;125(Suppl 11):S1–15. Epub 2015/08/11. eng.
36. Ongkasuwan J, Espinosa MCL, Hollas S, Devore D, Procter T, Bassett E, et al. Predictors of voice outcome in pediatric non-selective laryngeal reinnervation. Laryngoscope. 2020;130(6):1525–31. Epub 2019/09/10. eng.

37. Bouhabel S, Hartnick CJ. Current trends in practices in the treatment of pediatric unilateral vocal fold immobility: a survey on injections, thyroplasty and nerve reinnervation. Int J Pediatr Otorhinolaryngol. 2018;109:115–8. Epub 2018/05/08. eng.
38. Caloway CL, Bouhabel S, Hartnick CJ. Lessons learned to aid the successful outcome of pediatric recurrent laryngeal nerve reinnervation. Int J Pediatr Otorhinolaryngol. 2020;128:109,742. Epub 2019/11/05. eng.
39. van den Boer C, Wiersma AL, Marie JP, van Lith-Bijl JT. Treatment of unilateral vocal fold paralysis with ansa cervicalis to recurrent nerve anastomosis in a young adolescent: European case report. J Laryngol Otol. 2018;132(7):661–4. Epub 2018/06/30. eng.
40. Faoury M, Frampton S, Allen D, Burgess A, Heathcote K, Ismail-Koch H. Non-selective laryngeal reinnervation in a child with unilateral left vocal fold palsy utilizing laryngeal electromyography. J Surg Case Reports. 2019;2019(2):rjz039. Epub 2019/02/26. eng.
41. Aires MM, Marinho CB, Vasconcelos SJ. Surgical interventions for pediatric unilateral vocal fold paralysis: A systematic review and meta-analysis. Int J Pediatr Otorhinolaryngol. 2021;141:110,553. Epub 2020/12/18. eng.
42. Ab Rani A, Azman M, Ubaidah MA, Mohamad Yunus MR, Sani A, Mat BM. Nonselective laryngeal reinnervation versus type 1 thyroplasty in patients with unilateral vocal fold paralysis: a single tertiary centre experience. J Voice. 2019;12. Epub 2019/11/17. eng.
43. Paniello RC. Laryngeal reinnervation with the hypoglossal nerve: II. Clinical evaluation and early patient experience. Laryngoscope. 2000;110(5 Pt 1):739–48.
44. Wang W, Chen S, Chen D, Xia S, Qiu X, Liu Y, et al. Contralateral ansa cervicalis-to-recurrent laryngeal nerve anastomosis for unilateral vocal fold paralysis: a long-term outcome analysis of 56 cases. Laryngoscope. 2011;121(5):1027–34. Epub 2011/04/27. eng.
45. Graham ME, Smith ME. The nerve to thyrohyoid muscle as a novel donor nerve for laryngeal reinnervation. Ann Otol Rhinol Laryngol. 2020;129(4): 355–60. Epub 2019/11/19. eng.
46. Crampon F, Duparc F, Trost O, Marie JP. Selective laryngeal reinnervation: can rerouting of the thyrohyoid nerve simplify the procedure by avoiding the use of a nerve graft? Surg Radiol Anat. 2019;41(2):145–50. Epub 2018/10/31. eng.
47. Tucker HM. Human laryngeal reinnervation: long experience with neuromuscular pedicle technique. Laryngoscope. 1978;88:598–604.
48. Tucker HM. Long term results of nerve-muscle pedicle reinnervation for laryngeal paralysis. Ann Otol Rhinol Laryngol. 1989;1989(98):674–6.
49. Tucker HM. Long-term preservation of voice improvement following surgical medialization and reinnervation for unilateral vocal fold paralysis. J Voice. 1999;13(2):251–6.
50. Tucker HM. Combined laryngeal framework medialization and reinnervation for unilateral vocal cord paralysis. Ann Otol Rhinol Laryngol. 1990;90:778–81.
51. Chhetri DK, Gerratt BR, Kreiman J, Berke GS. Combined arytenoid adduction and laryngeal reinnervation in the treatment of vocal fold paralysis. Laryngoscope. 1999;109(12):1928–36. Epub 1999/12/11. eng.
52. Kodama N, Sanuki T, Kumai Y, Yumoto E. Long-term vocal outcomes of refined nerve-muscle pedicle flap implantation combined with arytenoid adduction. Eur Arch Oto-Rhino-Laryngol. 2015;272(3):681–8. Epub 2014/12/17. eng.
53. El-Kashlan HK, Carroll WR, Hogikyan ND, Chepeha DB, Kileny PR, Esclamado RM. Selective cricothyroid muscle reinnervation by muscle-nerve-muscle neurotization. Arch Otolaryngol Head Neck Surg. 2001;127(10):1211–5. Epub 2001/11/01. eng.
54. Hogikyan ND, Johns MM, Kileny PR, Urbanchek M, Carroll WR, Kuzon WM Jr. Motion-specific laryngeal reinnervation using muscle-nerve-muscle neurotization. Ann Otol Rhinol Laryngol. 2001;110(9):801–10. Epub 2001/09/18. eng.
55. Blumin JH, Ye M, Berke GS, Blackwell KE. Recovery of laryngeal sensation after superior laryngeal nerve anastomosis. Laryngoscope. 1999;109(10):1637–41.
56. Bouchetemble P, Marcolla A, Lacoume Y, Verin E, Dehesdin D, Marie JP. Laryngeal sensation recovery by reinnervation in rabbits. Laryngoscope. 2007;117(5):897–902.
57. Marie JP, Lerosey Y, Dehesdin D, Jin O, Tadíe M, Andrieu-Guitrancourt J. Experimental reinnervation of a strap muscle with a few roots of the phrenic nerve in rabbits. Ann Otol Rhinol Laryngol. 1999;108(10):1004–11. Epub 1999/10/20. eng.
58. Fayoux P, Maltezeanu A, Broucqsault H, Daniel SJ. Experience with laryngeal reinnervation using nerve-muscle pedicle in pediatric patients. Int J Pediatr Otorhinolaryngol. 2020;138:110,254. Epub 2020/11/04. eng.
59. Crumley RL. Experiments in laryngeal reinnervation. Laryngoscope. 1982;92(suppl 30):1–27.
60. Crumley RL. Phrenic nerve graft for bilateral vocal cord paralysis. Laryngoscope. 1983;93(4):425–8.
61. Rice DH. Laryngeal reinnervation. Laryngoscope. 1982;92:1049–59.
62. Mahieu HF, Lith-Bijl Van JT, Groenhout C, Tonnaer JAD, Wilde De P. Selective laryngeal abductor reinnervation in cats using phrenic nerve transfer and ORG 2766. Arch Otolaryngol Head Neck Surg. 1993;119:772–6.
63. van Lith-Bijl JT, Stolk RJ, Tonnaer JADM, Groenhout C, Konings PNM, Mahieu HF. Laryngeal abductor reinnervation with a phrenic nerve transfer after a 9-month delay. Arch Otolaryngol Head Neck Surg. 1998;124:393–8.
64. Crumley RL. Selective reinnervation of vocal cord adductors in unilateral vocal cord paralysis. Ann Otol Rhinol Laryngol. 1984;93:351–6.

65. Marie JP, Dehesdin D, Ducastelle T, Senant J. Selective reinnervation of the abductor and adductor muscles of the canine larynx after recurrent nerve paralysis. Ann Otol Rhinol Laryngol. 1989;98:530–6.
66. van Lith-Bijl JT, Stolk RJ, Tonnaer JADM, Groenhout C, Konings PNM, Mahieu HF. Selective laryngeal reinnervation with separate phrenic and ansa cervicalis nerve transfers. Arch Otolaryngol Head Neck Surg. 1997;123(4):406–11.
67. Zheng H, Zhou S, Li Z, Chen S, Zhang S, Huang Y, et al. Reinnervation of the posterior cricoarytenoid muscle by the phrenic nerve for bilateral vocal cord paralysis in humans. Zhonghua er bi yan hou ke za zhi. 2002;37(3):210–4. Epub 2003/05/30. chi.
68. Li M, Chen S, Zheng H, Chen D, Zhu M, Wang W, et al. Reinnervation of bilateral posterior cricoarytenoid muscles using the left phrenic nerve in patients with bilateral vocal fold paralysis. PLoS One. 2013;8(10):e77233. Epub 2013/10/08. eng.
69. de Corgnol AC, Guérout N, Duclos C, Vérin E, Marie JP. Olfactory ensheathing cells in a rat model of laryngeal reinnervation. Ann Otol Rhinol Laryngol. 2011;120(4):273–80. Epub 2011/05/19. eng.
70. Marie JP, Laquerrière A, Lerosey Y, Bodenant C, Tardif C, Hémet J, et al. Selective resection of the phrenic nerve roots in rabbits. Part I: Cartography of the residual innervation. Respir Physiol. 1997b;109:127–38.
71. Marie JP, Tardif C, Lerosey Y, Gibon JF, Hellot MF, Tadié M, et al. Selective resection of the phrenic nerve roots in rabbits. Part II: respiratory effects. Respir Physiol. 1997c;109:139–48.
72. Marie J-P, Laquerriere A, Choussy O, Lacoume Y, Dehesdin D, Andrieu-Guitrancourt J. Thyrohyoid branch of the hypoglossal nerve in the canine ; perspectives for larynx reinnervation. Eur Arch Oto Rhino Laryngol. 2000;257(S1):S11.
73. Song SA, Marie JP. Assessment of bilateral vocal fold immobility prior to selective bilateral laryngeal reinnervation. Clin Otolaryngol. 2020;45(3):432–5. Epub 2020/02/23. eng.
74. Selim J, Maquet C, Djerada Z, Besnier E, Compère V, Crampon F, et al. Anesthetic management for awake tubeless suspension microlaryngoscopy. Laryngoscope. 2021. Epub 2021/04/22. eng.
75. Lee JW, Bon-Mardion N, Smith ME, Marie JP. Bilateral selective laryngeal reinnervation for bilateral vocal fold paralysis in children. JAMA Otolaryngol Head Neck Surg. 2020;146(5):401–7. Epub 2020/03/20. eng.
76. Chhetri DK, Mendelsohn AH, Blumin JH, Berke GS. Long-term follow-up results of selective laryngeal adductor denervation-reinnervation surgery for adductor spasmodic dysphonia. Laryngoscope. 2006;116(4):635–42. Epub 2006/04/06. eng.
77. Hydman J, Remahl S, Björck G, Svensson M, Mattsson P. Nimodipine improves reinnervation and neuromuscular function after injury to the recurrent laryngeal nerve in the rat. Ann Otol Rhinol Laryngol. 2007;116(8):623–30. Epub 2007/09/13. eng.
78. Mattsson P, Björck G, Remahl S, Bäckdahl M, Hamberger B, Hydman J, et al. Nimodipine and microsurgery induced recovery of the vocal cord after recurrent laryngeal nerve resection. Laryngoscope. 2005;115(10):1863–5. Epub 2005/10/14. eng.
79. Lin RJ, Klein-Fedyshin M, Rosen CA. Nimodipine improves vocal fold and facial motion recovery after injury: a systematic review and meta-analysis. Laryngoscope. 2019;129(4):943–51. Epub 2018/11/20. eng.
80. Guérout N, Duclos C, Drouot L, Abramovici O, Bon-Mardion N, Lacoume Y, et al. Transplantation of olfactory ensheathing cells promotes axonal regeneration and functional recovery of peripheral nerve lesion in rats. Muscle Nerve. 2011;43(4):543–51. Epub 2011/02/10. eng.
81. Paviot A, Guérout N, Bon-Mardion N, Duclos C, Jean L, Boyer O, et al. Efficiency of laryngeal motor nerve repair is greater with bulbar than with mucosal olfactory ensheathing cells. Neurobiol Dis. 2011;41(3):688–94. Epub 2010/12/21. eng.
82. Bense F, Montava M, Duclos C, Bisson A, Delarue Q, Mardion NB, et al. Syngeneic transplantation of rat olfactory stem cells in a vein conduit improves facial movements and reduces synkinesis after facial nerve injury. Plastic Reconstr Surg. 2020;146(6):1295–305. Epub 2020/11/26. eng.
83. Toll EC, Seifalian AM, Birchall MA. The role of immunophilin ligands in nerve regeneration. Regener Med. 2011;6(5):635–52. Epub 2011/09/16. eng.
84. Gorphe P, Guerout N, Birchall M, Terenghi G, Marie JP. Tacrolimus enhances the recovery of normal laryngeal muscle fibre distribution after reinnervation. J Laryngol Otol. 2012;126(11):1155–8. Epub 2012/09/06. eng.
85. Pothion H, Jehan C, Tostivint H, Cartier D, Bucharles C, Falluel-Morel A, et al. Selenoprotein T: an essential oxidoreductase serving as a guardian of endoplasmic reticulum homeostasis. Antioxid Redox Signal. 2020;33(17):1257–75. Epub 2020/06/12. eng.

22 Preoperative Assessment of Laryngeal Cancer

Anastasios G. Hantzakos and Hans Edmund Eckel

Key Points

- Proper description and accurate staging are key factors for designing the treatment strategy for laryngeal carcinoma.
- Advances in imaging and optics have significantly improved the diagnostic accuracy of laryngeal tumors.
- Imaging with FDG PET-CT is the preferred method of choice for more accurate staging and follow-up of head and neck neoplasms.

22.1 Epidemiology of Laryngeal Cancer

Laryngeal cancer remains the most common head and neck malignancy. It is the nineteenth most common cause of death worldwide with 1% of the total cancer deaths [1]. Men are affected more frequently than women at a ratio of 4.8:1 [2]. In 2016, an estimated 13,430 new cases of laryngeal cancer will be diagnosed, with approximately 3620 patients dying from the disease [3]. The cancer of the larynx could possibly metastasize to the bone, brain, lung, and liver, causing a shorter survival, thus leading to the certain burden of disease on public health.

With the current trend, the American Cancer Society estimates a total of 12,370 new cases with 3750 estimated deaths from laryngeal cancer for 2020 in the USA. The incidence rates for 2012–2016 are 5.7/100,000 in men and 1.3/100,000 in women, with death rates being 1.7/100,000 and 0.4/100,000, respectively [4]. The probability of developing cancer is higher at the age over 50 years (0.1%) and highest over 70 years (0.2%) [4]. The most pertinent epidemiologic data from the EUROCARE-5 study indicate a European average relative 5-year survival of 58.99% in men and 59.57% in women, with the lower being in Eastern Europe in men over 75 years old (39.64%) [5]. In 2010, an estimated 20,272 new cases were diagnosed with laryngeal cancer in China, including 17,703 men and 2569 women. The crude incidence rate of laryngeal cancer was 1.54/100,000 in 2010, accounting for 0.66% of overall new cancer cases, with age-standardized mortality rates of the Chinese population and world population being 0.28/105 and 0.35/105, respectively [6].

A. G. Hantzakos (✉)
Department of Otolaryngology Head & Neck Surgery, Surgical Subspecialties Institute, Cleveland Clinic Abu Dhabi, Abu Dhabi, UAE

Cleveland Clinic Lerner College of Medicine, Case Western Reserve University, Cleveland, OH, USA
e-mail: HantzaA@ClevelandClinicAbuDhabi.ae

H. E. Eckel
Department of Otorhinolaryngology, Klinikum Klagenfurt am Wörthersee, Klagenfurt, Austria
e-mail: Hans.Eckel@kabeg.at

M. Remacle, H. E. Eckel (eds.), *Textbook of Surgery of Larynx and Trachea*,
https://doi.org/10.1007/978-3-031-09621-1_22

The highest world age-standardized incidence and mortality rates for laryngeal cancer are both in the Republic of Cuba [1]. Unfortunately, laryngeal cancer is one of a few oncologic diseases in which the 5-year survival rate has decreased over the past 40 years, from 66% to 63%, although the overall incidence is declining [3].

Tobacco and alcohol have long been recognized as the leading causes of head and neck cancer [7]. This association has not changed throughout the years. Although tobacco and alcohol are independent risk factors, it is often difficult to separate their contribution since they usually coexist and appear to have a synergistic effect in multiplying the incidence of laryngeal cancer. Smoking has been shown to have a linear association with the development of laryngeal cancer. The risk for smokers is 10–15 times higher than the risk for nonsmokers, with that of heaviest smokers rising as much as 30 times [8]. Several occupational exposures, such as strong acid mists [9], asbestos [10], and chlorinated solvents [11], are recognized risk factors for laryngeal cancer.

Gastroesophageal and laryngopharyngeal reflux diseases (GERD and LPR) have also been speculated to induce laryngeal malignancy. In a recent systematic review and meta-analysis conducted by Parsel et al., reflux disease was shown to increase the risk of malignancy with an odds ratio of 2.47 (95% CI = 1.90–3.21), whereas there was no statistical difference between patients with GERD and LPR [12]. A most pertinent systematic review and meta-analysis confirmed this association for laryngeal cancers with and odds ratio of 1.95 (95% CI = 1.33–2.86) [13].

Human papilloma virus (HPV) is detected in approximately 21%–27% of laryngeal cancer patients [14–16]. There is conflicting evidence in regards to prognosis, with some studies advocating a favorable one with good response to conservative management with chemoradiotherapy [17, 18], while some showed no difference in survival or locoregional control [14, 19]. Although elevated tumor expression of p16 (INK4A), a cyclin-dependent kinase-4 inhibitor, is strongly correlated with HPV in oropharyngeal cancer, an etiologic role in laryngeal cancer has not been established. In a population-based study by Hernandez et al. [14] evaluating the genotype-specific prevalence of HPV in invasive laryngeal cancer cases diagnosed in the USA, 13 different genotypes of HPV DNA were detected in 31 of 148 (21%) invasive laryngeal cancers; however, a causative relation was not proven. Another study by the same group [20] did not support a correlation between p16 and HPV infection, showing only a fraction (2%) of laryngeal cancers positive for both p16 and HPV DNA. These results are in contrast to others [21, 22], who showed common positivity in 65% and 86% of laryngeal cancers, respectively, however without establishing a causative relationship, since p16 positivity is also observed in laryngeal carcinogenesis due to somatic chromosomal alterations unrelated to HPV [23, 24].

22.2 Staging

Accurate staging is of paramount importance for the decision-making process, since it allows for a uniform description and diagnosis which leads to treatment. Despite its imperfections, the World Health Organization TNM classification system is widely accepted (Tables 22.1 and 22.2), which is determined by the size and extent of the tumor and the presence of nodal and distal metastases. The updated fourth edition does not contain any changes from the previous one in regards to laryngeal cancer staging [25]. For glottal cancer, the American Joint Committee on Cancer clinical staging system is also widely accepted in the US practice and literature.

Upon clinical suspicion of a lesion in the larynx, indirect laryngoscopy and careful fiber-optic endoscopic examination are of paramount importance for further investigation. Inspection of the problem will initiate further workup. Direct laryngoscopy accompanied by pharyngoesophagoscopy under general anesthesia permits closer inspection of the lesion with its local spread and allows for biopsy taking.

While direct laryngoscopy has been routinely applied since the emergence of endolaryngeal

Table 22.1 WHO TNM classification of carcinomas of the larynx [35]

T—primary tumor	
Tx	Primary tumor cannot be assessed
T0	No evidence of primary tumor
Tis	Carcinoma in situ
Supraglottis	
T1	Tumor limited to one subsite of the supraglottis with normal vocal cord mobility
T2	Tumor invades mucosa of more than one adjacent subsite of the supraglottis or glottis or region outside the supraglottis (e.g., mucosa of the base of the tongue, vallecula, medial wall of the pyriform sinus) without fixation of the larynx
T3	Tumor limited to the larynx with vocal cord fixation and/or invades any of the following: Postcricoid area, preepiglottic tissues, paraglottic space, and/or with minor thyroid cartilage erosion (e.g., inner cortex)
T4a	Tumor invades through the thyroid cartilage and/or invades tissues beyond the larynx, e.g., trachea, soft tissues of the neck including the deep/extrinsic muscle of the tongue (genioglossus, hyoglossus, palatoglossus, and styloglossus), strap muscles, thyroid, esophagus
T4b	Tumor invades the prevertebral space or mediastinal structures, or encases the carotid artery
Glottis	
T1	Tumor limited to the vocal cord(s) (may involve anterior or posterior commissure) with normal mobility
T1a	Tumor limited to one vocal cord
T1b	Tumor involves both vocal cords
T2	Tumor extends to the supraglottis and/or subglottis, and/or with impaired vocal cord mobility
T3	Tumor limited to the larynx with vocal cord fixation and/or invades the paraglottic space, and/or with minor thyroid cartilage erosion (e.g., inner cortex)
T4a	Tumor invades through the thyroid cartilage, or invades tissues beyond the larynx, e.g., trachea, soft tissues of the neck including the deep/extrinsic muscle of the tongue (genioglossus, hyoglossus, palatoglossus, and styloglossus), strap muscles, thyroid, esophagus
T4b	Tumor invades the prevertebral space or mediastinal structures, or encases the carotid artery
Subglottis	
T1	Tumor limited to the subglottis
T2	Tumor extends to the vocal cord(s) with normal or impaired mobility
T3	Tumor limited to the larynx with vocal cord fixation
T4a	Tumor invades through the cricoid or thyroid cartilage and/or invades tissues beyond the larynx, e.g., trachea, soft tissues of the neck including the deep/extrinsic muscle of tongue (genioglossus, hyoglossus, palatoglossus, and styloglossus), strap muscles, thyroid, esophagus
T4b	Tumor invades the prevertebral space or mediastinal structures, or encases the carotid artery
N—Regional lymph nodes	
NX	Regional lymph nodes cannot be assessed
N0	No regional lymph node metastasis
N1	Metastasis in a single ipsilateral lymph node, 3 cm or less in greatest dimension
N2	Metastasis as specified in N2a, 2b, 2c below
N2a	Metastasis in a single ipsilateral lymph node, more than 3 cm but not more than 6 cm in greatest dimension
N2b	Metastasis in multiple ipsilateral lymph nodes, none more than 6 cm in greatest dimension
N2c	Metastasis in bilateral or contralateral lymph nodes, none more than 6 cm in greatest dimension
N3	Metastasis in a lymph node more than 6 cm in greatest dimension
	Note: Midline nodes are considered ipsilateral nodes.
M—Distant metastasis	
MX	Distant metastasis cannot be assessed
M0	No distant metastasis
M1	Distant metastasis

Table 22.2 Staging of laryngeal cancer

Stage grouping			
Stage 0	Tis	N0	M0
Stage I	T1	N0	M0
Stage II	T2	N0	M0
Stage III	T1 T2 T3	N1 N0 N1	M0
Stage IVa	T1 T2 T3 T4a	N2 N0 N1 N2	M0
Stage IVb	T4b ANY T	ANY N N3	M0
Stage IVc	ANY T	ANY N	M1

surgery by Kleinsasser [26], newer tools have been recently added to the diagnostic armamentarium. Systematic use of rigid endoscopes of different angles (0°, 30°, 70°, 120°) can provide a more accurate view of the larynx and hypopharynx and complements topographic assessment of the lesion. Narrowband imaging (NBI) has been introduced as an optical modality to detect precancerous- and cancerous lesions. Contrary to white light, a special camera mode allows for only two wavelengths, specifically 415 nm and 540 nm, corresponding to the peak absorption of hemoglobin, therefore visualizing highly vascular tissues with better definition. Since premalignant and malignant lesions have increased vascularity, this method claims higher diagnostic accuracy both in early detection and during surveillance follow-ups by enhancing visualization of mucosal microvasculature, the so-called intraepithelial papillary capillary loops (IPCLs). A meta-analysis by Sun et al. showed a pooled sensitivity of 94% of NBI in the diagnosis of laryngeal cancer [27].

Contact endoscopy, as this was founded and mastered by M. Andrea [28], claims to offer in vivo and in situ evaluation of the mucosal surface for the detection of potential malignant pathology. As another diagnostic tool, direct autofluorescence laryngoscopy has been applied in the assessment of suspected precancerous and cancerous laryngeal lesions and is claimed to have a sensitivity rate of 97.3% and a specificity of 83.8%. Autofluorescence diagnosis is based on the ability of oxidized flavin mononucleotide (FMN) in normal cells to emit green fluorescence when exposed to blue light. Neoplastic cells have a significantly lower concentration of FMN and therefore do not have fluorescence to the same degree [29]. Fluorescence spectroscopy, a technique for evaluating the physical and chemical properties of a substance by analyzing the intensity and character of light emitted in the form of fluorescence, emerged as a promising refinement of autofluorescence endoscopy [30]. Additionally, optical coherence tomography (OCT), a high-resolution optical imaging technique that produces cross-sectional images of living tissues using light, is claimed to reliably identify invasion of the basement membrane in patients with laryngeal cancer [31]. Although promising, these additional diagnostic tools lack an adequate number of cases to justify their value in the diagnostic workup as of today.

22.3 Imaging

An increasing number of imaging modalities are available for more accurate assessment. However, these are largely dependent on the special interest of the radiologist. It is, therefore, important that the most specialized available neck radiologist be consulted prior to final staging. Computed tomography (CT) with intravenous contrast enhancement and magnetic resonance imaging (MRI) of the neck in axial and coronal sections allow for more precise imaging of soft tissue involvement, i.e., dissemination of the tumor to the preepiglottic and paraglottic spaces and presence of enlarged neck lymph nodes. For better imaging of the endolarynx, CT during inspiration is preferred. In that way, laryngeal surface anomalies are more accurately visualized. For bony or cartilaginous involvement, however, CT appears to be superior to MRI [32]. After initial assessment and upon establishment of diagnosis, 2-[18F]-fluoro-2-deoxy-D-glucose (FDG) positron emission tomography (PET) is preferred for the staging and follow-up of patients with head and neck cancer. PET with FDG is a functional imaging modality that uses abnormal tissue metabolism to detect neoplasms. The radioactive glucose analog FDG is metabolized in normal tissue and neoplastic tissues in proportion to the rate of tissue glucose metabolism. FDG is metabolically trapped in the intracellular space. This occurs more in tumors than in normal tissues and can be used to identify tumors based on accelerated glycolytic rates using PET. This method when coupled with CT or MRI can serve as reliable examinations for defining local resectability of head and neck cancer [33]. A masked prospective cohort study by Rohde et al. comparing chest X-ray/head and neck MRI, chest CT/head and neck MRI, and FDG-PET/CT showed a significantly higher detection rate of distant metastasis or synchronous cancer with FDG-PET/CT in current clinical imaging guidelines, of which European ones primarily recommend chest X-ray/MRI, whereas US guidelines preferably point to chest CT/head and neck MRI in patients with head and neck squamous cell carcinoma [34].

References

1. Ferlay J, Soerjomataram I, Dikshit R, Eser S, Mathers C, Rebelo M, et al. Cancer incidence and mortality worldwide: sources, methods and major patterns in GLOBOCAN 2012. Int J Cancer. 2015;136(5):E359–86.
2. Baselga J. Why the epidermal growth factor receptor? The rationale for cancer therapy. Oncologist. 2002;7(Suppl 4):2–8.
3. Siegel RL, Miller KD, Jemal A. Cancer statistics, 2016. CA Cancer J Clin. 2016;66(1):7–30.
4. American Cancer Society. Cancer Statistics Center. [Online]; 2020 [cited 2020 November 20. https://cancerstatisticscenter.cancer.org/?_ga=2.39553190.406516419.1605593839-190728790.1605593839#!/cancer-site/Larynx.
5. EUROCARE. Survival of cancer patients in Europe. [Online]; 2020 [cited 2020 November 20. Available from: https://w3.iss.it/site/EU5Results/forms/SA0007.aspx.
6. Du L, Li H, Zhu C, Zheng R, Zhang S, Chen W. Incidence and mortality of laryngeal cancer in China, 2011. Chin J Cancer Res. 2015;27(1):52–8.
7. Wynder EI, Bross IJ, Feldman RM. A study of the etiological factors in cancer of the mouth. Cancer. 1957;10(6):1300–23.
8. Kuper H, Boffetta P, Adami HO. Tobacco use and cancer causation: association by tumour type. J Intern Med. 2002;252(3):206–24.
9. IARC Working Group on the Evaluation of Carcinogenic Risks to Humans. Chemical agents and related occupations. Monograph. Lyon: World Health Organization, International Agency for Research on Cancer; 2012. Report No.: 100F.
10. Peng WJ, Mi J, Jiang YH. Asbestos exposure and laryngeal cancer mortality. Laryngoscope. 2016;126(5):1169–74.
11. Barul C, Carton M, Radoï L, Menvielle G, Pilorget C, Bara S, et al. Occupational exposure to petroleum-based and oxygenated solvents and hypopharyngeal and laryngeal cancer in France: the ICARE study. BMC Cancer. 2018;18(1):388.
12. Parsel SM, Wu EL, Riley CA, McCoul ED. Gastroesophageal and laryngopharyngeal reflux associated with laryngeal malignancy: a systematic review and meta-analysis. Clin Gastroenterol Hepatol. 2019;17(7):1253–64.
13. Eels AC, MacIntosh C, Marks L, Marino MJ. Gastroesophageal reflux disease and head and neck cancers: a systematic review and meta-analysis. Am J Otolaryngol. 2020;41(6)
14. Hernandez BY, Goodman MT, Lynch CF, Cozen W, Unger ER, Steinau M, et al. Human papillomavirus prevalence in invasive laryngeal cancer in the United States. PLoS One. 2014;9(12)
15. Li X, Gao L, Li H, Yang Y, Zhou F, Gao C, et al. Human papillomavirus infection and laryngeal cancer risk: a systematic review and meta-analysis. J Infect Dis. 2013;207(3):479–88.
16. Isayeva T, Li Y, Maswahu D, Brandstein-Gesler M. Human papillomavirus in non-oropharyngeal head and neck cancers: a systematic literature review. Head Neck Pathol. 2012;6(Suppl 1):S104–20.
17. Shaughnessy JN, Farghaly H, Wilson L, Redman R, Potts K, Bumpous K, et al. HPV: a factor in organ preservation for locally advanced larynx and hypopharynx cancer? Am J Otolaryngol. 2014;35(1):19–24.
18. Clayman GL, Stewart MG, Weber RS, El-Naggar AK, Grimm EA. Human papillomavirus in laryngeal and hypopharyngeal carcinomas. Relationship to survival. Arch Otolaryngol Head Neck Surg. 1994;120(7):743–8.
19. Hughes RT, Bauerlein WJ, O'Neill SS, Porosnicu M, Lycan TW, Waltonen J, et al. Human papillomavirus-associated squamous cell carcinoma of the larynx or hypopharynx: clinical outcomes and implications for laryngeal preservation. Oral Oncol. 2019;98:20–7.
20. Hernandez BY, Rahman M, Lynch CF, Cozen W, Unger ER, Steinau M, et al. p16(INK4A) expression in invasive laryngeal cancer. Papillomavirus Res. 2016;2:52–5.
21. Chernock RD, Wang X, Gao G, Lewis JS Jr, Zhang Q, Thorstad WL, et al. Detection and significance of human papillomavirus, CDKN2A(p16) and

CDKN1A(p21) expression in squamous cell carcinoma of the larynx. Mod Pathol. 2013;26(2):223–31.
22. Ndiaye C, Mena M, Alemany L, Arbyn M, Castellsagué X, Laporte L, et al. HPV DNA, E6/E7 mRNA, and p16INK4a detection in head and neck cancers: a systematic review and meta-analysis. Lancet Oncol. 2014;15(12):1319–31.
23. Combes JD, Franceschi S. Role of human papillomavirus in non-oropharyngeal head and neck cancers. Oral Oncol. 2014;50(5):370–9.
24. Larque AB, Conde L, Hakim S, Alos L, Jares P, Vilaseca I, et al. p16INK4a overexpression is associated with CDKN2A mutation and worse prognosis in HPV-negative laryngeal squamous cell carcinomas. Virchows Arch. 2015;466(4):375–82.
25. Slootweg PJ, El-Naggar AK. World Health Organization 4th edition of head and neck tumor classification: insight into the consequential modifications. Virchows Arch. 2018;472(3):311–3.
26. Kleinsasser O. Die Laryngomikroskopie (Lupenlaryngoskopie) und ihre Bedeutung für die Erkennung der Vorerkrankungen und Fröhformen des Stimmlippenkarzinoms. Arch Ohren Nasen Kehlkopfheilkd. 1962;180:724–7.
27. Sun C, Han X, Li X, Du X. Diagnostic performance of narrow band imaging for laryngeal cancer: a systematic review and meta-analysis. Otolaryngol Head Neck Surg. 2017;156(4):589–97.
28. Andrea M, Dias O, Santos A. Contact endoscopy during microlaryngeal surgery: a new technique for endoscopic examination of the larynx. Ann Otol Rhinol Laryngol. 1995;104(5):333–9.
29. Baletic N, Petrovic Z, Pendjer I, Malicevic H. Autofluorescent diagnostics in laryngeal pathology. Eur Arch Otorhinolaryngol. 2004;261(5):233–7.
30. Arens C, Reussner D, Neubacher H, Woeckenhaus J, Glanz H. Spectrometric measurement in laryngeal cancer. Eur Arch Otorhinolaryngol. 2006;263(11):1001–7.
31. Armstrong WB, Ridgway JM, Vokes DE, Guo S, Perez J, Jackson RP, et al. Optical coherence tomography of laryngeal cancer. Laryngoscope. 2006;116(7):1107–13.
32. DeSanto L. Current concept in otolaryngology: the options in early laryngeal carcinoma. N Engl J Med. 1982;306(15):910–2.
33. Sekine T, De Galiza BF, Delso G, Burger IA, Stolzmann P, Ter Voert EE, et al. Local resectability assessment of head and neck cancer: positron emission tomography/MRI versus positron emission tomography/CT. Head Neck. 2017;39(8):1550–8.
34. Rohde M, Nielsen AL, Johansen J, Sorensen JA, Nguyen N, Diaz A, et al. Head-to-head comparison of chest X-ray/head and neck MRI, chest CT/head and neck MRI, and 18F-FDG PET/CT for detection of distant metastases and synchronous cancer in Oral, pharyngeal, and laryngeal cancer. J Nucl Med. 2017;58(12):1919–24.
35. El-Naggar AK, Chan JK, Grandis JR, Slootweg PJ, editors. WHO classification of head and neck tumours. In WHO classification of Tumours. Lyon: IARC Press; 2017.

HPV and Laryngeal Cancer

23

Claus Wittekindt and Jens Peter Klussmann

Early studies on HPV are primarily characterized by the fact that widely varying prevalence rates have been published from less than 5% to over 50% in the cases studied. In a systematic review published in 2005 on HPV-DNA detection in over 5000 head and neck tumor cases (pooled analysis of over 50 studies from over 25 different countries), the overall prevalence rate was reported to be 24%, considering 10 different HPV types in 1435 cases with LSCC [1]. An important finding in this early work was significant regional differences (less than 15% HPV-positive in the United States, nearly 40% HPV-positive in Asia). Another feature of the published work is that the HPV-16-type DNA detection rate varied from 10% to just under 50% in the study material. In the work summarized in this review, it is remarkable that high-risk HPV types that are significant in carcinomas of the uterine cervix were often selectively included (HPV type 18). Notably, non-HPV-16 types can often be detected in LSCC patients (Fig. 23.1). Furthermore, it is important to note that the identification of viral genomes in a tumor sample alone does not provide sufficient evidence for virus-driven carcinogenesis, as can be well exemplified by the early published works. This is due to the fact that the PCR technique does not allow differentiation between a transient infection and an oncogenic/transforming HPV infection. Extensive analyses of oncogenic HPV infection in LSCC specimens using the p16 test, mRNA detection as an adjunct to HPV PCR, were generally not included in early published works. Furthermore, it can be considered that prior to 2005, the role of the p16 protein as a surrogate marker for oncogenic transformation was controversial and no uniform classification of the p16 staining pattern in terms of significance for HPV-driven carcinogenesis was available.

Thus, it appears that in early studies, the techniques of the examinations were the most important source of error for the reported divergent HPV prevalence rates in LSCC. Furthermore, small sample sizes and a high proportion of non-HPV-16 types influenced the outcome quality. Nearly 10 years later, an in-depth analysis of over 100 patients with LSCC was presented in which formalin-fixed and fresh-frozen tissues were evaluated for the presence of over 50 mucosal HPV types, E6 mRNA transcripts, and p16 expression. This demonstrated a positive DNA test in over one-third of patients, but only one-third of these samples were then reproducibly HPV-DNA-positive and only under 10% of patients had HPV-16-positive DNA tests and a

C. Wittekindt (✉)
Hals-Nasen-Ohrenklinik, Klinikum Dortmund gGmbH, Dortmund, Germany
e-mail: claus.wittekindt@klinikumdo.de

J. P. Klussmann
Department of Otorhinolaryngology, Head and Neck Surgery, University Hospital of Cologne, Cologne, Germany
e-mail: jens.klussmann@uk-koeln.de

M. Remacle, H. E. Eckel (eds.), *Textbook of Surgery of Larynx and Trachea*,
https://doi.org/10.1007/978-3-031-09621-1_23

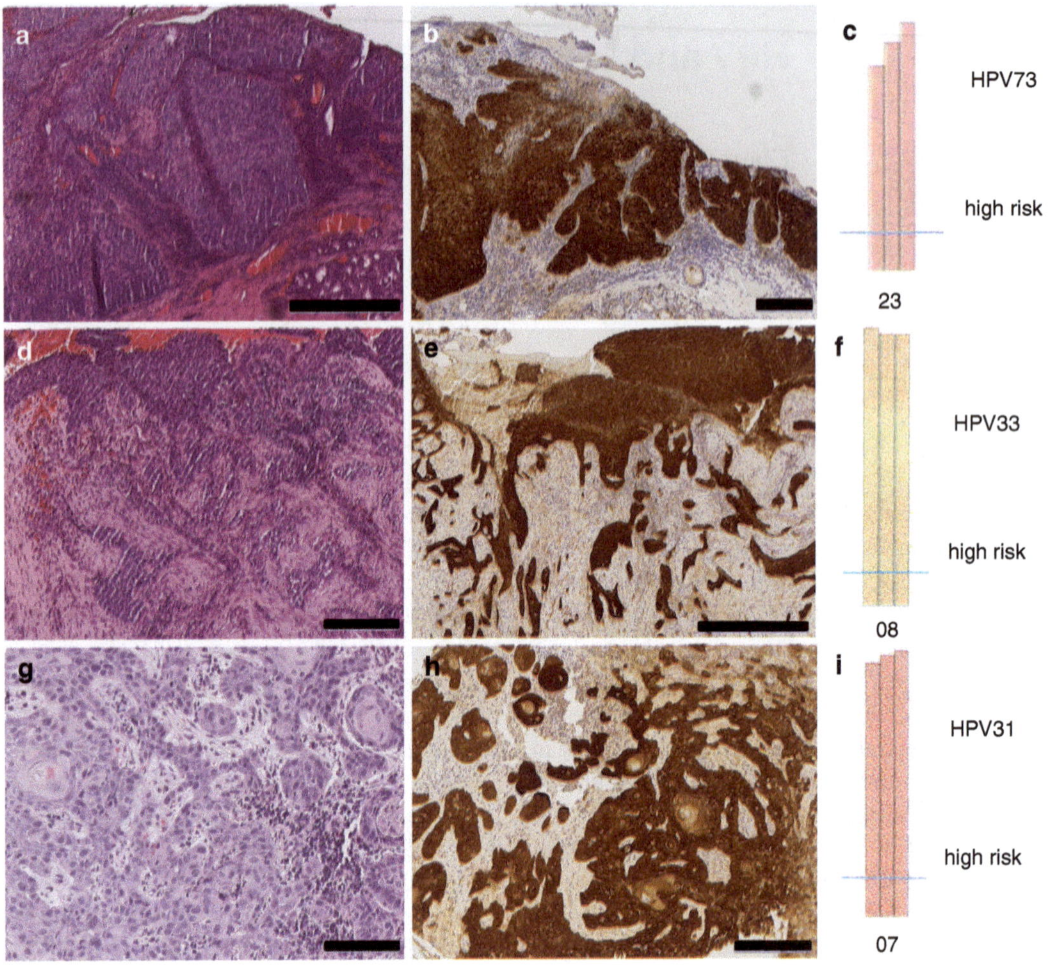

Fig. 23.1 Non-HPV-16 types are frequent: squamous cell carcinomas with molecular pathologically proven HPV-73 (**a–c**), HPV-33 (**d–f**), and HPV-31 association (**g–i**). The tumor cells show a continuous strong p16 stain. HPV test using primer to the E1 region of HPV with subsequent hybridization (AID HPV-DNA array). Bar 500 μm (**a**), 200 μm (**b**, **d**, **h**), 100 μm (**g**)

high viral load. After pooling all test results, only 3 of 92 patients with LSCC could be classified as HPV-driven [2].

Key Points

- Early studies on HPV overrated the true rate of HPV-driven LSCC.
- A positive HPV PCR test alone cannot prove oncogenic transformation.
- Test combinations are necessary to prove HPV-driven carcinogenesis.

23.1 p16 Immunohistochemistry as Surrogate Marker

HPV-related carcinogenesis may be visualized by the overexpression of the p16 protein by a simple immunohistochemistry assay on formalin-fixed tissue slides from biopsies. This is because overexpression of the p16 protein goes hand in hand with oncogenic HPV infection, followed by degradation of the retinoblastoma protein through the oncoprotein E7, from which p16 upregulation immediately follows [3]. For carcinomas of the oropharynx in particular, a significant correlation to survival after therapy has been shown for the p16 test in numerous studies [4]. In 2010, the clear correlation between p16 test and HPV positivity, in combination with favorable outcome, led to the implementation test routine for oropharyngeal carcinoma, and consequently, the p16 test also found its way into the eighth edition of the TNM staging system. The same has been shown for carcinomas without known primary tumor (CUP syndrome) in the head and neck region, because the p16 test then has similar prognostic value [5]. Although the p16 test is established as a surrogate marker for transcriptionally active oncogenic HPV infection in oropharyngeal carcinoma, there is no such association for head and neck tumors other than oropharyngeal carcinomas [6]. In addition, recent work has been published that also questions the significance of the p16 test alone for oropharyngeal carcinomas, since a significant proportion of oropharyngeal carcinoma patients with p16 test positivity differ in the outcome, particularly if the HPV-DNA test is negative [7].

Patterns of p16 staining do not correlate with HPV status in laryngeal papilloma [8]. Notably, no convincing studies outside the oropharynx in head and neck tumors are available on the prognostic value of the p16 test. Epithelial lesions of the larynx with proven HPV association typically show only scattered, weak, or moderate p16 expression (Fig. 23.2). In a recent publication, no association between p16 expression and patient

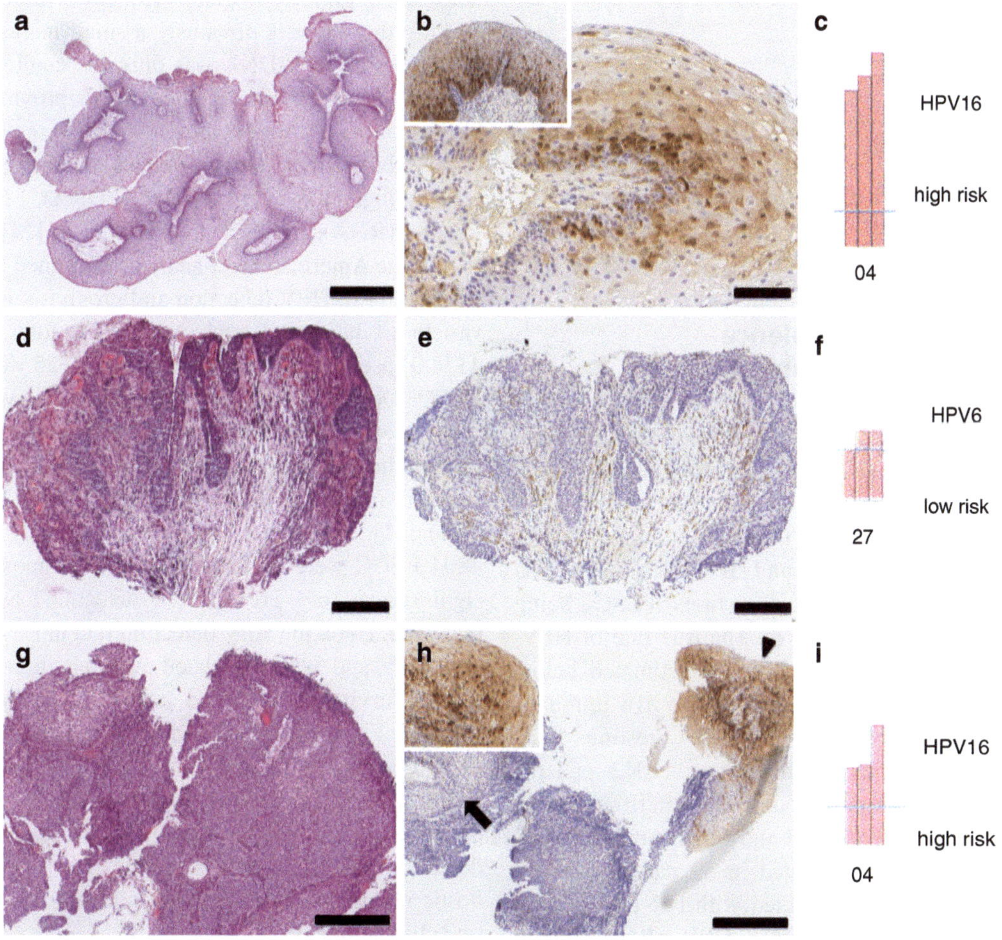

Fig. 23.2 Benign papilloma with HPV-16 (high-risk) association (**a**, **c**). The p16 staining is scattered with weak to moderate positivity (**b**). Severe dysplasia with HPV-6 (low-risk) association (**d**, **f**). The p16 stain is negative (**e**). Squamous cell carcinoma with HPV-16 (high-risk) association (**g**, **i**). The tumor cells show a focal and weak to moderate p16 staining; some invasive parts of the squamous cell carcinoma even exhibit no p16 expression (**h**)

outcome was seen in over 300 LSCC samples, and less than 50% of the p16-positive samples were mRNA-positive [9]. Accordingly, no correlation between HPV positivity and the outcome in LSCC has been published in 2020 [10]. In this recent work, the limitation of significance is also evident because the sum of p16- and HPV-DNA-positive LSCC continued to be reported as less than 5%. It can be noted that especially young patients more frequently test positive for HPV; therefore, a trend can possibly be read here that HPV prevalence in LSCC will increase in the next years. Regarding p16 significance, the evaluation of three RTOG studies can be further cited, where an association between survival and p16 testing could not be shown in LSCC patients [11].

Key Points

- The p16 test alone is unable to detect HPV-driven carcinogenesis in LSCC.
- p16 test results do not correlate with the outcome in LSCC.

23.2 HPV Prevalence and Prognostic Value

The identification of the transcripts of the viral oncogenes E6/E7, through mRNA techniques, is accepted as the gold standard test to detect HPV-attributed oncogenic transformation. The comparison of HPV-DNA and HPV-mRNA detection reveals HPV attributable fractions of LSCC being below 10% (Table 23.1). The true rate of HPV-associated LSCC can also be estimated below 5% when based on simultaneous p16 immunohistochemistry and HPV-DNA testing [12]. Castellsague et al. investigated 1042 patients with LSCC from 29 countries (49% from Europe and 35% from Central and South America), and HPV-DNA was detected in 59 patients (5.7%) and 51 patients presented with HR-HPV. Using simultaneously HPV-DNA, HPV-mRNA, or p16, the rates of true HPV association was only 3.5% (36/1042). The percentage was even lower with 1.5% (16/1042) when positivity was defined by detection of all three markers [13]. However, it is striking that there is obviously a small increase over time, as HPV-DNA was only detectable in later samples [13]. In a meta-analysis provided by Fusconi et al., four studies with triple testing (DNA/RNA/p16) were reviewed and positive test results ranged from 5.6% to 34.7% (DNA), 1.5% to 8.6% (RNA), and 3.2% to 27.6% (p16) [14].

Table 23.1 Published HPV-DNA versus HPV-mRNA prevalence in LSCC (adapted according to [14])

No. of cases	DNA (%)	mRNA (%)	Author (year)
31	6.5	3.2	Lewis (2012) [15]
64	1.6	1.6	Bishop (2012) [16]
76	17.1	5.3	Chernock (2013) [17]
102	31.4	5.9	Halec (2013) [2]
2739	22.1	8.6	Ndiaye (2014) [18]
43	9.3	4.7	Gheit (2014) [19]
1042	5.6	4.8	Castellsague (2016) [13]
404	13.4	1.7	Taberna (2016) [20]

A large American meta-analysis examined the association of HPV detection and prognosis in a variety of head and neck cancers. A total of 41,900 cases were included. Of these, 7725 were LSCC. Detection of a high-risk HPV type was considered HPV-positive. For LSCC, HPV tumors showed approximately 10% better overall survival and the difference was significant (HR 0.71) [21]. In another large database analysis, 4804 LSCC were evaluated and the prognostic significance of HPV-DNA detection was reviewed. Here, the HPV detection rate in LSCC was 11% and was associated with an inferior overall survival in advanced stages [22]. A prospective European study included 604 LSCC; here, no prognostic difference was shown for LSCC using p16 expression, HPV-16 DNA, or a combination of both [23]. In sum, therefore, HPV detection in LSCC to date is of little, if any, prognostic significance and thus not relevant in routine clinical practice.

Key Points
- The combination of two test results is necessary, e.g., DNA and RNA.
- The true HPV prevalence in LSCC is below 5%.
- HPV has no prognostic significance.

23.3 Serologic Testing

The presence of HPV-specific antibodies in patients with cancer may also indicate an HPV association. In an early study of serology against HPV antibodies in relation to the incidence of head and neck cancer, no significant association was found in LSCC [24]. In more recent studies, the relative risk of laryngeal carcinoma in patients with HPV-16 E6 antibodies was 4.18 (confidence interval 1.54–11.32). No significant difference was observed for antibodies to the E7 protein of HPV16. In the presence of both antibodies, there was a relative risk of 30.8, whereas there was almost a 900-fold risk for oropharyngeal carcinoma [25]. Interestingly, in contrast, an increased risk of LSCC was found in relation to antibodies to low-risk-type HPV-6. This might be related to a rare transformation in recurrent laryngeal papillomatosis [26]. In an American study, no association was found between the presence of HPV antibodies (on E6 and E7) and the risk of LSCC [25]. Serologic testing is not available for daily routine.

Take-Home Messages
- In contrast to the oropharynx, the p16 test is not valid for HPV detection.
- The DNA test often detects transient HPV infection unrelated to carcinogenesis.
- Only 5% or less are HPV-driven LSCC and the outcome seems unsatisfactory.
- Routine testing to date seems not to be warranted in LSCC.

References

1. Kreimer AR, Clifford GM, Boyle P, et al. Human papillomavirus types in head and neck squamous cell carcinomas worldwide: a systematic review. Cancer Epidemiol Biomark Prev. 2005;14(2):467–75.
2. Halec G, Holzinger D, Schmitt M, et al. Biological evidence for a causal role of HPV16 in a small fraction of laryngeal squamous cell carcinoma. Br J Cancer. 2013;109(1):172–83.
3. Klussmann JP, Gultekin E, Weissenborn SJ, et al. Expression of p16 protein identifies a distinct entity of tonsillar carcinomas associated with human papillomavirus. Am J Pathol. 2003;162(3):747–53.
4. Wagner S, Wittekindt C, Sharma SJ, et al. Human papillomavirus association is the most important predictor for surgically treated patients with oropharyngeal cancer. Br J Cancer. 2017;116(12):1604–11.
5. Vent J, Haidle B, Wedemeyer I, et al. p16 expression in carcinoma of unknown primary: diagnostic indicator and prognostic marker. Head Neck. 2013;35(11):1521–6.
6. Isayeva T, Li Y, Maswahu D, et al. Human papillomavirus in non-oropharyngeal head and neck cancers: a systematic literature review. Head Neck Pathol. 2012;6(Suppl 1):S104–20.
7. Wagner S, Prigge ES, Wuerdemann N, et al. Evaluation of p16(INK4a) expression as a single marker to select patients with HPV-driven oropharyngeal cancers for treatment de-escalation. Br J Cancer. 2020;123(7):1114–22.
8. Mooren JJ, Gultekin SE, Straetmans JM, et al. P16(INK4A) immunostaining is a strong indicator for high-risk-HPV-associated oropharyngeal carcinomas and dysplasias, but is unreliable to predict low-risk-HPV-infection in head and neck papillomas and laryngeal dysplasias. Int J Cancer. 2014;134(9):2108–17.
9. Young RJ, Urban D, Angel C, et al. Frequency and prognostic significance of p16(INK4A) protein overexpression and transcriptionally active human papillomavirus infection in laryngeal squamous cell carcinoma. Br J Cancer. 2015;112(6):1098–104.
10. Tagliabue M, Mena M, Maffini F, et al. Role of human papillomavirus infection in head and neck cancer in Italy: the HPV-AHEAD study. Cancers (Basel). 2020;12(12)
11. Chung CH, Zhang Q, Kong CS, et al. p16 protein expression and human papillomavirus status as prognostic biomarkers of nonoropharyngeal head and neck squamous cell carcinoma. J Clin Oncol. 2014;32(35):3930–8.
12. Wittekindt C, Wuerdemann N, Gattenlohner S, et al. The role of high-risk human papillomavirus infections in laryngeal squamous cell carcinoma. Eur Arch Otorhinolaryngol. 2017;274(11):3837–42.

13. Castellsague X, Alemany L, Quer M, et al. HPV involvement in head and neck cancers: comprehensive assessment of biomarkers in 3680 patients. J Natl Cancer Inst. 2016;108(6):djv403.
14. Fusconi M, Campo F, Gallo A, et al. Laryngeal cancer, HPV DNA vs E6/E7 mRNA test: a systematic review. J Voice. 2017;31(2):248 e241–5.
15. Lewis JS Jr, Ukpo OC, Ma XJ, et al. Transcriptionally-active high-risk human papillomavirus is rare in oral cavity and laryngeal/hypopharyngeal squamous cell carcinomas--a tissue microarray study utilizing E6/E7 mRNA in situ hybridization. Histopathology. 2012;60(6):982–91.
16. Bishop JA, Ma XJ, Wang H, et al. Detection of transcriptionally active high-risk HPV in patients with head and neck squamous cell carcinoma as visualized by a novel E6/E7 mRNA in situ hybridization method. Am J Surg Pathol. 2012;36(12):1874–82.
17. Chernock RD, Wang X, Gao G, et al. Detection and significance of human papillomavirus, CDKN2A(p16) and CDKN1A(p21) expression in squamous cell carcinoma of the larynx. Mod Pathol. 2013;26(2):223–31.
18. Ndiaye C, Mena M, Alemany L, et al. HPV DNA, E6/E7 mRNA, and p16INK4a detection in head and neck cancers: a systematic review and meta-analysis. Lancet Oncol. 2014;15(12):1319–31.
19. Gheit T, Abedi-Ardekani B, Carreira C, et al. Comprehensive analysis of HPV expression in laryngeal squamous cell carcinoma. J Med Virol. 2014;86(4):642–6.
20. Taberna M, Resteghini C, Swanson B, et al. Low etiologic fraction for human papillomavirus in larynx squamous cell carcinoma. Oral Oncol. 2016;61:55–61.
21. Li H, Torabi SJ, Yarbrough WG, et al. Association of Human Papillomavirus Status at head and neck carcinoma subsites with overall survival. JAMA Otolaryngol Head Neck Surg. 2018;144(6):519–25.
22. Tian S, Switchenko JM, Jhaveri J, et al. Survival outcomes by high-risk human papillomavirus status in nonoropharyngeal head and neck squamous cell carcinomas: a propensity-scored analysis of the National Cancer Data Base. Cancer. 2019;125(16):2782–93.
23. Abrahao R, Anantharaman D, Gaborieau V, et al. The influence of smoking, age and stage at diagnosis on the survival after larynx, hypopharynx and oral cavity cancers in Europe: the ARCAGE study. Int J Cancer. 2018;143(1):32–44.
24. Mork J, Lie AK, Glattre E, et al. Human papillomavirus infection as a risk factor for squamous-cell carcinoma of the head and neck. N Engl J Med. 2001;344(15):1125–31.
25. Anantharaman D, Gheit T, Waterboer T, et al. Human papillomavirus infections and upper aero-digestive tract cancers: the ARCAGE study. J Natl Cancer Inst. 2013;105(8):536–45.
26. Kreimer AR, Johansson M, Yanik EL, et al. Kinetics of the human papillomavirus type 16 E6 antibody response prior to oropharyngeal cancer. J Natl Cancer Inst. 2017;109(8)

24 Transoral Approach for Early Laryngeal Cancers

Cesare Piazza, Hans Edmund Eckel, Marc Remacle, Pamela Dela Cruz, Giorgio Peretti, and Claudio Sampieri

Abbreviations

AC Anterior commissure
CT Computed tomography
ELS European Laryngological Society
MR magnetic resonance
NBI Narrowband imaging
OPHL Open partial horizontal laryngectomies
RT Radiotherapy
SCC Squamous cell carcinoma
SI Saline infusion
TOLMS Transoral laser microsurgery
VLS Videolaryngostroboscopy

The original version of the chapter has been revised. A correction to this chapter can be found at https://doi.org/10.1007/978-3-031-09621-1_36

C. Piazza (✉)
Department of Otolaryngology—Head and Neck Surgery, ASST Spedali Civili di Brescia, University of Brescia, Brescia, Italy
e-mail: Cesare.piazza@unibs.it

H. E. Eckel
Department of Oto-Rhino-Laryngology, A.ö. Landeskrankenhaus Klagenfurt, HNO, Klagenfurt, Austria
e-mail: hans.eckel@kabeg.at

M. Remacle
Department of Oto-Rhino-Laryngology, Centre Hospitalier de Luxembourg (CHL), Luxembourg, Luxembourg

P. Dela Cruz
Department of Otorhinolaryngology, Philippine General Hospital, University of the Philippines, Metro Manila, Philippines

G. Peretti · C. Sampieri
Department of Otolaryngology—Head and Neck Surgery, IRCCS Ospedale Policlinico San Martino, University of Genoa, Genoa, Italy
e-mail: giorgio.peretti@unige.it

Key Points

- Transoral laser microsurgery (TOLMS) is suited for the curative treatment of most T1–T2 carcinomas of the glottic and supraglottic larynx.
- The main advantage of this mini-invasive surgical approach is the minimization of perioperative morbidity and hospital stay. Tracheotomy is rarely required.
- TOLMS of laryngeal tumors requires a meticulous preoperative evaluation in order to precisely define their superficial and deep extension. The diagnostic workup encompasses in-office transnasal videolaryngoscopy with the implementation of bioendoscopic techniques like narrowband imaging to obtain an "optical biopsy" of the lesion's nature, videolaryngostroboscopy, computed tomography and/or magnetic resonance in selected cases, preoperative assessment of laryngeal exposure, and rigid angled telescope evaluation under gen-

M. Remacle, H. E. Eckel (eds.), *Textbook of Surgery of Larynx and Trachea*, https://doi.org/10.1007/978-3-031-09621-1_24

eral anesthesia to define the precise superficial extension of the lesion.
- Classification systems for glottic and supraglottic TOLMS procedures have helped to standardize interventions, improve outcomes research, and ensure reproducible results.
- Dental injuries, mucosal tears, minor bleeding, postoperative aspiration following wider resections for supraglottic tumors, and glottic synechiae for major transcommissural resections are the most common complications and sequelae.
- Comprehensive technical equipment, including high-performance optical and carbon dioxide laser systems, focusing devices, operating laryngoscopes, multiple suction devices, and specifically designed instruments are required for successful TOLMS.
- TOLMS is not suited for tumors with arytenoid fixation. Anterior transcommissural tumors with vertical extension can be managed by TOLMS but are associated with worse oncological and vocal outcomes.
- With very rare exemptions, subglottic carcinomas are not suited for TOLMS.

24.1 Introduction

The higher frequency of laryngeal cancers is observed at the glottic level (approximately two-thirds), followed by the supraglottic area, while purely subglottic tumors are extremely rare. Among all laryngeal cancers, 53% are diagnosed when still limited to their local extension, when 5-year relative survival is estimated to be 78% (SEER data 2010–2016). Thus, these malignances can be potentially treated at an early stage when treatments can offer sound oncological and good functional outcomes.

Particularly for glottic cancer, hoarseness is often present from the very beginning of the neoplastic process, when the delicate multilayered structure of the vocal folds can be easily altered even by the presence of quite small lesions. Moreover, the predilection site for tumor origin at the level of the vocal cord is represented by its free margin, where the impact of tumor growth on mucosal vibration and its undulatory pattern may be even greater, causing a quite evident dysphonia. This peculiarity of glottic cancers, together with their low propensity to nodal spreading, means that nearly 75% of them are usually diagnosed at an early stage, in contrast with patients affected by supraglottic carcinomas who have, in the majority of cases, intermediate to advanced diseases at their first medical consultation. The distribution of laryngeal cancer burden varies consistently among different countries: the highest incidence is observed in Europe (5.45 new cases per 100,000), especially in the Southern and Mediterranean areas where, by far, the highest incidence of laryngeal cancer in men is reported [1]. Also for this reason, in European countries, surgery for laryngeal cancer has a long and well-established history, with a ratio between death and incidence of this type of cancer reported to be one of the lowest in the world (0.47) [2] (Fig. 24.1).

In contrast to the multimodal approaches usually needed for the management of more advanced stages, for early laryngeal carcinomas (Tis–T2), unimodal treatment (surgery or radiation) is strongly recommended. In the past, to preserve speech and swallowing while avoiding tracheostomy, early-staged cancers were treated by external radiation therapy (RT), keeping surgery (mainly total laryngectomy and open partial laryngectomies) in reserve for salvage. However, over the course of the past 30 years, advances in technology and instrumentation have offered transoral laser microsurgery (TOLMS) as an alternative for the upfront treatment of early laryngeal tumors. With technical advances in transoral surgery achieved during the 1960s by Kleinsasser [3] and his microlaryngoscopic technique of endolaryngeal surgery and the implementation of medical laser systems by Strong and Jako in the 1970s [4], things gradually changed beginning from the early 1980s. Clinical pioneers such as Grossenbacher, Motta,

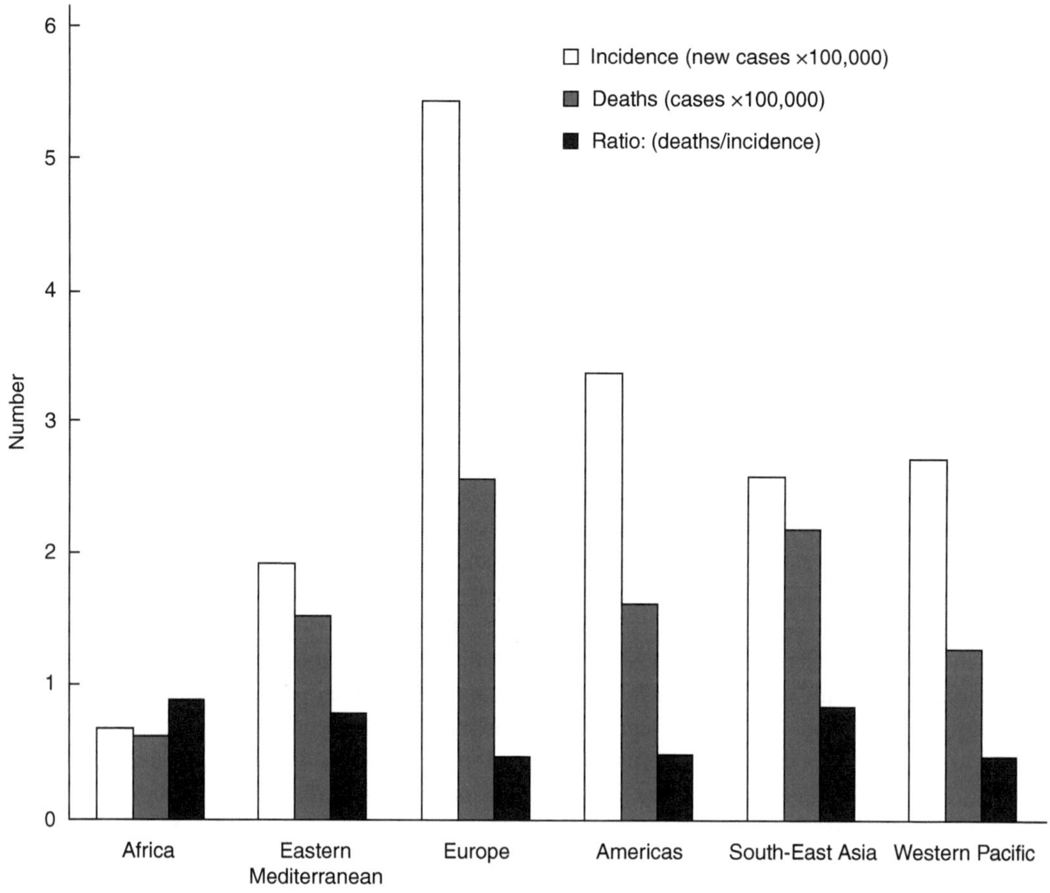

Fig. 24.1 Incidence and mortality of laryngeal cancer across different geographic areas. (Reproduced from Nocini et al. 2020)

Rudert, and Steiner in Europe and Vaughn, Davis, and Shapshay in North America were able to demonstrate that highly selected malignant lesions of the upper aerodigestive tract could now be treated transorally within narrow margin to preserve the maximal amount of surrounding healthy tissues thus achieving the best possible functional outcomes. The data presented in their studies demonstrated that carbon dioxide (CO_2) laser surgery causes minimal morbidity, offers good functional results, and provides an oncologically sound and cost-effective alternative to open surgical procedures and RT. Therefore, CO_2 TOLMS (as defined by Remacle and colleagues [5]) is now a widely accepted surgical approach to glottic and supraglottic T1–T2 carcinomas [6, 7]. Nevertheless, CO_2 TOLMS for laryngeal cancer is far from being worldwide established, as it encompasses the integration of specific individual clinical expertise and the availability of cutting-edge surgical devices. Notwithstanding, with the advent of new technological devices, CO_2 TOLMS is evolving and taking advantage of modern 3D exoscopes, capable to provide a widescreen 3D-magnified vision of the surgical field, that may one day substitute the more traditional operating microscopes [8].

24.2 Preoperative Diagnostic Procedures

A meticulous patient selection is an essential prerequisite in order to successfully treat early laryngeal cancers by CO_2 TOLMS. A rigorous preoperative diagnostic workup allows to correctly select cases and minimize intraoperative unexpected findings. This protocol aims not only to define the nature of the lesion but to provide a solid preoperative surgical plan by precisely delineating its superficial and deep extension. In this light, the possibility of intraoperatively tailoring the resection based on the endoscopic evaluation of the tumor provides the surgeon with an additional degree of freedom not conceivable with the traditional open-neck approaches.

The first step of preoperative evaluation starts in the office by a flexible transnasal videolaryngoscopy. The white light endoscopic appearance of laryngeal epithelial abnormalities is highly nonspecific, and preoperative clinical assessment is not reliable in regard to their true final pathology. The same macroscopic appearance can in fact correspond to a large spectrum of possible lesions, ranging from keratosis with or without atypia to invasive carcinoma. Therefore, this initial examination should also encompass a videostroboscopy and bioendoscopy by advanced light filters to enhance the vascular patterns of the lesion. Among the latter, narrowband imaging (NBI) is an established optical technique that enhances the diagnostic capability of endoscopes in characterizing tissues by using narrow bandwidth filters. These filters cut all wavelengths of white light except two narrow wavelengths corresponding to the peak of absorption of hemoglobin and therefore emphasize the darker framework of the capillary vessels on a blue-green mucosal background. Malignant lesions are identified by neoangiogenetic changes in their vascularity, shifting from a parallel course to a perpendicular one, enriched by the presence of intrapapillary capillary loops, designing dark spots that can be spotted within the lesion (Fig. 24.2). On the other hand, the loss of the vocal fold's mucosal wave at videolaryngostroboscopy (VLS) in a nonpreviously operated/radiated larynx is particularly suspicious for an invasive carcinoma that has transgressed the basal membrane and invaded the underlying vocal ligament, thus impairing the vocal fold vibratory properties [9]. Modern high-definition television devices may deliver clear, magnified images providing a superbly defined delineation of the superficial extent of the lesion. Moreover, this examination, conducted in the awake patient, exploits the precious opportunity to assess laryngeal mobility and sensibility. To date, there is no standard objective measurement

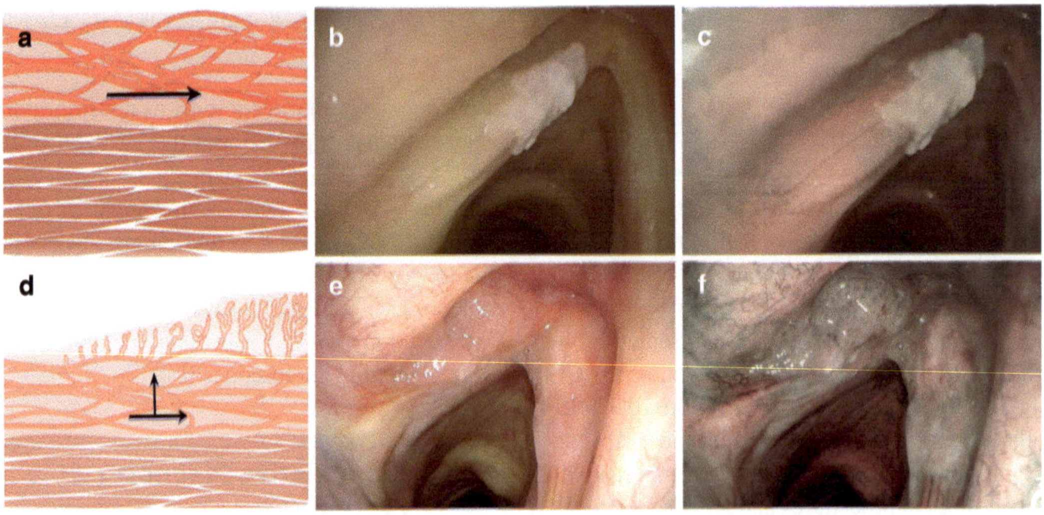

Fig. 24.2 (**a**) Longitudinal vascular changes parallel to the surface of the mucosa, (**b**) longitudinal vascular changes at the margins of a leukoplakia in white light, (**c**) longitudinal vascular changes at the margins of a leukoplakia in NBI, (**d**) development of perpendicular vascular changes in neoplasms, (**e**) glottic erythroplakia in white light, (**f**) intrapapillary capillary loops in the context on the glottic erythroplakia. (Reproduced from Arens et al. 2016)

of vocal fold/arytenoid range of motion; thus, it can only be subjectively expressed by generic terms ranging from impaired vocal cord mobility (due to tumor mass or vocal muscle invasion) to arytenoid fixation (for posterior paraglottic space invasion, cricoarytenoid joint infiltration, or recurrent nerve involvement). Last but not least, in this clinical setting, a comprehensive examination of the upper aerodigestive tract through oral examination and with the aid of a transnasal flexible videoendoscopy should be always undertaken in order to rule out any synchronous primary tumor.

The next step of the clinical examination of a laryngeal tumor includes rigid endoscopy under general anesthesia during microlaryngoscopy. With this method, a more detailed multiperspective endoscopic view of the larynx can be obtained by 0° and angled (30°, 45°, 70°, and 120°) rigid telescopes (Fig. 24.3). In this way, particular zones of the larynx and hypopharynx (anterior and posterior commissures, bottom and roof of the ventricle, subglottis, apex of the piriform sinus, and postcricoid area) that are difficult to explore during awake transnasal fiber-optic laryngoscopy can be adequately visualized. At

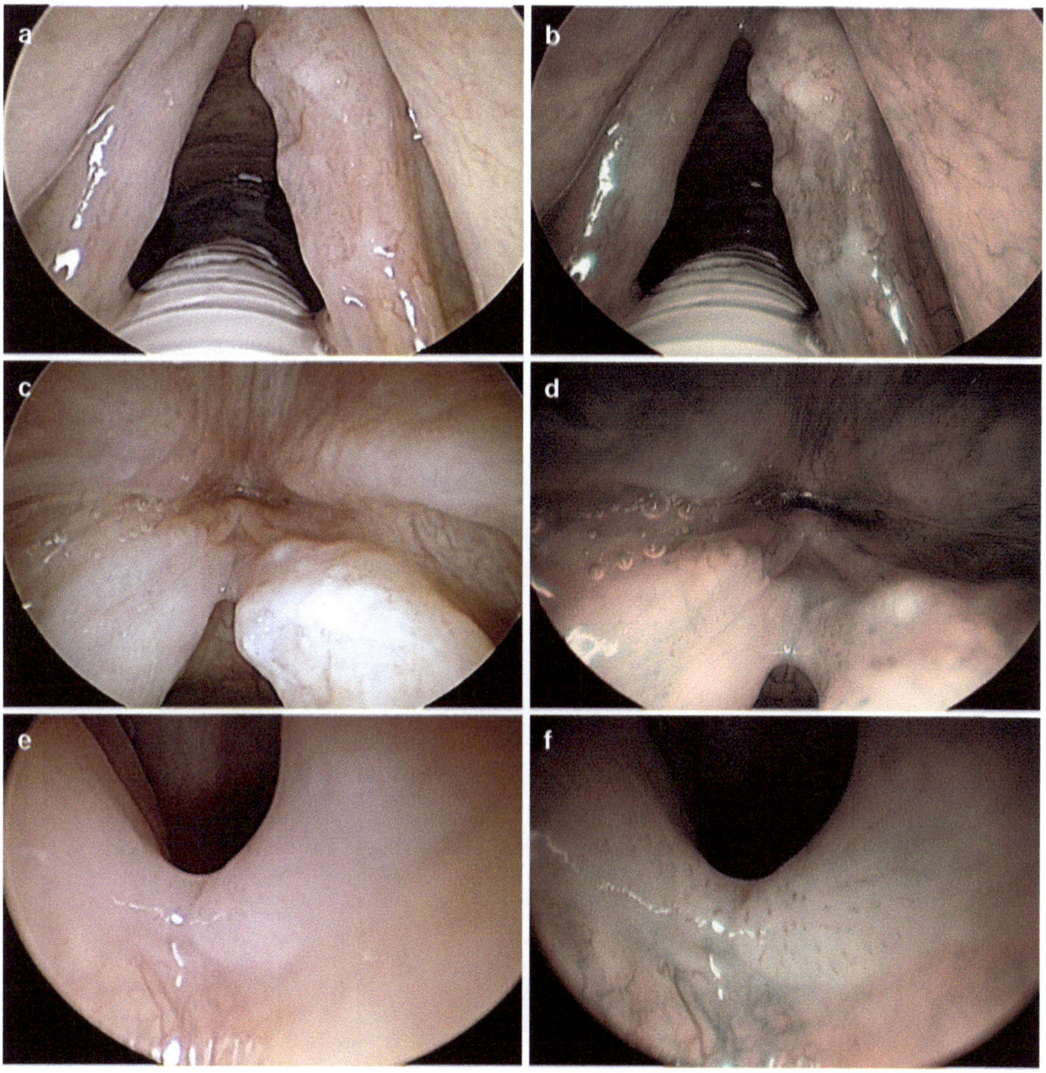

Fig. 24.3 Intraoperative evaluation with rigid telescopes: (**a**) 0° view in white light, (**b**) 0° view in NBI, (**c**) 70° view in white light, (**d**) 70° view in NBI, (**e**) 120° view in white light, (**f**) 120° view in NBI

this step, with rigid telescopes, the highest definition in the visualization of the larynx can be now achieved and, with the help of angulated optics and NBI evaluation, the superficial margins of the lesions can be thoroughly assessed. Adjunctive information can be obtained by combining the use of angled telescopes with special probes and microinstrumentation to evert and palpate the free edge of the true vocal cords, lift the false vocal folds to inspect the ventricle, and divaricate the arytenoids.

In this setting, another useful maneuver is represented by saline infusion (SI). In case of glottic cancer limited to the true vocal cord, SI using an appropriately angled needle allows further confirmation of preoperative stroboscopic findings (such as impairment of mucosal wave) regarding involvement of the lamina propria by the neoplastic growth (Fig. 24.4). Complete SI hydrodissection of the mucoligamentous plane, with consequent ballooning and lifting of the lesion from the underlying intermediate layer of the lamina propria, suggests purely intraepithelial confinement of the neoplastic nests. Moreover, the mechanical expansion of Reinke's space after SI facilitates subsequent removal of the lesion itself, serving as a plane for laser dissection and protecting the vocal ligament by excessive thermal damage when performing a subepithelial dissection. On the other hand, an incomplete or absent SI mucoligamentous hydrodissection has the same implications of a reduced or absent mucosal wave at VLS, and it is associated with the transgression of the basal membrane by neoplastic cells fixing it to the underlying vocal ligament. The results of intraoperative SI should always be integrated with those of preoperative VLS. If these two tests deliver conflicting results, especially in case of NBI-positive vascular pattern, the ensuing cordectomy should be tailored according to the more pessimistic scenario (i.e., as if they were both positive for vocal ligament involvement). Applying such a simple diagnostic algorithm, adequacy of surgical treatment can be obtained in 89% of cases [10].

Applying such a comprehensive pre- and intraoperative diagnostic workup makes, in most cases, incisional biopsy superfluous in the preoperative setting. As a matter of fact, even multiple biopsies (with or without frozen section analysis) can be frequently inadequate in obtaining a precise diagnosis. Furthermore, multiple sampling may cause undue damage and fibrosis to the multilayered and delicate microanatomy of the vocal

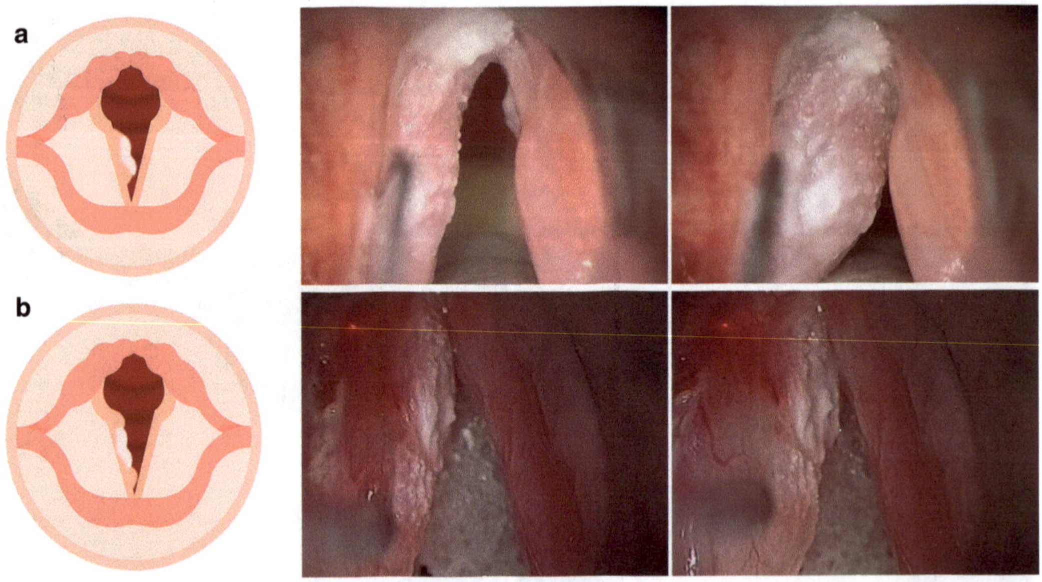

Fig. 24.4 (**a**) Positive ballooning after saline infusion in the left vocal fold, (**b**) negative ballooning after saline infusion in the left vocal fold

cord, forcing the surgeon to subsequently perform a wider and deeper resection to excise the tumor and surrounding cicatricial tissues. Several studies [11] showed not only that an accurate pre- and intraoperative diagnostic workup allows to avoid any preemptive biopsy, directly treating a given glottic lesion by a single-stage CO_2 TOLMS session, but that it is possible to minimize the rates of over- and undertreatments in terms of cordectomy extension, adequately treating 90% of patients in a single-stage operation [12]. In summary, if an accurate preoperative workup is conducted, the most adequate extension of surgery is selected so that the tumor can be completely excised within ultranarrow, free surgical margins in a single-step operation. This "en bloc" tailored removal of the tumor provides a reliable histopathologic diagnosis and a high local control rate with minimal morbidity and without the sacrifice of an undue amount of surrounding healthy tissue. This phonomicrosurgical approach to early laryngeal cancer has demonstrated its efficacy in several case series [9, 10, 12, 13]. However, some exceptions may require a preoperative histologic evaluation, like in the presence of submucosal lesions, doubt of persistence/recurrence in the irradiated larynx, or unconventional histotypes. Squamous cell carcinoma (SCC) is in fact reported to represent around 98% of laryngeal malignances [2]: it arises from the laryngeal mucosa and is characterized by the presence of altered superficial intrapapillary capillary loops, usually well detectable at NBI. Conversely, other histologies, especially those arising from submucosal structures such as adenocarcinomas and sarcomas, or hematologic neoplasm such as lymphomas, can turn out negative at NBI evaluation and may require different, nonsurgical treatments. In case of suspicious non-mucosal lesions, tomographic imaging should be always required as, in many cases, it can orientate towards the correct diagnosis or confirm the need for an incisional biopsy.

Integration of endoscopic findings with those from radiological imaging is mandatory in some cases even for early laryngeal cancer. Magnetic resonance (MR) has gradually emerged as the preferred method of investigation in such a field due to its superior capability of space and tissue density resolution. Dedicated laryngeal radiofrequency coils may be unavailable in the majority of centers; however, standard MR may provide additional information to conventional computed tomography (CT), especially when cartilage invasion is suspected. However, CT presents some unique advantages: its reduced examination time, especially valuable in the presence of claustrophobic patients with minimal compliance, and its wide availability make it a sound diagnostic tool. When CT findings are unclear, such as in the presence of minimal thyroid cartilage erosion and/or paraglottic space involvement, further insight by MR can increase diagnostic accuracy. The European Laryngological Society (ELS) has recently published an imaging checklist for the preoperative evaluation of laryngeal tumors to be treated by CO_2 TOLMS [14] (Table 24.1). The evaluation of the majority of small-volume early laryngeal cancers can rely on the endoscopic preoperative workup described above and will not need a radiological assessment in the first place. However, some locations are more subtle due to a higher risk of deeper infiltration that cannot be uncovered otherwise. Glottic tumors that infiltrate the anterior commissure (AC), particularly those with vertical transglottic extension, should always be evaluated with tomographic imaging as the preepiglottic and paraglottic spaces are almost virtual here and the thyroid cartilage may be infiltrated, therefore excluding the possibility of an adequate CO_2 TOLMS treatment. For the same reasons, a tumor that infiltrates the bottom of the laryngeal ventricle may preclude the estimation of its real deep extension at fiber-optic transnasal laryngeal endoscopy and should therefore undergo proper radiological evaluation. Supraglottic cancers, except for limited superficial tumors (such as those of the free edge of the epiglottis), should always be evaluated radiologically as the risk of arytenoid or thyroid cartilage erosion or preepiglottic space invasion is concrete. Moreover, CT and MR also allow evaluation of the regional lymph node status. This should be assessed before planning the most appropriate treatment by simultaneous or delayed

Table 24.1 ELS checklist for the preoperative evaluation of laryngeal tumors with tomographic imaging (Chiesa-Estomba et al. 2020)

Parameters	Check	CT/MR plane(s) of evaluation
Vocal fold involvement Anterior third Middle third Posterior third	Yes: ___ No: ___ Yes: ___ No: ___ Yes: ___ No: ___ Yes: ___ No: ___	Axial
Anterior commissure involvement	Yes: ___ No: ___ Vertical extension: Supraglottis: ___ Subglottis: ___	Axial and sagittal
Laryngeal ventricle/false vocal fold involvement	Yes: ___ No: ___	Coronal
Subglottic extension	Yes: ___ No: ___ Lateral: ___ Anterior: ___	Axial, coronal, and sagittal
Cartilage(s) involvement Epiglottis Thyroid Cricoid Arytenoid	Yes: ___ No: ___ Yes: ___ No: ___ Yes: ___ No: ___ Yes: ___ No: ___	Axial, coronal, and sagittal
Cricoarytenoid unit involvement	Yes: ___ No: ___	Axial, coronal, and sagittal
Posterior commissure involvement	Yes: ___ No: ___	Axial
Deep extension Anterior PGS Posterior PGS Inferior PGS PES	Yes: ___ No: ___ Yes: ___ No: ___ Yes: ___ No: ___ Yes: ___ No: ___ Yes: ___ No: ___	Axial and coronal Axial and coronal Axial and coronal Axial and sagittal Axial and sagittal
Extralaryngeal extension		

PGS Paraglottic space, *PES* Preepiglottic space

neck dissection. The N category plays a definitive role in terms of prognosis of these tumors, particularly when dealing with supraglottic lesions. Combining clinically evident and occult lymph node metastases from intermediate T2 supraglottic tumors, around 20% of them can be expected to present regional disease at the time of diagnosis [15]. Therefore, if tomographic imaging is not planned, neck lymph node ultrasound is strongly recommended in these patients: if suspicious lymph nodes are detected, fine-needle aspiration cytology should be complemented. Systematic and thorough research of distant metastasis is not indicated for early laryngeal cancers. However, taking into consideration patient's history and smoking habit, chest CT in these patients may rule out the presence of a pulmonary synchronous primary tumor.

Difficult laryngeal exposure represents the main limiting factor for CO_2 TOLMS, affecting the chance to obtain free resection margins and consequently adequate tumor control. For this reason, when considering CO_2 TOLMS, it is essential to preliminarily assess appropriate visualization of the surgical field through the available operating laryngoscopes. The AC is the most difficult area to properly visualize through the laryngoscope. In 2014, Piazza et al. developed the Laryngoscore, a preoperative predictive score, aimed at anticipating the degree of glottic visualization for each individual patient [16]. The Laryngoscore took into account 11 parameters: the sum of the preoperative score (range, 0–17) was found to be correlated with different ways of AC visualization. In particular, when the Laryngoscore was <6, good laryngeal exposure was obtained in 94% of patients. When the Laryngoscore was ≥6, the exposure was satisfying only in 60% of cases. When the total score was ≥9, a difficult exposure was found in 67% of patients. As stated above, complete tumor visualization is essential in obtaining an adequate CO_2 TOLMS resection, and the correlation between laryngeal exposure, assessed using the Laryngoscore, and the postoperative surgical margin status demonstrated that patients with difficult laryngeal exposure based on the Laryngoscore had a

Table 24.2 Mini-version of the "Laryngoscore." Possible final scores are associated with the rate of good laryngeal exposure (Incandela et al. 2019)

Parameters	Scores
Interincisor gap	
≥4 cm	0
<4 cm	1
Thyromental distance	
>6.5 cm	0
6–6.5 cm	0
<6 cm	1
Upper jaw dental status	
Edentulous	0
Partially edentulous	0
Normal teeth	1
Prominent teeth	2
Frequency of good exposure	Possible total score
97%	0
85%	1
65%	2
20%	3
<20%	4

higher rate of positive surgical margins [17]. In 2019, the same group published a mini-version of the Laryngoscore, a simplified, less subjective, three-item evaluation score taking into consideration just the interincisor gap, thyromental distance, and upper jaw dental status and demonstrating a similar efficacy in predicting adequate laryngeal exposure [18] (Table 24.2).

24.3 Surgical Technique

Under general anesthesia, a laser-safe endotracheal tube is inserted in the trachea. Shielding the endotracheal tube and cuff by cottonoids imbued with saline solution is essential to avoid serious airway complications (ignition of oxygen, perforation of the cuff with possible intraoperative blood inhalation) and a small-caliber tube is usually preferred especially for the management of glottic lesions. For posterior commissure and bulky tumors, jet ventilation might represent an adequate complementary approach [19]. Laryngeal structures are exposed by the largest operating laryngoscope available, with a built-in smoke evacuator channel. Another suction device is handled by the surgeon throughout the intervention and is used to evacuate mucus, saliva, blood, and plume and manipulate endolaryngeal tissues. The appropriate choice of laryngoscopes should meet the demands of different configurations of larynges and tumor locations. For easy exposures, large-bore laryngoscope (i.e., Dedo) allows a comfortable view and use of instruments. Narrow-caliber laryngoscopes (i.e., Ossoff-Karlan-Dedo) serve the purpose for difficult exposures, at the expense of instrument maneuverability and binocular vision. Finally, bivalved devices (i.e., Hinni or Steiner) offer a comprehensive view of the supraglottic region. Moreover, the assistant's external manipulation of the larynx, by mobilizing it using a hand on the neck, may be necessary to reach an appropriate exposure in anteriorly located lesions.

The most common laser used is the CO_2 laser beam, in the infrared region of the light spectrum, with a wavelength of 10.6 μm. This straight laser beam is directed in the surgical field by pairing the micromanipulator with the microscope in a coaxial way and offers several advantages, such as minimal scatter, minimal reflection, and strong absorption by water. The area of surrounding necrosis is less than 0.5 μm with an absorption depth of 0.2 mm. For these reasons, so far, the CO_2 surgical laser clearly represents the gold standard tool for the oncological surgery of the larynx. For this purpose, it is generally set at an output power of 2–6 watts in a superpulse, ultrapulse, or continuous mode, at a spot size of approximately 0.8 mm^2.

The principle of laser surgery is complete tumor removal, but, unlike open surgery, access to the lesion does not require opening of the laryngeal framework box with the ensuing risk of sacrificing normal tissues such as prelaryngeal muscles, neurovascular bundles, and unaffected laryngeal or pharyngeal mucosa. Therefore, tumor resection is precisely customized and tailored to each individual patient following the specific size and pathways of diffusion of the lesion to be treated. However, in every case, tumors must be resected with sufficiently safe surgical margins (at least 1 mm in width at definitive histopathology is the generally accepted rule for confirmation of an R0 resection). Specimens are excised in one piece whenever possible: while the "en bloc" technique is ideal for limited superficial lesions, on the other hand, due to the small operative field, it is often required to transect larger tumors to assess their depth of invasion and create the necessary visualization and space for piecemeal (or multi-bloc) tumor disassembling and composite resection. Removal of a tumor in two or more portions (a concept first introduced by Wolfgang Steiner, Göttingen, Germany) apparently does not comply with the generally accepted basics of oncologic surgery but is usually reserved for more advanced tumors and has been largely legitimized in other endoscopic surgical procedures like transnasal skull base tumor resections. After removal, however, specimens should be carefully oriented and marked with ink, to facilitate histopathological examination of the most meaningful margins (Fig. 24.5). The value of frozen sections in such a

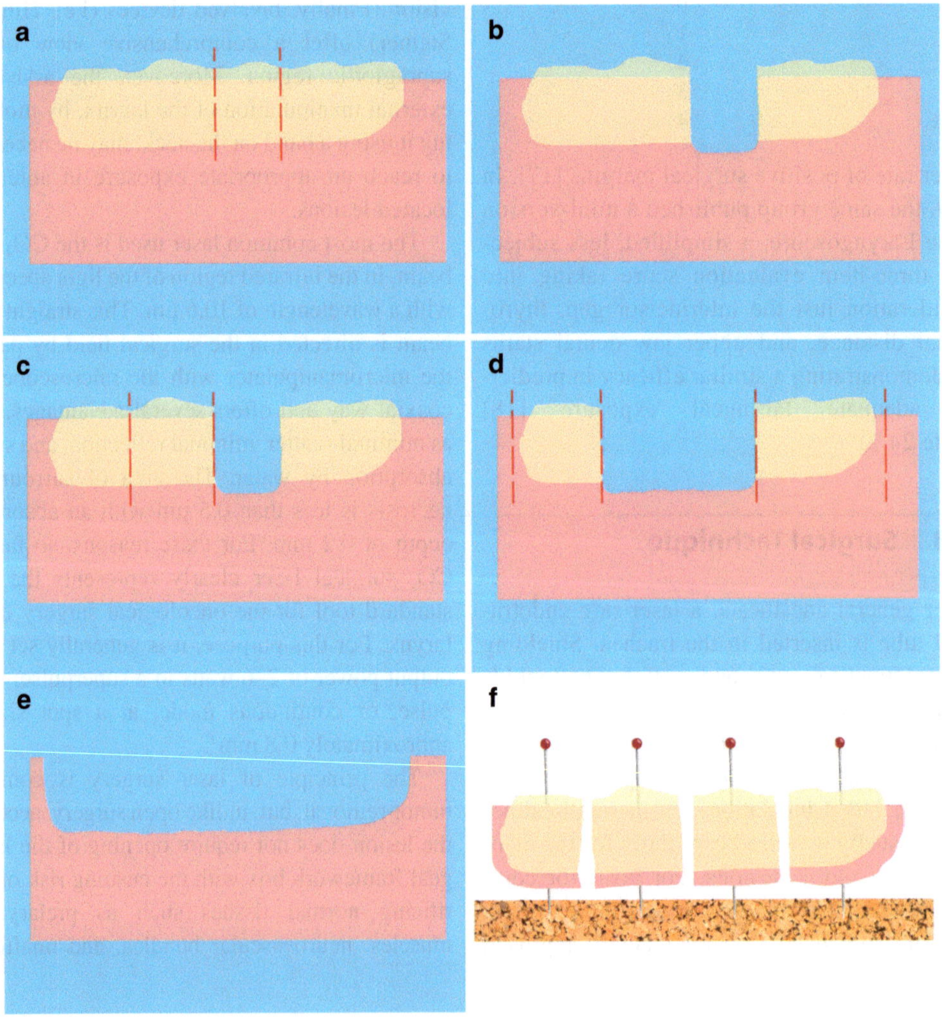

Fig. 24.5 Scheme of a multiblock excision: (**a**) transtumoral incisions are made in order to assess the depth of infiltration, (**b**) the first piece is removed, (**c**) the deep margins of the residual tumor can be assessed, (**d**) the step is repeated with the adjacent blocks, (**e**) the final result after the tumor has been excised completely, (**f**) the blocks are carefully oriented for the pathological evaluation

context remains unclear to date, and not all experienced laser surgeons use them routinely.

In early-stage glottic cancer, elective treatment of the neck lymph nodes is not justified as the rate of occult metastases usually does not exceed 8%: this makes these lesions particularly suitable for one-step CO_2 TOLMS. By contrast, in supraglottic cancers, treatment of both sides of the neck by selective neck dissection or with RT is strongly warranted, at least for T2 lesions, due to the higher incidence (around 20% of cases) of occult metastases detected [15]. However, the need for an elective neck treatment does not preclude the chance to manage the primary tumor by a transoral approach, possibly associating concomitant or 15-day delayed uni- or bilateral neck dissection according to the relationship of the lesion with the midline.

For what concerns subglottic carcinomas, apart from being very rare, they are generally not suitable for CO_2 TOLMS due to exposure issues, being RT or open-neck surgery the preferred treatment options.

24.3.1 Classification of Procedures for Glottic Carcinoma

In 2000, the ELS Working Committee on Nomenclature proposed a classification of endoscopic procedures for the treatment of glottic dysplasia and carcinoma. They did so intending to reach better agreement and uniformity concerning the extent and depth of resection among different cordectomies by offering reproducibility to laryngologists and allow relevant comparisons with the literature when presenting/publishing their oncological and functional outcomes [20]. The classification described eight types of cordectomy: subepithelial (type I), subligamental (type II), transmuscular (type III), total (type IV), and extended cordectomies including the extension to the contralateral vocal fold and the AC (type Va), one arytenoid cartilage (type Vb), subglottic structures (type Vc), or the ventricle and paraglottic space (type Vd). This classification was subsequently widely used internationally by many surgeons to describe their endoscopic procedures. A new cordectomy, encompassing the AC, the anterior part of both true and false vocal folds, and the petiole of the epiglottis (type VI), was later introduced by the ELS Working Committee on Nomenclature in 2007 [21]. A synthesis of the 2000 classification and its 2007 modification is given here (Fig. 24.6).

24.3.1.1 Subepithelial Cordectomy (Type I)

It involves the resection of the vocal fold epithelium, passing through the superficial layer of the lamina propria. This surgical procedure spares the deeper layers of the lamina propria and thus the vocal ligament. Subepithelial cordectomy is performed for cases of vocal fold lesions suspected of premalignant transformation. Ideally, the lesion intended to be treated by type I cordectomy should not be suspicious for malignancy at NBI and should present an intact mucosal wave at VLS. In this circumstance, SI finds its role as it ensures that no infiltration of the vocal ligament is present while facilitating the individuation of the most adequate resection plane. The amount of tissue resected with this procedure makes it inadequate for oncologic purposes: therefore, the main role of type I cordectomy is diagnostic. It can also play a therapeutic role whenever histological results confirm hyperplasia, dysplasia, or, at most, carcinoma in situ without signs of microinvasion. Indeed, by definition, these lesions are in fact limited to the epithelium. On the other hand, if microinvasive carcinoma is identified, subepithelial resection may not achieve safe deep resection margins, and thus, a further procedure (e.g., type II cordectomy) is required.

24.3.1.2 Subligamental Cordectomy (Type II)

It involves the resection of the epithelium, Reinke's space, and underlying vocal ligament up to the very superficial fibers of the vocal muscle. It is performed by cutting along the interface between the vocal ligament and muscle. The latter is however preserved as much as possible. The resection may extend from the vocal process to the anterior macula flava and may be performed

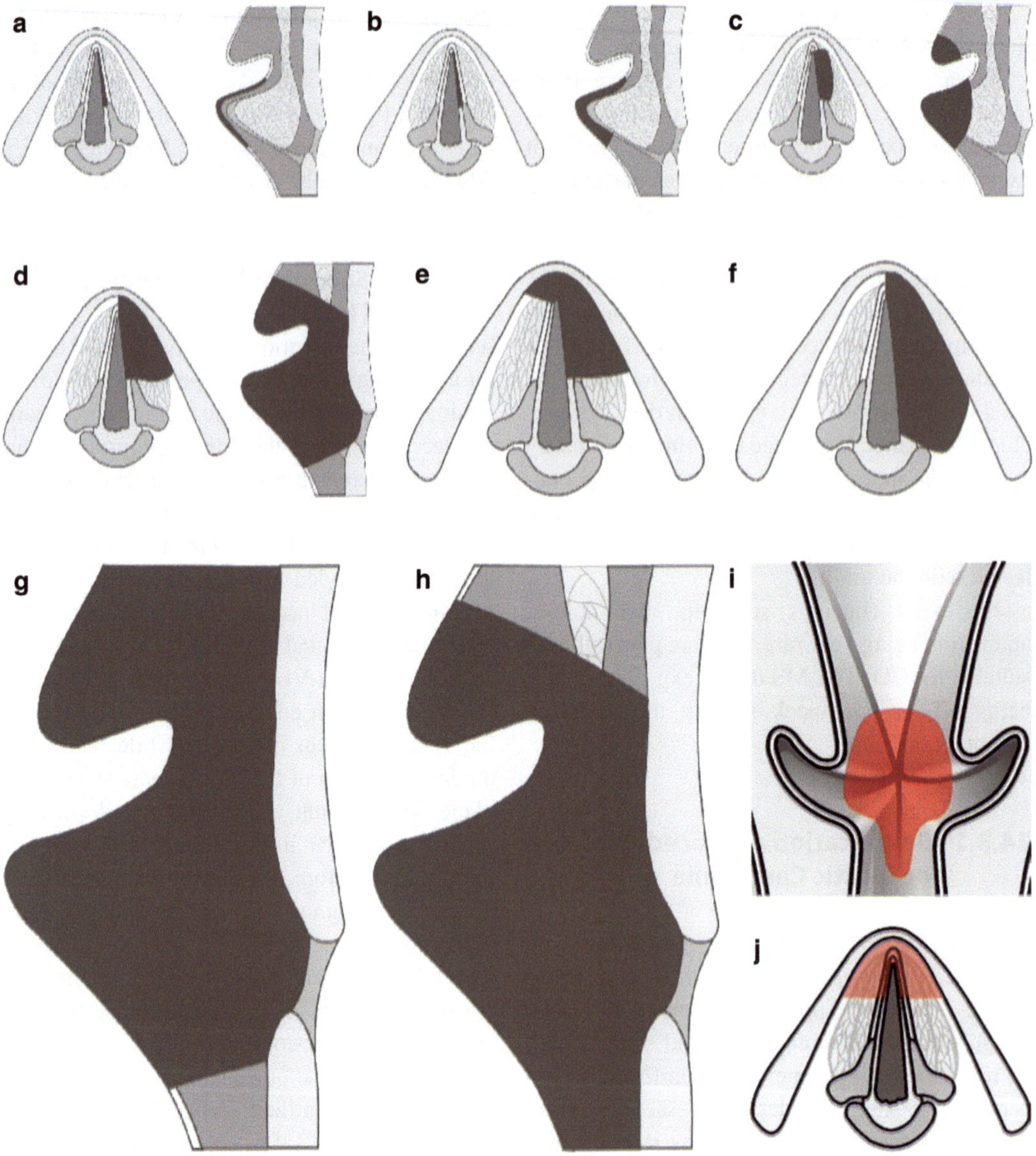

Fig. 24.6 ELS classification for endoscopic cordectomies: (**a**) type I, (**b**) type II, (**c**) type III, (**d**) type IV, (**e**) type Va, (**f**) type Vb, (**g**) type Vc, (**h**) type Vd, (**i**) type VI coronal view, (**j**) type VI axial view. (Reproduced from Remacle et al. 2000 and Remacle et al. 2007)

bilaterally if needed. This procedure is indicated whenever a lesion shows clinical signs of neoplastic transformation, especially at NBI, and VLS examination indicates deep infiltration, or impairment/absence of mucosal wave ("vibratory silence"). SI displays no mucoligamentous hydrodissection (absent or incomplete ballooning). When palpated, the vocal cord feels thickened and the mucosa cannot be freely moved over the underlying structures. At a therapeutic level, subligamental cordectomy is indicated for microinvasive or invasive glottic carcinoma (cT1), the latter being limited to the vocal ligament in 95% of cases [11, 13].

24.3.1.3 Transmuscular Cordectomy (Type III)

It is performed by cutting through the vocalis muscle. The resection encompasses the epithelium, lamina propria, and medial portion of the vocalis muscle. The resection may extend from the vocal process to the AC. Partial resection of the ventricular fold may be necessary to expose the lateral extent of the entire vocal fold at the level of the floor of the ventricle, up to the point of its reflection into the bottom and roof of the ventricular cavity. Transmuscular cordectomy is indicated for bulky T1 of the vocal fold causing reduced mobility for a mass effect (without the possibility to precisely evaluate a limited vocal muscle infiltration) or in true T2 lesions infiltrating the vocal muscle itself. In the authors' hands, however, type III cordectomy is the ideal tool to manage previously biopsied lesions whenever the dissection planes and neoplasm margins are difficult to be ascertained due to the presence of scar tissue. In this scenario, the sacrifice of part of the vocal muscle, at the expense of the vocal outcome, will result in safer resection margins without the need for further reinterventions, which would have a higher cost in terms of vocal muscle volume loss and oncologic outcomes.

24.3.1.4 Total or Complete Cordectomy (Type IV)

It longitudinally extends from the arytenoid to the AC. The depth of the surgical margins reaches the internal perichondrium of the thyroid cartilage ala. Sometimes the perichondrium is included within the resection. Anteriorly, the incision is made in the midline of the AC detaching the macula flava and the Broyle's ligament from the inner surface of the thyroid cartilage. Total cordectomy is reserved for glottic cancer infiltrating the vocal muscle with impairment of vocal fold mobility (T2) or with limited involvement of the anterior paraglottic space at the glottic level (T3). This condition should be however clearly differentiated from arytenoid hypomobility/fixation due to massive posterior paraglottic space encroachment which, instead, is considered an absolute contraindication to CO_2 TOLMS.

24.3.1.5 Extended Cordectomy Encompassing the Contralateral Vocal Fold (Type Va)

Extended cordectomies were meant to describe a heterogeneous array of possible procedures extending beyond the confines of one vocal fold. In particular, type Va is a complete cordectomy extended to the AC and, according to the extent of the tumor, possibly to a segment or the entire length of the contralateral vocal fold. This procedure is somewhat controversial because resection around the AC may be technically demanding, especially in patients with suboptimal laryngeal exposure, and usually leads to poor phonatory results. In case of intraoperative detection of minor thyroid cartilage erosion, CO_2 TOLMS should be abandoned in favor of an open-neck procedure (open partial laryngectomies or total laryngectomy according to the different clinical scenarios) or nonsurgical organ preservation attempts.

24.3.1.6 Extended Cordectomy Encompassing the Arytenoid (Type Vb)

It is a complete cordectomy encompassing the arytenoid and is indicated for vocal fold carcinoma involving the vocal process or superficially extending to the arytenoid cartilage posteriorly. The cartilage is thus partially or totally resected. The posterior arytenoid mucosa may be preserved if this decision is oncologically sound. The arytenoid should be mobile and posterior paraglottic space not infiltrated. Otherwise, CO_2 TOLMS is usually contraindicated for the high risk of positive surgical margins. The necessary full exposure of the posterior commissure and arytenoid may be reached by either dislodging the orotracheal tube anteriorly and intercalating the operating laryngoscope in between the tube and the posterior commissure or using jet ventilation through a small transglottic catheter [17, 19].

24.3.1.7 Extended Cordectomy Encompassing the Ventricular Fold (Type Vc)

Total cordectomy can be also extended to the mucosa of the laryngeal ventricle, ventricular fold, and paraglottic fat pad. This procedure is indicated for ventricular or transglottic cancers spreading to the bottom and roof of the ventricle (cT2–cT3).

24.3.1.8 Extended Cordectomy Encompassing the Subglottis (Type Vd)

If necessary, an extended cordectomy can be enlarged to include the structures below the glottic plane to expose the cricothyroid membrane and cricoid cartilage. In selected cases, this procedure may be indicated for the removal of cT2 carcinoma with limited subglottic extension without cartilage invasion and/or extension through the cricothyroid and crico-tracheal membranes.

24.3.1.9 Extended Cordectomy for Cancers Arising from the Anterior Commissure (Type VI)

Type VI cordectomy is indicated for tumors originating from the AC, extended (or not) to one or both true and false vocal folds, to the petiole of the epiglottis and/or anterior subglottis, without infiltration of the thyroid cartilage. This procedure includes resection of the AC with the anterior thirds of the true and false vocal cords, Broyle's tendon, and conoid ligament. To remove the entire AC area within safe margins, the incision should be started above the plane of the false vocal folds, at the level of the epiglottic insertion on the thyroid notch, and then extended downwards through the Broyle's ligament, at least until the inferior margin of the thyroid cartilage. Inclusion of the subglottic mucosa and cricothyroid membrane into the surgical specimen is justified since AC cancers tend to spread towards the anterior subglottic lymphatic vessels. This technique is the ideal tool for treating AC cancers with vertical extension (anterior transcommissural tumors) and properly clear the inside aspect of the anterior laryngeal box.

24.3.2 Classification of Procedures for Supraglottic Carcinoma

Among the indications of CO_2 TOLMS for laryngeal cancer, supraglottic laryngectomies for early-stage supraglottic lesions definitively play a prominent role. This is mainly due to the oncological outcomes described, comparable to those obtained by other therapeutic options, and to the better functional results (especially when compared to those achieved by OPHL) [22]. Of course, there remain various indications for conservative open neck approaches like, for example, OPHL type I which is, again, a good reason why head and neck surgeons should be trained in the wide field of transoral and open laryngeal surgery, not focusing uniquely on one treatment method, especially when dealing with oncologic issues. The main advantage of CO_2 TOLMS for supraglottic tumors is that the resection can be personalized and tailored to the precise extent of a given tumor. Moreover, hospitalization times are shorter, and morbidity is lower, as it avoids tracheostomy in the vast majority of cases [23]. "En bloc" resection is mainly possible for small (cT1 to small-volume cT2), circumscribed carcinomas of the supraglottis. Surgical technique is comparable to resection of early glottic cancer even though tumors in this area should be resected with wider margins since they are well known to have a more aggressive biologic behavior than glottic tumors, a higher tendency of lymphatic spread, and such increased surgical aggressiveness usually do not compromise vocal outcomes and swallowing. If multi-bloc (or piecemeal) resection is needed (especially in large-volume cT2–cT3 lesions), it mandates a high accuracy in the precise orientation of the specimen, close cooperation with the pathologist to accurately assess the adequacy of the resection margins, and true multidisciplinary teamwork in understanding the three-dimensional tumor volume and nature of surgical margins in order to appropriately select those patients needing adjuvant treatments.

Tumor extension of infrahyoid epiglottic carcinomas is rather difficult to determine preoperatively, particularly in the petiolar area. Thus, it is often difficult to differentiate between superficial T1 and deeper T3 carcinomas before surgery, even in the presence of a state-of-the-art imaging. However, clinical experience shows that preepiglottic space infiltration should be anticipated for all tumors of the infrahyoid region. However, in the case of the demonstrated deep involvement of such a visceral space, CO_2 TOLMS is not contraindicated, but the treating surgeon should be prepared to comprehensively manage a cT3 lesion. Bleeding of vessels in this area is usually well controlled by conventional electrocautery and titanium clips, which have proved to be appropriate especially when the superior laryngeal pedicle is encountered at the level of the lateral portion of the pharyngoepiglottic fold. Depending on the extent of planned resection, unilateral arytenoid sacrifice can be considered, knowing that it will cause the highest degree of postoperative swallowing difficulties encountered after CO_2 TOLMS [24]. However, resection of both arytenoids must be avoided to prevent persistent severe postoperative dysphagia with massive aspiration.

In contrast to open neck surgery, nasogastric feeding tube, when needed, can be maintained for a few days only, and temporary tracheostomy can be generally avoided. In the authors' experience, nasogastric feeding tube is mainly indicated for those procedures involving wider supraglottic resections, especially when one arytenoid has been (sub)totally resected. Of course, this does not mean that supraglottic partial laryngectomy by CO_2 TOLMS is a risk-free method: there are cases with significant postoperative bleeding or persistent functional deficits such as swallowing difficulties with aspiration. Therefore, as for every other therapeutic approach, proper patient selection with respect to age, functional status, and extent of surgical resection should be always taken into account, as postoperative rehabilitation may be demanding. Regarding the risk of postoperative bleeding, it should be ensured that patients remain under continuous supervision, with daily fiber-optic transnasal endoscopies, at least during the first 5–6 postoperative days, so they can be adequately treated in case of an emergency, including rapid intubation if required.

Several complications, regarding around 30% of the overall procedures, have been reported for CO_2 TOLMS of supraglottic carcinomas: local infection, chondronecrosis, subcutaneous emphysema, salivary fistula, bleeding, respiratory distress due to stenosis or edema, swallowing difficulties, and aspiration pneumonia [25]. The complication rate is determined mainly by the surgeon's experience and extent of resection. This is the reason why clinical training should start with procedures for circumscribed supraglottic lesions and, later, after gaining adequate experience, the treatment spectrum can be enlarged to more extended supraglottic carcinomas.

In 2009, the ELS Working Committee on Nomenclature proposed a classification for endoscopic supraglottic partial laryngectomies [26]. A synthesis of this classification is herein discussed (Fig. 24.7).

24.3.2.1 Limited Excision (Type I)

This type of supraglottic resection entails the excision of small superficial tumors on the free border of the epiglottis, aryepiglottic fold, arytenoid or ventricular fold, or any other part of the supraglottis.

24.3.2.2 Medial Supraglottic Laryngectomy with Partial Resection of the Preepiglottic Space (Type II)

In the case of small and superficial T1 tumors of the laryngeal surface of the epiglottis, located above the hyoid bone, the resection may include half of the suprahyoid epiglottis (type IIa). For tumors extending below the hyoid bone, a total epiglottectomy may be needed (type IIb). The section line goes through the preepiglottic space without its complete excision. The pharyngoepiglottic, aryepiglottic, and ventricular folds are preserved.

24.3.2.3 Medial Supraglottic Laryngectomy with Resection of the Preepiglottic Space (Type III)

Resection of T2 tumors extending to the petiole of the epiglottis must include the preepiglottic space (type IIIa). The surgical incision is carried along the valleculae until the hyoid bone is reached. The dissection then moves caudally from the hyoid bone towards the thyrohyoid membrane until the upper border of the thyroid

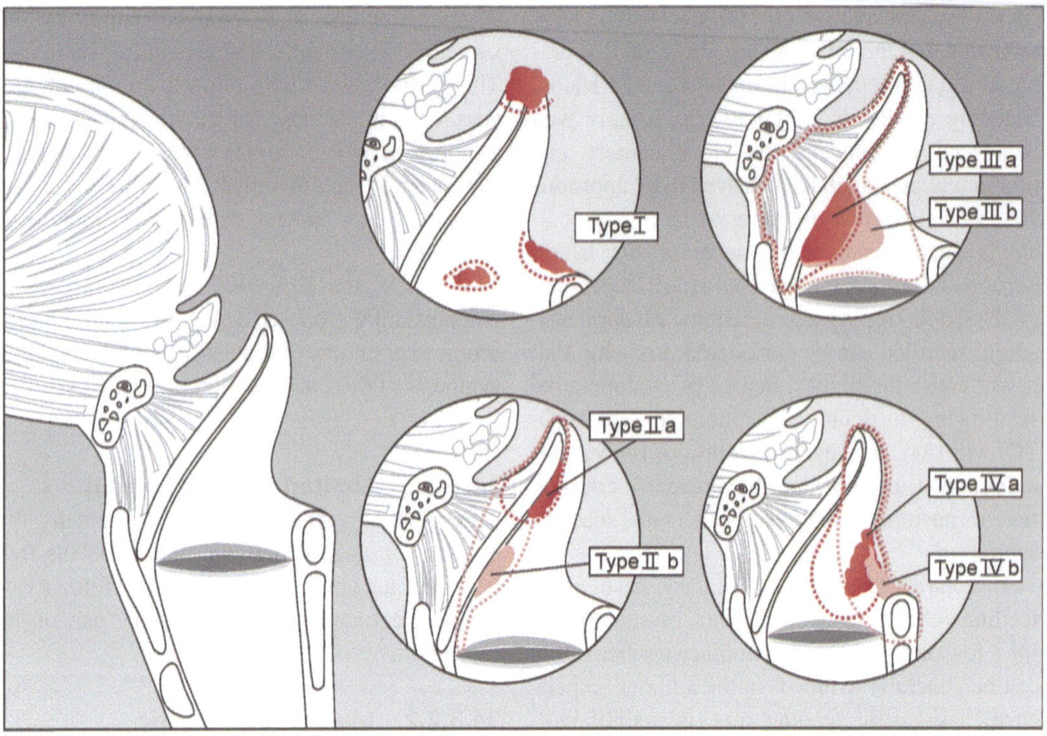

Fig. 24.7 ELS classification for endoscopic supraglottic laryngectomies. (Reproduced from Remacle et al. 2009)

cartilage is exposed. From this point, the whole entity of the preepiglottic space is removed along the inner surface of the thyroid laminae together with the epiglottis towards the anterior commissure of the vocal folds. T2 tumors of the infrahyoid epiglottis extending to the ventricular fold can be resected with the same technique (type IIIb). The ventricular folds can be completely dissected from the thyroid cartilage along the inner surface towards the laryngeal ventricle.

24.3.2.4 Lateral Supraglottic Laryngectomy (Type IV)

In case of tumors of the three-folds' region, which includes the lateral free edge of the epiglottis, the aryepiglottic, and the pharyngoepiglottic folds with possible extension to the ventricular bands, the resection includes the free edge of the epiglottis, the medial wall of the piriform sinus, and the ventricular fold (type IVa). In case of extension to the arytenoid, the resection will encompass the most advanced and aggressive form of supraglottic resection, potentially including a significant portion of the adjacent piriform sinus (type IVb).

Since its publication, the ELS classification system has been cited hundreds of times in the literature [27]. Numerous centers in various countries have adopted this system to describe the type of resection made. This classification allows reproducibility of the technique and serves to improve the teaching and training of inexperienced surgeons in endoscopic cordectomy and supraglottic partial resections.

24.4 Recurrence: Follow-Up, Diagnosis, and Management

One essential prerequisite for the transoral management of laryngeal tumors is ensuring adequate patient compliance to a compulsive postoperative follow-up. Tailored endoscopic resections are often performed within millimetric safe margins and such an ultraconservative approach is potentially dangerous if patients escape regular controls. Detection of early recurrence is, in fact, important since transoral procedures can still be an option for managing recurrences in these patients. Therefore, the rationale behind the need for a postoperative follow-up includes evaluation of treatment response, early identification of recurrence, possible detection of further metachronous tumors, management of complications, and optimization of voice/swallowing rehabilitation.

In this context, ventricular fold resection before approaching every glottic lesion gives not only the advantage to enhance the exposure during primary surgery, but it also facilitates subsequent transnasal fiber-optic laryngoscopy control during follow-up. Particularly when dealing with tumors at high risk of recurrence (e.g., T2 glottic lesions with anterior transcommissural extension, or supraglottic tumors with lateral extension to the bottom of the ventricle and paraglottic space), an even closer clinical follow-up is strongly recommended. In particular, when dealing with such intermediate to advanced tumors, a CT and/or MR follow-up should be also combined and scheduled twice a year for the first 2 years after surgery, even in case of a negative clinical evaluation [28].

In 2014, a working group of the Head and Neck Cancer Committee of the ELS published a paper containing evidence-based recommendations regarding laryngeal cancer follow-up [29]. According to their work, patients should be followed up for a minimum of 5 years with prolonged surveillance for those with a high risk of late recurrence (e.g., active smokers). When the risk of locoregional recurrence is high, patients should be followed up at least bimonthly in the first 2 years and quarterly to every 6 months in the subsequent years. However, longer intervals can be proposed for smaller lesions (i.e., glottic T1) with clear margins. Clinical assessment should be conducted by a dedicated otolaryngologist and it should include an adequate examination of the entire mucosal lining of the upper aerodigestive tract (in order to detect possible second primary tumors) and neck palpation. Seriated video-recorded examinations using high-resolution flexible endoscopes are of paramount value for sharing opinions between different examiners, storing images of individual patients, and making comparisons during the entire posttherapeutic period. NBI, possibly associated with high-definition television technology, can enhance the chance of detecting superficial persistence/recurrences or second primary tumors (Fig. 24.8). A second-look microlaryngoscopy should be reserved to selected cases, as for uncertain (close or altered for iatrogenic artifacts) surgical margins, granulomas, webs, or other post-excisional abnormal tissue growth at the level of the primary resection site, and should not be performed before 8 weeks from surgery for possible confounding factors due to the ongoing healing process.

As previously described in the preoperative setting, strict cooperation between the surgeon

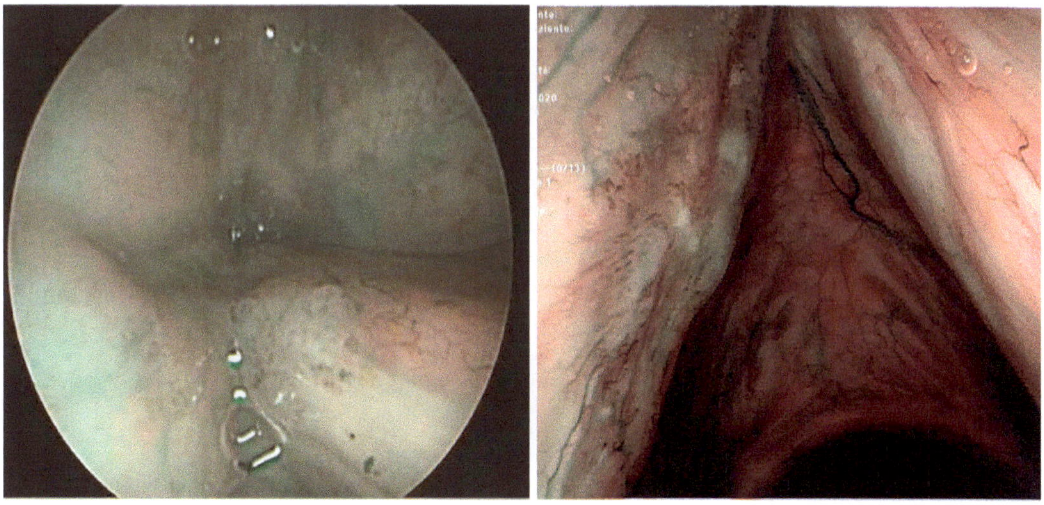

Fig. 24.8 Glottic recurrences enhanced by NBI evaluation

and an experienced radiologist is mandatory during follow-up. The authors' policy encompasses periodic CT and/or MR (even in the absence of endoscopic abnormalities) in patients with T2 or more advanced glottic and supraglottic tumors. Any endoscopic abnormalities deemed not related to normal postoperative sequelae and hiding possible deep patterns of disease progression should be immediately evaluated by the appropriate imaging modality. Neck monitoring can be performed simply with clinical examination for early glottic tumors, especially considering their low propensity for nodal involvement. An ultrasonography every 4 months during the first 2 years, when not performing CT, is indicated in patients with T2 supraglottic tumors submitted to a "wait and see" policy of the neck, while longer intervals (i.e., once a year) can be adopted for patients treated by elective neck dissection. In case of suspicious ultrasonographic findings, fine-needle aspiration cytology is strongly recommended. For early glottic cancer, imaging for distant metastasis detection may not be required, even though monitoring of the chest in the quest of metachronous lung tumors is strongly warranted, especially in active smokers. This type of surveillance may be also indicated for T2 supraglottic cancers, especially if nodal involvement was present at the time of treatment.

Recurrences after transoral surgery can follow completely different patterns of progression. Aside from superficial persistence/recurrence of mucosal dysplasia with possible progression to invasive cancer, directly detectable by endoscopic evaluation, the main concerns of follow-up examination should always be directed to early diagnosis of deep submucosal progression to the visceral spaces, laryngeal framework, and/or soft tissues of the neck (Fig. 24.9). Symptoms such as worsening dysphonia and progressive dysphagia with

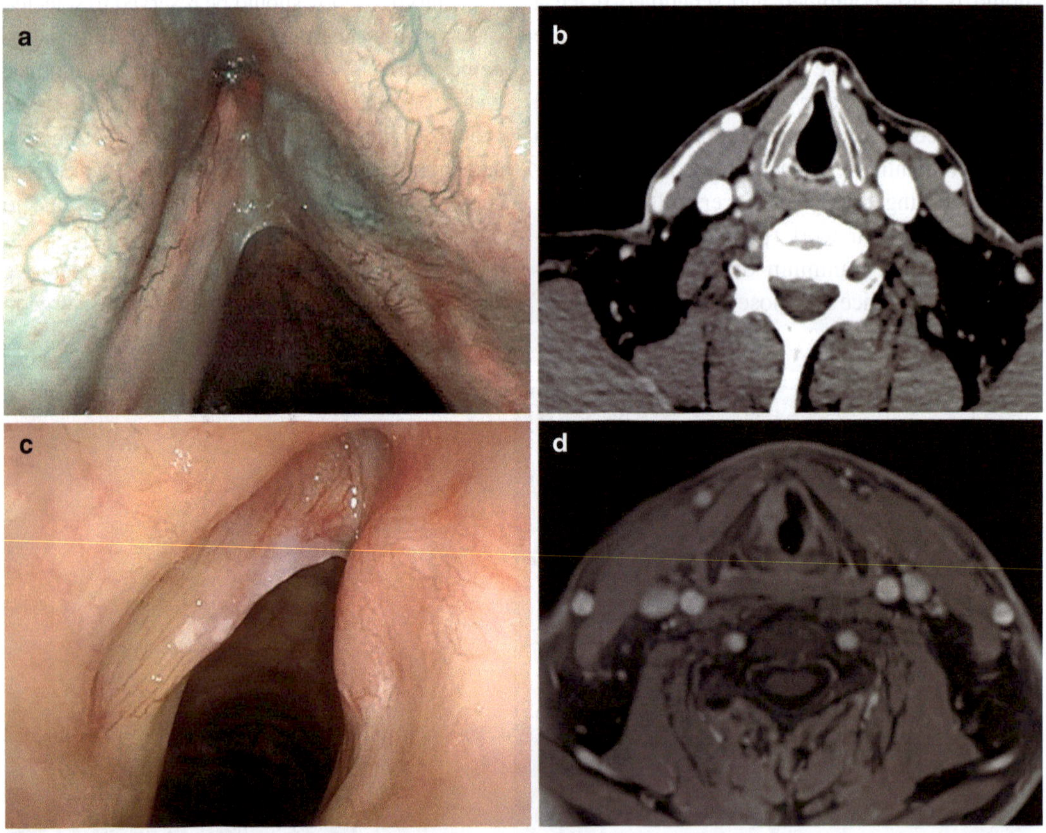

Fig. 24.9 Examples of glottic recurrence: (**a–b**) superficial recurrence on the right vocal fold in NBI endoscopy and CT, (**c–d**) submucosal recurrence of the right vocal fold with anterior paraglottic space involvement and initial thyroid cartilage erosion in WL endoscopy and MR

associated otalgia should always be taken into account, with a prompt, careful search for submucosal laryngo-hypopharyngeal bulging, impaired vocal cord and/or arytenoid mobility, or subglottic mass. The presence of any of these clinical features should require immediate evaluation by neck CT or MR.

If local recurrence is detected, a larger number of retreatment options are still available after initial CO_2 TOLMS than after initial RT or OPHL. In fact, after transoral surgery, no increased rate of wound complications was reported for redo-CO_2 TOLMS, different from what was observed after previous RT. Moreover, in this case, the laryngeal framework is still intact, thus preventing early extralaryngeal spread of local failures. These characteristics make local recurrences after transoral surgery still manageable either by CO_2 TOLMS again or open surgery: however, when detected early, local recurrences can be safely treated by organ preservation surgery or radiotherapy [30]. If superficial recurrence occurs, the oncological outcomes are usually not worsened in such a salvage scenario, being comparable to those observed in the primary therapeutic setting. By contrast, a submucosal progression of residual neoplastic cells towards the deep visceral spaces is certainly burdened by worse prognosis, even if still manageable by salvage treatments. In fact, previous transoral removal of some natural barriers to the tumor spread (Broyle's ligament, conus elasticus, vocal ligament, quadrangular membrane, and epiglottis) makes the subsequent patterns of tumor diffusion somewhat unpredictable. However, preservation of the cartilaginous laryngeal framework during initial laser surgery usually prevents recurrences from spreading beyond the larynx for a long time.

24.5 Oncological Outcomes

Oncological data on CO_2 TOLMS for T1–T2 carcinomas of the larynx are exclusively based on retrospective studies and meta-analyses (level III and IV evidence). Prospective randomized trials comparing oncological outcomes of different therapeutic approaches are currently not available.

24.5.1 Glottic Cancer

The existing data on T1 glottic carcinomas reveal a good 5-year local control ranging from 85% to 100% after transoral surgery, open partial laryngectomies, or RT with no significant difference between these treatment modalities. Slightly lower control rates (66%–100%) are reported after transoral surgery for T2 glottic carcinomas, with results comparable to OPHL and RT as well [31, 32]. Similarly, the meta-analyses present in the literature do not show a significant difference in terms of local control after CO_2 TOLMS or RT [33, 34]: nevertheless, a trend towards better laryngectomy-free survival for transoral surgery was observed in some studies [33, 35]. This can be explained by the fact that, when RT is used as the primary treatment modality, if recurrence occurs, patients can only be further treated surgically, by total laryngectomy as the gold standard treatment for salvage. On the other hand, when CO_2 TOLMS is applied as the first-line treatment, in case of recurrence, RT can still be used as salvage therapy. Moreover, one final advantage of transoral surgery is that, in contrast to OPHL, age does not represent a contraindication.

24.5.2 Supraglottic Cancer

As for glottic carcinoma, when discussing the optimal treatment option for supraglottic cancer, it must be considered that the primary tumor can be successfully treated either by CO_2 TOLMS, OPHL, or RT in most cases. For what concerns transoral surgery, the reported 5-year local control rates range from 66% to 92% for T1–T2 supraglottic carcinomas, with laryngeal preservation obtainable in 85%–90% of cases [23, 36, 37]. A 2016 meta-analysis by Patel et al. suggests that patients undergoing primary organ-preservation surgery have better survival than those treated by primary RT [38]: in this review, OPHLs were also included; however, long-term oncologic outcomes comparing CO_2 TOLMS and open surgery suggest that their results are similar [39]. From the oncological point of view, one of the advantages of transoral surgery combined with neck dissection compared to RT is the ability of the former approach to identify patients with occult nodal metastasis in the neck. This is an important consideration given that up to 20% of patients with early supraglottic cancer may have occult nodal metastasis [15]. Thus, although these patients are early staged at the time of recruitment, the discovery of positive nodal metastases after elective neck dissection can result in upstaging and adjuvant therapy may be recommended as needed.

24.5.3 Transoral Laser Microsurgery Excision Margins

The development of modern laser systems permits laser application with lower power settings, so that charring and artifacts at the level of the specimen margins are greatly reduced in comparison to what was observed in the past using older laser systems. Thus, it is nowadays easier for pathologists to properly evaluate the resection margins. It is widely accepted that ≥1 millimeter free resection margins, especially at the level of the glottic plane, should be considered as negative. Below this threshold, a close resection margin is usually defined [40]. As every narrow margin surgery, CO_2 TOLMS may present close and positive margins in around 50% of the cases at the final histopathologic report: nevertheless, up to 80% of close and positive margins may result negative at a subsequent second-look, being indeed false positives [40–42]. Post-resection and postfixation shrinkage of the surgical specimen and artifacts caused by the CO_2 laser thermal effect may alter the histological evaluation and are at least partially responsible for the high incidence of apparently unsafe surgical margins. Therefore, contrary to conventional open surgery, the report of a final close/positive margin after transoral laser surgery may not always require a reexcision. Indeed, the impact of margin status on survival rates remains controversial: whereas some authors found close and positive margins to be independent risk factors for recurrence and poorer survival rates, others did not find any significant variations compared with negative ones.

On a retrospective multi-institutional series of 634 patients by Fiz and coworkers, close and positive single superficial margins did not negatively affect DSS in respect to negative ones (98.7%, 100%, and 100%). However, positive multiple superficial, as well as positive deep margins, determined a slight, but significant, reduction of DSS compared with the negative ones (93.6% and 97% vs. 100%, respectively) [43]. Therefore, the authors' policy is to perform a watchful waiting in patients with close superficial and positive single superficial margins. Instead, a second-look microlaryngoscopy seems preferable in case of deep and positive multiple superficial margins. Finally, according to some authors, intraoperative assessment of margins by means of frozen section can limit the need for second-look surgeries. Remacle and colleagues assessed the reliability of this method by comparing frozen section outcomes with the results of the final histology in 97 patients submitted to CO_2 TOLMS for glottic carcinomas at different stages: 94.8% of the frozen sections were later histologically confirmed at definitive examination after formalin fixation [44]. This surgical technique may be indeed time-consuming if implemented routinely but offer a reliable aid in selected complex cases.

24.5.4 Anterior Commissure Involvement and Vocal Fold Mobility Impairment

Among early glottic cancers, several tumors with different locations and sizes are sometimes grouped together. Recent publications have underlined that not all sites and subsites of the larynx, when involved, share the same prognosis when treated by CO_2 TOLMS. As such, we designed a 3D map of the larynx characterizing diverse zones with different oncologic outcomes [45]. According to this approach, there are two broad categories of early glottic tumors burdened by a potentially worse prognosis: tumors involving the AC with vertical extension towards the supra- and/or subglottis and tumors deeply invading the vocal muscle.

The oncological meaning of neoplastic AC invasion has been repeatedly debated throughout the literature. From the most recent systematic review on the theme by Hendriksma and Sjögren, no consistent results emerge analyzing the series present in the literature, though a trend towards poorer outcomes can be observed [46]. This might be explained by the fact that no standard definition and reporting on AC exist. In the authors' opinion, the AC should not be considered a single spot in the glottis but, instead, a 3D space in close relation with the adjacent visceral spaces (i.e., the preepiglottic upwards and the anterosuperior paraglottic spaces laterally). Several studies have shown that AC involvement is a significant variable affecting both local control and organ preservation rate, and therefore, they all propose a more aggressive treatment for these kinds of tumor [45, 47, 48]. It is the authors' opinion that particular attention should be paid when vertically AC-involving tumors are managed by CO_2 TOLMS (Fig. 24.10): in these cases, a type VI cordectomy should be used to clear all the anterior laryngeal compartment, potentially from the mid-true and false cords to the epiglottic petiole, cricoid arch, and inner perichondrium of the thyroid laminae. To achieve safe oncological results, standard requirements should include a proper diagnostic workup with optical biopsy (to correctly assess the tumor margins) and tomographic imaging (to exclude cartilage involvement), complete tumor exposure, and adequate surgical expertise [49]. The latter has been demonstrated to significantly increase the outcomes in this kind of tumors [47, 50]. The slightly worse results offered by CO_2 TOLMS for AC-infiltrating tumors in respect to OPHL may be due to the higher difficulty to completely expose the AC in many patients and the close proximity of the underlying cartilage that, if infiltrated, offers low chances to be controlled by laser alone. Therefore, in fit patients, supracricoid OPHL may be more appropriate for these lesions, as consistent data in the literature demonstrate that satisfying local control rates can be achieved with this technique [51, 52].

Vocal fold mobility impairment should be clearly distinguished from vocal fold fixation. The latter is, in fact, the result of the arytenoid fixation and therefore defines a posterior-invading T3 carcinoma not suitable for CO_2 TOLMS resection. On the other hand, vocal fold hypomobility, which clinically defines a T2 tumor, arises when the vocal muscle is deeply infiltrated [53]. Nevertheless, also tumors superficially spreading to the supraglottis and subglottis are categorized as T2 (formerly T2a in older versions of the TNM as distinguished from T2b for vocal cord mobility impairment), but according to some authors, these two subsets of patients may still have different outcomes and should be distinguished along with all the statistical analysis on the sub-

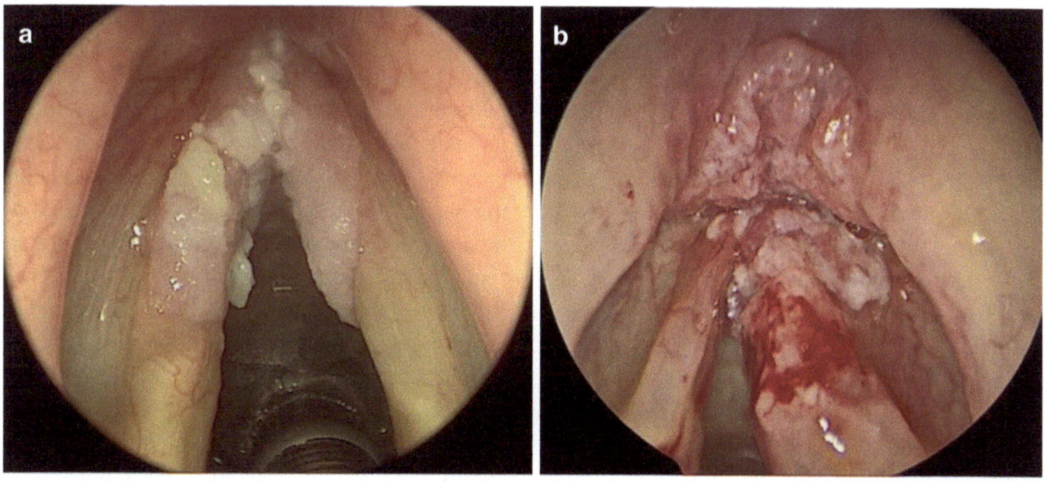

Fig. 24.10 Patterns of anterior commissure cancer invasion: (**a**) horizontal invasion, (**b**) vertical invasion

ject. According to the latest review on the topic [54], the few studies reporting separately oncologic outcomes of T2a and T2b demonstrated poorer outcomes of the latter category. In this regard, T2 for impaired mobility should be treated more aggressively with at least a type IV cordectomy in order to fully resect all the vocal muscle. Moreover, considering that no clear boundaries exist between the vocal muscle and the paraglottic space as the muscle fibers gradually fade in the adipose tissue, some authors have argued that all the lateral paraglottic compartment up to the vocal process of the arytenoid should be surgically cleared for these tumors. One of the remaining problems concerning the definition of the T2 category in case of vocal cord hypomobility is the difficulty in clinically quantifying it in an objective way. During pathological evaluation, however, significant invasion of the thyroarytenoid muscle (up to its half in depth or more) might define a pT2 carcinoma [55], as it has been demonstrated that vocal muscle infiltration is almost absent in the histological evaluation of T1 lesions [13].

24.6 Functional Outcomes

Functional preservation during the treatment of early glottic cancer should aim to guarantee the best vocal and swallowing outcomes. Swallowing is usually not impaired after standard cordectomies. However, an impairment may arise when the surgeon embraces more extended (type V and VI cordectomies) procedures to treat more advanced glottic tumors or those with significant supraglottic extension. On the other hand, voice quality after CO_2 TOLMS mainly depends on the grade of glottic gap resulting from the loss of vocal fold volume after the operation. However, it should be noted that also other areas of the larynx might work as a glottis substitute after surgery. Thus, voice quality may vary significantly despite similar interventions in different patients. For early glottic cancer, both CO_2 TOLMS and RT are recognized as the gold standard treatment. While the oncologic outcomes of both modalities are similar, controversy exists as to which treatment leads to better functional preservation, especially in terms of voice quality. One of the historical arguments supporting RT for early glottic cancer has always been better vocal function when compared to cordectomy through thyrotomy and vertical partial laryngectomies [56]. However, different transoral procedures can vary a lot in terms of volume of vocal cord resected and thus several studies missed the chance to draw precise comparisons between CO_2 TOLMS and RT regarding vocal outcomes. In this light, the ELS classification allows defining and clearly distinguishing the extent of excision, which facilitates making meaningful comparisons between vocal outcomes after different types of cordectomy [58]. Another consequence of such a classification is the possibility to compare vocal outcomes after endoscopic surgery with those achieved after RT. The University of Brescia retrospectively analyzed the functional outcomes after different types of cordectomy performed for early glottic cancer [57, 59]. In those patients, no statistically significant difference in the voice after type I and II cordectomy compared to a group of normal subjects was observed. Significant and persistent dysphonia was documented only after type III, IV, and V resections, mainly due to two key factors: anterior commissure synechiae (particularly after type Va cordectomy) and substantial glottic gap after removal of a significant amount of vocal muscle (more than one-third of its depth), necessitating further phonosurgical procedures in order to improve voice quality. For T1b tumors involving the anterior thirds of both vocal folds or the AC in a horizontal fashion, a staged surgery separately conducted on both sides may be considered for selected patients to maximize vocal outcomes reducing the risk of anterior synechiae. A silicon keel may be also positioned at the glottic level but its removal invariably requires a second surgery. Revision phonosurgery procedures can be undertaken in patients with severe dysphonia after the histological report with negative margins. Finally, when compared to OPHL, CO_2 TOLMS offers the best advantages in terms of functional outcomes: tracheotomy is avoided, vocal outcome is superior, swallowing function is intact, and the patient can restart oral diet from the day after surgery [60]. Functional preservation for the supraglottic larynx aims to maintain airway patency and oral feeding. In this regard, functional results after CO_2 TOLMS are highly satisfactory with very rare sequelae [61]. Moreover, especially when compared to open surgery, transoral procedures result in a reduced incidence of dysphagia, shorter hospitalization, and a low incidence of gastrostomies and tracheostomies [60]. However, to date, no head-to-head studies are available confronting CO_2 TOLMS, RT, and transoral robotic surgery in terms of functional outcomes for supraglottic cancers due to the well-known difficulties in the design and performance of prospective randomized controlled surgical trials.

24.7 Conclusions

- CO_2 TOLMS is a cost-effective and time-sparing treatment providing sound oncologic results and favorable functional outcomes with low complication rates in early glottic and supraglottic carcinomas.
- An accurate preoperative and intraoperative workup, including the use of videolaryngostroboscopy and biologic endoscopy techniques, ensure a customized, oncologically safe resection with minimal sacrifice of surrounding healthy tissue.
- Adequate laryngeal exposure is an essential prerequisite especially for the treatment of glottic tumors, and it should be assessed during in-office evaluation whenever possible.
- Adequate imaging of the larynx should be performed in the presence of AC-involving glottic lesions and vocal cord mobility-impairing carcinomas and most supraglottic lesions, to assess the true extent of the tumor before planning endoscopic surgery.
- In the absence of clinically evident metastasis, elective neck dissection is not necessary for early glottic carcinoma, while bilateral neck dissection is advised for T2 supraglottic carcinoma involving the midline.
- With rare exceptions, subglottic carcinomas are not suited for transoral surgery.
- En bloc resection is feasible in most cases of early laryngeal cancer. For bulkier tumors, a multi-bloc or piecemeal resection with meticulous orientation for pathological assessment is recommended.
- Patient compliance to a compulsive postoperative follow-up is mandatory as CO_2 TOLMS consists of tailored transoral microsurgery often performed within millimetric safe margins.
- The incidence of positive margins in CO_2 TOLMS is high but its real impact on oncologic outcomes is debated. In this scenario, a second-look procedure is the safest option, but it may reveal no tumor left in up to 80% of cases. A watchful waiting policy can be viable for selected cases.
- Tumors arising from the AC, especially on a vertical plane, are particularly difficult to expose and may offer poorer outcomes if treated by CO_2 TOLMS especially when not properly staged and evaluated. In these cases, open partial laryngectomies may be considered as a sound surgical alternative.

References

1. Bradley PJ, Piazza C, Paderno A. A roadmap of six different pathways to improve survival in laryngeal cancer patients. Curr Opin Otolaryngol Head Neck Surg. 2021;29(2):65–78. https://doi.org/10.1097/MOO.0000000000000684.
2. Nocini R, Molteni G, Mattiuzzi C, Lippi G. Updates on larynx cancer epidemiology. Chinese J Cancer Res. 2020;32(1):18–25. https://doi.org/10.21147/j.issn.1000-9604.2020.01.03.
3. Kleinsasser O. Laryngomicroscopy (lens laryngoscopy) and its importance in the diagnosis of premorbid diseases and early forms of carcinoma of the labium vocale. Arch fur Ohren-Nasen- und Kehlkopfheilkd. 1962;180:724–7.
4. Strong MS, Jako GJ. Laser surgery in the larynx. Early clinical experience with continuous CO 2 laser. Ann Otol Rhinol Laryngol. 1972;81(6):791–8. https://doi.org/10.1177/000348947208100606.
5. Remacle M, Arens C, Eldin MB, et al. Laser-assisted surgery of the upper aero-digestive tract: a clarification of nomenclature. A consensus statement of the European Laryngological Society. Eur Arch Oto-Rhino-Laryngol. 2017;274(10):3723–7. https://doi.org/10.1007/s00405-017-4708-3.

6. Ambrosch P. The role of laser microsurgery in the treatment of laryngeal cancer. Curr Opin Otolaryngol Head Neck Surg. 2007;15(2):82–8. https://doi.org/10.1097/MOO.0b013e3280147336.
7. Piazza C, Peretti G, Vander PV. Editorial: Advances in transoral approaches for laryngeal cancer. Front Oncol. 2018;8(OCT):1–3. https://doi.org/10.3389/fonc.2018.00455.
8. Alberto, Paderno Alberto, Deganello Davide, Lancini Cesare, Piazza. Is the exoscope ready to replace the operative microscope in transoral surgery?. Curr Opin Otolaryngol Head Neck Surg. 2022;30(2):79–86. https://doi.org/10.1097/MOO.0000000000000794.
9. Arens C, Piazza C, Andrea M, et al. Proposal for a descriptive guideline of vascular changes in lesions of the vocal folds by the committee on endoscopic laryngeal imaging of the European laryngological society. Eur Arch Oto-Rhino-Laryngol. 2016;273(5):1207–14. https://doi.org/10.1007/s00405-015-3851-y.
10. Peretti G, Piazza C, Berlucchi M, Cappiello J, Giudice M, Nicolai P. Pre- and intraoperative assessment of mid-cord erythroleukoplakias: a prospective study on 52 patients. Eur Arch Oto-Rhino-Laryngol. 2003;260(10):525–8. https://doi.org/10.1007/s00405-003-0584-0.
11. Mora F, Carta F, Missale F, et al. Laryngeal mid-cord erythroleukoplakias: how to modulate the transoral co2 laser excisional biopsy. Cancers (Basel). 2020;12(8):1–10. https://doi.org/10.3390/cancers12082165.
12. Peretti G, Cappiello J, Nicolai P, Smussi C, Antonelli AR. Endoscopic laser excisional biopsy for selected glottic carcinomas. Laryngoscope. 1994;104(10):1276–9. https://doi.org/10.1288/00005537-199410000-00017.
13. Hamzany Y, Shoffel-Havakuk H, Devons-Sberro S, Shteinberg S, Yaniv D, Mizrachi A. Single stage transoral laser microsurgery for early glottic cancer. Front Oncol. 2018;8(AUG):1–8. https://doi.org/10.3389/fonc.2018.00298.
14. Pittore B, Ismail-Koch H, Davis A, et al. Thyroarytenoid muscle invasion in T1 glottic carcinoma. Eur Arch Oto-Rhino-Laryngol. 2009;266(11):1787–91. https://doi.org/10.1007/s00405-009-0929-4.
15. Chiesa-Estomba CM, Ravanelli M, Farina D, et al. Imaging checklist for preoperative evaluation of laryngeal tumors to be treated by transoral microsurgery: guidelines from the European laryngological society. Eur Arch Oto-Rhino-Laryngol. 2020;277(6):1707–14. https://doi.org/10.1007/s00405-020-05869-0.
16. Sanabria A, Shah JP, Medina JE, et al. Incidence of occult lymph node metastasis in primary larynx squamous cell carcinoma, by subsite, t classification and neck level: a systematic review. Cancers (Basel). 2020;12(4) https://doi.org/10.3390/cancers12041059.
17. Piazza C, Mangili S, Del Bon F, et al. Preoperative clinical predictors of difficult laryngeal exposure for microlaryngoscopy: the laryngoscore. Laryngoscope. 2014;124(11):2561–7. https://doi.org/10.1002/lary.24803.
18. Piazza C, Paderno A, Grazioli P, et al. Laryngeal exposure and margin status in glottic cancer treated by transoral laser microsurgery. Laryngoscope. 2018;128(5):1146–51. https://doi.org/10.1002/lary.26861.
19. Incandela F, Paderno A, Missale F, et al. Glottic exposure for transoral laser microsurgery: proposal of a mini-version of the laryngoscore. Laryngoscope. 2019;129(7):1617–22. https://doi.org/10.1002/lary.27525.
20. Mora F, Missale F, Incandela F, et al. High frequency jet ventilation during transoral laser microsurgery for Tis-T2 laryngeal cancer. Front Oncol. 2017;7(NOV):1–5. https://doi.org/10.3389/fonc.2017.00282.
21. Remacle M, Eckel HE, Antonelli A, et al. Endoscopic cordectomy. A proposal for a classification by the Working Committee, European Laryngological Society. Eur Arch Oto-Rhino-Laryngol. 2000;257(4):227–31. https://doi.org/10.1007/s004050050228.
22. Remacle M, Van Haverbeke C, Eckel H, et al. Proposal for revision of the European Laryngological Society classification of endoscopic cordectomies. Eur Arch Oto-Rhino-Laryngol. 2007;264(5):499–504. https://doi.org/10.1007/s00405-007-0279-z.
23. Rudert HH, Werner JA, Höft S. Transoral carbon dioxide laser resection of supraglottic carcinoma. Ann Otol Rhinol Laryngol. 1999;108(9 I):819–27. https://doi.org/10.1177/000348949910800901.
24. Canis M, Martin A, Ihler F, et al. Results of transoral laser microsurgery for supraglottic carcinoma in 277 patients. Eur Arch Oto-Rhino-Laryngol. 2013;270(8):2315–26. https://doi.org/10.1007/s00405-012-2327-6.
25. Piazza C, Barbieri D, Del Bon F, et al. Functional outcomes after different types of transoral supraglottic laryngectomy. In: Laryngoscope, vol. 126. John Wiley and Sons Inc.; 2016. p. 1131–5. https://doi.org/10.1002/lary.25562.
26. Vilaseca-González I, Bernal-Sprekelsen M, Blanch-Alejandro JL, Moragas-Lluis M. Complications in transoral CO2 laser surgery for carcinoma of the larynx and hypopharynx. Head Neck. 2003;25(5):382–8. https://doi.org/10.1002/hed.10207.
27. Remacle M, Hantzakos A, Eckel H, et al. Endoscopic supraglottic laryngectomy: a proposal for a classification by the working committee on nomenclature, Eur Laryngological Society. Eur Arch Oto-Rhino-Laryngol. 2009;266(7):993–8. https://doi.org/10.1007/s00405-008-0901-8.
28. Mendelsohn AH, Remacle MJ. Vocal fold cancer transoral laser microsurgery following European Laryngological Society laser cordectomy classification. Front Oncol. 2018;8(JUN):1–8. https://doi.org/10.3389/fonc.2018.00231.
29. Marchi F, Piazza C, Ravanelli M, et al. Role of imaging in the follow-up of T2–T3 glottic cancer treated by transoral laser microsurgery. Eur Arch Oto-

Rhino-Laryngol. 2017;274(10):3679–86. https://doi.org/10.1007/s00405-017-4642-4.
30. Simo R, Bradley P, Chevalier D, et al. European Laryngological Society: ELS recommendations for the follow-up of patients treated for laryngeal cancer. Eur Arch Oto-Rhino-Laryngol. 2014;271(9):2469–79. https://doi.org/10.1007/s00405-014-2966-x.
31. Eckel HE. Local recurrences following transoral laser surgery for early glottic carcinoma: frequency, management, and outcome. Ann Otol Rhinol Laryngol. 2001;110(1):7–15. https://doi.org/10.1177/000348940111000102.
32. Cesare, Piazza Alberto, Paderno Francesca, Del Bon Davide, Lancini Milena, Fior Giulia, Berretti Paolo, Bosio Alberto, Deganello Giorgio, Peretti. Long-term Oncologic Outcomes of 1188 Tis-T2 Glottic Cancers Treated by Transoral Laser Microsurgery. Otolaryngology–Head and Neck Surgery. 2021;165(2):321–28. https://doi.org/10.1177/0194599820983727.
33. Hartl DM, Ferlito A, Brasnu DF, et al. Evidence-based review of treatment options for patients with glottic cancer. Head Neck. 2011;33(11):1638–48. https://doi.org/10.1002/hed.21528.
34. Abdurehim Y, Hua Z, Yasin Y, Xukurhan A, Imam I, Yuqin F. Transoral laser surgery versus radiotherapy: systematic review and meta-analysis for treatment options of T1a glottic cancer. Head Neck. 2012;34(1):23–33. https://doi.org/10.1002/hed.21686.
35. Higgins KM, Shah MD, Ogaick MJ, Enepekides D. Treatment of early-stage glottic cancer: meta-analysis comparison of laser excision versus radiotherapy. J Otolaryngol Head Neck Surg. 2009;38(6):603–12. https://doi.org/10.2310/7070.2009.080235.
36. Yoo J, Lacchetti C, Hammond JA, Gilbert RW. Role of endolaryngeal surgery (with or without laser) versus radiotherapy in the management of early (T1) glottic cancer: a systematic review. Head Neck. 2014;36(12):1807–19. https://doi.org/10.1002/hed.23504.
37. Giorgio, Peretti Cesare, Piazza Mohssen, Ansarin Luigi, De Benedetto Daniela, Cocco Augusto, Cattaneo Piero, Nicolai Fausto, Chiesa. Transoral CO2 laser microsurgery for Tis-T3 supraglottic squamous cell carcinomas. European Archives of Oto-Rhino-Laryngology. 2010;267(11):1735–42. https://doi.org/10.1007/s00405-010-1284-1.
38. Motta G, Esposito E, Testa D, Iovine R, Motta S. CO2 laser treatment of supraglottic cancer. Head Neck. 2004;26(5):442–6. https://doi.org/10.1002/hed.10395.
39. Patel KB, Nichols AC, Fung K, Yoo J, MacNeil SD. Treatment of early stage Supraglottic squamous cell carcinoma: meta-analysis comparing primary surgery versus primary radiotherapy. J Otolaryngol Head Neck Surg. 2018;47(1):1–8. https://doi.org/10.1186/s40463-018-0262-2.
40. Cabanillas R, Rodrigo JP, Llorente JL, Suárez C. Oncologic outcomes of transoral laser surgery of supraglottic carcinoma compared with a transcervical approach. Head Neck. 2008;30(6):750–5. https://doi.org/10.1002/hed.20778.
41. Fiz I, Koelmel JC, Sittel C. Nature and role of surgical margins in transoral laser microsurgery for early and intermediate glottic cancer. Curr Opin Otolaryngol Head Neck Surg. 2018;26(2):78–83. https://doi.org/10.1097/MOO.0000000000000446.
42. Canis M, Ihler F, Martin A, Matthias C, Steiner W. Transoral laser microsurgery for T1a glottic cancer: review of 404 cases. Head Neck. 2015;37(6):889–95. https://doi.org/10.1002/hed.23688.
43. Jumaily M, Faraji F, Osazuwa-Peters N, Walker RJ, Ward GM. Prognostic significance of surgical margins after transoral laser microsurgery for early-stage glottic squamous cell carcinoma. Oral Oncol. 2019;97:105–11. https://doi.org/10.1016/j.oraloncology.2019.08.005.
44. Fiz I, Mazzola F, Fiz F, et al. Impact of close and positive margins in transoral laser microsurgery for TIS-T2 glottic cancer. Front Oncol. 2017;7(OCT):1–9. https://doi.org/10.3389/fonc.2017.00245.
45. Remacle M, Matar N, Delos M, Nollevaux MC, Jamart J, Lawson G. Is frozen section reliable in transoral CO2 laser-assisted cordectomies? Eur Arch Oto-Rhino-Laryngol. 2010;267(3):397–400. https://doi.org/10.1007/s00405-009-1101-x.
46. Piazza C, Filauro M, Paderno A, et al. Three-dimensional map of isoprognostic zones in glottic cancer treated by transoral laser microsurgery as a unimodal treatment strategy. Front Oncol. 2018;8(MAY):1–7. https://doi.org/10.3389/fonc.2018.00175.
47. Hendriksma M, Sjögren EV. Involvement of the anterior commissure in early glottic cancer (tis-T2): a review of the literature. Cancers (Basel). 2019;11(9):1–15. https://doi.org/10.3390/cancers11091234.
48. Vilaseca I, Nogués-Sabaté A, Avilés-Jurado FX, et al. Factors of local recurrence and organ preservation with transoral laser microsurgery in laryngeal carcinomas; CHAID decision-tree analysis. Head Neck. 2019;41(3):756–64. https://doi.org/10.1002/hed.25422.
49. Carta F, Bandino F, Olla AM, Chuchueva N, Gerosa C, Puxeddu R. Prognostic value of age, subglottic, and anterior commissure involvement for early glottic carcinoma treated with CO2 laser transoral microsurgery: a retrospective, single-center cohort study of 261 patients. Eur Arch Oto-Rhino-Laryngol. 2018;275(5):1199–210. https://doi.org/10.1007/s00405-018-4890-y.
50. Peretti G, Piazza C, Mora F, Garofolo S, Guastini L. Reasonable limits for transoral laser microsurgery in laryngeal cancer. Curr Opin Otolaryngol Head Neck Surg. 2016;24(2):135–9. https://doi.org/10.1097/MOO.0000000000000240.
51. Blanch JL, Vilaseca I, Caballero M, Moragas M, Berenguer J, Bernal-Sprekelsen M. Outcome of

transoral laser microsurgery for T2-T3 tumors growing in the laryngeal anterior commissure. Head Neck. 2011;33(9):1252–9. https://doi.org/10.1002/hed.21605.

52. Allegra E, Saita V, Azzolina A, et al. Impact of the anterior commissure involvement on the survival of early glottic cancer treated with cricohyoidoepiglottopexy: a retrospective study. Cancer Manag Res. 2018;10:5553–8. https://doi.org/10.2147/CMAR.S182854.
53. Del Bon F, Piazza C, Lancini D, et al. Open partial horizontal laryngectomies for T3–T4 laryngeal cancer: Prognostic impact of anterior vs. posterior laryngeal compartmentalization. Cancers (Basel). 2019;11(3) https://doi.org/10.3390/cancers11030289.
54. Hirano M, Kurita S, Matsuoka H, Tateishi M. Vocal fold fixation in laryngeal carcinomas. Acta Otolaryngol. 1991;111(2):449–54. https://doi.org/10.3109/00016489109137418.
55. Hendriksma M, Heijnen BJ, Sjögren EV. Oncologic and functional outcomes of patients treated with transoral CO 2 laser microsurgery or radiotherapy for T2 glottic carcinoma: a systematic review of the literature. Curr Opin Otolaryngol Head Neck Surg. 2018;26(2):84–93. https://doi.org/10.1097/MOO.0000000000000438.
56. Lionello M, Bertolin A, Nardello E, et al. Could the infiltration of the thyroarytenoid muscle define the pT2 glottic carcinoma? Head Neck. 2019;41(10):3639–46. https://doi.org/10.1002/hed.25893.
57. Bron LP, Soldati D, Zouhair A, et al. Treatment of early stage squamous-cell carcinoma of the glottic larynx: endoscopic surgery or cricohyoidoepiglottopexy versus radiotherapy. Head Neck. 2001;23(10):823–9. https://doi.org/10.1002/hed.1120.
58. Elisabeth, Sjogren Martine, Hendriksma Cesare, Piazza Dana M., Hartl Carlos, Suarez Oded, Cohen Remco, de Bree Miquel, Quer Vincent Vander, Poorten Juan Pablo, Rodrigo Francisco, Civantos Eric, Genden Luiz P., Kowalski Antti, Makitie Ashok, Shaha Robert P., Takes Alvaro, Sanabria Orlando, Guntinas-Lichius Alessandra, Rinaldo Alfio, Ferlito. Voice Outcome After Carbon Dioxide Transoral Laser Microsurgery for Glottic Cancer According to the European Laryngological Society Classification of Cordectomy Types – A Systematic Review. Journal of Voice. 2022: S0892199722000698. https://doi.org/10.1016/j.jvoice.2022.03.003.
59. Peretti G, Mensi MC, Piazza C, Rossini M, Balzanelli C, Antonelli AR. Preoperative and postoperative voice in Tis-T1 glottic cancer treated by endoscopic cordectomy: an additional issue for patient counseling. Ann Otol Rhinol Laryngol. 2003;112(9 I):759–63. https://doi.org/10.1177/000348940311200903.
60. Peretti G, Piazza C, Cantarella G, Balzanelli C, Nicolai P. Vocal outcome after endoscopic cordectomies for tis and T1 glottic carcinomas. Ann Otol Rhinol Laryngol. 2003;112(2):174–9. https://doi.org/10.1177/000348940311200212.
61. Peretti G, Piazza C, Cattaneo A, De Benedetto L, Martin E, Nicolai P. Comparison of functional outcomes after endoscopic versus open-neck supraglottic laryngectomies. Ann Otol Rhinol Laryngol. 2006;115(11):827–32. https://doi.org/10.1177/000348940611501106.
62. Davis RK, Kriskovich MD, Buntin CS, Galloway EB, Jepsen MC. Endoscopic supraglottic laryngectomy with postoperative irradiation. Ann Otol Rhinol Laryngol. 2004;113(2):132–8. https://doi.org/10.1177/000348940411300210.

25 Transoral Approach for Extended Cancers (T3–T4a)

Isabel Vilaseca and Manuel Bernal-Sprekelsen

Key Points

- Transoral surgery strategies have shown its validity in selected advanced laryngeal tumors with adequate exposure.
- Intraoperative frozen sections may be necessary to ensure a margin-free resection.
- Tumors involving the posterior compartment have a worse exposure and a lower larynx preservation rate than those involving anterior compartments.
- Treatment of the neck has to be planned as in open partial or total laryngectomies.
- In supraglottic tumors, make sure to properly address the vascular supply in order to avoid postoperative bleeding.

25.1 Introduction

Transoral surgery (TOS) is a minimally invasive surgical approach to a tailored cancer resection that has been proved effective and safe for early and intermediate laryngeal cases. Although not systematically widespread in locally advanced tumors, experience with TOS is increasing progressively and series are being published in different countries. International guidelines recognize transoral surgery as one of the recommended treatments for selected T3 laryngeal tumors, as a way to achieve surgical organ preservation [1].

The most used transoral technique for larynx cancer resection is transoral laser microsurgery (TOLMS), which combines the magnified microscopic view with the precise cut and coagulation capability of the CO_2 laser. The experience with this technique overcomes 30 years and has been spread around the world [2]. More recently, new transoral approaches have been developed, replacing the microscopic view for the endoscopic view, with or without the assistance of robotic platforms. These techniques, which have their main indication in the oropharynx, can be also implemented in the larynx, especially in the supraglottic area, among them, the transoral videoendoscopic surgery (TOVS) [3], transoral ultrasonic surgery (TOUSS) [4], and transoral robotic surgery (TORS) [5, 6].

One of the advantages of the transoral approach is the tailored resection, which provides preservation of healthy tissue and the avoidance of external cervical disruption with preservation of sensitive nerves among other anatomical structures. Moreover, the preservation of prelaryngeal muscles and the reduced need of a tracheotomy

I. Vilaseca (✉) · M. Bernal-Sprekelsen
Department of Otorhinolaryngology, Hospital Clínic, University of Barcelona, Barcelona, Spain
e-mail: ivila@clinic.cat; mbernal@clinic.cat

M. Remacle, H. E. Eckel (eds.), *Textbook of Surgery of Larynx and Trachea*,
https://doi.org/10.1007/978-3-031-09621-1_25

reduce the postoperative morbidity, favor patient recovery, and shorten hospital stay.

Among the drawbacks of the transoral approaches for extended cancers are the difficulties for an adequate exposure, especially in the anterior commissure of the larynx or in the case of bulky tumors with reduced mobility. The need to transect the tumor in the TOLMS approach represents also a difficulty in the assessment of tumor margins. In addition, the extended resected areas have to heal by second intention and the lack of reconstruction may preclude, in part, the functional recovery.

25.2 Indications

The authors agree that selection of patients for transoral surgery is crucial for an oncologic and functional sound resection and that achievement of negative margins is a must to obtain favorable results. Moreover, according to the results published in the literature, a long learning curve is required in order to manage this type of tumors [7].

In the TNM eighth edition, a locally advanced laryngeal tumor is determined by the presence of a fixed vocal cord (with or without cricoarytenoid joint involvement), the invasion of the preepiglottic or paraglottic spaces, the infiltration of the thyroid cartilage, or the extension to the soft tissues of the neck [8].

Peretti et al. published an article describing the reasonable limits of transoral resection according to oncologic and functional expectatives [9]. These limits included bilateral involvement of the posterior commissure or the cricoid cartilage, extensive subglottic growth, and marked extralaryngeal tumor. For the majority of experienced surgeons, the best candidates are T3 laryngeal tumors located in the supraglottis or the anterior compartments of the glottis. T4 tumors are generally excluded from the transoral approach and also those T3 tumors with a depth of infiltration in the posterior commissure or lower extension towards the subglottis, mainly in the posterior area [10].

One of the difficulties in the indication of surgery relies in the preoperative assessment of T3 cancers, specially the accurate diagnosis of cartilage infiltration and the knowledge of the underlying causes of vocal cord fixation. Regarding the immobility of the vocal cord, the endoscopic evaluation may be somewhat subjective and the impairment be due to a mass effect, muscle infiltration, or cricoarytenoid joint involvement. These three scenarios carry a different prognosis in terms of functional and oncologic outcomes.

Another difficulty is the radiological evaluation of the lesion. Contrast-enhanced CT scan, the most used imaging technique for staging and treatment planning, has some limitations in the paraglottic space, where the tumor can be confounded with other normal soft tissues, or in its capacity to diagnose with precision cartilage infiltration [11]. Magnetic resonance imaging allows a better definition of tumor infiltration in the paraglottic space (specificity 96.9% and sensitivity 78.6%) but still has limitations in the cartilage assessment (specificity 70%) [12].

Other aspects also play a role in the treatment decision making. The presumed need of postoperative radical adjuvant treatment may favor an upfront nonsurgical strategy, whereas younger age, possibility to avoid adjuvant treatment, or comorbidities that contraindicate chemotherapy may favor the indication of surgery.

25.3 Exposure and Resection

Whatever the chosen technique, an adequate exposure is crucial for an oncologic sound resection with tumor-free margins. In the supraglottic area, double-valve laryngoscopes or specific laryngopharyngoscope retractors may be used to facilitate exposure. In the glottis, rigid laryngoscopes are recommended, starting with the largest possible diameter and moving to smaller ones in areas difficult to expose. This is the case in the anterior commissure of the glottis or the posterior part of the larynx, where the coincidence with the anesthetic tube makes the resection more tricky.

At present, the majority of glottic tumors are treated with TOLMS, because it provides the best exposure and a highly precise resection with the minimum thermal damage. In the case of TORS, TOUSS, or TOVS, the current experience is mainly limited to early tumors of the supraglottic area [3, 6]. In these techniques specific oropharynx retractors are used for exposure and visualization, with some difficulties, secondary to the lack of space, in the lower areas. It makes the positioning of the robotic arms difficult and limits the instrument maneuverability deep within the laryngopharyngeal complex. From this point of view, the MedRobotics Flex system [13], or the new generation of the single-port da Vinci system (preclinical data) [14], has been developed to facilitate exposure and resection.

As a concept, to perform a resection of advanced tumors of the larynx with TOLMS, laser incisions are made to the tumor to assess the depth of infiltration and to create more manageable units. In the glottis, incisions are carried out laterally onto the thyroid cartilage, removing the inner perichondrium when the muscle is infiltrated. In case of unexpected focal infiltration of the cartilage, the involved portion of the cartilage can be removed with the laser. One of the most complex areas is the posterior paraglottic space, which has to be completely removed to avoid tumor persistence. The vocal process of the arytenoid may be excised with the tumor and the fat of the paraglottic space is cleaned up to the cricoid cartilage (Figs. 25.1 and 25.2). Cricoarytenoid joint

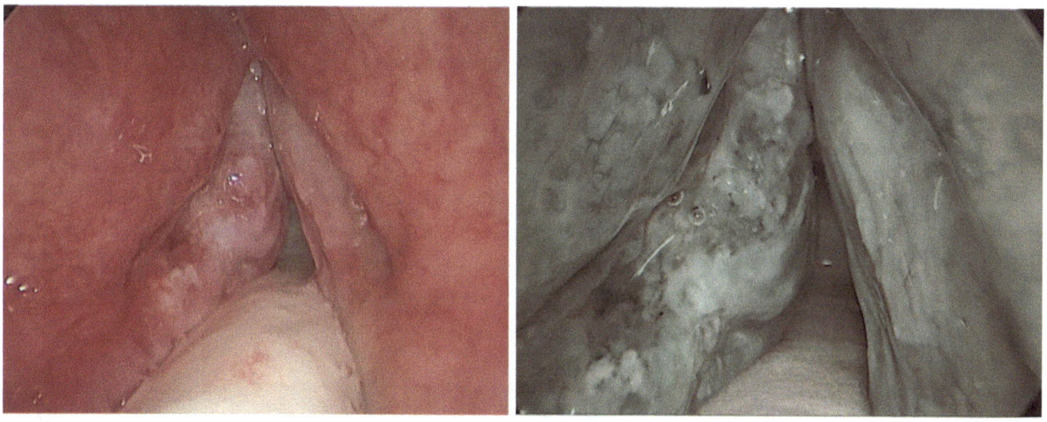

Fig. 25.1 Endoscopic view of a deeply infiltrating tumor of the left vocal fold with white light and SPIES filter (Spectra A)

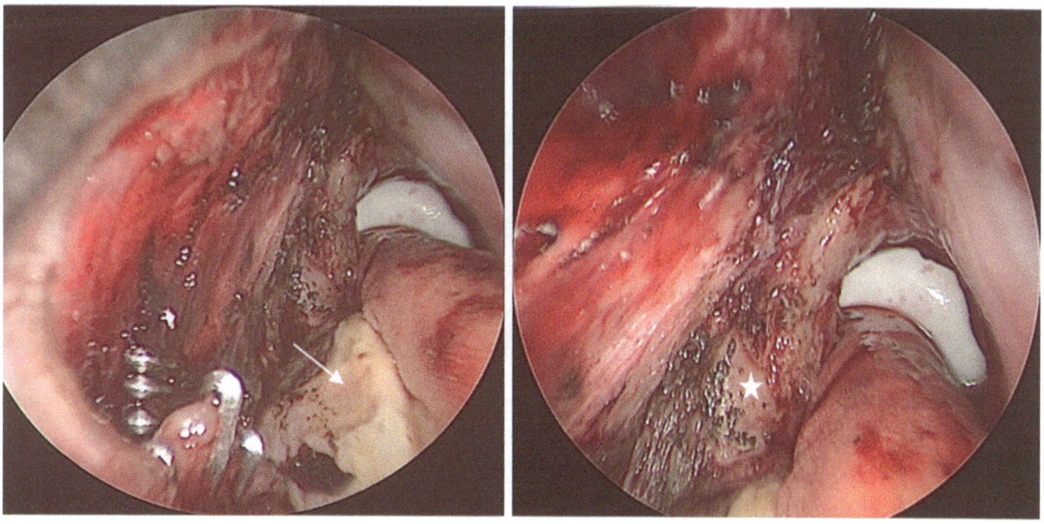

Fig. 25.2 Endoscopic view of the final resection of the tumor presented in Fig. 25.1. Details of the posterior paraglottic resection with several vascular clips in the posterior area. Left vocal process of the arytenoid completely denudated (white arrow). Inferior detail of the cricoid cartilage (asterisk). Note that no tracheotomy has been performed

involvement is considered a limit of transoral resection for a majority of authors since it requires a total arytenoidectomy, with the functional implications that this entails.

In the supraglottic region, resection is usually tailored following the size and extension of the tumor and favoring the preservation of tissue in lateralized tumors. After dividing the epiglottis, it may be resected completely or partly, but as a norm, in those infrahyoid tumors, the preepiglottic fat should be completely removed even in the absence of a radiologic evidence of a tumor. Special attention is needed when dividing the pharyngoepiglottic and aryepiglottic folds to achieve adequate hemostasia. Ideally, the superior pedicle has to be dissected and secured with hemostatic clips and/or cautery.

Treatment of tumors involving the vertical plane of the anterior commissure with TOLMS is somewhat controversial and a large learning curve is required to approach this area without jeopardizing outcomes [15]. Reduced local control has been published in this location in comparison with other external partial techniques [16], even in cases with negative margins [17]. In locally advanced tumors, exposure may be very difficult, and the location does not facilitate working adequately with a laser on a perpendicular axis. Moreover, the absence of the perichondrium in the central part or the focal infiltration of the cartilage hinders the detachment of the perichondrium, requiring superficial ablation of the thyroid cartilage to increase the safety margin of the resection [10].

The recommended technique for advanced tumors of the anterior commissure consists of a wide excision of the lesion with a top-down approach systematically including the resection of the lower epiglottis, the ventricular folds, and the accompanying preepiglottic fat. This aforementioned approach enables a better identification of potential in-depth infiltration and creates a hole in the petiole area that is very useful for postoperative fiberendoscopic follow-up (Figs. 25.3 and 25.4).

Once the tumor has been resected, the neck has to be treated following the same criteria as in open surgery.

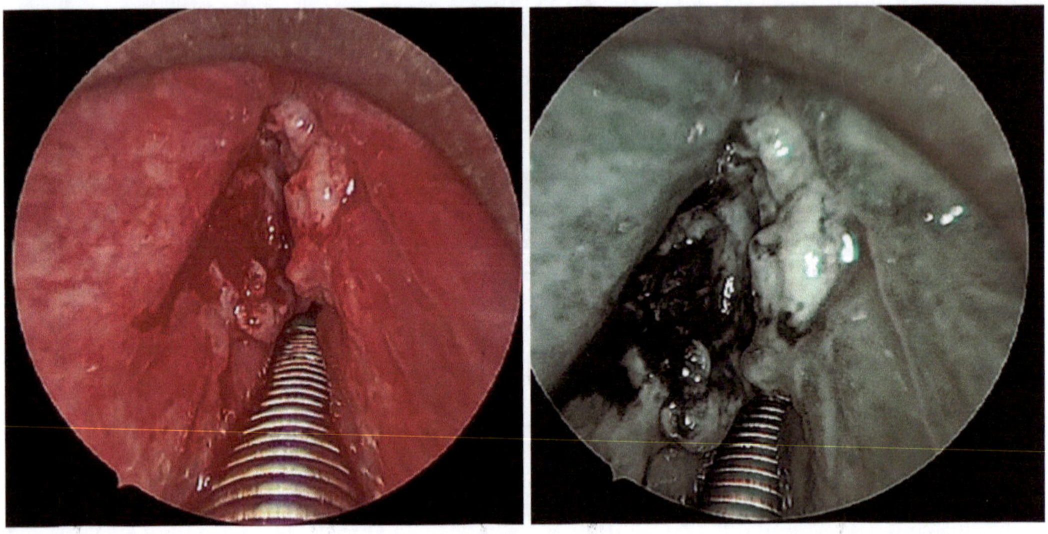

Fig. 25.3 Endoscopic view of a tumor involving the anterior commissure of the larynx in the vertical plane. White light (left) and SPIES Spectra A (right) views

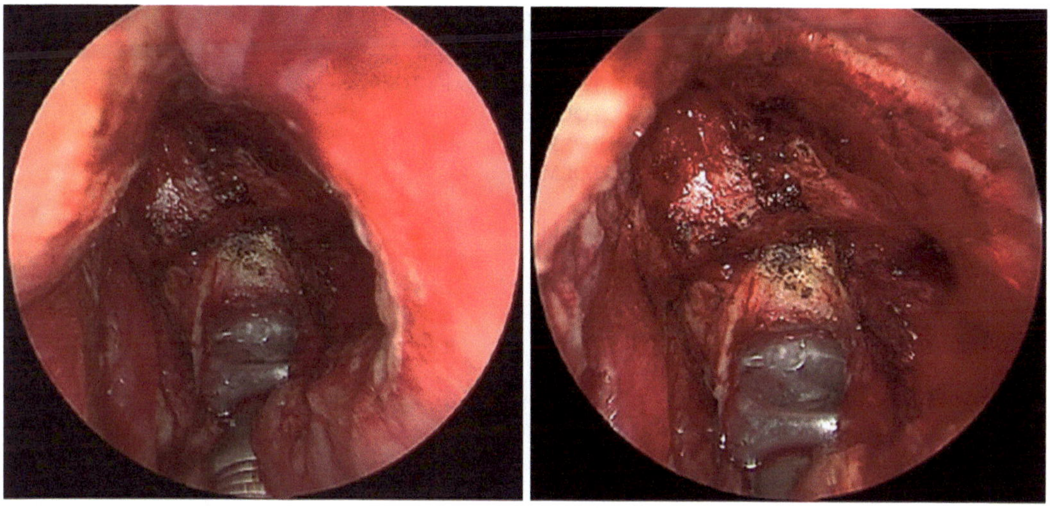

Fig. 25.4 Endoscopic view of the final resection of the lesion presented in Fig. 25.3. Supraglottic section at the level of the lower epiglottis and false cords (left). Glottic-subglottic resection with exposure of the thyroid lamina and cricothyroid membrane (right). Note that no tracheotomy has been performed

25.4 Surgical Margins

Negative surgical margins are key to reduce the risk of local relapse, to avoid the need for adjuvant treatment, and to obtain the best possible oncologic and functional result. Ideally, margins should be representative of the entire resection which is not always easy in the case of large tumors. In TOLMS, piecemeal resection may compromise specimen orientation and therefore create uncertainty in the final assessment of the margins. For this reason, the majority of authors obtain the margins from the tumor bed itself and enlarge the resection with additional laser ablation, whenever possible. This (extra) ablation usually pursues a double purpose: regularization of the surgical bed to facilitate a uniform reepithelialization of the area and the systematic expansion of the margin, which tends to be overestimated when performing surgery under microscopic magnification. Detaching the inner perichondrium of the thyroid cartilage provides a safety deep margin in case the cartilage is not infiltrated. For bordering areas, intraoperative frozen sections, studied by a dedicated pathologist, facilitates an oncologic safe resection and are therefore highly recommended.

Conversely, in TORS, TOVS, or TOUSS, the authors recommend a resection of the tumor in en bloc with the use of monopolar spatula, ultrasonic energy, or CO_2 fiber laser. The en bloc resection facilitates the orientation and margin assessment of the main specimen in comparison with TOLMS, but the type of energies used (monopolar, ultrasounds) increases the thermal damage, which means that the margins have to be broader from the beginning [18].

At present, TORS, TOVS, and TOUSS have demonstrated to be feasible in early and in some advanced supraglottic tumors mainly of the suprahyoid area, being the resection of the infrahyoid epiglottis more difficult in infiltrating tumors [3–6, 13]. The combination of techniques, instruments, and energies, applied on demand, is an option in cases with a difficult access and will probably gain importance in the future.

25.5 Oncologic Outcomes

Since the publication in 1993 of the first series of locally advanced cases treated with TOLMS by Wolfgang Steiner [19], many other authors have published their experiences (see Tables 25.1 and 25.2). Globally, the best local control is achieved

Table 25.1 Oncologic outcomes of transoral surgery for locally advanced glottic cancers

Author	N	T	Technique	Local control with TOS	5y DSS/DFS	5y OS
Motta (1997) [20]	37	T3	TOLMS	–	67% DSS	55%
Ambrosch (2001) [21]	70	T3a	TOLMS	68%	62% DFS	
Motta (2005) [22]	51	T3	TOLMS	–	72% DSS 60% [b] DFS	64% [b]
Hinni (2007) [23]	41	T3/T4	TOLMS	74%	68% DFS	55%
Grant (2007) [24]	10	T3/T4	TOLMS	45%	40% DSS	62%
Peretti (2010) [25]	11	T3	TOLMS	71.6%	100% DSS 40.9% DFS	–
Canis (2013) [26]	31	T4a	TOLMS	66.6%	75.4% DSS 62.2% DFS	65.3%
Canis (2013) [27]	122	pT3	TOLMS	–	84.1% DSS 57.8% DFS	58.6%
Breda (2015) [28]	40	T3–T4a	TOLMS	–	90.8% DSS	–
Pantazis (2015) [29]	19	T3	TOLMS	52.7%	63.2% DSS	63.2%
Vilaseca (2016) [2]	82	T3/T4a	TOLMS	LPR: 55% (74% for survivors)	75.8% DSS	53.1%
Peretti (2016) [30]	34	T3	TOLMS	70%	72.9% DFS	65.2%
Day (2016) [31]	12	T3	TOLMS	58%	60% DSS 38% DFS	46%
Chang (2019) [32]	14	T3–T4	TOLMS	–	88% DSS 62% DFS	71%
Chien (2021) [33]	44	T3	TOLMS	78% LPR: 82%	84% DSS	75%

TOS Transoral surgery, *DSS* Disease-specific survival, *DFS* Disease-free survival, *OS* Overall survival, *TOLMS* Transoral laser microsurgery, *LPR* Larynx preservation rate

Table 25.2 Oncologic outcomes of transoral surgery for locally advanced supraglottic cancers

Author	N	TNM	Technique	5y LC with TOS	5y DSS	OS
Ambrosch (2001) [21]	50	T3	TOLMS	86%	71%	–
Motta (2004) [34]	18	T3	TOLMS	77%	81%	81%
Cabanillas (2008) [35]	15	T3	TOLMS	70%	80%	–
Peretti (2010) [36]	20	T3	TOLMS	83%	59.6%	–
Canis (2013) [26]	48	T4a	TOLMS	–	62.9%	49.9%
Canis (2014) [37]	159	T3/T4	TOLMS	T3: 82% T4: 76%	Stage III + IVA: 81%	Stage III + IVA: 59%
Vilaseca (2016) [38]	154	T3/T4a	TOLMS	73.8%	67.6%	55.6%
Ambrosch (2018) [39]	34	T3–T4a	TOLMS	67%	64%	58%

LC Local control, *TOS* Transoral surgery, *DSS* Disease-specific survival, *OS* Overall survival, *TOLMS* Transoral laser microsurgery

in the supraglottic tumors regardless of the technique employed, and the best disease-specific survival is found in the glottic subsite. Of course, the nodal status is determinant in this last matter. In Tables 25.1 and 25.2, the 5-year local control and survival rates of locally advanced glottic and supraglottic tumors are summarized.

In 2010, we evaluated the prognostic factors of local recurrence and larynx preservation in a series of T3 tumors. Cartilage infiltration and vocal cord fixation were negative independent factors for larynx preservation [40]. In that study, the underlying cause of vocal cord fixation was not analyzed. On the opposite, the best local control was achieved in those patients with preepiglottic involvement, suggesting that supraglottic tumors were those that fit best in a transoral approach. More recently, an analysis with a

CHAID decision tree analysis of 1119 consecutive patients treated with TOLMS confirmed that paraglottic and anterior commissure involvement, as well as the margin status, were the most important factors for local control [41].

In the absence of a randomized trial, a recent systematic review highlighted the difficulties to find a consensus for an optimal organ-preserving treatment in T3 laryngeal carcinomas [42]. According to the review, the 5-year disease-specific survival is around 60% for chemoradiation protocols, 70%–85% for TOLMS, and 85%–94% for open partial laryngectomies.

More recently, the classification of larynx tumors based on the compartments has been emphasized as an important point to establish the indications of partial surgery of the larynx [43]. The creation of a perpendicular plane to the thyroid lamina at the level of the vocal process allows to differentiate between anterior and posterior paraglottic spaces. From this point of view, the anterior compartments have demonstrated to be best suited for the resection of advanced tumors in the case of external partial surgery [44], showing worse outcomes in those tumors with posterior involvement.

We recently reviewed a series of 203 consecutive locally advanced laryngeal tumors treated with TOLMS and analyzed our outcomes according to the compartmental concept of the larynx as proposed by Succo et al. [44]. Better outcomes in terms of local relapse and larynx preservation were found in those tumors involving the anterior compartments of the larynx (Table 25.3). Independent factors of local relapse were anterior and posterior paraglottic involvement and cartilage infiltration. Independent negative factors of larynx preservation were impaired/fixed vocal cord, impaired/fixed arytenoid, anterior paraglottic involvement, and reduced surgeon's experience (unpublished data).

25.6 Complications

Although TOS is a minimally surgical approach, postoperative complications may occur especially in locally extended resections. The complication rate is about 10%, with severe hemorrhage being the most fearsome, with a reported rate of mortality ranging between 0% and 0.3% [45]. Of importance, the majority of patients are treated without a tracheotomy, and thus, they are kept in a potentially risky situation during the postoperative period. For these reasons some authors recommend a prophylactic tracheotomy or an overnight, 24-h intubation in case no on-call doctor is available.

Postoperative bleeding tends to occur in the first 24–48 h or delayed, 7–10 days after surgery, and its management ranges from conservative measures to endoscopic cautery in the operation theatre, external carotid artery ligation, or embolization. All authors agree that the best way to manage the bleeding is preventing it. For this reason, systematic dissection of the laryngeal vessels in the pharyngoepiglottic or arytenoepiglottic folds is recommended, in order to coagulate or clip them before being transected.

Other complications of TOS include postoperative pneumonia, local infection, dyspnea, or emphysema. Although their rates are much lower,

Table 25.3 Local relapse and larynx preservation rates according to pT classification and involved compartments of the larynx clinically assessed by arytenoid mobility

	Local relapse		Total laryngectomy	
	No	Yes	No	Yes
Anterior pT3 with normal arytenoid mobility	102 (70.8%)	42 (29.2%)	114 (79.2%)	30 (20.8%)
Posterior pT3 with impaired/absent mobility	8 (38.1%)	13 (61.9%)	8 (38.1%)	13 (61.9%)
Anterior pT4 with normal arytenoid mobility	16 (66.7%)	8 (33.3%)	18 (72%)	7 (28%)
Posterior pT4 with impaired/absent mobility	0	1 (100%)	0	1 (100%)

they should be taken into account in extended resections, particularly aspiration pneumonia after extensive resections of the supraglottis. The site of the primary tumor and the surgeon's experience have significant influence in the complication rate [7], the supraglottic being the more risky area [45].

25.7 Functional Outcomes

In the case of locally extended TOS, postoperative rehabilitation is crucial to obtain the best functional results. Fiber-optic endoscopic evaluation of swallowing is very useful to assess laryngopharyngeal remnant structures and to decide the timing of oral intake and nasogastric feeding tube removal. Testing the swallowing function with different volumes and textures, stained with methylene blue, allows a precise assessment of swallowing and facilitates a tailored swallowing rehabilitation program for each patient. The latter may include environmental modifications, adaptation of volumes and textures, postural strategies, and specific swallowing maneuvers. In general, glottic tumors have the lowest risk of aspiration and no feeding tube is needed in the majority of patients, whereas supraglottic tumors have a fourfold increased risk of dysphagia [46].

Advanced malignant tumors of the glottis require type IV-V-VI cordectomies [47], which may end in a permanent postoperative dysphonia. Tumor location and criteria for locally advanced tumors will determine different scenarios. For example, if the conus elasticus is preserved, the fibrin exudation on top may lead to the formation of a structure resembling a new fold facilitating the glottic closure with the contralateral vocal fold after rehabilitation. When the anterior commissure is removed, a synechia is to be expected after healing. This synechia usually allows a glottic voice, but reduces the vibratory part of the vocal fold, leading to an increased fundamental frequency. In lateral tumors extending to the subglottis, a complete paraglottic resection is needed, resulting in glottic insufficiency with a breathy voice. Voice rehabilitation will be addressed to reduce fibrosis, enable a more elastic scar tissue to facilitate vibration in cases of glottic closure, or favor a ventricular or supraglottic closure in cases of a significant gap.

Even considering all these issues, TOS achieves high larynx preservation rates in adequately selected cases, with a very low percentage of patients in need of a definitive tracheotomy or gastrostomy [2]. Moreover, very good QOL outcomes have been reported in different centers, with neck dissection, the need of postoperative adjuvant treatment, and age being independent negative predictors of overall QOL [48].

In conclusion, TOLMS is an organ-preservation strategy for locally advanced laryngeal cancers that achieves oncologic outcomes and larynx preservation rates that are comparable to open partial surgeries or organ-preservation options in adequately selected patients. Other transoral approaches (assisted or not with robotic platforms) are promising, but outcomes are mainly limited to early tumors. More research is needed to evaluate its role in locally advanced tumors.

References

1. Pfister DG, Spencer S, Adelstein D, et al. Head and neck cancers, version 2.2020, NCCN clinical practice guidelines in oncology. J Natl Compr Cancer Netw. 2020;18(7):873–98. https://doi.org/10.6004/jnccn.2020.0031.
2. Bernal-Sprekelsen M, Vilaseca I. Transoral laser microsurgery of benign and malignant lesions. Thieme Publishers Stttgart; 2015. ISBN: 9783131723918.
3. Tomifuji M, Araki K, Yamashita T, Shiotani A. Transoral videolaryngoscopic surgery for oropharyngeal, hypopharyngeal, and supraglottic cancer. Eur Arch Otorhinolaryngol. 2014;271(3):589–97. https://doi.org/10.1007/s00405-013-2575-0.
4. Fernández-Fernández MM, Montes-Jovellar L, Parente Arias PL, Ortega Del Alamo P. TransOral endoscopic UltraSonic Surgery (TOUSS): a preliminary report of a novel robotless alternative to TORS. Eur Arch Otorhinolaryngol. 2015;272(12):3785–91. https://doi.org/10.1007/s00405-014-3423-6.
5. Doazan M, Hans S, Morinière S, et al. Oncologic outcomes with transoral robotic surgery for supraglottic squamous cell carcinoma: Results of the French Robotic Surgery Group of GETTEC. Head Neck. 2018;40(9):2050–9. https://doi.org/10.1002/hed.25199.
6. Lechien JR, Fakhry N, Saussez S, et al. Surgical, clinical and functional outcomes of transoral robotic

surgery for supraglottic laryngeal cancers: a systematic review. Oral Oncol. 2020;109:104,848. https://doi.org/10.1016/j.oraloncology.2020.104848. Epub ahead of print.

7. Bernal-Sprekelsen M, Blanch JL, Caballero-Borrego M, Vilaseca I. The learning curve in transoral laser microsurgery for malignant tumors of the larynx and hypopharynx: parameters for a levelled surgical approach. Eur Arch Otorhinolaryngol. 2013;270(2):623–8. https://doi.org/10.1007/s00405-012-2181-6. Epub 2012 Sep 21.
8. Lydiatt WM, Patel SG, O'Sullivan B, et al. Head and neck cancers-major changes in the American Joint Committee on cancer eighth edition cancer staging manual. CA Cancer J Clin. 2017;67(2):122–37.
9. Peretti G, Piazza C, Mora F, Garofolo S, Guastini L. Reasonable limits for transoral laser microsurgery in laryngeal cancer. Curr Opin Otolaryngol Head Neck Surg. 2016;24(2):135–9. https://doi.org/10.1097/MOO.0000000000000240.
10. Vilaseca I, Bernal-Sprekelsen M. Transoral laser microsurgery for locally advanced laryngeal cancer. Acta Otorrinolaringol Esp. 2013;64(2):140–9. English, Spanish. https://doi.org/10.1016/j.otorri.2012.01.013.
11. Agnello F, Cupido F, Sparacia G, Midiri F, Miroddi M, Grassedonio E, Galia M. Computerised tomography and magnetic resonance imaging of laryngeal squamous cell carcinoma: a practical approach. Neuroradiol J. 2017;30:197–204.
12. Tokat T, Adibelli ZH, Koc AM, Muderris T, Atsal G, Ozkok G. Impact of magnetic resonance on the decision of conservative surgery in advanced larynx cancer. Am J Otolaryngol. 2021;42(2):102855. https://doi.org/10.1016/j.amjoto.2020.102855.
13. Hussain T, Lang S, Haßkamp P, Holtmann L, Höing B, Mattheis S. The flex robotic system compared to transoral laser microsurgery for the resection of supraglottic carcinomas: first results and preliminary oncologic outcomes. Eur Arch Otorhinolaryngol. 2020;277(3):917–24. https://doi.org/10.1007/s00405-019-05767-0.
14. Orosco RK, Tam K, Nakayama M, Holsinger FC, Spriano G. Transoral supraglottic laryngectomy using a next-generation single-port robotic surgical system. Head Neck. 2019;41(7):2143–7. https://doi.org/10.1002/hed.25676.
15. Blanch JL, Vilaseca I, Caballero M, Moragas M, Berenguer J, Bernal-Sprekelsen M. Outcome of transoral laser microsurgery for T2---T3 tumors growing in the laryngeal anterior commissure. Head Neck 2011;33:1252–1259.
16. Eckel HE. Local recurrences following transoral laser surgery for early glottic carcinoma: frequency, management, and outcome. Ann Otol Rhinol Laryngol. 2001;110:7–15.
17. Steiner W, Ambrosch P, Rödel RMW, Kron M. Impact of anterior commissure involvement on local control of early glottic carcinoma treated by laser microresection. Laryngoscope. 2004;114:1485–91.
18. Benazzo M, Canzi P, Mauramati S, et al. Transoral robot-assisted surgery in Supraglottic and oropharyngeal squamous cell carcinoma: laser versus monopolar electrocautery. J Clin Med. 2019;8(12):2166. https://doi.org/10.3390/jcm8122166.
19. Steiner W. Results of curative laser microsurgery of laryngeal carcinomas. Am J Otolaryngol. 1993;14(2):116–21. https://doi.org/10.1016/0196-0709(93)90050-h.
20. Motta G, Esposito E, Cassiano B, Motta S. T1-T2-T3 glottic tumors: fifteen years experience with CO2 laser. Acta Otolaryngol Suppl 1997;527:155–159. doi: https://doi.org/10.3109/00016489709124062.
21. Ambrosch P, Rödel R, Kron M, Steiner W. Die Transorale Lasermikrochirurgie des Larynkarzinoms. Onkologe. 2001;5:505–12.
22. Motta G, Esposito E, Motta S, Tartaro G, Testa D. CO2 laser surgery in the treatment of glottic cancer. Head Neck. 2005;27(8):733. https://doi.org/10.1002/hed.20266.
23. Hinni ML, Salassa JR, Grant DG, et al. Transoral laser microsurgery for advanced laryngeal cancer. Arch Otolaryngol Head Neck Surg. 2007;133(12):1198–204. https://doi.org/10.1001/archotol.133.12.1198.
24. Grant DG, Salassa JR, Hinni ML, Pearson BW, Hayden RE, Perry WC. Transoral laser microsurgery for untreated glottic carcinoma. Otolaryngol Head Neck Surg. 2007;137(3):482–6. https://doi.org/10.1016/j.otohns.2007.05.064.
25. Peretti G, Piazza C, Cocco D, et al. Transoral CO(2) laser treatment for T(is)-T(3) glottic cancer: the University of Brescia experience on 595 patients. Head Neck. 2010;32(8):977–83. https://doi.org/10.1002/hed.21278.
26. Canis M, Ihler F, Martin A, Wolff HA, Matthias C, Steiner W. Organ preservation in T4a laryngeal cancer: is transoral laser microsurgery an option? Eur Arch Otorhinolaryngol. 2013;270(10):2719–27. https://doi.org/10.1007/s00405-013-2382-7.
27. Canis M, Martin A, Ihler F, Wolff HA, Kron M, Matthias C, Steiner W. Transoral laser microsurgery in treatment of pT2 and pT3 glottic laryngeal squamous cell carcinoma—results of 391 patients. Head Neck. 2014;36(6):859–66. https://doi.org/10.1002/hed.23389.
28. Breda E, Catarino R, Monteiro E. Transoral laser microsurgery for laryngeal carcinoma: survival analysis in a hospital-based population. Head Neck. 2015;37(8):1181–6. https://doi.org/10.1002/hed.23728.
29. Pantazis D, Liapi G, Kostarelos D, Kyriazis G, Pantazis TL, Riga M. Glottic and supraglottic pT3 squamous cell carcinoma: outcomes with transoral laser microsurgery. Eur Arch Otorhinolaryngol. 2015;272(8):1983–90. https://doi.org/10.1007/s00405-015-3611-z.
30. Peretti G, Piazza C, Penco S, et al. Transoral laser microsurgery as primary treatment for selected T3 glottic and supraglottic cancers. Head Neck.

2016;38(7):1107–12. https://doi.org/10.1002/hed.24424.
31. Day AT, Sinha P, Nussenbaum B, Kallogjeri D, Haughey BH. Management of primary T1-T4 glottic squamous cell carcinoma by transoral laser microsurgery. Laryngoscope. 2017;127(3):597–604. https://doi.org/10.1002/lary.26207.
32. Chang BA, Lott DG, Nagel TH, Howard BE, Hayden RE, Hinni ML. Outcomes following transoral laser microsurgery with resection of cartilage for laryngeal cancer. Ann Otol Rhinol Laryngol. 2019;128(10):978–82. https://doi.org/10.1177/0003489419851521.
33. Chien PJ, Hung LT, Wang LW, Yang MH, Chu PY. Oncologic results and quality of life in patients with T3 glottic cancer after transoral laser microsurgery. Eur Arch Otorhinolaryngol. 2021;278:2983. https://doi.org/10.1007/s00405-020-06445-2.
34. Motta G, Esposito E, Testa D, Iovine R, Motta S. CO2 laser treatment of supraglottic cancer. Head Neck. 2004;26(5):442–6. https://doi.org/10.1002/hed.10395.
35. Cabanillas R, Rodrigo JP, Llorente JL, Suárez C. Oncologic outcomes of transoral laser surgery of supraglottic carcinoma compared with a transcervical approach. Head Neck. 2008;30(6):750–5. https://doi.org/10.1002/hed.20778.
36. Peretti G, Piazza C, Ansarin M, De Benedetto L, Cocco D, Cattaneo A, Nicolai P, Chiesa F. Transoral CO2 laser microsurgery for tis-T3 supraglottic squamous cell carcinomas. Eur Arch Otorhinolaryngol. 2010;267(11):1735–42. https://doi.org/10.1007/s00405-010-1284-1.
37. Canis M, Ihler F, Martin A, Wolff HA, Matthias C, Steiner W. Results of 226 patients with T3 laryngeal carcinoma after treatment with transoral laser microsurgery. Head Neck. 2014;36(5):652–9. https://doi.org/10.1002/hed.23338.
38. Vilaseca I, Blanch JL, Berenguer J, Grau JJ, Verger E, Muxí Á, Bernal-Sprekelsen M. Transoral laser microsurgery for locally advanced (T3-T4a) supraglottic squamous cell carcinoma: sixteen years of experience. Head Neck. 2016;38(7):1050–7. https://doi.org/10.1002/hed.24408.
39. Ambrosch P, Gonzalez-Donate M, Fazel A, Schmalz C, Hedderich J. Transoral laser microsurgery for Supraglottic cancer. Front Oncol. 2018;8:158. https://doi.org/10.3389/fonc.2018.00158.
40. Vilaseca I, Bernal-Sprekelsen M, Luis BJ. Transoral laser microsurgery for T3 laryngeal tumors: prognostic factors. Head Neck. 2010;32:929–38.
41. Vilaseca I, Nogués-Sabaté A, Avilés-Jurado FX, et al. Factors of local recurrence and organ preservation with transoral laser microsurgery in laryngeal carcinomas; CHAID decision-tree analysis. Head Neck. 2019;41(3):756–64. https://doi.org/10.1002/hed.25422.
42. Riga M, Chelis L, Danielides V, Vogiatzaki T, Pantazis TL, Pantazis D. Systematic review on T3 laryngeal squamous cell carcinoma; still far from a consensus on the optimal organ preserving treatment. Eur J Surg Oncol. 2017;43(1):20–31. https://doi.org/10.1016/j.ejso.2016.05.030.
43. Piazza C, Filauro M, Paderno A, et al. Three-dimensional map of isoprognostic zones in glottic cancer treated by transoral laser microsurgery as a unimodal treatment strategy. Front Oncol. 2018;8:175. https://doi.org/10.3389/fonc.2018.00175.
44. Succo G, Crosetti E, Bertolin A, et al. Treatment for T3 to T4a laryngeal cancer by open partial horizontal laryngectomies: prognostic impact of different pathologic tumor subcategories. Head Neck. 2018;40(9):1897–908. https://doi.org/10.1002/hed.25176.
45. Vilaseca-González I, Bernal-Sprekelsen M, Blanch-Alejandro JL, Moragas-Lluis M. Complications in transoral CO2 laser surgery for carcinoma of the larynx and hypopharynx. Head Neck. 2003;25(5):382–8. https://doi.org/10.1002/hed.10207.
46. Bernal-Sprekelsen M, Vilaseca-González I, Blanch-Alejandro JL. Predictive values for aspiration after endoscopic laser resections of malignant tumors of the hypopharynx and larynx. Head Neck. 2004;26(2):103–10. https://doi.org/10.1002/hed.10363.
47. Remacle M, Van Haverbeke C, Eckel H, et al. Proposal for revision of the European Laryngological Society classification of endoscopic cordectomies. Eur Arch Otorhinolaryngol. 2007;264(5):499–504. https://doi.org/10.1007/s00405-007-0279-z.
48. Vilaseca I, Bernal-Sprekelsen M, Him R, Mandry A, Lehrer E, Blanch JL. Prognostic factors of quality of life after transoral laser microsurgery for laryngeal cancer. Eur Arch Otorhinolaryngol. 2015;272(5):1203–10. https://doi.org/10.1007/s00405-014-3030-6.

Open Neck Approaches: Partial and Reconstructive Laryngectomies

26

Dominique Chevalier and Giovanni Succo

Key Points

- The endoscopic approach is a safe surgical technique, more and more performed, and considered as routinely indicated. Therefore, in particular situations, open partial surgery should be solely performed. We consider those techniques as still necessary in our surgical arsenal.
- We would like to focus on workup, surgical technique, post-op course, and follow-up as important steps integrated in the process.

26.1 Introduction

The larynx and pharynx are both important for the three functions of swallowing, voice, and breathing. Any surgery at this level may have a negative impact. Many of these require a temporary tracheotomy and nasogastric tube. Decision making is based on evaluation of the patient, the tumor, the local resources and expertise, and the possibility of functional salvage if any [1].

26.2 The Preoperative Workup

The examination of the larynx in indirect laryngoscopy is carried out using a flexible nasopharyngolaryngoscope or 70°/90° angled telescopes. The main goals of this endoscopy, in addition to a general overview of the aerodigestive tract and a first assessment of the extent of the neoplasm, is the dynamic evaluation of the motility of the vocal cord and arytenoid. These parameters are extremely useful in the preoperative assessment of a patient candidate for a partial open laryngectomy, especially arytenoid fixation often identifying the invasion of the posterior paraglottic space by cancer. The use of stroboscopic light and methods of submucosal vascularization enhancement (NBI, SPIES) are useful for assessing the superficial extension of the disease [2].

26.2.1 Direct Pharyngolaryngoscopy

Direct endoscopic examination of the pharynx, larynx, and esophagus is performed under general anesthesia. It is conducted with 0°–30° and 70° rigid telescopes to improve the quality of the

D. Chevalier (✉)
ENT Head Neck Surgery, Huriez Hospital, University of Lille, Lille, France
e-mail: dominique.chevalier@chru-lille.fr

G. Succo
Head and Neck Oncology Unit, Candiolo Cancer Institute, FPO-IRCCS, Candiolo, Italy

Department of Oncology, University of Turin, Turin, Italy
e-mail: giovanni.succo@unito.it

M. Remacle, H. E. Eckel (eds.), *Textbook of Surgery of Larynx and Trachea*,
https://doi.org/10.1007/978-3-031-09621-1_26

mucosal assessment particularly in the case of a small cancer [3]. It is an indispensable diagnostic tool and has several goals:

- It allows for multiple mucosal biopsies for histological examination.
- It provides an accurate evaluation of the superficial tumor spread.
- The systematic examination of the entire upper aerodigestive tract and the esophagus allows for detection of synchronous cancers.

During this step careful palpation of the true vocal cord and the tumor is important for the evaluation of the depth of the lesion. In addition, if available, drawings, pictures, and/or videos of the tumor are helpful to the clinician in decision making at time of the multidisciplinary meeting.

26.2.2 Imaging

Imaging techniques are becoming more precise and are routinely used to compliment the clinical and the endoscopic assessment of patients with laryngeal and hypopharyngeal carcinomas.

Computed tomography (CT) is currently the most useful imaging modality [4]. The goal of CT is to accurately assess the location and size of the primary cancer and to evaluate extension to the neck either directly or through lymphatic metastasis. CT examination must be performed from the nasopharynx to the upper mediastinum with and without intravenous contrast enhancement. In case of a small laryngeal tumor, CT is preferably performed before the endoscopy and the biopsies, to avoid inflammation, which may result in an overestimation of the cancer infiltration. CT also allows for the use of dynamic maneuvers such as the Valsalva and phonation.

Knowing the natural course of the tumor, it is important to assess carefully the different anatomic areas of the larynx and hypopharynx. A cancer of the vocal cord or the ventricle may extend into the paraglottic space, and a supraglottic cancer can extend to into the preepiglottic space. Preepiglottic extension is easily detected after image reconstruction in the sagittal plane. Laterally laryngeal cancer may extend to the thyroid cartilage, which acts as a temporary barrier against extension in the neck. The CT scan technique allows exploring in the same session the upper aerodigestive tract and the lung as well.

Metastatic lymph nodes are frequently encountered with carcinoma of the supraglottis. The probability of metastatic involvement of a lymph node is associated with the following criteria seen on imaging:

- Size greater than 10 mm (12 mm in the subdigastric area)
- Central necrosis with heterogeneity and peripheral enhancement
- Circular shape

In the evaluation of carcinoma of the subglottis, CT scan yields important information regarding superior mediastinal and retropharyngeal lymph nodes where clinical examination is not feasible.

Magnetic resonance imaging (MRI) is performed with the use of an anterior neck coil and application or use of a protocol, which consists of axial T2-weighted fast spin echo and T1-weighted spin echo images. Then following intravenous administration of gadolinium, axial, sagittal, and coronal T1-weighted spin echo images are obtained. MRI is more sensitive in detecting minimal neoplastic invasion to the cartilage than CT [5], whereas CT is more specific. MRI shows superior resolution for demonstrating soft tissue details, initial cartilage involvement, and differential diagnosis between tumor and peritumoral edema [6]. Nevertheless, due to its susceptibility to motion-induced artefact, MRI is not routinely performed in the staging of cancer of the larynx.

Ultrasonography is helpful for the assessment of cervical lymph nodes. It is a simple, noninvasive, rapid, and high-sensitivity technique for the detection of subclinical lymph node metastasis but its reliability is operator-dependent. It is a useful method for follow-up and can be combined with fine-needle aspiration to confirm histological invasion.

26.3 Partial Surgery for Laryngeal Cancer

The larynx is divided in into three different sites:

- Supraglottis, which includes the lingual and laryngeal surfaces of the epiglottis, the aryepiglottic folds, the arytenoid cartilages, the false vocal folds, and the ventricle
- Glottis, which includes the true vocal cords and the anterior and posterior commissures
- Subglottis, which is the area of the larynx inferior to the glottis (1 cm below the free edge of the vocal cord to the lower edge of the cricoid cartilage)

Many different partial procedures have been described which provide a wide choice of conservative treatments with the goal to cure with preservation of laryngeal functions. We select in this chapter the most used and published procedures.

26.3.1 Cordectomy

26.3.1.1 Core Messages

Most of the patients are treated through an endoscopic approach which is considered safe and is routinely performed.

26.3.1.2 Indications

When an endoscopic procedure is not feasible due to anatomic or technical considerations, the external approach is still possible. The main indication is T1 glottic cancer involving the mild true vocal cord without extension to the anterior commissure.

26.3.1.3 Surgical Technique

After a horizontal incision, the thyroid cartilage is exposed and a midline thyrotomy is performed. The larynx is opened after sectioning of the cricothyroid membrane and the anterior commissure. The inner perichondrium is elevated on the tumor side and the true vocal cord is removed under direct vision. The anterior commissure is reconstructed by anchorage of the remaining vocal cord to the thyroid cartilage which is sutured on the midline. The strap muscles and the external perichondrium are closed [7].

We recommend, for this procedure, to assess carefully the local extension. It is not indicated in case of deep extension into the vocal muscle. This condition, often characterized by an impaired mobility of the true vocal cord, can hide an early involvement of the paraglottic space and is responsible for a higher risk of local recurrence.

Patient can swallow easily the day after the procedure and be discharged from the hospital quickly as no tracheotomy is performed.

26.3.1.4 Results

Few publications are available since the development of the endoscopic procedure. Lefebvre [8] reported a 5-year local control rate of 94% and a 5-year survival rate of 87%.

26.3.1.5 Tips and Pearl to Avoid Complications

- The most important thing is to confirm the indication; it is important to be sure that the tumor does not involve the vocal muscle. In that case there is a higher risk of local recurrence.
- The thyrotomy must be strictly median in order not to risk sectioning the true vocal cord, especially on the side not involved by the tumor. As no tracheotomy is performed, a small drain is necessary to avoid subcutaneous emphysema.

26.3.2 Frontolateral Vertical Laryngectomy

This procedure was described by Leroux-Robert and consists a vertical laryngectomy with removal of the anterior commissure and corresponding thyroid cartilage.

26.3.2.1 Core Message

- Like open neck cordectomy, this procedure is less performed nowadays.
- It is therefore considered as an alternative in case of exposition failure during transoral laser procedure due to unfavorable anatomic conditions.

26.3.2.2 Indications

This procedure is indicated to surgically treat T1b glottic cancer with extension close to the anterior commissure but without deep invasion of the same.

26.3.2.3 Surgical Technique

After a horizontal incision, the thyroid cartilage is exposed and a lateral thyrotomy is performed on both sides close to the midline The larynx is opened after sectioning of the cricothyroid membrane on the tumor-free side. The inner perichondrium is elevated on the tumor side and the true vocal cord with the anterior commissure attached to the thyroid cartilage is removed under direct vision of the tumor. The remaining vocal cord is sutured anteriorly to the thyroid cartilage which is then sutured at the level of the midline. The strap muscle and the external perichondrium are closed.

26.3.2.4 Specific Recommendations According to the Technique

It is important to suture anteriorly the petiole of the epiglottis to the remnant thyroid cartilage to avoid its displacement determining postop stenosis.

26.3.2.5 Results

In our experience, results are good: the 5-year survival rate was 83% and the local control rate was 96%. In a review, Brumund [9] reported the results of a series of 270 patients in the ENT and Head and Neck Surgery Department of Georges Pompidou European Hospital. He confirmed the excellent results: the 5-year actuarial survival rate was 83.1% in T1 and 67.2% in T2. He also found that the actuarial local control ranged from 96.2% (T1) to 68.2% (T2).

26.3.2.6 Tips and Pearl to Avoid Complications

This surgical technique is safe and as mentioned can be performed without tracheotomy. Therefore, careful hemostasis must be done at the time of closure.

26.3.3 Frontal Anterior Laryngectomy with Epiglottoplasty

Bouche [10] and Sedlacek in 1965 and Kambic in 1977 pointed the interest of the epiglottis to reconstruct the larynx. Tucker [11] in 1979 published a series of patients who underwent a "near-total laryngectomy" which was in fact a frontal anterior resection of the larynx using the epiglottis to close the larynx anteriorly.

26.3.3.1 Core Message

- This procedure allows resection of both false and true vocal cords with the anterior part of the thyroid cartilage.
- The reconstruction is done anteriorly to close the remaining larynx with the epiglottis.
- Functional results are usually good and such a procedure can be performed in the elderly.

26.3.3.2 Indications

This procedure is indicated to treat glottic cancer classified T1b or T2. It is still indicated in case of superficial anterior commissure involvement.

26.3.3.3 Surgical Technique

A tracheotomy is necessary. The thyroid cartilage is exposed and two lateral thyrotomies are performed at least 1.5 cm from the midline. The larynx is opened superiorly through the petiole of the epiglottis. Inferiorly, the cricothyroid membrane is transected at level of the superior border of the cricoid cartilage. The inner perichondrium is elevated on both sides and then both false and true vocal cords are removed with the anterior commissure attached to the thyroid cartilage. The epiglottis is then pulled downward, its anterior face is dissected close to the cartilage, and the hyoepiglottic ligament is transected. The epiglottis is sutured laterally to the remaining thyroid cartilage and inferiorly to the cricoid cartilage. The strap muscle and the external perichondrium are closed.

26.3.3.4 Specific Recommendations According to the Technique

- The hyoepiglottic ligament must be transected to allow the suture of the petiole with the cricoid cartilage mucosa without any tension.
- Both ventricles must be removed with the specimen.

26.3.3.5 Recommendations for Follow-up

The tracheostomy tube is removed when the laryngeal respiratory space is sufficient. Usually it can be done at day 4 but sometimes edema can occur after this time and it is careful to keep a tracheotomy tube (smallest size as possible) until the beginning of swallowing. The nasogastric tube is removed when the patient is able to swallow liquids, which means at least between days 12 and 18.

26.3.3.6 Results

Local control and survival rates are also excellent. Giovanni [12] reported a 5-year survival and local control rates of 86% and 92%, respectively. Mallet [13] confirmed those results in a population of 65 patients with 5-year survival and local control rates of 82% and 94%, respectively. As with other partial laryngectomies, all patients presented hoarseness and weakness of the voice. Aspiration can occur during the postoperative course and speech therapy is mandatory.

26.3.3.7 Tips and Pearl to Avoid Complications

- It is necessary to suture the epiglottis to the thyroid cartilage laterally. If not, there is a possible risk of stenosis

26.3.4 Open Partial Horizontal Laryngectomies (OPHLs)

A model for the rational classification of open partial horizontal laryngectomies (OPHLs) was proposed in 2014 by the European Laryngological Society (ELS), based on the cranio-caudal extent of laryngeal resection, and it defined three types: supraglottic laryngectomy (type I, SGPL), supracricoid laryngectomy (type II, SCPL), and supratracheal laryngectomy (type III, STPL) [14].

26.3.4.1 Supraglottic Laryngectomy

Supraglottic laryngectomy was described by Alonso [15]. It consists of the resection of the whole supraglottic part of the larynx including both ventricular folds and the epiglottis. Extensions of this procedure have been described particularly in case of superior tumor extension with a partial resection of the base of the tongue or lateral extension with partial resection of the pyriform sinus.

26.3.4.2 Supracricoid Laryngectomy with CHEP

- Supraglottic partial laryngectomy is the most classical technique and is widely performed.
- This technique allows resection of supraglottic cancer without deep extension into the preepiglottic space.
- Oncologic and functional results are good when properly indicated and performed.

26.3.4.3 Supracricoid Laryngectomy with CHP

The main indications are tumor of the epiglottis and the anterior part of the ventricular folds. Contraindications are invasion of the glottis and/or the ventricle, thyroid cartilage extension, impaired motion of the vocal cord, and consistent tongue base extension.

26.3.4.4 Supratracheal Partial Laryngectomy with Tracheohyoidoepiglottopexy (THEP) and Tracheohyoidopexy

After incision and elevation of the skin, a bilateral neck dissection is performed first.

The infrahyoid muscles are transected at the level of the hyoid bone and reflected inferiorly to expose the superior edge of the thyroid cartilage. The superior cornu is transected. The external perichondrium of the thyroid cartilage is elevated and reflected inferiorly at the level of the true vocal cords, located exactly halfway between the thyroid notch and the lower edge of the thyroid. Then the thyroid cartilage is transected horizontally on both sides. The larynx is entered superiorly in the valleculae after elevation of the mucosa from the inferior edge of the hyoid bone. Then the surgeon moves close to the midline to have a large view of the operating field, and then the incision is enlarged laterally and inferiorly to expose the larynx. Both aryepiglottic folds are transected and incision is continued into the ventricles and anteriorly above the anterior commissure and true vocal cords.

Closure is performed by impaction of the remaining thyroid cartilage to the base of the tongue and, if spared, the hyoid bone using 3 or 4 sutures (Vicryl® 2–0).

At the end, the perichondrium is sutured to the hyoid bone and the infrahyoid muscles are sutured superiorly covering the surgical field.

26.3.4.5 Specific Recommendations

It is important to save both true vocal cords and to avoid injury at the time of tumor resection. The inferior and superior laryngeal nerves must be protected and spared.

26.3.4.6 Results

Oncologic results are good with a low recurrence rate of 5–15% for T1 and T2 supraglottic carcinomas. Survival is excellent and one of the main causes of failure is second primary.

26.3.4.7 Recommendations for Follow-Up

The tracheostomy tube is removed as soon as the laryngeal respiratory space is sufficient. Usually it can be done at day 4.

The nasogastric tube is removed when the patient is able to swallow liquids, which means at least between days 10 and 16. Aspiration can occur but is less frequent than after supracricoid partial laryngectomy.

26.3.4.8 Tips and Pearl to Avoid Complications

At the time of specimen removal, it is important to keep in mind the exact level of the glottis. In case of injury, the functional result could be worse.

26.3.5 Supracricoid Partial Laryngectomy with Cricohyoidoepiglottopexy (CHEP): OPHL Type IIa

After the publications by Majer [19] and Labayle, Piquet [16] published the first report of a series of patients with glottic cancer treated with this surgical technique. The aim was to perform a large or subtotal resection of the larynx to decrease the local recurrence rate of glottic cancer which was initially treated with transcartilaginous techniques. In the seventies this techniique was frequently used in France and Italy and then gained popularity throughout Europe and overseas countries. The main problem consists of the postoperative course and the higher risk of aspiration in comparison with other partial laryngectomies.

26.3.5.1 Core Message

- This technique allows removal of a large part of the larynx.
- The epiglottis is useful to improve functional results.
- At least one functional cricoarytenoid unit must be preserved.
- Subglottic extension is associated with a higher risk of recurrence.

26.3.5.2 Indications

CHEP is indicated to surgically treat glottic carcinomas with deep invasion into the vocal muscle, close to the thyroid cartilage or involving the inner cortex but without extension through it. CHEP is indicated in case of impaired motion of the true vocal cord, but the arytenoid cartilage must be still mobile.

Subglottic extension must be carefully assessed, and when it is more than the superior border of the cricoid cartilage, it is considered a contraindication. Therefore, posterior subglottic extension is considered much more at risk than the anterior one.

CHEP is also indicated in bilateral glottic cancer and/or with anterior commissure invasion but without extension to the petiole of the epiglottis.

Using the UICC classification, CHEP is indicated for T2 and selected T3 glottic cancers.

26.3.5.3 Surgical Technique

After elevation of the apron flap, the midline raphe of the strap muscles is divided. The sternohyoid and thyrohyoid muscles are transected close to the hyoid bone. The superior border of the thyroid cartilage is dissected, and the inferior constrictor muscles are transected at the posterior border of both thyroid cartilage ala. To avoid injury of the inferior laryngeal nerve, the inferior cornu of the thyroid cartilage is transected and left in place on the side(s) of remaining arytenoid(s) cartilage(s). With the same intent, concerning the superior laryngeal nerves, both superior cornu are preserved. The superior border of the cricoid cartilage is dissected; on the tumor side, the mucosa and the inner perichondrium can be elevated to enlarge the margins at the time of resection. The larynx is opened by a transepiglottic laryngotomy placed horizontally at the level of the superior edge of the thyroid cartilage through the preepiglottic space. The resection is extended through the upper part of the aryepiglottic fold and the false vocal cord anteriorly to the arytenoid cartilage; both true and false vocal cords are removed. When necessary, the (T3) arytenoid cartilage can be removed; it is important to spare the posterior mucosa, which is then sutured anteriorly and can be useful to improve the vocal result. Inferiorly, the cricothyroid membrane is transected at the level of the upper edge of the cricoid cartilage and the specimen is then removed.

Closure is performed by impaction of the cricoid cartilage to the hyoid bone using 3 or 4 sutures (Vicryl® 2–0). The needle is passed under the cricoid cartilage, through the inferior part of the epiglottis and around the hyoid bone with part of the base of the tongue. Care must be done superiorly to avoid injury of both hypoglossal nerves and the needle is grasped close to the midline of the hyoid bone. The strap muscles are sutured, tracheostomy is carried out, the skin flap is closed over a drain, and the tracheotomy tube is inserted.

26.3.5.4 Specific Recommendations According to the Technique

It is important to save at least one mobile cricoarytenoid unit.

Inferior and superior laryngeal nerves must be protected and spared.

At the time of resection, both ventricles must be totally removed to avoid a cyst which can create a laryngeal stenosis.

26.3.5.5 Recommendations for Follow-up

The tracheotomy tube is removed as soon as the laryngeal respiratory space is sufficient. Usually it can be done at day 4 but sometimes edema can occur after this time and it is careful to keep a tracheotomy tube (smallest size as possible) until the beginning of swallowing. Some authors advocate for an early decannulation but care must be done to avoid severe dyspnea and we think it is better to do it when the risk of edema disappears.

The nasogastric tube is removed when the patient is able to swallow liquids, which means at least between days 12 and 18.

Aspiration frequently occurs and decreases progressively. Speech therapy is always mandatory and should continue when the patient is discharged from hospital.

26.3.5.6 Results

As the goal is to decrease the risk of local recurrence, it is clear that the wide resection of the larynx provides excellent oncologic results. In our experience results are good with a 5-year survival rate of 78% and a local control rate of 94.3%. Those results are confirmed by other teams with a local control rate which ranges between 90% and 96% [17, 18].

26.3.5.7 Tips and Pearl to Avoid Complications

- At the time of closure, superior stitches encircle the base of the tongue and the hyoid bone. These stitches must be close to the midline to avoid injury of both the hypoglossal nerves and lingual artery.
- At the time of closure, the needle of the median stitch runs through the submucosa at the level of the petiole of the epiglottis to avoid an epiglottis posterior displacement determining soft tissue stenosis.

26.3.6 Supracricoid Partial Laryngectomy with Cricohyoidopexy (CHP): OPHL Type IIb

Following the principles first described by Majer and Rieder [19], this technique was described by Labayle and is very similar with the CHEP technique but allows the total removal of the supraglottis. It is one of the partial surgery techniques allowing for the widest resection of the larynx. Due to the risk of aspiration, selection of patient is important and attention must be paid to the patient's general health status [20].

26.3.6.1 Core Message

- The CHP technique is similar to the CHEP.
- The preepiglottic space and the whole epiglottis are removed.
- Functional results are less good than with other techniques.

26.3.6.2 Indication

The CHP technique is indicated to surgically treat the following:

- Supraglottic cancer without extension to the upper part of the preepiglottic space.
- Glottic cancer invading the supraglottis, particularly when the site of origin is the anterior commissure. In that case there is a high risk of extension to the inferior part of the preepiglottic space and its removal is mandatory.
- Transglottic and supraglottic cancers with vocal cord fixation but without arytenoid cartilage fixation.

26.3.6.3 Surgical Technique

It is very similar to the CHEP technique which was previously described. A neck dissection is routinely performed prior to laryngeal surgery. The main difference is the removal of the epiglottis with the preepiglottic space. That means that at the time of dissection, the hyoepiglottic ligament is detached from the hyoid bone allowing the total removal of the preepiglottic space with the specimen. If possible at least one arytenoid cartilage is preserved. At the time of reconstruction, there is no difference and the pexy is performed with four stiches crossing under the cricoid cartilage and the hyoid bone with the base of the tongue. The strap muscles are sutured, tracheostomy is carried out, the skin flap is closed over a drain, and the tracheotomy tube is inserted.

26.3.6.4 Specific Recommendations

As the resection is large, aspiration occurs frequently. If possible it is better to spare both arytenoid cartilages. Speech therapy must be performed and continued after hospital discharge. The goals are swallowing first and optimizing voice result second. Inferior and superior laryngeal nerves must be protected and spared.

26.3.6.5 Results

As it is indicated to surgically treat supraglottic cancer, oncologic results are good. Survival ranges between 68% and 84%. Local recurrence rate is low, between 0% and 16% [21].

26.3.6.6 Recommendations for Follow-Up

Recommendations are similar with the CHEP technique. The tracheostomy tube is removed as soon as the laryngeal respiratory space is sufficient. Usually it can be done at day 4 but sometimes edema can occur after this time and it is careful to keep a tracheotomy tube (smallest size as possible) until the beginning of swallowing.

26.3.6.7 Tips and Pearl to Avoid Complications

As the larynx is very large, the impaction of the cricoid cartilage and the hyoid bone must be done at the same level. If the cricoid cartilage is located backward, the risk of aspiration is higher.

26.3.7 Supratracheal Partial Laryngectomy with Tracheohyoidoepiglottopexy (THEP) and Tracheohyoidopexy (THP): OPHL Type III

This technique described by Serafini [22] and later by Lacourreye [23] is very similar to the CHEP/CHP techniques allowing the enlargement of the resection to the cricoid ring +/– one cricoarytenoid unit.

The introduction of the OPHL type III has opened a useful window into function-sparing surgical protocols. In fact, during a planned supracricoid laryngectomy, in case of positive inferior intraoperative margins, the resection can be easily enlarged from a supracricoid to a supratracheal laryngectomy.

Also in this case, due to the risk of aspiration, patient selection is important and attention must be paid to the patient's general health status.

26.3.7.1 Core Message

- The THEP technique is similar to the CHEP, while the THP technique is similar to the CHP technique.
- The subglottic site is removed sparing at least one functioning cricoarytenoid unit.
- Functional results are similar than with other techniques.

26.3.7.2 Indication

The THEP/THP technique is indicated to surgically treat the following:

- Glottic cancer with extension to the subglottic site reaching the level of the cricoid cartilage
- Glottic cancer with arytenoid fixation and extension to the posterior paraglottic space
- Transglottic cancer with arytenoid fixation

26.3.7.3 Surgical Technique

It is very similar to the CHEP/CHP techniques which were previously described. A neck dissection is routinely performed prior to laryngeal surgery. Level VI dissection is strongly recommended due to the high risk of metastases by a cancer involving the subglottic site. The main difference is the removal of the cricoid ring +/– one cricoarytenoid unit (arytenoid + hemicricoid plate + cricoarytenoid muscles). At the time of reconstruction, the pexy is performed with four to five stiches crossing under the first tracheal ring and the hyoid bone with the base of the tongue. The strap muscles are sutured, tracheostomy is carried out, the skin flap is closed over a drain, and the tracheotomy tube is inserted.

26.3.7.4 Specific Recommendations

As the resection is wide, aspiration occurs frequently. If possible it is better to spare both cricoarytenoid units. Speech therapy must be performed and continued after hospital discharge. The goals are decannulation and swallowing first and optimizing voice result second. Inferior and superior laryngeal nerves must be protected and spared.

26.3.7.5 Results

As it is indicated to surgically treat glottic/transglottic cancer with subglottic involvement, oncologic results are quite good. In our experience, survival is about 78% for selected cT3–cT4a, while locoregional recurrence is about 26.2% [24, 25].

26.3.7.6 Recommendations for Follow-Up

Recommendations are similar with the CHEP/CHP techniques. The tracheostomy tube is removed as soon as the laryngeal respiratory space is sufficient. Usually it can be done at days 4–7 but sometimes soft tissue edema can occur after this time and it is careful to keep a tracheotomy tube (smallest size as possible) until the beginning of swallowing.

26.3.7.7 Tips and Pearl to Avoid Complications

The impaction of the trachea and the hyoid bone must be done as much as possible at the same level. If the tracheal ring is stretched, the risk of neoglottis stenosis is high.

26.4 Partial Surgery for Hypopharyngeal Cancer

By comparison with laryngeal surgery, less partial pharyngectomy procedures are available for the surgical treatment of hypopharyngeal cancers with preservation of laryngeal and pharyngeal function. Because occult cervical metastasis is frequent, neck dissection should be performed systematically. Only a few patients are amenable to partial pharyngectomy. These procedures are associated with good local control of the disease, but patients have a poor prognosis due to the high incidence of second primary tumors, comorbidities, and metastasis.

26.4.1 Posterior Partial Pharyngectomy

26.4.1.1 Core Messages

- As diagnosis is done late, there are few indications.
- Small and superficial tumors can be treated with an endoscopic resection.

26.4.1.2 Indications

This procedure is indicated for tumors which are limited to the posterior and lower wall of the pharynx without extension to the piriform sinus and the larynx. Such tumors are routinely treated by radiotherapy.

26.4.1.3 Specific Assessment

During workup, it is essential to assess the exact local extension because if the defect of the posterior wall is too large, it is necessary to perform immediate reconstruction.

26.4.1.4 Surgical Technique

The pharynx can be opened anteriorly, through a transhyoid approach. It is necessary to detach the suprahyoid muscles from the hyoid bone. The mucosa of the vallecula is then incised to open the surgical field and provide a direct access to the tumor. After excision of the tumor, the surgical defect is left open and the mucosal edge is sutured to the prevertebral fascia using resorbable sutures. The pharynx can be opened laterally, when tumors are larger and need a reconstruction. In such situation, bilateral neck dissection is performed first. The posterior wall of the hypopharynx is exposed and the larynx and the base of the tongue are elevated to open the surgical field. The posterior wall mucosa is dissected from the prevertebral fascia. After opening of the pharynx, the tumor is removed under direct vision in a monobloc specimen. Reconstruction is then performed using either a radial forearm free flap or a pectoralis major myocutaneous flap, which is less employed due to its size [26].

26.4.2 Partial Lateral Pharyngectomy (Trotter)

Using a lateral approach, the posterior two-thirds of the thyroid cartilage and the greater cornu of the hyoid bone are resected. Then the lateral wall of the pyriform sinus is resected as well as the deep fascia and the thyrohyoid muscle. Primary closure is usually possible but reconstruction with a local muscular flap is sometimes necessary. This procedure is indicated for limited cancer to the lateral wall of the pyriform sinus.

26.4.3 Supracricoid Hemipharyngolaryngectomy

26.4.3.1 Core Messages

- It allows for the surgical treatment of large tumors of the upper part of the pyriform sinus.
- Oncologic results are good when properly indicated.

26.4.3.2 Indications

This procedure is indicated for tumors of the medial wall of the pyriform sinus without impaired mobility of the larynx and located above the level of the superior border of the cricoid cartilage.

26.4.3.3 Surgical Technique

Ipsilateral neck dissection is performed first. Using a lateral approach, the ipsilateral thyroid ala and half of the hyoid bone are resected. The infrahyoid muscles are reflected inferiorly and the larynx is entered through the vallecula. The preepiglottic space and the epiglottis are vertically transected. Resection is continued inferiorly above the superior border of the cricoid cartilage, and the vocal cord is removed with the ventricle. At this point the lateral margin and the pyriform sinus are visualized and vertical posterior resection is performed under direct vision. The defect is covered by apposition of the edges, after mobilization of the prevertebral muscle insertions that are sutured to the posterior border of the infrahyoid muscles.

Superiorly, the pharynx is closed by suturing the remaining mucosa of the pharyngeal wall to the vallecula. Then the edges of the previously spared infrahyoid muscles are sutured externally to the constrictor muscles. The entire pyriform sinus and the ipsilateral hemilarynx above the cricoid cartilage are removed with the tumor.

26.4.3.4 Recommendations for Follow-up

The postoperative course is often marked by the slow recovery of swallowing ability and a risk of aspiration and bronchopulmonary infections. Patients begin oral feeding by the tenth postoperative day very carefully.

26.4.3.5 Results

Laccourreye [27] in a series of 34 patients with cancer of the pyriform sinus staged as T2 confirmed the reliability of this technique with 5-year actuarial local and 5-year actuarial regional control rates of 96.6% and 93.7%, respectively.

26.4.3.6 Tips and Pearl to Avoid Complications

At the time of closure of the pharynx, stitches must be done without tension to avoid misfunction of the cricopharyngeal muscle and aspiration.

26.4.4 Supraglottic Hemipharyngolaryngectomy

26.4.4.1 Core Message

This is a variant from the previous one only in that both true vocal cords are conserved.

Functional results are better than with the supracricoid hemipharyngolaryngectomy.

26.4.4.2 Indications

The procedure is indicated for tumors of the upper part of the pyriform sinus extending to the aryepiglottic fold particularly in the case of ulceration or infiltration.

26.4.4.3 Surgical Technique

Neck dissection is performed first. The infrahyoid muscles are transected from the lower border of the hyoid bone. Half of this hyoid horn is resected. The infrahyoid muscles are reflected inferiorly and the thyroid cartilage is exposed. The ipsilateral superior two-thirds of the thyroid cartilage is resected to allow for exposure of the ipsilateral vocal cord. The larynx is entered through the vallecula, and the preepiglottic space and the epiglottis are vertically transected. Resection is continued inferiorly above the floor of the ventricle, and the vocal cord is spared. At this point the lateral margin and the pyriform sinus are visualized and vertical posterior resection is performed under direct vision. Superiorly, the pharynx is closed by suturing the remaining mucosa of the pharyngeal wall to the vallecula and to the medial laryngeal remnant taking care not to suture the remaining half of the epiglottis. Then the edges of the previously spared infrahyoid muscles are sutured externally to the constrictor muscles, medially to the contralateral infrahyoid muscles, and superiorly to the mylohyoid muscle.

Closure is achieved by apposition of the mucosal edges or use of a subhyoid muscle flap.

26.4.4.4 Recommendations for Follow-up

The tracheotomy tube is plugged by the eighth postoperative day. Patients can begin to phonate after day 8, and oral feeding can begin by the tenth postoperative day.

26.4.4.5 Results

In a series of 45 patients [28] who underwent this procedure in association with postoperative radiotherapy, a high local control rate (97.8%) was reported.

26.4.4.6 Tips and Pearl to Avoid Complications

- At the time of closure of the pharynx, stitches must be done without tension to avoid misfunction of the cricopharyngeal muscle and aspiration.
- If radiotherapy is performed, it is better to keep the tracheotomy to avoid obstruction of the larynx due to edema.

References

1. Lefebvre JL, Coche-Dequeant B. Treatment of laryngeal cancer : the permanent challenge. Expert Rev Anticancer Ther. 2004;4:913–20.
2. Eckel HE, Simo R. European laryngological society position paper on laryngeal dysplasia part II: diagnosis, treatment, and follow-up. Eur Arch Otorhinolaryngol. 2020;278:1723. https://doi.org/10.1007/s00405-020-06406-9.
3. Chevalier D, Fayoux P. Endoscopic evaluation of glottic cancer. Ann Otolaryngol Chir Cervicofac (Paris). 1997;114:197–8.
4. Piquet JJ, Desaulty A. Crico-hyoido-épiglotto-pexie. Technique opératoire et résultats fonctionnels (1974). Ann Otolaryngol Chir Cervicofac. 1974;91:681–9.
5. Castelijns JA, Gerritsen GJ. Invasion of laryngeal cartilage by cancer: comparison of CT and MRI imaging. Radiology. 1998;167:199–206.
6. Maroldi R, Ravanelli M. Magnetic resonance for laryngeal cancer. Curr Opin Otolaryngol Head Neck Surg. 2014;2014(22):131–9. https://doi.org/10.1097/moo.0000000000000036.
7. Kacker A, Wolden S. Cancer of the larynx. Shah J Head and neck surgery and oncology. Mosby New-York; 2003.
8. Lefebvre JL, Vankemmel B. La cordectomie dans le traitement des cancers de corde vocale. A propos de 200 cas. Journal Français d'ORL. 1987;36:415–21.
9. Brumund K, Gutierrez-Fonseca R. Frontolateral vertical partial laryngectomy for invasive squamous cell carcinoma of the true vocal cord : a 25 year experience. Ann Otol Rhinol Laryngol. 2005;114:314–22.
10. Bouche J, Freche C. L'hémilaryngectomie avec epiglottoplastie. Ann Otolaryngol Chir Cervico Fac. 1965;82:421–4.
11. Tucker HM, Wood BJ. Glottic reconstruction after near total laryngectomy. Laryngoscope. 1979;89:609–17.
12. Giovanni A, Guelfucci B. Partial frontolateral laryngectomy with epiglottic reconstruction in the management of early-stage glottic carcinoma. Laryngoscope. 2001;111:663–8.
13. Mallet Y, Chevalier D. Near total laryngectomy with epiglottic reconstruction, our experience of 65 cases. Eur Arch Otorhinolaryngol. 2001;258:488–91.
14. Succo G, Peretti G. Open partial horizontal laryngectomies: a proposal for classification by the working committee on nomenclature of the European Laryngological Society. Eur Arch Otorhinolaryngol. 2014;2014:2489–96.
15. Alonso JM. La chirurgie conservatrice pour le cancer du larynx et de l'hypopharynx. Ann Otolaryngol Chir Cervicofac. 1951;68:689–96.
16. Piquet JJ. Functional laryngectomy (cricohyoidopexy). Clin Otolaryngol. 1976;1:7–16.
17. Chevalier D, Laccourreye O. Cricohyoidoepiglottopexy for glottic carcinoma with fixation or impaired mobility of the true vocal cord : 5-year oncologic results with 112 patients. Ann Otol Rhinol Laryngol. 1997;106:364–9.
18. Laccourreye H, Laccourreye O. Supracricoid laryngectomy with cricohyoidoepiglottopexy: a partial laryngeal procedure for glottic carcinoma. Ann Otol Rhinol Laryngol. 1990;99:421–6.
19. Majer H, Rieder A. Technique de laryngectomie permettant de conserver la perméabilité respiratoire: la crico-hyoido-pexie. Ann Otolaryngol Chir Cervicofac. 1959;76:677–83.
20. Naudo P, Laccourreye O. Functional outcome and prognosis factors after supracricoid partial laryngectomy with cricohyoidopexy. Ann Otol Rhinol Laryngol. 1997;106(4):291–6.
21. Laccourreye H, Laccourreye O. Supracricoid laryngectomy with cricohyoidopexy: a partial laryngeal procedure for selected supraglottic and transglottic carcinomas. Laryngoscope. 1990;100(7):735–41.
22. Serafini I. Reconstructive laryngectomy. Rev Laryngol Otol Rhinol. 1972;1972:23–32.
23. Laccourreye O, Brasnu D, Jouffre V, et al. Supracricoid partial laryngectomy extended to the anterior arch of the cricoid with tracheo-crico-hyoido-epiglottopexy. Oncologic and functional results. Ann Otolaryngol Chir Cervicofac. 1996;113:15–9.
24. Rizzotto G, Crosetti E, Lucioni M, et al. Oncologic outcomes of supratracheal laryngectomy: critical analysis. Head Neck. 2015:1417–24.
25. Succo G, Fantini M. Supratracheal partial laryngectomy: indications, oncologic and functional results. Curr Opin Otolaryngol. 2017;25:127.
26. Silver CE, Moisa I. Surgical therapy. In: Ferlito A, editor. Neoplasm of the larynx. London: Churchill Livingstone; 1993.
27. Laccourreye O, Merite-Drancy A. Supracricoid hemilaryngopharyngectomy in selected pyriform carcinoma. Laryngoscope. 1993;103:1373–9.
28. Chevalier D, Watelet JB. Supraglottic hemipharyngolaryngectomy plus radiation for the treatment of early lateral margin and pyriform sinus carcinoma. Head Neck. 1997;19:1–5.

Total Laryngectomy

27

Małgorzata Wierzbicka and Joanna Jackowska

Abbreviations

CT	Chemotherapy
DFS	Disease-free survival
ECS	Extracapsular spread
EGF	Epidermal growth factor
ETL	Extended total laryngectomy
FGF-1 and FGF-2	Fibroblast growth factors,
FU	Follow-up
HME	Heat and moisture exchange system
HRQoL	Health-Related Quality of Life
LCA	Lateral cervical approach
OPL	Open partial laryngectomy
OS	Overall survival
PCF	Pharyngocutaneous fistula
PM	Pectoralis major
PMMF	Pectoralis major myocutaneous flap
PNI	Perineural invasion VFSS - videofluoroscopic swallowing study
POD	Postoperative delirium
RFFF	Radial forearm free flaps
RT	Radiotherapy
RT/CT	Radio-chemotherapy
SCM	Sternocleidomastoid muscle
STL	Salvage total laryngectomy
TGF	Transforming growth factor
TL	Total laryngectomy
TOLM	Transoral laser microsurgery
TORS TL	Transoral Robotic Total Laryngectomy
TORS	Transoral Robotic Surgery
TOUSS	Transoral ultrasonic surgery
TOUSS-TL	The transoral endoscopic ultrasonic total laryngectomy
TPFF	Temporoparietalis fascia flap
VEGF	Vascular endothelial growth factors

M. Wierzbicka · J. Jackowska (✉)
Department of Otolaryngology and Oncological Laryngology, Poznan University of Medical Sciences, Poznan, Poland
e-mail: otosk2@ump.edu.pl; joanna.jackowska@ump.edu.pl

27.1 Selected Details of Larynx Anatomy

Laryngeal cancer, which initially develops on the epithelium lining within individual layers of the larynx, infiltrating deep into or beyond the larynx, spreads in a characteristic way, conditioned

M. Remacle, H. E. Eckel (eds.), *Textbook of Surgery of Larynx and Trachea*,
https://doi.org/10.1007/978-3-031-09621-1_27

by the structure of intralaryngeal ligament structures, connective tissue membranes, or cartilages of the laryngeal scaffold. Key to the pathology of laryngeal cancer is infiltration of the preglottic space, periglottic spread, and anterior infiltration of the cancer from the anterior commissure (into the thyroid cartilage and prelaryngeal area).

The pre-epiglottic space filled with connective tissue and adipose tissue is limited at the top by the hyoid-epiglottic ligament and in part by the mucosa of the lingual wells. Anteriorly it is bound by the thyroid-hyoid membrane, posteriorly by the anterior surface of the epiglottis. This space is the pathway for cancer to spread within the supraglottic floor. The epiglottic cartilage is not a sufficient barrier as it is usually perforated in many places, especially in its lower portion. Therefore, almost 50% of carcinomas developing on the subglottic part of the epiglottis pass into the preglottal space (box).

The symmetrical periglottic space, filled in part by connective and adipose tissue, in part by the vocal muscle, is more difficult to define. It is laterally bound by the inner cartilage of the thyroid cartilage and partially, in its upper part, by the thyroid-hyoid membrane. The upper part of the medial limitation is a quadrangular membrane, reaching with its lower edge to the vestibular fold. Dorsally, this space is limited only by the mucosa of the pyriform recess. The medial and anterior limitation in the lower part is the membranous structure of the elastic cone.

The anterior commissure ligament (Broyles ligament) is a band of fibrous tissue approximately 1 mm wide and approximately 10 mm long, running perfectly in the midline and connecting the symmetrical vocal ligaments that join in the anterior commissure, with the inner surface of the thyroid cartilage in its upper third. The Broyles ligament contains small blood and lymph vessels, and its attachment to the discoid cartilage is a place devoid of internal cartilage. In this way, cancer infiltration in the anterior commissure spreads easily not only to the cartilage, but also to the soft tissues of the prelaryngeal region, and thus metastasizes to the prelaryngeal node (Delphian node).

The consequence of the differentiated embryological development of the epiglottic (from the oropharyngeal) and subglottic (from the tracheopulmonary) part of the larynx is a clearly separated lymph outflow from both parts. The lymphatic anatomy and the patterns of nodal metastasis reflect the location and extent of invasion of the primary tumor. The vocal folds themselves have a sparse network of lymph vessels, which clinically translates to a lower tendency to metastasize to regional lymph nodes than in the other two levels of the larynx. In turn, the layout of the lymphatic network in the upper layer (epiglottis), with a tendency to bilateral tumor spreading through the lymphatic pathways, often necessitates bilateral nodal surgeries in upper laryngeal cancer [1, 2].

27.1.1 Lymphatic Network

27.1.1.1 Glottis

- The vocal folds have a sparse lymphatic system, only the upper surface of the vocal fold and the bottom of the laryngeal sack contain individual lymph vessels, otherwise the vocal fold is devoid of any absorbent vascularity. Infiltrates in the area of the anterior commissure may spread to prelaryngeal and visceral nodes of level VI, and then bilaterally to levels II and III. The overall incidence of node metastases is less than 10% and occurs in stages T3 and T4 [3].

27.1.1.2 Supraglottis

- It has a very rich, dense system of lymph vessels, most of which are located in the vestibular fold and laryngeal sack.
- Lymphatic drainage takes place on the frontal surface of the aryoepiglottic folds, leaving the larynx through vessels along the vascular-nerve bundles to the deep upper and lower neck lymph nodes. The lymph nodes exit from the larynx through the thyrohyoid membrane and drain to the upper and midjugular chain, mainly to the upper, middle, and lower lymph node groups II, III, and IV. Tumors located near the

midline may metastasize bilaterally. Supraglottic lesions frequently metastasize to the neck even in early stages. The frequency of metastasis ranges from 25% to over 40% [4, 5].

27.1.1.3 Subglottis

- The system of lymphatic vessels is not as abundant as in the supraglottic area.
- Lymphatic drainage takes place through the pre- and peritracheal nodes, it is also possible to provide additional lymphatic drainage to the peritracheal and mediastinal nodes, which is of great clinical importance. Penetration into the subglottic region causes the risk of metastasis to paratracheal lymph nodes to increase, from where lymphatic drainage drains to regions III and IV [6].

The numerous submucosal and preglottic junctions in the midline of the larynx play an important role in bilateral and contralateral cancer metastasis. The posterior commissure is an important point that connects the lymphatic vessels from different places in the larynx. The laryngeal lymph is eventually collected in the upper and lower deep neck lymph nodes.

It is important to note that external capsular infiltration worsens the prognosis by more than half [7].

27.1.2 Vessels Supply

Angiogenesis is one of the originally constituted hallmarks of cancer. It is an intricate multistep process of endothelial migration and proliferation, capillary maturation, anastomosis, and lumen development, along with extracellular matrix remodeling. It is well known that highly vascularized tumors show a greater likelihood to produce metastases compared to less angiogenic neoplasms. Angiogenesis requires the activation of many receptors, like vascular endothelial growth factors (VEGFs), fibroblast growth factors (FGF-1 and FGF-2), and epidermal growth factor/transforming growth factor-α (EGF/TGF-α) [8].

27.1.3 Nerves Supply

Perineural invasion (PNI), also known as neurotropic carcinomatous spread, is a process predominantly characterized by neoplastic invasion of the nerves. In PNI, the propagation of neoplastic cells to the primitive site of the tumor does not occur via lymphatic dissemination, but through molecular mediators that guide these cells during the invasion of the nerve sheath. The diffusion of laryngeal cancer cells in the perineural space is a parameter associated with a negative prognosis, high locoregional recurrence, and low disease-free survival rates. The spread of tumor cells on the perineural sheath highlights the histopathologically and clinically aggressive behavior of this type of tumor. Therefore, it is important to complement the surgical therapeutic treatment with adjuvant RT. [9]

27.1.4 Surrounding Structures Important for Surgical Anatomy

- Platysma
- Cervical fascia
- Sternocleidomastoid muscle
- Omohyoid muscle
- Carotid artery
- Jugular vein
- Vagus nerve
- Hyoid bone
- Thyroid gland with thyroid isthmus
- Suprahyoid muscles: mylohyoid, geniohyoid, digastric, hyoglossus
- Infrahyoid muscles: sternohyoid, thyrohyoid
- Hypoglossal nerve
- Inferior and superior thyroid artery (Fig. 27.1)

27.1.5 Directions of Extralaryngeal Spread

Patterns of regional spread from the primary:

27.1.5.1 Supraglottis

The tumor invades one or more of the structures that make up the upper level of the larynx, that is, the epiglottis, vestibular folds, aryo-epiglottic folds, arytenoids, laryngeal sack, and the epiglottic pedicle.

This region may be subdivided into

- The anterior marginal region, suprahyoid epiglottis—in this part of larynx, spread occurs outside the endolarynx along mucosal pathways into the piriform sinus or postcricoid area
- The midline infrahyoid epiglottis—the spread occurs in the pre-epiglottic space
- The lateral infrahyoid areas—the spread occurs across the anterior commissure tendon or through the paraglottic space inferiorly to the subglottic space [10]

27.1.5.2 Glottis

Tumors developing in the anterior commissure or reaching it more often penetrate the thyroid cartilage. When the infiltration reaches the anterior commissure, it spreads submucosally to the opposite side, penetrating the supraglottic, subglottic, or extralaryngeal regions. By infiltrating deeply, the neoplasm causes various degrees of immobilization of the vocal fold. When symptoms of deep infiltration appear, including immobilization of the intralaryngeal muscles and involvement of the arytenoid cartilage, the risk of infiltration of the thyroid cartilage and further spread beyond the anatomical limits of the larynx increases.

The infiltration of the discoid cartilage occurs in large tumors and is most common in the ossified areas of cartilage. Through the ossified parts of cartilage, and also through the cricothyroid membrane and laterally through the cricothyroid space, there is an extralaryngeal passage of cancer. Vocal cord immobilization may occur in relatively small tumors and is prognostically significant. In advanced cancers, invasion to the paraglottic and subglottic space with egress through the cricothyroid is common. The other route of spread is via the ventricle. Invasion of laryngeal cartilage (thyroid) is very common [11].

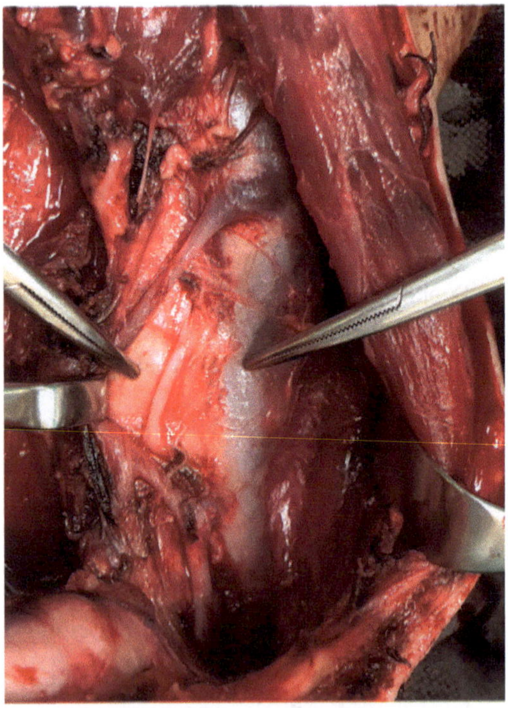

Fig. 27.1 Important anatomical structures of the neck: (1) Carotid artery, (2) Jugular vein, (3) Vagus nerve

27.1.5.3 Subglottis

The pathway of invasion of this area begins with the thyroarytenoid muscle. The tumor invades the cricothyroid membrane or inferiorly, the trachea. Invasion of the inferior margin of the thyroid cartilage, which is situated nearby the cricothyroid membrane or cricoid space, provides a direct passage for extralaryngeal spread. Subglottic cancer invades the laryngeal part of the pharynx, esophagus, and the thyroid gland more often, and metastasizes to the paratracheal lymph nodes.

27.1.6 Pattern of Metastasis

Regional metastasis to the cervical lymph nodes is the most important prognostic factor of laryngeal carcinoma, next to tumor localization and tumor size. The number and size of involved nodes, extracapsular spread, and nodal fixation are very important characteristics of the metastatic lymph nodes. Survival rate in patients with cervical metastases decreases with the increasing number of involved nodes, as well as with the presence of capsular rupture.

Nodal metastases are also associated with a high rate of regional recurrence. Distant metastases are rare but occur in a small percentage of cases (2–5%) and are most often located in the lungs, less often in the liver, bones, and brain [12].

27.2 General Principles of Surgical and Combined Treatment in the Advanced Stages of Disease

In the treatment of laryngeal cancer, surgery and radiotherapy are used as independent methods, as combined treatment methods, or as complementary methods in the treatment of failures. Radiotherapy can be performed with radical intention as an independent treatment or in combination with chemotherapy. It can be part of combined treatment after laryngectomy as an adjuvant therapy. In a number of clinical cases, the efficacy of radiotherapy and the efficacy of surgery as stand-alone options are similar, which makes the two methods competitive with each other. Chemotherapy is not used as a self-treatment method for laryngeal cancer. Induction or adjuvant chemotherapy, combined with radiotherapy, is the subject of clinical trials, mainly in "organ-sparing" programs. In patients who are not eligible for chemotherapy, the combination of RT with cetuximab remains an alternative to RT / CT. Cetuximab is a monoclonal antiepidermal growth factor antibody, a cell-surface Epidermal Growth Factor Receptor (EGFR).

Currently, in addition to the cure rates, more and more importance is attached to the quality of life (QL). Hence, when choosing equivalent therapies in terms of oncological outcomes, we are primarily guided by the possibility of maintaining laryngeal function. For 2 decades, "Organ preservation treatment" programs have been implemented, extending the indications for radiotherapy and radio-chemotherapy. At the same time, the methods of partial resections with preservation or reconstruction of the respiratory, phonative, and defensive functions of the larynx are constantly being improved. The multitude of methods of partial laryngeal resection allows the individualization of the techniques used, depending on the specific location, tumor characteristics, experience, and preferences of the surgeon. The range of methods of laryngeal surgery includes procedures of an extremely diverse scope: microinvasive phonosurgical procedures with endoscopic CO2 laser access, endoscopic partial laryngectomy, external partial and reconstructive surgeries, and amputation operations: total laryngectomy, total laryngectomy extended with tissues (thyroid, soft tissues of the neck, esophagus). At the same time, reconstruction is performed with the restoration of the continuity of the alimentary tract (free intestinal transplant with a microanastomosis, free skin transplant with a microanastomosis, pedicle skin flaps) and replacement of skin and neck tissue defects. An integral part of the surgical treatment is surgical speech rehabilitation in patients deprived of the larynx, currently almost exclusively carried out by implanting a unilateral tracheoesophageal valve fistula [13].

27.3 Total Laryngectomy

Despite the constant improvement of the methods of partial resections, classic total laryngectomy still remains the basic therapeutic standard in surgery for advanced stages of laryngeal cancer.

Total laryngectomy is the surgical procedure in which the larynx is totally removed, the airway and upper part of alimentary tract is interrupted, with respiration being performed through a tracheal stoma resulting from bringing the trachea to the skin in the lower cervical area. This provides a complete and permanent separation of the superior part of the airway from the inferior one, and also permanent separation of respiratory and digestive tracts. After total laryngectomy, the patient experiences a loss of smell and taste due to anatomical changes [1, 2].

27.3.1 History

The first total laryngectomy for a malignant tumor was performed by Billroth in Vienna on the December 31, 1873. The postoperative course was complicated by a significant fistula between the pharynx and skin, but in the end, the patient resumed oral nutrition. The patient survived for 7 months.

In 1875, Bottini from Turin conducted a total laryngectomy in a patient who survived for 10 years after surgery.

In 1880, Gluck, according to a retrospective study, reported that the best results were achieved, when the surgery was divided into two stages: initially, a separation of the trachea from the larynx, followed by, in the second stage 2 weeks later, a total laryngectomy.

In 1890, Sorenson presented a new total laryngectomy technique in one step: the retrograde laryngectomy.

Crile and Jawdynski from Poland, independently, were the first who recognized the important role of the radical neck dissection routine in the same intervention with the total laryngectomy.

In 1950, Martin and Ogura standardized total laryngectomy with neck dissection [14].

27.3.2 Indications and Contraindications

27.3.2.1 Common Indications

- Advanced laryngeal cancer or hypopharynx with the invasion of
  - Thyroid or cricoid cartilage (perichondium, focal cortical layer, high volume)
  - Extra laryngeal soft tissue
  - With massive subglottic extension
- After failed response to RT, RT/CT, induction CT, or in the case of relapse after oncological treatment
- Tumor recurrence after conservative treatment with TOLM or OPL, when recurrence occurs with cartilage infiltration or tumors invading adjacent organs: pharynx, esophagus, thyroid gland
- Histopathological subtypes of extensive tumors that have proven resistant to RT or RT/CT: soft tissue sarcomas, chondrosarcomas, melanomas, adenocarcinomas, large cell neuroendocrine tumors, tumors of the minor salivary glands [14]

27.3.2.2 Rare Indications

- After laryngeal trauma, where the organ cannot be reconstructed to restore function, followed by necrosis and aspiration
- No voice and chronic aspiration due to palsy of the ninth, tenth, and eleventh cranial nerves
- After extensive OPL, when the patient cannot achieve a sufficient recovery to normal swallowing and develops aspiration pneumonia [15]
- Severe recurrent laryngeal papillomatosis with an increased risk of tracheal and pulmonary invasion [14]

27.3.2.3 Contraindications

General

- The presence of incurable synchronous tumors
- The presence of incurable distant metastases
- Severe systemic general disease or poor general condition resulting in high anesthetic risk

27.3.2.4 Nonresectable Disease

- Tumor invading the deep parts of the tongue
- Tumor that exceeds the prevertebral fascia
- Tumor or metastasis that encases the common or internal carotid artery [16, 14].

27.3.3 Technique

The division of operations into individual stages not only explains the technical details, but also allows for a more efficient procedure, including modifications and deviations from the basic standard in the operating protocol, and constant improvement of own solutions at individual stages of the operation.

Stage I—The prepared operating field should extend from the top to the edge of the mandible, laterally from the tops of the mastoid processes, along the posterior edges of the sternocleidomastoid muscle (SCM), from the bottom along the edges of the clavicles, revealing the entire central skin above the suprasternal notch.

A U-shaped skin incision (called the Gluck–Sorenson U-shaped incision) extending bilaterally to the palpable horns of the hyoid bone is one of the most often used. The inferior edge of the incision should be led approximately 1–2 cm above the suprasternal notch or, if a tracheotomy had been performed previously, the skin around the tracheostomy should be cut in the form of a wide horizontal lens. Such an incision can be extended, if necessary, if a decision is made intraoperatively to extend the resection of regional lymph nodes to include selective or radical nodal surgery. Skin incisions are subject to various modifications depending on the extent of the tumor and the direction of infiltration of external tissues as well as the operator's experience. Besides the U-shaped skin incision, the most commonly used incisions are

- The vertical midline incision: from the body of the hyoid bone to the tracheal stoma
- Transverse in the skin fold: from the posterior border of the SCM on one side to the one on the other side, at the level of the thyroid cartilage, completed with a circular incision to account for the tracheotomy
- Y incisions: described by Crile
- rarely J, H V, T shaped, and horizontal.

The dermal and tissue flap, which contains, apart from the skin and subcutaneous tissues, the broad neck muscle, is raised along with the superficial lamina of the neck fascia (almost bloodless) up to the level of the hyoid bone, exposing the lateral corners of the bones. After cutting the thyroid node and exposing the anterior wall of the trachea to a large extent, an incision is made transversely (minimum ½ of the circumference), and below the 1st–third ring (depending on the location of the tumor in the larynx), the anterior wall is sutured with three definitive skin sutures. The sterile intubation tubes are changed. If an initial tracheotomy has been performed previously, the tracheostomy canal with the tracheal ring underneath the surgical specimen is excised and the trachea sewn into the skin *(as above)* (Fig. 27.2).

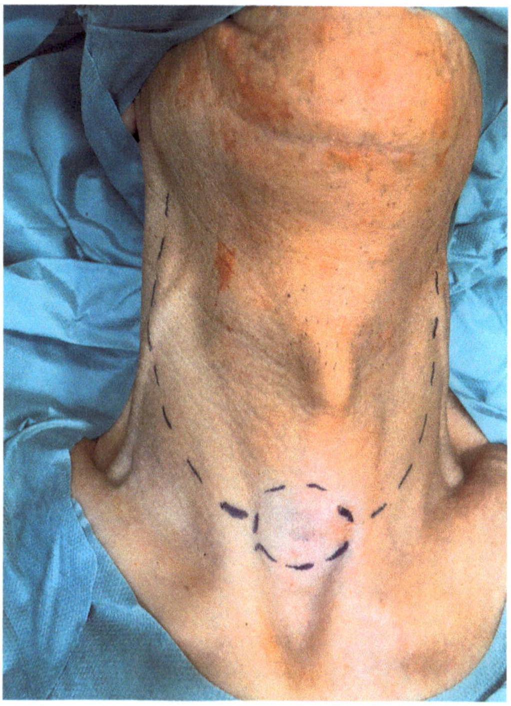

Fig. 27.2 U-shaped skin incision, called the Gluck - Sorenson U-shaped incision

Stage II—The front edge of the SCM muscle along its entire length is exposed, moved slightly to the side in the lower part and a blunt dissection below the prelaryngeal muscles covered by the fascia plate (the pretracheal plate of the neck fascia) is done. Parallel to the edge of the SCM, the prelaryngeal muscles are cut, thus revealing the thyroid gland and upper disc vessels. If indicated, at this stage, subtotal removal of the thyroid lobe or the medial parts (1/3–1/2) of both lobes is done. The thyroid is dissected to the sides so that it does not cover the lower pharynx and the cervical part of the esophagus in this part. At this stage, as a rule, coagulation or lancing and ligation of cricothyroid vascular branches branching from the thyroid vessels is necessary (Fig. 27.3).

Stage III—With a sharp hook, the laryngeal box is rotated to the side opposite to the operated side and the lower pharyngeal sphincter muscle is cut from the edge of the thyroid cartilage, revealing upward the entire upper corner of the cartilage. At this stage, care should be taken not to damage the superior thyroid artery. After

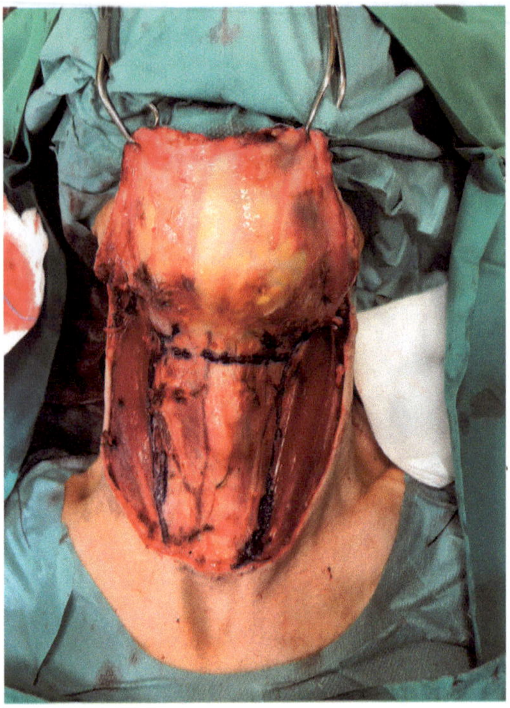

Fig. 27.3 Exposure of the front edge of the SCM and the pre-laryngeal muscles after the lifting of the skin flap

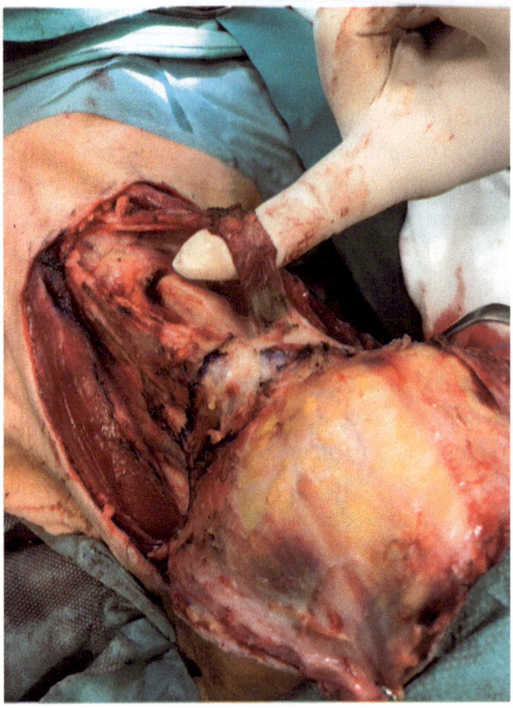

Fig. 27.4 Exposure of the laryngeal cartilages and infrahyoid muscles

bilateral "skeletonization" of the larynx from the sides, the mucosa of the piriform recesses is bluntly separated (if not infiltrated by the tumor) from the inner surface of the thyroid cartilage plates, using an electric knife to cut the suprahyoid muscle attachments; first from the hyoid bone shaft, and then along the greater horns. Using a partly blunt, partly sharp dissection, the corner of the hyoid bone is exposed, cutting off its upper ligamentous attachments. At this stage, care must be taken not to damage the lingual artery (Fig. 27.4).

Stage IV—After the maximum rotation of the larynx to the opposite side, pulling the corner of the hyoid bone upward, and the corner of the upper thyroid cartilage downward, it is relatively easy to identify the vascular-nerve bundle of the larynx (nerve, vein, and superior laryngeal artery) and ligate it in the peripheral part (Fig. 27.5).

Stage V—The first step in removing the larynx begins with cutting it from the bottom by cutting the trachea around its entire circumference, leaving a larger part of the posterior wall, in relation to the remaining tracheal ring, which will ensure better functional sewing of the tracheal stump to the skin. By pulling the larynx up with a hook, the trachea and the cricoid cartilage are separated partly bluntly, partly sharply, along with the posterior cricothyroid muscle, which is visible on its posterior surface from the mucosa of the postcricoid area, and the lower pharynx is opened in the midline. Under the control of a finger inserted through the created opening, the mucosa of the laryngeal part of the pharynx is cut, along the arytenoid cartilage and further upward, circumscribing, through the lingual pits to the opposite side. At this stage, if the tumor has infiltrated toward the pyriform recess, the larynx is cut, first on the opposite side, and in the last stage, fully under visual control, from the side of the tumor. It is now that the places of the smallest margin are marked and additionally the marginal fragment of the leftover mucosa are collected for a separate examination. The same process is repeated in cases where the tumor infiltrates the base of the tongue (Figs. 27.6 and 27.7).

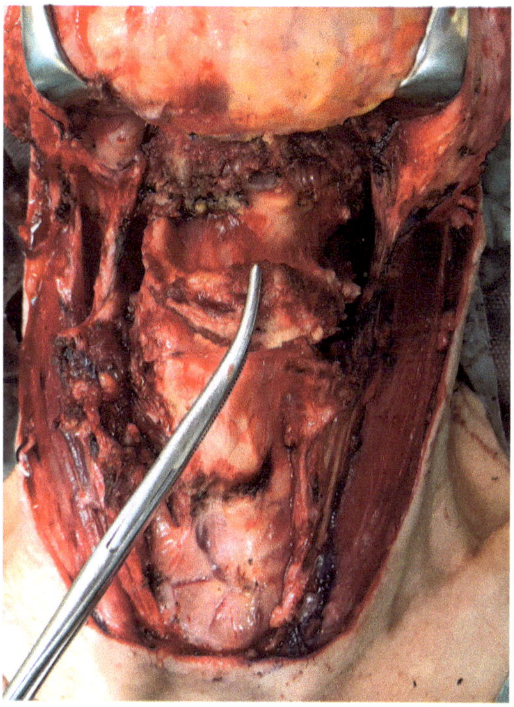

Fig. 27.5 Exposure of the hyoid bone and suprahyoid muscles

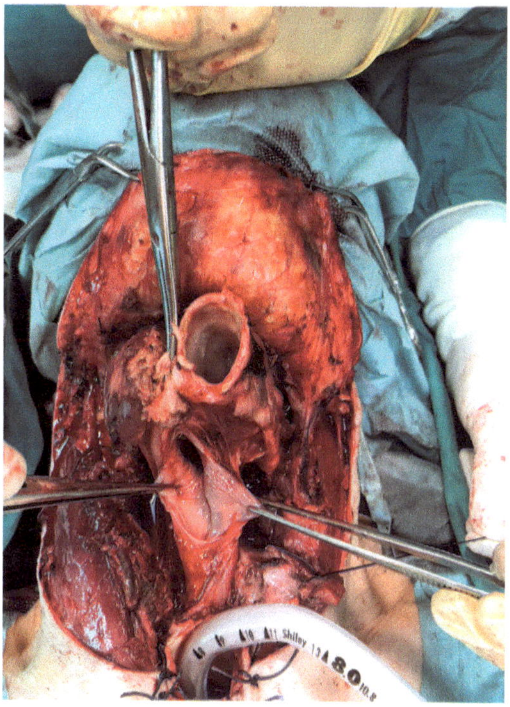

Fig. 27.6 Visualization of the esophagus after dissection of the larynx from the trachea

Stage VI—After the larynx has been removed, the voice prosthesis is placed, and then the nasogastric feeding tube is inserted through the nose, placing it with its end in the lower esophagus. At this stage, some operators perform a lateral myotomy in the lower section of the lower pharyngeal sphincter muscle and the cervical muscle of the esophagus. Cutting the inferior SCM muscle in the medial quarter results in flattening of the skin around the tracheostomy after the final healing. This facilitates closing the tracheostomy opening with a finger for the patient. This should be taken under consideration when referring to using sticky overlays on the tracheostomy area (breathing air heat and moisture exchange system (HME system). The throat is sutured in two layers, vertically, from the top. The first layer is a single absorbable 3–0 suture, or 4–0, covered. Suturing this layer is completed with a pouch suture. The second layer, sewn with a similar material, connects the suprahyoid muscles from above to the lower pharyngeal sphincter muscle further downward. (Povidone-Iodine).

Stage VII—Depending on the location of the primary tumor and the degree of local advancement, unilateral or bilateral lymph node removal surgery is performed along the vascular bundle of the cervical vessels. Therefore, it is an incomplete elective operation of the II, III, and IV nodal region. If, at the very beginning of the operation, an enlarged lymph node along the vascular bundle under the SCM muscle is palpated, intraoperative histological examination must be taken and then, a continuation of the laryngeal resection can continue. If the result of the examined nodes is positive, the scope of nodal resection is to be extended to radical surgery according to Crile -Jawdyński, or to a radical modified resection.

Stage VIII—An active suction drain is inserted from a separate incision on one or both sides and the skin is sutured in two layers, with the first layer joining the edges of the broad neck muscles. Using a circular suturing technique for attaching the trachea to the skin, it is attached subcutaneously and superficially to the skin flap.

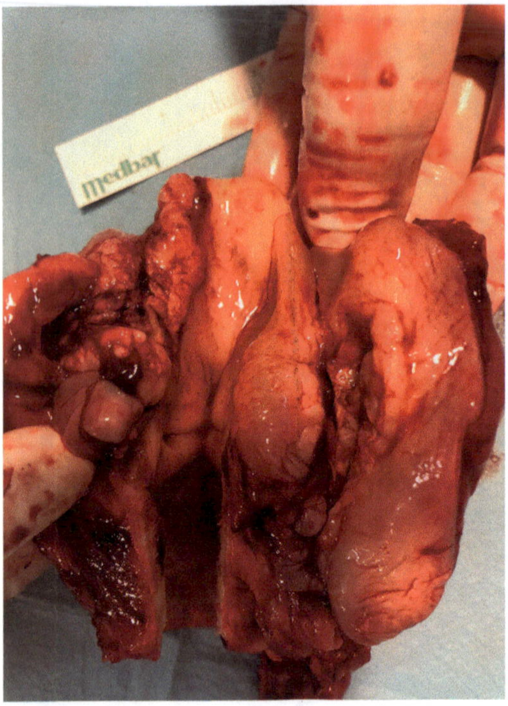

Fig. 27.7 Larynx after removal, visualization of the tumor

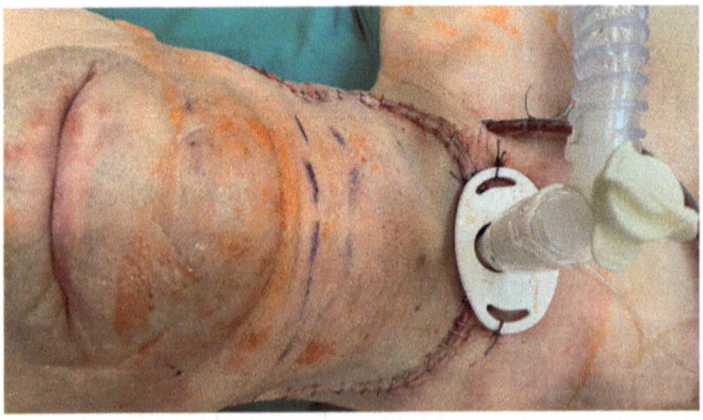

Fig. 27.8 Skin sutures and the tracheotomy tube

Replacing the endotracheal tube with a tracheotomy tube and a light pressure bandage completes the operation (Fig. 27.8).

27.3.4 Salvage Total Laryngectomy after Conservation Laryngeal Surgery (TOLM, Open Partial Laryngectomy OPL)

Recurrence rates for laryngeal cancer range from 16% to 40%. The most common salvage surgery is a total laryngectomy. Salvage surgery results in acceptable oncologic outcomes. Stage, disease site, perineural invasion, and margins are associated with inferior DSS [17]. One the other hand, oncological and functional outcomes of TL performed as first-line treatment are significantly better than after salvage TL [18].

STL is very often an aggressive surgical technique characterized by removing the whole larynx or neolarynx in addition to prelaryngeal soft tissue, strap muscles, and the skin area overlying the larynx. It is used in cases of recurrence after conservative surgical techniques performed for treatment of laryngeal cancer to preserve the organ like TOLM, and reconstructive laryngectomies. After conservative treatment failure in many cases, it was observed that the neoplastic infiltration spread to the preglottal area as

- a local recurrent tumor inside the neolarynx (visible as submucosal recurrence) in continuity with extralaryngeal spread;
- an extralaryngeal recurrence, due to extracapsular spread (ECS) from Delphian lymph node or level VI nodes;
- a tumor involving and destroying the remnant laryngeal framework with extralaryngeal extension.

27.3.5 Salvage Total Laryngectomy after RT or RT/CT Failure

Oncological and functional outcomes of TL performed as first-line treatment are significantly better than after salvage TL. If salvage TL is performed after conservative surgery has failed, the oncological and functional results are better than after the failure of organ-preserving protocols [18]. The stage of recurrence of the primary (rT) and details of cancer spread determine the extent of resection. The time from treatment, the dose that the patient received, and the severity of the tissue radioreaction determine the technical difficulties of the procedure [cytowanie]. There are pronounced differences between STL after surgical and radiotherapy, and chemoradiotherapy failures [19, 20].

Radiotherapy and CRT not only kill tumor cells but also cause damage to other tissues, including blood vessels. Postirradiation increases intima thickness, proteoglycan deposition, and inflammatory cell infiltration into medium-sized arteries and arteries, which are normally resistant to the natural atherosclerosis process.

Factors that can affect success of STL after RT or RT/ CT:

- Patients' general status
- Vascularization of irradiated tissues [19]
- Healing properties of mucosa
- Skin quality

Weak points: skin defects and pharyngo-esophageal fistulas.

27.3.6 The Indications to Plan a Reconstruction After TL Can Be Divided into

1. The need of supporting irradiated tissues.
2. The necessity to cover the defect not eligible for primary sutures [21]. The reconstruction method/flaps can be divided into local, transpositional, and microvascular, all harvested from distant regions of the body.
3. Protection of the suture line of the neopharynx after a laryngectomy with vascularized tissues is of utmost importance in preventing a wound-related complication. Pedicled infrahyoid muscle, myofascial or myoperichondrial flap is a simple quick and reliable option to protect the fashioned neopharynx [22].

27.3.6.1 The Flap Techniques Used in Closure of the Defect

In the case when the resection is very extensive and requires removal of the skin, subcutaneous, fascial, and muscular planes overlying the laryngeal lodge, the surgical defect has to be reconstructed. Extended total laryngectomy with en bloc resection of overlying cervical skin is indicated in cases with infiltration of the prelaryngeal soft tissues [23–25].

(a) **Temporoparietal fascia flap (TPFF)**—it represents a reliable alternative to other flaps, with minor donor-site morbidity and good functional outcomes comparing rates of postoperative pharyngocutaneous fistula (PCF) and functional outcomes with those of pectoralis major myocutaneous flap (PMMF) use and primary closure of the pharynx, in STL [26].
(b) **Pectoralis major myocutaneous flap (PMMF)**—a pectoral flap may be considered in the absence of good vessel perfusion.
(c) **Radial forearm free flap (RFFF)**—it is an excellent option demonstrating the lowest rates of postoperative fistula and enteral feeding tube dependence; majority of patients will not require long-term enteral support. But, in other experiences, vascularized tissue augmentation did not significantly prevent clinical PCF [27].
(d) **Free thigh flap**—it is a good option for extensive resections, especially those involving the base of the tongue.

27.3.6.2 Other Surgical Tips

Stapler use benefits salvage total laryngectomy in terms of surgical time, hospitalization length, oral feeding time, and occurrence of pharyngocutaneous fistula, as well as aids in the risk factor evaluation for fistula onset. Using a stapler shortened operative time and hospitalization, while also providing a faster return to oral feeding. Moreover, mechanical pharyngeal suturing seems to decrease fistula formation rate even though its preventative role in salvage laryngectomy should be taken into consideration.

The surgical outcomes in terms of postoperative wound complications in patients treated with the lateral cervical approach (LCA) for STL without prophylactic use of the pectoralis major myocutaneous flap (PMMF) or free flaps are good. The technique is feasible and seems to be effective in terms of prevention of local complications [28].

27.3.7 Cost-Effectiveness

Between flaps, a free flap is cost-effective over a pectoralis flap [29]. Despite significant costs and longer hospitalization, the use of flap techniques seems to be effective in terms of prevention of local complications [28]. Primary closure is less expensive than both pectoralis or free flaps [29].

Key Points

- Before starting the operation, the patient should be properly positioned.
- U-shaped skin incision and preparation of subcutaneous flap.
- Bilateral "skeletonization" of the larynx from the sides.
- Dissection of the muscles inserted into the hyoid bone.
- Identification and ligation of the vascular-nerve bundle of the larynx (nerve, vein, and superior laryngeal artery).
- Removal of the larynx and entry into the pharynx, with pharyngeal mucosa preservation as much as possible, in order to achieve a tension-free suture, which will prevent fistulas and will allow a rapid healing.
- The tension in the pharyngeal sutures should be moderate as sutures, which are too tight, may tear the mucosa or produce its necrosis, and those that are too loose may cause the formation of a fistula or dehiscence.
- The trachea should be anchored to the skin with thick threads sutured in a radial pattern.
- Depending on the location of the primary tumor and the degree of local advancement, unilateral or bilateral lymph node removal surgery along the vascular bundle of the cervical vessels may be required.
- Insertion of tracheotomy tube and a light pressure bandage end the operation.

27.3.8 The Transoral Endoscopic Ultrasonic Total Laryngectomy (TOUSS-TL)

Transoral ultrasonic surgery (TOUSS) has been used as a transoral endoscopic approach initially for oropharyngeal, hypopharyngeal, and supraglottic tumors. The main advantage of TOUSS is the achievement of the same output as TORS without the costs of a robotic platform [30].

Indications for TOUSS-TL:

- Laryngeal cancer with indication for total laryngectomy
- Laryngeal cancer without indication for neck dissection
- Salvage TL after radiotherapy

Contraindications:

- Invasion through the thyroid cartilage or soft tissues of the neck (T4a)
- Major extralaryngeal invasion (T4b)

The Tools Required for TOUSS:

- The Feyh-Kastembauer retractor—it is used for the transoral exposition of the larynx.
- Videoendoscopes used in combination with the Martin's arm scope holder.
- The 35 cm ThunderbeatTM, an integrated ultrasonic and bipolar cutting-coagulating device, used as a resection tool. This is an ultrasonic scissor, integrated with a bipolar vascular sealing system approved for safely sealing vessels up to 7 mm.

27.3.9 Transoral Robotic Total Laryngectomy (TORS)

The treatment of larynx cancer has changed greatly in the last years and continues to evolve. The goal of many of the changes has been to decrease morbidity and increase function without decreasing survival. For years, minimally invasive treatment methods have been sought, especially in advanced forms of pharynx, oral cavity, and laryngeal cancers. Transoral robotic surgery (TORS), utilizing the DaVinci robotic surgery system, has begun to play a larger role in the surgery of the pharynx and larynx. TORS has proven to be safe, feasible, and a minimally invasive method of treatment [20, 31].

Indications for TORS-TL:

- Laryngeal cancer with indication for total laryngectomy
- Salvage TL after radiotherapy or radio and chemotherapy
- Larynx dysfunction and chronic aspiration

Contraindications

- Invasion through the thyroid cartilage or soft tissues of the neck (T4a)
- Major extralaryngeal invasion (T4b)

The Tools Required for TORS:

- The Feyh-Kastembauer retractor—used for the transoral exposition of the larynx
- Crowe-Davis mouth gag—used to expose the pharyngolaryngeal structures
- Martin's arm retractor
- The DaVinci Surgical Robot
- The 30-degree telescope—placed into the central arm
- 5-mm Schertel or Maryland forceps—placed through the left robotic arm
- The spatula monopolar cautery—placed through the right robotic arm

TOUSS and TORS-TL are new endoscopic surgery techniques using a transoral approach. These seem to be the direction of the development of new techniques in the treatment of head and neck cancers.

27.3.10 Postoperative Complications

1. Bleeding (hematoma in the wound or bleeding into the lumen of the throat) may be a significant complication after total laryngectomy, requiring reoperation.
2. Neck abscess, wound breakdown—when bacterial inflammation of the wound occurs, targeted antibiotic therapy is required.
3. Postoperative delirium (POD) in patients undergoing laryngectomy for laryngeal cancer accounted for nearly 10% of POD, with most episodes occurring during the first 3 postoperative days; intraoperative dexmedetomidine use can reduce POD occurrences [32].
4. Dysphagia—it is a problem that is observed in up to 30% of patients after total laryngectomy during follow-up [27, 33]. Factors predisposing to the occurrence of dysphagia are
   (a) combined treatments, surgery and adjuvant radiotherapy (vs. radiotherapy alone);
   (b) TL after chemoradiotherapy treatment failure [34];
   (c) advanced stage of the disease [34];
   (d) PCF;
   (e) STL;
   (f) flap reconstruction (PMC or free flap) [35]; and,
   (g) a free jejunum flap [36].

5. Fistula development—A complication, especially in patients who had previously undergone chemoradiotherapy or radiotherapy. Age, smoking, COPD, CAD, T-stage, previous radiotherapy, preoperative albumin level, preoperative hemoglobin level, tumor size, and treatment method are considered as the main risk factors of PCF [37, 38]. The prevalence of PCF varies between 23% and 34% [27, 39], and is highest in patients after major surgery, for example, extended total laryngectomy with en bloc resection of overlying cervical skin [23]. A fistula is the connection between the pharynx and the skin or between the esophagus and trachea. This results in the leakage of saliva and pharyngeal contents into the neck. If the infection in the fistula is resolved, it can be closed in most cases. If the fistula persists for more than 2–3 weeks, a temporary gastrostomy or PEG should be considered, which greatly facilitates conservative management and is also a significant facilitation where it is decided to surgically close the fistula. Most infections in the postoperative laryngectomy wound are caused by pathogens of the patient's own bacterial flora from the patient's mouth and throat. In the preopera-

tive period, treatment of sick teeth should be performed, and the oral cavity should be rinsed with hibitane solution, which should be continued until the nasogastric tube is removed postoperatively and the inflammation of the paranasal sinuses is treated. 5–6 days of postoperative use of antibiotics: cefuroxime or amoxicillin with clavulanic acid + metronidazole is the standard procedure. It should be remembered that the main factor contributing to infection in the postoperative wound is the residual discharge in the wound. Properly inserted active drainage, maintained for 2–3 days, is of key importance here. An important element, during the operation, after suturing the throat, is rinsing the wound several times with saline containing Povidone Iodine. The use of platelet-rich fibrin (PRF) in the repair of the pharynx during TL enhances the healing process and thus reduces the incidence of PCF [40]. Fibrin tissue glue is an easily applied, and cost-effective, adjunct that may reduce pharyngocutaneous fistula risk [41]. Also the low-pressure vacuum drain method is effective in reducing the incidence of PCF after total laryngectomy [42]. In some patients, a Montgomery tube is used to prevent pharyngocutaneous fistula formations after total laryngectomy [43]. Finally, early oral hydration seems to be significantly associated with a decreased risk of PCF after total laryngectomy (TL) or total pharyngolaryngectomy (TPL) [44].

6. Airway problems—in patients who undergo total laryngectomy, excessive secretions and crusting mucus can occlude the trachea and cause problems with breathing. Inflammation of the trachea and lower airways is especially often seen a few months after surgery. The lack of airway protection may result in increased risk of aspiration.
7. Cranial nerve injury—during neck dissection, some cranial nerves are at a potential risk of injury: the marginal mandibular branch of VII nerve, IX, X, XI, and XII nerves. Injury of these nerves causes the following complications: asymmetric smile, impairment of tongue mobility, swallowing difficulties, shoulder drop, and range of motion limitation.
8. Loss of taste and smell—anatomical changes after larynx removal result in a lack of airflow through the nose and mouth, which causes loss of smell.
9. Hypothyroidism—a loss of thyroid function can occur as a result of partial thyroid removal during laryngectomy or after radiation. That is why thyroid hormone monitoring is required periodically for adequate supplementation. Severe hypothyroidism may be responsible for poor healing of flaps and fistula formation [45].
10. Hypoparathyroidism occurs in a significant number of patients who underwent laryngectomy with concomitant hemithyroidectomy and is associated with significant short- and long-term morbidities [46].

Key Points

1. Complications after total laryngectomy can be divided into early (e.g., bleeding or hematoma in the wound) and late (e.g., loss of taste and smell).
2. In the postoperative period, the status of thyroid hormones and calcium levels should be monitored, especially in patients after partial or complete thyroid resection.
3. It should be noted that the occurrence of postoperative complications as well as positive lymph node status, preoperative chemotherapy, comorbidity grade, and delayed adjuvant therapy independently predicted shorter OS and DFS [47].
4. Patient optimization and timely management of postoperative complications may play a critical role in long-term survival. Although adjuvant therapy is significant, the occurrence of pharyngocutaneous fistula (PCF), neck abscess, wound breakdown, and postoperative pneumonia is associated

with a delay in initiation of adjuvant radiation [48, 49].

5. Interestingly, in an multivariable model, lower preoperative hemoglobin (<12.5 g/dL) was identified as an independent prognostic factor for a higher overall complication rate [33].

27.4 Swallowing Rehabilitation After Total Laryngectomy

Total laryngectomy (TL) is a surgical procedure involving the resection of the entire larynx and separation of the respiratory and digestive tracts. A neopharynx is created by closing the surgical defect of the pharynx, either directly, or if necessary with different types of pedicled or free flaps. Preservation of the swallowing function is a very important goal. Subjective dysphagia was reported by 31.3% of patients during follow-up [27].

Factors that Increase the Risk of Dysphagia Include

- salvage TL after RT;
- salvage TL with flap reconstruction;
- primary TL with flap reconstruction;
- fistula occurrence; and,
- voice prosthesis leakage.

When primary closure is achievable, there are improved swallowing outcomes with better tolerance of oral diet and shorter pharyngeal transit times compared to PMC or free flap treatments [35]. The moment in which a PCF forms greatly impacts oral functionality, such that, patients with positive section margins, patients initially treated with surgery combined with adjuvant RT (vs. radiotherapy alone), and those developing PCF after STL are less likely to achieve total peroral intake. Postoperative dysphagia proved more likely in patients who developed a PCF postoperatively, and less likely in patients who underwent STL without partial pharyngectomy and in patients with pectoralis major myocutaneous (PMMF) flap reconstruction, compared to muscle only PM flap.

The Main Symptoms of Oropharyngeal Dysphagia Are

- impaired bolus transport;
- food "sticking" in the throat;
- regurgitation;
- globus sensation;
- prolonged mealtime.

Tools Used to Evaluate Swallowing Function Are

- videofluoroscopic swallowing study (VFSS);
- videomanometry;
- Swallowing Quality-of-Life questionnaire (SWAL-QoL) – to evaluate this problem from the patients' perspective.

Treatment

- Endoscopic dilatation of neopharynx.
- Radiological guided balloon dilatation.
- CO_2 laser therapy;
- Botulinum toxin A injections.

If rehabilitation does not bring satisfactory results, for a long time, a feeding tube or PEG is required.

Patients undergoing TL after treatment failure with chemoradiotherapy, with advanced stage disease, were the most often dependent on a feeding tube [34]. A free jejunum flap repair and requiring chemoradiation are the only two variables that added significantly to the model of worse self-reported swallowing outcomes in patients who reported swallowing difficulties after total laryngectomies [36]. It is important to note that swallowing gradually improves in the first 18 months after surgery.

27.5 Speech Rehabilitation After Total Laryngectomy

The loss of speech is a profound disability that should be rehabilitated either by teaching the patient to replace esophageal speech or, which is currently becoming a standard, by implanting the so-called vocal prosthesis:

1. **Esophageal speech**—the esophagus is used as the air source and the mouth of the esophagus

as the pseudoglottis, 65–80% of patients are able to produce esophageal voice. It is natural speech with some form of control over pitch/loudness and hands are free for greater independence for a more active lifestyle. Learning esophageal speech is difficult and that is why high motivation and hard work are required in achieving functional speech. Postradiation fibrosis, pharyngeal scarring, esophageal stenosis, and defects in neural innervation preclude the use of esophageal speech. Some studies show that development of a functional voice is not significantly different between salvage and primary TL patients, with a majority achieving laryngeal speech [50, 51]. Patients after total laryngectomy may develop poor speech because of hypertonicity or spasm of the pharyngoesophageal segment (PES). Conventional PES dilation, pharyngeal neurectomy, and myotomy [52] are used as a treatment for hypertonicity PES spasm, but endoscopic dilatation increasing UOS diameter may provide a new approach to treat unsuccessful TE phonation [53]. An alternative to such invasive treatment is the use of botox as an effective treatment for pharyngoesophageal segment (PES) hypertonicity or spasm in laryngectomies with poor tracheoesphageal puncture (TEP) speech [54, 55].
2. **Surgical speech restoration**—it is a unidirectional valve placed in the created tracheoesophageal fistula. Formation of a fistula and implantation of a voice prosthesis may be performed primarily during laryngectomy, as a stage preceding pharyngeal closure after dissection of the larynx, or secondarily, for example, in patients in whom rehabilitation by developing esophageal speech skills has not been successful. Secondary implantation consists in creating a fistula between the posterior wall of the tracheal stump (approx. 1 cm) below the tracheostomy and the cervical esophagus, with the help of a special bent trocar, inserted from the side of the trachea, under the control of a rigid esophagoscope, inserted with the tip into the puncture site and turned by 180 ° so that the oblique cut of the tube protects against accidental injury to the posterior esophageal wall with the trocar. The disadvantages of the voice prosthesis are the necessity of its periodic replacement (on an outpatient basis or in a one day surgery), the cost of the voice prosthesis, and a few complications (granulation tissue around the prosthesis, or leakage of saliva and fluids around the prosthesis). Management of late complications represents the main reason for the reluctance in using voice prosthesis rehabilitation. Leakage through the prosthesis is the most common cause for requiring access to a doctor in an emergency setting, but, on the other side, radiotherapy or modality (primary or secondary) of the puncture does not influence the number of medical visits per year in long-term outpatient management or the prosthesis lifetime [56]. Another problem connected with VP is biofilm colonization. It is one of the main reasons for VP degradation that can lead to VP dysfunction. The development of methods to prevent or inhibit biofilm formation on the VP surface would translate into an increase in their durability and safety [57]. Nevertheless, patients with tracheoesophageal prosthesis reported a better quality of life, compared to patients using an electrolarynx or esophageal voice [58, 59].
3. **Electronic larynx**—this generates sound vibrations outside the body, which are then transmitted through the tissues of the neck, cheek, or intraorally through a tube, so that

Key Points

1. Speech rehabilitation following laryngectomy is a key part of improving the quality of life in laryngectomy patients.
2. A speech therapist familiar with postlaryngectomy voice rehabilitation is an essential member of the care team for patients undergoing total laryngectomy.
3. Esophageal speech is a recognized and well-tolerated method of rehabilitation of the voice after laryngeal removal.
4. The undeniable advantage of surgical rehabilitation of speech is easier and faster rehabilitation and incomparably better effectiveness of the "prosthetic"

speech. This results from much more readily available air, necessary for pseudophonation, which is directed from the lungs to the throat by the patient with the prosthesis, compared to the air previously aspirated into the esophagus available to the patient learning esophageal speech for pseudophonation [60].

they can be shaped into speech with the use of the resonating cavities and articulators.

27.6 General Care After Total Laryngectomy

Patients after removal of the larynx, often combined with lymphadenectomy, require long-term postoperative care. This care includes not only postoperative wound management but also internist care. Most of the patients require intensive care in the postoperative ward with monitoring of vital functions.

1. In the first days after the surgery, it is crucial to check the levels of: morphology, electrolytes, thyroid hormone levels, calcium and parathyroid hormone level, albumin, total protein, and inflammatory markers. The level of these parameters is significantly associated with postoperative hospital stay [61].
2. Empirical antibiotic therapy, according to the established protocol, is required in the perioperative period. In patients with previous tracheotomy and evidence of local infection, targeted treatment should be initiated with antibiotics not included within prophylaxis protocols.
3. Daily change of the pressure dressing of the neck and keeping the area around the tracheostomy in good hygiene is necessary to avoid wound infection.
4. During the first 2 weeks after surgery, patients receive nutrition through a nasogastric tube [44].
5. Use of heat and moisture exchangers (HMEs) is crucial to help reduce the production of secretions from the tracheobronchial tree [62].
6. High-volume hospital care for laryngectomy has been shown to be associated with reduced morbidity, mortality, and costs [63].

27.7 Prognosis

The treatment outcomes for laryngeal cancer depend primarily on the stage of clinical advancement, with treatment failures being associated more with the occurrence of regional lymph node metastases than with local recurrence. Favorable oncologic outcomes are reported after STL. Increasing clinical tumor stage, increasing number of metastatic cervical lymph nodes, hypopharyngeal and supraglottic tumor location, positive section margins, and perineural invasion are identified as independent negative prognosticators for all oncologic outcome measures [33, 64].

Distant metastases without the presence of nodal metastases are rare. While in T1–T2, N0 tumors, both glottal and supraglottic 5-year survival rates reach 80–90%, both with radical radiotherapy and surgical treatment, in advanced cases T3–T4/N0–N + oscillates within 40–70% and they depend, to a greater extent, on the N feature more than on the T feature.

27.8 Neck Dissection

The metastatic capacity of laryngeal cancer depends on the degree of T classification and the location of the primary tumor. The network of lymphatic vessels varies greatly depending on their level:

- Supraglottic—rich in lymph vessels draining the lymph mainly to the upper, middle, and lower lymph nodes of groups II, III, and IV.
- Glottis—poor in lymphatic vessels; metastasizes less frequently, with the exception of infiltrates in the area of the anterior commissure, which spread to prelaryngeal and visceral nodes of level VI, and then bilaterally to level II and III.
- With penetration into the subglottic region below 10 mm, the risk of metastasis to

paratracheal lymph nodes increases, from where lymphatic drainage leads to regions III and IV.
- External capsular infiltration worsens the prognosis by more than a half.
- Micrometastases occur on average in about 30% of laryngeal cancer cases.
- Supraglottic carcinomas give hidden metastases in 20–25% of cases.
- Glottic carcinomas—in about 10% of cases, more clinically advanced glottic carcinomas in about 30% of cases.
- Distant metastases are rare, occur in a small percentage of cases (2–5%) and are most often located in the lungs, less often in the liver, bones, and brain.
- Management of the N0 neck (END during salvage) TL may reduce the rate of regional recurrence, but not at the expense of improving DSS or OS. Rates of occult metastases, regional recurrence, and "cure" through salvage neck dissection are not equivalent [65, 66].

27.9 Treatment Failures

Treatment failures can be predicted by the following pathologic factors:

- presence of subglottic extension,
- primary tumor size greater than 1.5 cm,
- metastases to regional lymph nodes,
- presence of lymph node metastasis in the laryngectomy and neck dissection specimen (pretracheal, Delphian, parathyroid, or tracheoesophageal), and
- distant metastases.

Recurrences around tracheostomy fluctuate in the range of 3–15%, and the risk factors are

- primary subglottic localization,
- urgent tracheotomy,
- high stage of primary tumor,
- metastases to region VI, and
- abandonment of adjuvant radiotherapy.

The prognosis and treatment planning depends on

- the stage, and
- location and direction of tumor spread, according to the Sisson classification.

Definition of the Sisson Classification:
- Type I—tumor located in the upper pole, tracheostomy; detected early gives the possibility of radical surgical treatment
- Type II—tumor invades the esophagus, but its location in the upper part of the neck is still resectable
- Type III—infiltration in the area of the lower pole of the tracheostomy, penetrating toward the mediastinum, unresectable type
- Type IV—reaches below the collarbone, nonresectable type

27.10 Health-Related Quality of Life Following Total Laryngectomy

The loss of the larynx, and the related loss of its basic functions, leads to a significant reduction in the quality of life of patients. A general perception is that TL has a significantly negative impact on the individual's life. Many studies have confirmed that people after TL have a worse HRQoL, than the male normative reference population. However, even though TL patients experience a clinically important difference in many domains when compared with normative data, their burden of symptoms is generally mild [67].

The occurrence of postoperative complications, such as a fistula, problems with swallowing, or the inability to rehabilitate speech quickly, intensifies the very low assessment of the patient's quality of life [60, 68].

The age of the patient who underwent laryngectomy has a large impact on the assessment of the quality of life. Younger patients have different problems compared to older patients.

Younger age is significantly associated with financial difficulties, whereas professional activity and lower education level is significant predictors of xerostomia and swallowing problems, respectively [69].

Many years of observations of patients after total laryngectomy show that the low assessment of the quality of life occurs in the first month after surgery and during adjuvant treatment. The noticeable effects of rehabilitation improve quality of life. The overall quality of life is considered good to excellent by 83.2% of the patients [58].

EORTEC—European Organization for Research and Treatment of Cancer is an organization whose main task is to provide international prospective and retrospective translational and clinical research to improve the standard of cancer treatment for patients. EORTEC tries to establish new standards of postoperative care, or show that the previous ones were ineffective or redundant. All these efforts lead to an improvement in the quality of life of patients during or after oncological treatment [70].

27.11 Long-Term Follow-Up

Patients after total laryngectomy should be examined during routine outpatient department visits in 4–6 week intervals. The value of the follow-up (FU) scheme is confirmed by a high rate of recurrence detected in medical examination (60%) and routine imaging studies (27%), as opposed to only 13% in spontaneous reports. Local recurrences are the most common within the group of patients with head and neck cancer, and in most cases, an effective initial diagnosis is made by a physical examination carried out by a specialist.

During these control visits, a complete laryngological examination must be performed, focusing on the signs of recurrence, but also screening for second primary malignant tumors. An ultrasound scan of the neck is required to identify a nodal recurrence. The follow-up scheme after oncological treatment in patients with laryngeal cancer should include regular visits in the outpatient department:

- during the first year, visits every 4 weeks,
- in the second year, visits every 2 months,
- in the third year one visit every 3–6 months, and
- in the fourth and fifth years one visit every 6 months.

Over the period of 5 years, some of oncology centers recommend visits once a year, and some end FU at this point. Minimum FU in patients with head and neck cancer should last at least 5 years [71].

The FU therapeutic profit in the form of high percentages of preclinical relapse and the human benefit in the form of high percentages of FU visits concluding with medical advice at a reasonable cost is justified medically and socially. Reportability to FU visits should be intensified through patients' education during and immediately after treatment.

27.12 Summary

Take-Home Messages

1. Total laryngectomy is the basic therapeutic standard in surgery of advanced stages of laryngeal cancer.
2. Loss of basic functions of the larynx, such as: breathing, swallowing, voice formation is also in some cases an indication for its removal.
3. The techniques of the procedure may be different, endoscopic operations with the use of the Da Vinci Robot, which seem to be a new direction of development in ENT oncology.
4. A variety of complications, both early and late, can occur after a total laryngectomy.
5. The loss of speech is a profound disability, which is why voice rehabilitation as soon as possible is required.
6. Tumor stage, number of metastatic cervical lymph nodes, hypopharyngeal and supraglottic tumor location, positive section margins,

and perineural invasion are independent negative prognostic factors.
7. The loss of the larynx, and the related loss of its basic functions, leads to a significant reduction in the quality of life of patients.
8. Regular follow-up is required for every patient after total laryngectomy.

References

1. Bozec A, Culié D, Poissonnet G, Dassonville O. Current role of total laryngectomy in the era of organ preservation. Cancers. 2020;3;12(3):584. https://doi.org/10.3390/cancers12030584.
2. Obid R, Redlich M, Tomeh C. The treatment of laryngeal cancer. Oral Maxillofac Surg Clin N Am. 2019;31(1):1–11. https://doi.org/10.1016/j.coms.2018.09.001.
3. Patel TR, Eggerstedt M, Toor J, Tajudeen BA, Husain I, Stenson K, et al. Occult lymph node metastasis in early-stage glottic cancer in the national cancer database. Laryngoscope. 2020;131(4):E1139–E1146. https://doi.org/10.1002/lary.28995.
4. Xu Y, Zhang Y, Xu Z, Liu S, Xu G, Gao L, et al. Patterns of cervical lymph node metastasis in locally advanced Supraglottic squamous cell carcinoma: implications for neck CTV delineation. Front Oncol. 2020;10:1596. https://doi.org/10.3389/fonc.2020.01596.
5. Ye LL, Rao J, Fan XW, Kong FF, Hu CS, Ying HM. The prognostic value of tumor depth for cervical lymph node metastasis in hypopharyngeal and supraglottic carcinomas. Head Neck. 2019;41(7):2116–2122. https://doi.org/10.1002/hed.25667.
6. Lucioni M, D'Ascanio L, De Nardi E, Lionello M, Bertolin A, Rizzotto G. Management of paratracheal lymph nodes in laryngeal cancer with subglottic involvement. Head Neck. 2018;40(1):24–33. https://doi.org/10.1002/hed.24905.
7. Ho AS, Kim S, Tighiouart M, Gudino C, Mita A, Scher KS, et al. Association of quantitativemetastatic lymph node burden with survival in hypopharyngeal and laryngeal cancer. JAMA Oncol. 2018;4(7):985–89. https://doi.org/10.1001/jamaoncol.2017.3852.
8. Popov TM, Dikov T, Goranova TE, Stancheva G, Kaneva RP, Todorov S, et al. Macrophageal infiltration and microvessel density in laryngeal carcinoma: study of 52 cases. Acta Otorhinolaryngol Ital. 2015;35(5):321–4. https://doi.org/10.14639/0392-100X-588.
9. Mesolella M, Iorio B, Misso G, Luce A, Cimmino M, Iengo M, et al. Role of perineural invasion as a prognostic factor in laryngeal cancer. Oncol Lett. 2016;11(4):2595–8. https://doi.org/10.3892/ol.2016.4265.
10. Coskun H, Mendenhall WM, Rinaldo A, Rodrigo JP, Suárez C, Strojan P, et al. Prognosis of subglottic carcinoma: is it really worse? Head and neck. 2019;41(2):511–21. https://doi.org/10.1002/hed.25172.
11. Zbären P, Nuyens M, Curschmann J, Stauffer E. Histologic characteristics and tumor spread of recurrent glottic carcinoma: analysis on whole-organ sections and comparison with tumor spread of primary glottic carcinomas. Head Neck. 2007;29(1):26–32. https://doi.org/10.1002/hed.20502.
12. Spector GJ. Distant metastases from laryngeal and hypopharyngeal cancer. ORL. 2001;63(4):224–8. https://doi.org/10.1159/000055746.
13. García Lorenzo J, Montoro Martínez V, Rigo Quera A, Codina Aroca A, López Vilas M, Quer Agustí M, et al. Modifications in the treatment of advanced laryngeal cancer throughout the last 30 years. Eur Arch Oto-Rhino-Laryngology. 2017;274(9):3449–55. https://doi.org/10.1007/s00405-017-4639-z.
14. Ceachir O, Hainarosie R, Zainea V. Total laryngectomy - past, present, future. Maedica (Buchar). 2014;9(2):210–6.
15. Wu MP, Goldsmith T, Holman A, Kammer R, Parikh A, Devore EK, et al. Risk factors for laryngectomy for dysfunctional larynx after organ preservation protocols: a case-control analysis. Otolaryngol Head Neck Surg. 2020;164(3):608-615. https://doi.org/10.1177/0194599820947702.
16. Verma SP, Mahboubi H. The changing landscape of total laryngectomy surgery. Otolaryngol Head Neck Surg. 2014;150(3):413–8. https://doi.org/10.1177/0194599813514515.
17. Mimica X, Hanson M, Patel SG, McGill M, McBride S, Lee N, et al. Salvage surgery for recurrent larynx cancer. Head Neck. 2019;41(11):3906–915. https://doi.org/10.1002/hed.25925.
18. Bertolin A, Lionello M, Zanotti C, Franz L, Giacomelli L, Rizzotto G, et al. Oncological and functional outcomes of primary and salvage total laryngectomy. Laryngoscope 2020,131(2):E569-E575. https://doi.org/10.1002/lary.28955.
19. Russell NS, Hoving S, Heeneman S, Hage JJ, Woerdeman LAE, de Bree R, et al. Novel insights into pathological changes in muscular arteries of radiotherapy patients. Radiother Oncol. 2009,92(3):477–83. https://doi.org/10.1016/j.radonc.2009.05.021.
20. Dowthwaite S, Nichols AC, Yoo J, Smith RV, Dhaliwal S, Basmaji J, Franklin JH, Fung K. Transoral robotic total laryngectomy: report of 3 cases. Head Neck. 2013;35(11):E338–42. https://doi.org/10.1002/hed.23226.
21. Elson NC, Martinez DC, Cervenka BP. Current opinions in otolaryngology and head and neck surgery: functional considerations in reconstruction after laryngectomy. Curr Opin Otolaryngol Head Neck Surg. 2020;28(5):355–364. https://doi.org/10.1097/MOO.0000000000000645.
22. Varghese BT. Bilateral infrahyoid muscle, myofascial and myoperichondrial flaps in laryngectomy. Oral Oncol. 2019;98:165–7. https://doi.org/10.1016/j.oraloncology.2019.09.002.
23. León X, López M, García J, Casasayas M, Rovira C, Quer M. Indications and results of extended

total laryngectomy with enbloc resection of overlying cervical skin. Eur Arch Oto-Rhino-Laryngology. 2019,276(11):3179–84. https://doi.org/10.1007/s00405-019-05573-8.
24. Gonzalez-Orús Álvarez-Morujo R, Martinez Pascual P, Tucciarone M, Fernández Fernández M, Souviron Encabo R, Martinez Guirado T. Salvage total laryngectomy: is a flap necessary? Braz J Otorhinolaryngol. 2020;86(2):228–36. https://doi.org/10.1016/j.bjorl.2018.11.007.
25. Piazza C, Paderno A, Del Bon F, Grammatica A, Montalto N, Bresciani L, et al. Fascio-cutaneous-free flaps as primary reconstruction in salvage total laryngectomy. Eur Arch Oto-Rhino-Laryngology. 2020;278(1):219–26. https://doi.org/10.1007/s00405-020-06137-x.
26. Pellini R, Zocchi J, Pichi B, Manciocco V, Marchesi P, Sperduti I, et al. Prevention of fistulas after salvage laryngectomy using temporoparietal fascia free flap. Acta Otorhinolaryngol Ital. 2020;40(3):181–9. https://doi.org/10.14639/0392-100X-N0411.
27. Meulemans J, Demarsin H, Debacker J, Batailde G, Mennes T, Laenen A, et al. Functional outcomes and complications after salvage Total laryngectomy for residual, recurrent, and second primary squamous cell carcinoma of the larynx and hypopharynx: a multicenter retrospective cohort study. Front Oncol. 2020;10:1390. https://doi.org/10.3389/fonc.2020.01390.
28. Ferreli F, Mercante G, De Virgilio A, Di Maio P, Iocca O, Pellini R, et al. Lateral cervical approach for salvage total laryngectomy without pharyngeal reinforcement with pedicled or free flaps: our preliminary experience in six patients. Eur Arch Oto-Rhino-Laryngology. 2020;277(6):1837–41. https://doi.org/10.1007/s00405-020-05942-8.
29. Acevedo JR, Yu JC, Cameron B, Nurimba M, Hay JW, Kokot NC. Reconstruction after salvage total laryngectomy: a costeffectiveness analysis. Otolaryngol Head Neck Surg. 2020;164(1):139–45. https://doi.org/10.1177/0194599820936264.
30. Fernández-Fernández MM, González LMJ, Calvo CR, Arias PP, Cabré FC, del Álamo PO. Transoral ultrasonic total laryngectomy (TOUSS-TL): description of a new endoscopic approach and report of two cases. Eur Arch Oto-Rhino- Laryngology. 2016; 273(9):2689–96. https://doi.org/10.1007/s00405-015-3784-5.
31. Wang CC, Wang CC, Wang CC, Wang CC, Lin WJ, De Virgilio A, et al. Long-term outcomes of transoral robotic surgeryassisted total laryngectomy for recurrent laryngeal cancers. Jpn J Clin Oncol. 2020;50(6):653–60. https://doi.org/10.1093/jjco/hyaa034.
32. Wang Y, Yu H, Qiao H, Li C, Chen K, Shen X. Risk factors and incidence of postoperative delirium in patients undergoing laryngectomy. Otolaryngol Head Neck Surg (United States). 2019;161(5):807–13. https://doi.org/10.1177/0194599819864304.
33. Meulemans J, Debacker J, Demarsin H, Vanclooster C, Neyt P, Mennes T, et al. Oncologic outcomes after salvage laryngectomy for squamous cell carcinoma of the larynx and hypopharynx: a multicenter retrospective cohort study. Ann Surg Oncol. 2020;28(3):1751–61. https://doi.org/10.1245/s10434-020-09017-0.
34. Balaji A, Thiagarajan S, Dhar H, Malik A, Bhattacharjee A, Chakraborthy A, et al. The results of sequential swallowing assessments after total laryngectomy for laryngeal and hypopharyngeal malignancies. Eur Arch Oto-Rhino-Laryngol. 2020;277(12):3469–77. https://doi.org/10.1007/s00405-020-06105-5.
35. Harris BN, Hoshal SG, Evangelista L, Kuhn M. Reconstruction technique following total laryngectomy affects swallowing outcomes. Laryngoscope Investig Otolaryngol. 2020;5(4):703–7. https://doi.org/10.1002/lio2.430.
36. Lee MT, Govender R, Roy PJ, Vaz F, Hilari K. Factors affecting swallowing outcomes after total laryngectomy: participant self-report using the swallowing outcomes after laryngectomy questionnaire. Head Neck. 2020;42(8):1963–69. https://doi.org/10.1002/hed.26132.
37. Wang M, Xun Y, Wang K, Lu L, Yu A, Guan B, et al. Risk factors of pharyngocutaneous fistula after total laryngectomy: a systematic review and meta-analysis. Eur Arch Otorhinolaryngol. 2020;277(2):585–99. https://doi.org/10.1007/s00405-019-05718-9.
38. Carsuzaa F, Capitaine AL, Ferrié JC, Apert V, Tonnerre D, Frasca D, et al. Pharyngocutaneous fistulas after total laryngectomy or pharyngolaryngectomy: place of video-fluoroscopic swallowing study. Head Neck. 2020;42(12):3638–46. https://doi.org/10.1002/hed.26429.
39. Okamoto I, Matsuki T, Sato H, Kondo T, Fushimi C, Okada T, et al. Post-operative complications due to salvage total laryngectomy for recurrent laryngeal cancer after radiotherapy–a multicentre retrospective study. Acta Otolaryngol. 2020;140(2):170–4. https://doi.org/10.1080/00016489.2019.1699251.
40. Eid AM, Ebada HA, El-Fattah AMA, Tawfik A. Platelet-rich fibrin: an autologous biomaterial for healing assistance of pharyngeal repair in total laryngectomy. Eur Arch Oto-Rhino-Laryngol. 2020;278(2):463–70. https://doi.org/10.1007/s00405-020-06404-x.
41. Park J, Chang C, Kwon D. Use of fibrin adhesive for preventing pharyngocutaneous fistula in total laryngectomy. Am J Otolaryngol Head Neck Med Surg. 2020;41(6):102674. https://doi.org/10.1016/j.amjoto.2020.102674.
42. Maleki Delarestaghi M, Ahmadi A, Dehghani Firouzabadi F, Roomiani M, Dehghani Firouzabadi M, Faham Z. Effect of lowpressure drainage suction on pharyngocutaneous fistula after total laryngectomy. Ann Otol Rhinol Laryngol. 2020;130(1):32–37. https://doi.org/10.1177/0003489420934506.
43. Torrico Román P, García Nogales A, Trinidad RG. Utility of the Montgomery salivary tubes for preventing pharyngocutaneous fistula in total laryngectomy. Am J Otolaryngol Head Neck Med Surg. 2020;41(4):102557. https://doi.org/10.1016/j.amjoto.2020.102557.

44. Le Flem M, Santini L, Boulze C, Alshukry A, Giovanni A, Dessi P, et al. Early oral hydration protects against pharyngocutaneous fistula after total laryngectomy or total pharyngolaryngectomy. Head Neck. 2020;42(8):1902–6. https://doi.org/10.1002/hed.26122.
45. McGuire JK, Viljoen G, Rocke J, Fitzpatrick S, Dalvie S, Fagan JJ. Does thyroid gland preserving Total laryngectomy affect oncological control in laryngeal carcinoma? Laryngoscope. 2020;130(6):1465–69. https://doi.org/10.1002/lary.28235.
46. Edafe O, Sandler LM, Beasley N, Balasubramanian SP. Systematic review of incidence, risk factors, prevention and treatment of post-laryngectomy hypoparathyroidism. Eur Arch Otorhinolaryngol. 2020;278(5):1337–44. https://doi.org/10.1007/s00405-020-06213-2.
47. Boukovalas S, Goepfert RP, Smith JM, Mecham E, Liu J, Zafereo ME, et al. Association between postoperative complications and long-term oncologic outcomes following total laryngectomy: 10-year experience at MD Anderson Cancer Center. Cancer. 2020;126(22):4905–16. https://doi.org/1002/cncr.33185.
48. Vimawala S, Topf MC, Savard C, Zhan T, Keane W, Luginbuhl A, et al. Risk factors for unplanned readmission in total laryngectomy patients. Laryngoscope. 2020;130(7):1725–32. https://doi.org/10.1002/lary.28255.
49. Pézier TF, Rijken JA, Tijink BM, Braunius WW, de Bree R. Time interval between (chemo)radiotherapy and subsequent laryngectomy is not prognostic for post operative complications and survival. Eur Arch Oto-Rhino-Laryngol. 2020;278(7):2511–6. https://doi.org/10.1007/s00405-020-06384-y.
50. Sullivan CB, Ostedgaard KL, Al-Qurayshi Z, Pagedar NA, Sperry SM. Primary laryngectomy versus salvage laryngectomy: a comparison of outcomes in the chemoradiation era. Laryngoscope. 2020;130(9):2179–85. https://doi.org/10.1002/lary.28343.
51. van Sluis KE, van Son RJJH, van der Molen L, McGuinness AJ, Palme CE, Novakovic D, et al. Multidimensional evaluation of voice outcomes following total laryngectomy: a prospective multicenter cohort study. Eur Arch Oto-Rhino-Laryngology. 2020;278(4):1209–22. https://doi.org/10.1007/s00405-020-06216-z.
52. Farlow JL, Birkeland AC, Hardenbergh A, Lyden T, Brenner JC, Shuman AG, et al. Speech and swallowing outcomes after laryngectomy for the dysfunctional irradiated larynx. Eur Arch Oto-Rhino-Laryngol. 2020;277(5):1459–65. https://doi.org/10.1007/s00405-020-05809-y.
53. Zhang T, Cook I, Szczęśniak M, Maclean J, Wu P, Nguyen DD, et al. The relationship between biomechanics of pharyngoesophageal segment and tracheoesophageal phonation. Sci Rep. 2019;9(1):9722. https://doi.org/10.1038/s41598-019-46223-7.
54. Zormeier MM, Meleca RJ, Simpson ML, Dworkin JP, Klein R, Gross M, et al. Botulinum toxin injection to improve tracheoesophageal speech after total laryngectomy. Otolaryngol Head Neck Surg. 1999;120(3):314–9. https://doi.org/10.1016/S0194-5998(99)70268-8.
55. Wypych A, Wierzchowska M, Burduk P, Zawada E, Nadolska K, Serafin Z. Cortical presentation of language functions in patients after total laryngectomy: a fMRI study. Neuroradiology. 2020;62(7):843-849. https://doi.org/10.1007/s00234-020-02407-x.
56. Parrilla C, Longobardi Y, Paludetti G, Marenda ME, D'alatri L, Bussu F, et al. A one-year time frame for voice prosthesis management. What should the physician expect? is it an overrated job? Acta Otorhinolaryngol Ital. 2020;40(4):270–6. https://doi.org/10.14639/0392-100X-N0587.
57. Spałek J, Deptuła P, Cieśluk M, Strzelecka A, Łysik D, Mystkowska J, et al. Biofilm growth causes damage to silicone voice prostheses in patients after surgical treatment of locally advanced laryngeal cancer. Pathogens. 2020;9(10):793. https://doi.org/10.3390/pathogens9100793.
58. Souza FGR, Santos IC, Bergmann A, Thuler LCS, Freitas AS, Freitas EQ, et al. Quality of life after total laryngectomy: impact of different vocal rehabilitation methods in a middle income country. Health Qual Life Outcomes. 2020;18(1):92. https://doi.org/10.1186/s12955-020-1281-z.
59. Azizli E, Alkan Z, Koçak I, Yiğit Ö. Voice onset time in patients using speech prosthesis after Total laryngectomy. J Voice. 2020;S0892-1997(20)30362–3. 10.1016/j.jvoice.2020.09.018.
60. Antin F, Breheret R, Goineau A, Capitain O, Laccourreye L. Rehabilitation following total laryngectomy: oncologic, functional, socio-occupational and psychological aspects. Eur Ann Otorhinolaryngol Head Neck Dis. 2020;138(1):19–22. https://doi.org/10.1016/j.anorl.2020.06.006.
61. Tsai MH, Chuang HC, Lin YT, Lu H, Fang FM, Huang TL, et al. Predictors of hospital expenses and hospital stay among patients undergoing total laryngectomy: cost effectiveness analysis. PLoS One. 2020;15(7):e0236122. https://doi.org/10.1371/journal.pone.0236122.
62. Beck AJCC, Retèl VP, Bunting G, Sethi RKV, Deschler DG, van den Brekel MWM, et al. Cost-effectiveness analysis of using the heat and moisture exchangers compared with alternative stoma covers in laryngectomy rehabilitation: US perspective. Head Neck. 2020;42(12):3720–34. https://doi.org/10.1002/hed.26442.
63. Gourin CG, Vosler PS, Mandal R, Pitman KT, Fakhry C, Eisele DW, et al. Association between hospital market concentration and costs of laryngectomy. JAMA Otolaryngol Head Neck Surg. 2019;145(10):939–47. https://doi.org/10.1001/jamaoto.2019.2303.
64. Debacker J, Meulemans J, Huvenne W, Vander Poorten V. ASO author reflections: salvage total laryngectomy, the last resort for patients with residual, recurrent or second primary laryngeal and hypopharyngeal cancer in times of nonsurgical organ preserving treatment strategies. Ann Surg Oncol. 2020;27(Suppl 3):905–6. https://doi.org/10.1245/s10434-020-09037-w.

65. Xiao CC, Imam SA, Nguyen SA, Camilon MP, Baker AB, Day TA, et al. Neck dissection does not add to morbidity or mortality of laryngectomy. World J Otorhinolaryngol Head Neck Surg. 2019;5(4):215–21. https://doi.org/10.1016/j.wjorl.2019.01.004.
66. Davies-Husband CR, Drinnan M, King E. Elective neck dissection for salvage total laryngectomy: a systematic review, metaanalysis and "decision-to-treat" approach. Clin Otolaryngol. 2020;45(4):558–73. https://doi.org/10.1111/coa.13520.
67. Wulff NB, Højager A, Wessel I, Dalton SO, Homøe P. Health-related quality of life following total laryngectomy: a systematic review. Laryngoscope. 2020; 131(4):820–31. https://doi.org/10.1002/lary.29027.
68. Kemps GJF, Krebbers I, Pilz W, Vanbelle S, Baijens LWJ. Affective symptoms and swallow-specific quality of life in total laryngectomy patients. Head Neck. 2020;42(11):3179–87. https://doi.org/10.1002/hed.26365.
69. Bozec A, Schultz P, Gal J, Chamorey E, Chateau Y, Dassonville O, et al. Evaluation of the information given to patients undergoing total pharyngolaryngectomy and quality of life: a prospective multicentric study. Eur Arch Oto-Rhino-Laryngol. 2019;276(9):2531–39. https://doi.org/10.1007/s00405-019-05513-6.
70. Iravani K, Jafari P, Akhlaghi A, Khademi B. Assessing whether EORTC QLQ-30 and FACT-G measure the same constructs of quality of life in patients with total laryngectomy. Health Qual Life Outcomes. 2018;16(1):183. https://doi.org/10.1186/s12955-018-1012-x.
71. Jackowska J, Abelak Y, Piersiala K, Wierzbicka M. The effectiveness of the follow-up of patients after surgery due to cancer of the head and neck. J Comp Eff Res. 2018;7(8):765–73. https://doi.org/10.2217/cer-2017-0096.

Principles of Salvage Laryngeal Surgery

28

Aina Brunet, Aleix Rovira, and Ricard Simo

Key Points

- SS is currently the only treatment option with curative intent for recurrent LC.
- Salvage TL is associated to a high risk of postoperative complications.
- Multidisciplinary team (MDT) approach, preoperative and postoperative optimization is imperative in LC recurrence.
- Patient selection is of upmost importance in SL setting.
- The use of flaps either free or pedicled should be considered when deciding to perform a TL in the salvage setting.

28.1 Introduction

In recent years, nonsurgical treatment strategies have allowed to successfully treat laryngeal cancer (LC) while preserving the larynx and its function [1]. When persistent or recurrent disease is identified, it is widely recognized that the most reliable treatment option with curative intent is salvage surgery (SS). In this setting, chemotherapy, reirradiation, and, more recently, immunotherapy are utilized with palliative intention or rarely as adjuvant therapy after SS [2, 3]. Treatment of LC is intrinsically challenging due to the potential functional impact through disruption of vital anatomy and function as well as the cosmetic impact, all affecting patient's quality of life. The term "salvage surgery" (SS) is used in head and neck cancer to describe surgical treatment for cancers showing lack of response after adequate management of the primary tumour [4], delayed neck metastasis, and even for lung metastasis [5]. However, the current definition includes the management of residual as well as recurrent tumors in patients who have undergone radical radiotherapy-based (with or without chemotherapy) treatments or radical surgery upfront.

In such patients, previous radiotherapy affects healing and increases the risk of postoperative complications [6–8], ranging from 23% to 86% [9]. Complications after laryngectomy such as pharyngocutaneous fistula (PCF), wound infection, chyle leak, neural injuries, swallowing dys-

A. Brunet (✉)
Department of Otorhinolaryngology Head and Neck Surgery, Head, Neck and Thyroid Cancer Unit, Guy's and St Thomas' Hospital NHS Foundation Trust, London, UK

Department of Otorhinolaryngology Head and Neck Surgery, Hospital Universitari Bellvitge, L'Hospitalet de Llobregat, Barcelona, Spain

A. Rovira · R. Simo
Department of Otorhinolaryngology Head and Neck Surgery, Head, Neck and Thyroid Cancer Unit, Guy's and St Thomas' Hospital NHS Foundation Trust, London, UK
e-mail: aleix.rovira@gstt.nhs.uk; ricard.simo@gstt.nhs.uk

M. Remacle, H. E. Eckel (eds.), *Textbook of Surgery of Larynx and Trachea*,
https://doi.org/10.1007/978-3-031-09621-1_28

function, and airway compromise have a significant impact on the patient's well-being, causing prolonged hospitalization and, inevitably, increased health-care costs [7]. However, data from a recent review regarding outcomes of SS is encouraging; it has been reported that patients with LC recurrence have 5-year overall survival rates ranging from 30% to 70% depending on staging [10].

28.2 Evaluation of Recurrence

Locally advanced head and neck cancer (HNC) carries a high risk of local recurrence (15–40% depending on location and staging) and distant metastasis, with a poor prognosis (5-year overall survival, <50%) after initial treatment [11]. It is therefore evident that the initial evaluation and subsequent follow-up of patients treated with radiotherapy-based protocols are a fundamental part of their care [12–14]. Follow-up is essential to ensure appropriate assessment of the response to the treatment, identify possible recurrences or secondary tumors, monitor complications, and provide support for patients and their families. Initial posttreatment response evaluation is normally conducted with a combination of clinical examination and structural and metabolical imaging that is also useful to establish a baseline [13, 15].

Following treatment, the intensity of follow-up is greatest in the first 2 years, when the majority of recurrences occur [15]. Pain complaints must be regarded as serious warning of recurrent disease even when recurrence is not obvious on examination, being the first symptom of recurrent disease in 70% [16]. Unfortunately, there is no evidence of any clinical value of tumor markers in laryngeal cancer as yet. Accordingly, one of the most important aspects that can improve early identification of recurrence is patient education including identification of symptoms and relevance of risk factors [15].

The first step when evaluating a patient with a possible recurrence is elucidating the details and chronology of any previous treatment as well as his/her fitness for any further treatment, either curative or palliative. The second step should include the evaluation of the recurrence both with clinical examination (Fig. 28.1) and imaging techniques (Fig. 28.2). Clinical examination,

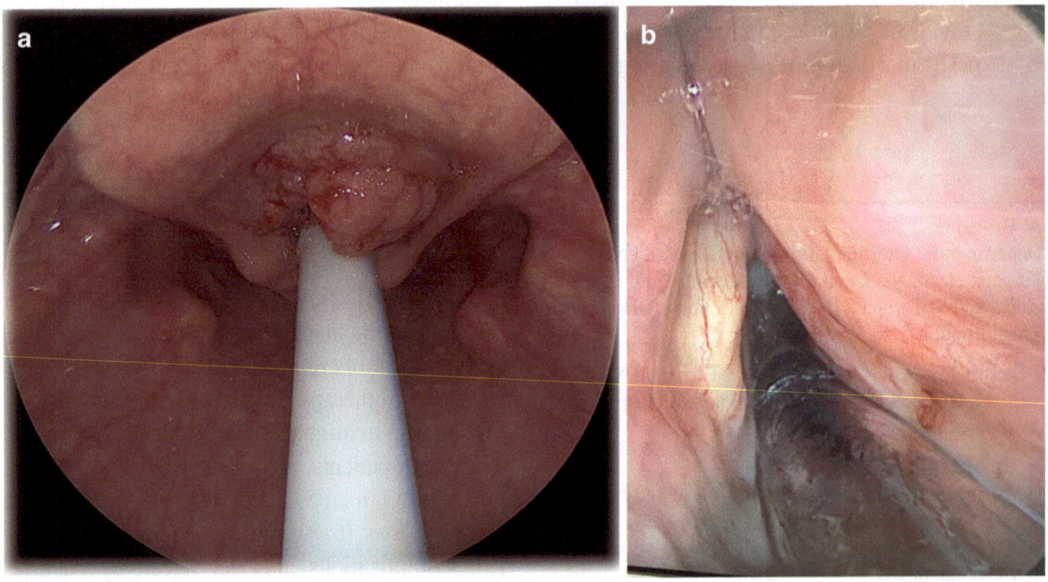

Fig. 28.1 (**a**) Clinical photograph from a patient that presents with an obvious supraglottic carcinoma. (**b**) Clinical photograph from a patient with a right vocal cord recurrent carcinoma in which the recurrence was not obvious clinically

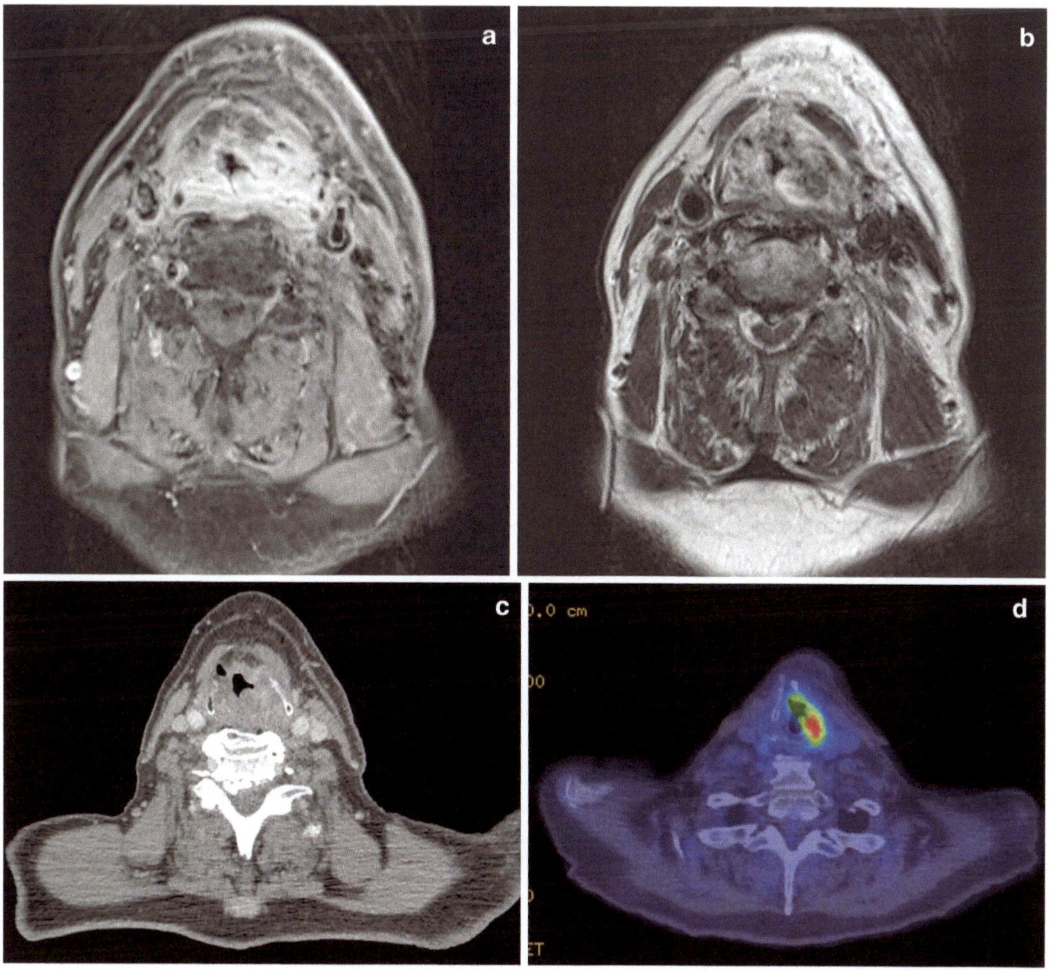

Fig. 28.2 MRI, CT, and PET-CT of a patient with a left transglottic tumor recurrence. (**a**) T2 MRI. (**b**) T1 post-contrast MRI. (**c**) CT with contrast. (**d**) PET-CT

however, has been reported to be challenging in this scenario, even when performed under general anesthesia, with very high false-negative rates [17].It is often necessary the use of multiple imaging techniques including CT with contrast, MRI scan and Ultrasound guided fine-needle aspiration cytology (US FNAC). Each modality provides specific information regarding the recurrence either on the primary site or the neck.

All patients with suspected recurrences or second primary tumors should be also evaluated for distant metastases prior to consideration of any radical treatment. Positron emission tomography combined with computed tomography (PET-CT) has proved to be very useful identifying local recurrence, regional and distant metastasis. The negative predictive value of PET-CT has been reported to be high for local and regional recurrence after HNC treated with radiotherapy-based treatment, with values between 93–95% and 94–100%, respectively [18]. A meta-analysis also showed high sensitivity and specificity for distant metastasis in this setting (92% and 95%, respectively) [19].

Palliative chemotherapy, immunotherapy, and/or supportive care are the most appropriate options for patients with locally recurrent and/or metastatic disease that is not amenable to definitive therapy, as well as for patients who have widely disseminated disease. Immunotherapy may lead to lengthy remissions in some patients.

28.3 Patient Selection

Patients with recurrent LC after nonsurgical organ preservation treatment represent significant challenge for the head and neck multidisciplinary team (MDT). Studies on outcomes and prognostic factors for the treatment of recurrent LC are retrospective and offer poor scientific evidence. Knowing the preoperative predictors having a significant impact on survival would have a major impact both on patient counselling and patient selection therefore being crucial information for patient and clinician decision making.

Table 28.1 Risk factors associated to worse survival outcomes

Patient	Tumor	Treatment
Poor performance status	Advanced stage	Previous radiotherapy
Comorbidities	Nonglottic tumor	Previous chemotherapy
Smoker	Neck disease	Toxicity from previous treatments
Alcohol excess	Extracapsular spread	Involved margins
No social support	Early recurrence	Postoperative complications

The following table summarizes the risk factors associated to worse survival outcomes (Table 28.1) [17, 20].

28.4 Setting

SS is best carried out in tertiary centers as its management requires experienced MDT input. The MDT plays a crucial role in selecting patients suitable for salvage laryngectomy, and it has been identified as an indicator of the value and quality of the treatment of HNC [21], and its importance and impact on outcomes is well recognized [22–25]. MDTs have been related to improved efficiency and completeness of care [26, 27].

28.5 Perioperative Optimization and Planning

Perioperative management is paramount for an optimal outcome of SS. Recently, the introduction of enhanced recovery after surgery programs (ERAS) has allowed to integrate and optimize perioperative care combining all relevant aspects of care in a single pathway [28]. Every individual case should be reviewed at the MDT meeting by experienced teams, with the results from the biopsies and combined multimodality imaging.

Table 28.2 Preoperative, intraoperative, and postoperative factors from the enhanced recovery after surgery programs. CNS: clinical nurse specialist, SALT: speech and language therapist

Preoperative	Intraoperative	Postoperative
Diagnostic planning	Patient assessed by the surgical team and anesthetist	Appropriate IV therapy
Optimized health/medical condition	CHO loading	Catheters removed early
Optimizing preoperative hemoglobin levels	Optimized fluid management	Regular oral analgesia
Patient information and decision making	Minimally invasive surgery	Avoidance of systemic opiate-based analgesia where possible
Preoperative therapy instruction as appropriate		Planned mobilization
Seen by a dentist if needed		
Plan made for a gastrostomy		
CNS/SALT/physiotherapists and dietitians		
ECG and preoperative bloods		
Alcohol and smoking assessment		

Surgical treatment planning should be discussed, determining tumor approach, adequate exposure, and anticipation of the anatomical surgical defect from the resection in order to define reconstructive options [27]. An Enhanced Recovery after Surgery (ERAS) protocol ensures patients are in optimal condition for treatment, have the best possible care during the operation, and experience optimal postoperative rehabilitation (Table 28.2). It improves patient experience and satisfaction, clinical outcomes, efficiency, capacity, and MDT working. It reduces the rate of complications, length of stay, stress, and costs [28].

28.5.1 The Use of Antibiotics

Salvage TL is a clean-contaminated procedure with described infection rates of up to 87% [29]. After radiotherapy, blood supply is compromised due to endarteritis obliterans [30]. Current evidence suggests providing cover for aerobic, anaerobic, and Gram-negative bacteria. Common bacteria include MRSA (43%) and *Pseudomonas aeruginosa* (36%) [31]. There is little evidence on the extent of antibiotic prophylactic treatment, although it is suggested that an anti-MRSA agent is used in addition to standard postoperative antibiotics for at least 3 days in all SS, as MRSA has also been identified as a factor contributing to PCF formation, pulmonary infections, risk of carotid blowout, and postoperative cellulitis after salvage TL [27, 32].

28.6 Surgical Management

Surgical options for recurrent LC include transoral surgeries (TSs) being the most commonly used one transoral laser surgery (TOLS), open partial laryngectomy (OPL), or TL (Table 28.3), which are described in detail in Chaps. 24–27, respectively. For T1 and T2 lesions, the first surgical option should be TS or OPL, except in cases where the tumor is multicentric or the larynx is already dysfunctional, in which a TL is preferred. In T3 tumors OPL should be considered in cases of localized tumors. In T4 recurrences, the first surgical option is a TL or extended TL [33–35].

28.6.1 Surgical Principles

In this section, we will address fundamentally TL.

Incisions. Single longitudinal incisions following Langer's tension lines separated from the stoma when possible. Moreover, T, H, or U flaps should be avoided in order to prevent necrosis of flap corners and further complications such as lymphoedema.

Excision Index Tumor. Tumor resection should start away from recurrent tumor side in order to facilitate tumor visualization during resection, decreasing rate of involved margins and increasing mucosal preservation (Fig. 28.3). Frozen section should be considered in order to better control tumor extent and a macroscopic margin of at least one centimeter should be target whenever it is possible [27].

28.6.2 Neck Management

The usefulness of elective neck dissection (END) in patients clinically and radiologically recurring as N0 is poorly defined. This is due to the variability reported both in terms of occult neck disease (OND) and its impact on complications and sur-

Table 28.3 Treatment options depending on tumor staging. Green: highly recommended. Orange: recommended. Red: Not recommended

	T1	T2	T3	T4
TS	+	+	+/-	+/-
OPL	+	+	+//-	+?
TL	+	+	+	+

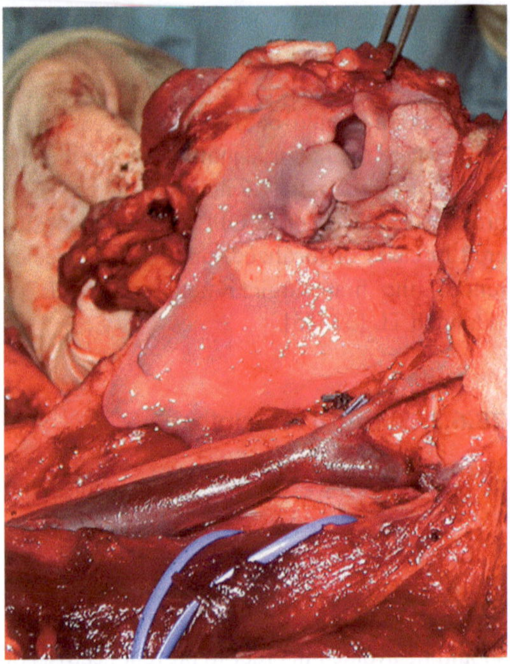

Fig. 28.3 Intraoperative image of a tumor involving the right pyriform fossa

vival. END is used for N0 patients whose primary cancer is associated with relative high risk (>20%) of OND [36]. Previous studies identified neck dissection (ND) as an independent factor for postoperative morbidity during SS after radiotherapy-based treatment, while others showed no association between the two variables.

In a systematic review analyzing the risk of complications during salvage TL, Hasan et al. studied the possible relation between ND and PCF fistula [33]. With 7 studies including 656 patients, ND was not associated to a significant increased incidence of PCF. Two studies specifically looked at complications of END in the N0 neck [37, 38]. Between these studies there was a total of 116 patients who had 29 (25%) PCF, 6 (5.2%) wound infections, 1 (0.9%) wound dehiscence, and 11 (9.5%) bleeding complications. The reported rate of OND in this series was very low (4–5%).

Lin et al. performed a systematic review analyzing the role of END during salvage TL in 2019 [39]. Data was available for 370 patients in 5 out of 19 studies for ND and complications. Overall, 51% of patients who underwent END and 34% who were observed suffered complications with a pooled relative risk of postoperative complications with END compared to observation was 1.72 ($p = 0.07$, 95% CI = 0.96–3.10). Hamoir et al. reported that patients undergoing salvage TL combined with ND are more at risk of developing complications than patients undergoing primary site surgery alone or ND alone [40]. The largest series advocating for the need of END was reported by Birkeland et al. in 2016 [43] with 203 recurrent or persistent LC recurrences classified as crN0 with CT scan. A total of 406 END were performed with 17% of cases having OND, being more prevalent in T4 (34%) and supraglottic tumors (28%). By performing bilateral ND to every patient independently of the staging, this study avoids the selection bias. However, not only the number of OND is below the 20%, restaging prior to salvage surgery was performed with PET scan in only 21% of the patients, avoiding the potential benefit of PET according to its reported accuracy [18, 19].

Other published series have promoted avoiding ND. The series with a largest number of patients includes 125 SL with 98 patient undergoing ND [42]. Although incurring into a potential selection bias, especially because there is no report of the proportion of patients with N+ disease at the time of initial diagnosis, the authors concluded that according to the lack of benefit of END in disease specific survival (DSS) and overall survival (OS), END is not recommended.

The only large series to date reporting the risk of OND in a specific neck level according to primary tumor location (but not recurrent stage) [41] showed that the risk of OND at levels I, IV, and V for supraglottic SCC and all levels for glottis SCC (except level VI) is less than 10%, while the risk of OND at levels II, III, and VI for supraglottic SCC is more than 10% even on the contralateral side. A systematic review fails to conclude with a strong recommendation regarding the indications of END stating that the rate of OND is higher with supraglottic and T3/T4 recurrences and therefore, END should be considered [39].

ND is typically performed for more advanced disease, involves large incisions, prolongs operating time, and puts several critical structures at risk of injury, which may explain the high complication rates in these patients. That being said, ND is indicated when there is confirmation or suspicion of neck disease on preoperative evaluation. When no sign of neck recurrence or persistence exists, there is consensus about not doing neck dissection for early stage glottic cancer recurred at an early stage; however, no agreement exists regarding all the other locations and advanced stages [43].

28.6.3 The Use of Flaps

Reconstruction with pedicled or microvascular flaps should be considered in patients undergoing SL. It provides healthy, vascularized, nonirradiated tissue, which will aid in healing (Fig. 28.4). It is especially important when a significant anatomical defect is expected in order to decrease the tension in the suture line and necessary when circular resections are performed. The use of flaps has been related to a reduced rate of infection and complications [20, 27, 37, 44]. It has shown to decrease PCF rates in cases where there is any tension on wound closure [45]. A meta-analysis showed that use of a vascularized flap to augment the circumference or support the repair reduces the risk of PCF formation by one third [46]. However, other authors reported that although it might reduce the size of the PCF, the use of flaps does not necessarily prevent its development. Nonetheless, the fact that it decreases its size makes it more likely that it will be able to heal with conservative treatment [27, 44]. Withrow et al. demonstrated that in patients who could have otherwise had their pharynx closed primarily, the addition of a free flap as a patch graft greatly reduced the fistula rate from 50% to 18% and lowered the stricture rate as well as feeding tube dependence [47, 48].

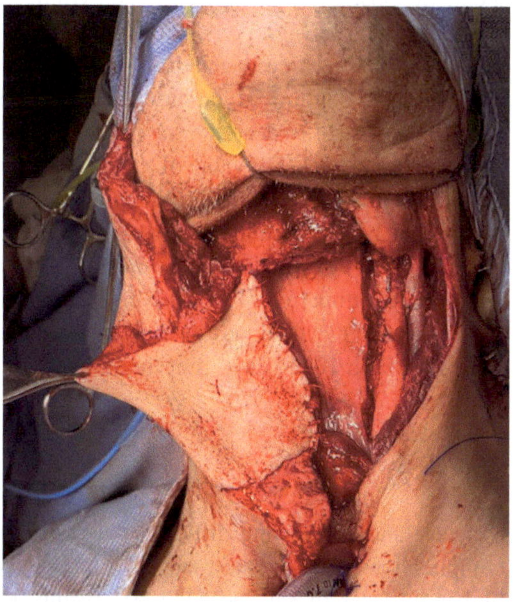

Fig. 28.4 Anterolateral tight free flap used insertion to reconstruct the anterior pharyngeal wall

28.6.4 Management of the Thyroid Gland

Albeit some authors have described the role of thyroidectomy in TL [49], there is few data regarding the need for thyroid surgery on the SS setting [50]. Although some authors have tried to define predictive factors of TGI, as T staging, presence of subglottic extension and CT evidence of TGI, there is need for further research in order to better establish these criteria [49, 51]. Our own unpublished data [52] shows that the incidence of thyroid gland invasion (TGI) on salvage laryngectomy is 7.8%. Moreover, total thyroidectomy adds a nonnegligible degree of morbidity especially in the salvage setting. Therefore, the extent of thyroidectomy should be carefully considered and total thyroidectomy should be limited and specifically considered in patients with radiological or intraoperative evidence of bilateral TGI.

28.6.5 The Use of Salivary Bypass Tubes

The use of silicone bypass salivary tubes to prevent PCF formation and stenosis has been advocated in SS. While some authors support that its use decreases PCF rates and is cost-effective in TL [18], others state that it does not appear to reduce the rate of PCF [53], but may help to reduce its severity and hospital stay. Salivary bypass tubes should be considered in SS as an adjunct [27].

28.6.6 Voice Rehabilitation

There is an increased risk of PCF in patients undergoing primary tracheoesophageal puncture (TOP) [17]. Infection and devascularization of inferior pharyngeal segment are predisposing factors of TOP. Delayed voice restoration achieves similar speech fluency compared to primary puncture, although it is obtained later [54]. Voice-related Quality of Life Measure (V-RQOL) score suggests that speech and swallowing functions are reasonable following free flap reinforcement [55].

28.7 Complications

Overall complication rates after TL in the literature range from 5% to 78% with the most common complication being PCF formation occurring in as many as 73% of cases in SS [10]. This wide variation in the rate of postoperative complications can be due to numerous factors, one being the lack of consistency in reporting complications. The importance of accurately collecting postoperative complications data using a widely accepted classification system [56] was recently highlighted in HNC surgery [57]. Depending on the definition of a complication, a single institution can significantly modify its reported complication rates. While some authors have found that the complication rate for salvage surgery after CRT is higher than that after RT alone [58–60], others report no significant differences [61–63]. Surgical complications after anti-EFGR based treatment have shown similar complication rates to those reported after platinum-based therapies [9, 64]. Boukovalas et al. recently published that postoperative complications following TL are associated with worse overall survival and disease-free survival in comparison to uncomplicated cases [65].

Apart from the previously mentioned ND, other variables have been associated to an increased risk of complications. The period of time between the end of the nonsurgical treatment and the time of SS, or disease-free interval (DFI) has been described to be a predictive factor for developing PCF [20, 66]. Multiple studies have cited an increased incidence of complications with a shorter DFI [47, 48, 67] while others failed to observe any association between DFI and complication rates [61, 62, 68].

No relevant studies have been conducted in order to assess the rate of postoperative complications during HNC SS depending on the type of radiotherapy (3D vs. IMRT) or comparing patient that received induction chemotherapy or not.

28.8 Postoperative Management

28.8.1 Postoperative Care

Hemoglobin, electrolytes, albumin, calcium, PTH, and thyroid levels should be routinely assessed due to the risk of anemia, malnourishment, hypoparathyroidism, and hypothyroidism associated with salvage TL [27]. Early cuff deflation should be achieved and the tracheostomy tube should be removed in order to optimize stoma healing and to decrease the risk of wound pressure ulcers [27]. The value of a water-soluble swallow study in order to detect potential anastomotic leaks before starting oral tolerance remains uncertain, and most studies have evaluated this in the primary setting [69–71]. However, the authors of this chapter would advise a water-soluble swallow within 10–14 days after the surgery.

28.8.2 Swallowing

Stricture and swallowing difficulties are known complications of TL, but their rates are even higher in cases of salvage TL [75]. Twenty to forty percent of the cases would have gastrostomy tube dependency related to difficulty swallowing [72–74]. Whereas some authors reported that the reconstruction of the pharynx with free flaps might improve swallow rates and [48] contribute to a lower rate of gastrostomy tube dependence [74], other authors consider that pharyngeal stenosis is generally increased in the setting of flap reconstruction [10]. One also needs to contemplate that a free flap is also normally contemplate when major resections are needed, hence the increased incidence of dysphagia. A gastrostomy tube will maximize preoperative nutrition and avoid erosion or irritation of the anastomotic margins. Swallowing difficulty is also among the most significant factors affecting quality of life after salvage TL [74].

28.9 Conclusions

Salvage surgery for laryngeal cancer is challenging. Surgical teams offering salvage surgery should be proficient in the management of such patients and be able to offer all relevant options of treatment. Transoral surgery for early recurrence, OPL for intermediate recurrence, and TL for advanced recurrences with or without reconstruction should be in their armamentarium. Salvage total laryngectomy is the ultimate procedure for recurrent laryngeal cancer but has a reported high rate of complications. Although increased survival rates have been reported, quality of life also has to be considered when counselling a patient with a laryngeal recurrence. With all that in mind, patient selection is one of the most important factors.

References

1. Department of Veterans Affairs Laryngeal Cancer Study Group, Wolf G, Fisher S, et al. Induction chemotherapy plus radiation compared with surgery plus radiation in patients with advanced laryngeal cancer. N Engl J Med. 1991;324(24):1685–90.
2. De Crevoisier R, Domenge C, Wibault P, et al. Full dose reirradiation combined with chemotherapy after salvage surgery in head and neck carcinoma. Cancer. 2001;91(11):2071–6.
3. Wong LY, Wei WI, Lam LK, Yuen APW. Salvage of recurrent head and neck squamous cell carcinoma after primary curative surgery. Head Neck. 2003;25(11):953–9.
4. Poncet P. Total laryngectomy for salvage in cancers of the glottic regions. Laryngoscope. 1975;85(9):1430–4.
5. Sanabria A, Kowalski LP, Shaha AR, et al. Salvage surgery for head and neck cancer: a plea for better definitions. Eur Arch Oto-Rhino-Laryngol. 2014;271(6):1347–50.
6. Tibbs MK. Wound healing following radiation therapy: a review. Radiother Oncol. 1997;42(2):99–106.
7. Goodwin WJ. Salvage surgery for patients with recurrent squamous cell carcinoma of the upper aerodigestive tract: when do the ends justify the means? Laryngoscope. 2000;110(3 Pt 2 Suppl 93):1–18.
8. Paydarfar JA, Birkmeyer NJ. Complications in head and neck surgery. A meta-analysis of postlaryngectomy pharyngocutaneous fistula. Arch Otolaryngol Neck Surg. 2006;132(1):67.
9. Rovira A, Tornero J, Oliva M, et al. Salvage surgery after head and neck squamous cell carcinoma treated with bioradiotherapy. Head Neck. 2017;39(1):116–21.
10. Silverman DA, Puram SV, Rocco JW, Old MO, Kang SY. Salvage laryngectomy following organ-preservation therapy – an evidence-based review. Oral Oncol. 2018;2019(88):137–44.
11. Braakhuis BJM, Brakenhoff RH, René leemans C. Treatment choice for locally advanced head and neck cancers on the basis of risk factors: biological risk factors. Ann Oncol. 2012;23(Suppl. 10):x173–7.
12. Simo R, Bradley P, Chevalier D, et al. European laryngological society: ELS recommendations for the follow-up of patients treated for laryngeal cancer. Eur Arch Oto-Rhino-Laryngol. 2014;271(9):2469–79.
13. Joshi A, Calman F, O'Connell M, Jeannon JP, Pracy P, Simo R. Current trends in the follow-up of head and neck cancer patients in the UK. Clin Oncol. 2010;22(2):114–8.
14. Kothari P, Trinidade A, Hewitt RJD, Singh A, O'Flynn P. The follow-up of patients with head and neck cancer: an analysis of 1,039 patients. Eur Arch Oto-Rhino-Laryngol. 2011;268(8):1191–200.
15. Simo R, Homer J, Clarke P, et al. Follow-up after treatment for head and neck cancer: United Kingdom National Multidisciplinary Guidelines. J Laryngol Otol. 2016;130(S2):S208–11.
16. Scharpf J, Karnell LH, Christensen AJ, Funk GF. The role of pain in head and neck cancer recurrence and survivorship. Arch Otolaryngol Head Neck Surg. 2009;135(8):789–94.
17. Mehanna H, Kong A, Ahmed S. United Kingdom national multidisciplinary guideliness. J Laryngol Otol. 2016;130
18. Gupta T, Master Z, Kannan S, et al. Diagnostic performance of post-treatment FDG PET or FDG PET/CT imaging in head and neck cancer: a systematic review and meta-analysis. Eur J Nucl Med Mol Imaging. 2011;38(11):2083–95.
19. Gao S, Li S, Yang X, Tang Q. 18FDG PET-CT for distant metastases in patients with recurrent head

and neck cancer after definitive treatment. A meta-analysis. Oral Oncol. 2014;50(3):163–7.
20. Scotton WJ, Nixon IJ, Pezier TF, et al. Time interval between primary radiotherapy and salvage laryngectomy: a predictor of pharyngocutaneous fistula formation. Eur Arch Oto-Rhino-Laryngol. 2014;271(8):2277–83.
21. Takes RP, Halmos GB, Ridge JA, et al. Value and quality of care in head and neck oncology. Curr Oncol Rep. 2020;22(9):92.
22. Liu JC, Kaplon A, Blackman E, Miyamoto C, Savior D, Ragin C. The impact of the multidisciplinary tumor board on head and neck cancer outcomes. Laryngoscope. 2020;130(4):946–50.
23. Kelly SL, Jackson JE, Hickey BE, Szallasi FG, Bond CA. Multidisciplinary clinic care improves adherence to best practice in head and neck cancer. Am J Otolaryngol Head Neck Med Surg. 2013;34(1):57–60.
24. Friedland PL, Bozic B, Dewar J, Kuan R, Meyer C, Phillips M. Impact of multidisciplinary team management in head and neck cancer patients. Br J Cancer. 2011;104(8):1246–8.
25. Marchi F, Filauro M, Missale F, et al. A multidisciplinary team guided approach to the management of cT3 laryngeal cancer: a retrospective analysis of 104 cases. Cancers (Basel). 2019;11(5):717.
26. Townsend M, Kallogjeri D, Scott-Wittenborn N, Gerull K, Jansen S, Nussenbaum B. Multidisciplinary clinic management of head and neck cancer. JAMA Otolaryngol Head Neck Surg. 2017;143(12):1213–9.
27. Pang L, Jeannon JP, Simo R. Minimizing complications in salvage head and neck oncological surgery following radiotherapy and chemo-radiotherapy. Curr Opin Otolaryngol Head Neck Surg. 2011;19(2):125–31.
28. Coyle MJ, Main B, Hughes C, et al. Enhanced recovery after surgery (ERAS) for head and neck oncology patients. Clin Otolaryngol. 2016;41(2):118–26.
29. Simo R, French G. The use of prophylactic antibiotics in head and neck oncological surgery. Curr Opin Otolaryngol Head Neck Surg. 2006;14(2):55–61.
30. Baselet B, Sonveaux P, Baatout S, Aerts A. Pathological effects of ionizing radiation: endothelial activation and dysfunction. Cell Mol Life Sci. 2019;76(4):699–728.
31. Scotton W, Cobb R, Pang L, et al. Post-operative wound infection in salvage laryngectomy: does antibiotic prophylaxis have an impact? Eur Arch Oto-Rhino-Laryngol. 2012;269(11):2415–22.
32. Harris R, Ofo E, Cope D, et al. Current trends in antibiotic prophylaxis for laryngectomy in the UK - a national survey. J Laryngol Otol. 2015;129(1):63–7.
33. Hasan Z, Dwivedi RC, Gunaratne DA, Virk SA, Palme CE, Riffat F. Systematic review and meta-analysis of the complications of salvage total laryngectomy. Eur J Surg Oncol. 2017;43(1):42–51.
34. Vaculik MF, MacKay CA, Taylor SM, Trites JRB, Hart RD, Rigby MH. Systematic review and meta-analysis of T1 glottic cancer outcomes comparing CO2 transoral laser microsurgery and radiotherapy. J Otolaryngol Head Neck Surg. 2019;48(1):1–11.
35. Cheraghlou S, Kuo P, Mehra S, Yarbrough WG, Judson BL. Salvage surgery after radiation failure in T1/T2 larynx cancer: outcomes following total versus conservation surgery. Otolaryngol Head Neck Surg. 2018;158(3):497–504.
36. Ferlito A, Rinaldo A, Silver CE, et al. Elective and therapeutic selective neck dissection. Oral Oncol. 2006;42(1):14–25.
37. Bohannon I, Desmond R, Clemanos L. Management of the N0 neck in recurrent laryngeal squamous cell carcinoma. Laryngoscope. 2010;120:58–61.
38. Basheeth N, O'Leary G, Sheahan P. Elective neck dissection for NO neck during salvage total laryngectomy: findings, complications, and oncological outcome. JAMA Otolaryngol Head Neck Surg. 2013;139(8):790–6.
39. Lin C, Puram SV, Bulbul MG, et al. Elective neck dissection for salvage laryngectomy: a systematic review and meta-analysis. Oral Oncol. 2019;96(July):97–104.
40. Hamoir M, Holvoet E, Ambroise J, Lengelé B, Schmitz S. Salvage surgery in recurrent head and neck squamous cell carcinoma: oncologic outcome and predictors of disease free survival. Oral Oncol. 2017;67:1–9.
41. Birkeland AC, Rosko AJ, Issa MR, et al. Occult nodal disease prevalence and distribution in recurrent laryngeal cancer requiring salvage laryngectomy. Otolaryngol Head Neck Surg. 2016;154(3):473–9.
42. Freiser ME, Ojo RB, Lo K, et al. Complications and oncologic outcomes following elective neck dissection with salvage laryngectomy for the N0 neck. Am J Otolaryngol Head Neck Med Surg. 2016;37(3):186–94.
43. Sanabria A, Silver CE, Olsen KD, et al. Is elective neck dissection indicated during salvage surgery for head and neck squamous cell carcinoma? Eur Arch Oto-Rhino-Laryngology. 2014;271(12):3111–9.
44. Patel UA, Moore BA, Wax M, et al. Impact of pharyngeal closure technique on fistula after salvage laryngectomy. JAMA Otolaryngol Head Neck Surg. 2013;139(11):1156–62.
45. Elson NC, Martinez DC, Cervenka BP. Current opinions in otolaryngology and head and neck surgery: functional considerations in reconstruction after laryngectomy. Curr Opin Otolaryngol Head Neck Surg. 2020;28(5):355–64.
46. Paleri V, Drinnan M, Van Den Brekel MWM, et al. Vascularized tissue to reduce fistula following salvage total laryngectomy: a systematic review. Laryngoscope. 2014;124(8):1848–53.
47. Hanasono MM, Lin D, Wax MK, Rosenthal EL. Closure of laryngectomy defects in the age of chemoradiation therapy. Head Neck. 2012;34:580–8.
48. Withrow KP, Rosenthal EL, Gourin CG, et al. Free tissue transfer to manage salvage laryngectomy defects after organ preservation failure. Laryngoscope. 2007;117(5):781–4.
49. Elliott MS, Odell EW, Tysome JR, et al. Role of thyroidectomy in advanced laryngeal and pharyngolaryngeal carcinoma. Otolaryngology. 2010;142(6):851–5.

50. Muhammad T, Dhanani R, Mohtasham S, et al. Incidence of thyroid gland invasion in advanced laryngeal cancers and its impact on disease-specific survival; a retrospective review at a tertiary care center. Acta Otolaryngol. 2020;140(10):882–5.
51. Gilbert RW, Cullen RJ, Van Nostrand AWP, Bryce DP, Harwood AR. Prognostic significance of thyroid gland involvement in laryngeal carcinoma. Arch Otolaryngol Neck Surg. 1986;112(8):856–9.
52. Brunet A, Tornari C, Ezebuiro A, et al. Role of thyroidectomy in recurrent laryngeal carcinoma. Otolaryngol Head Neck Surg. 2022;166(5):894–900. Epub 2021 Aug 17.
53. Hone RWA, Rahman E, Wong G, et al. Do salivary bypass tubes lower the incidence of pharyngocutaneous fistula following total laryngectomy? A retrospective analysis of predictive factors using multivariate analysis. Eur Arch Oto-Rhino-Laryngol. 2017;274(4):1983–91.
54. Emerick KS, Tomycz L, Bradford CR, et al. Primary versus secondary tracheoesophageal puncture in salvage total laryngectomy following chemoradiation. Otolaryngol Head Neck Surg. 2009;140(3):386–90.
55. Fung K, Teknos TN, Vandenberg CD, et al. Prevention of wound complications following salvage laryngectomy using free vascularized tissue. Head Neck. 2007;29(5):425–30.
56. Dindo D, Demartines N, Clavien PA. Classification of surgical complications: a new proposal with evaluation in a cohort of 6336 patients and results of a survey. Ann Surg. 2004;240(2):205–13.
57. Awad MI, Shuman AG, Montero PH, Palmer FL, Shah JP, Patel SG. Accuracy of administrative and clinical registry data in reporting postoperative complications after surgery for oral cavity squamous cell carcinoma. Head Neck. 2015;37(6):851–61.
58. Agra IMG, Carvalho AL, Pontes E, et al. Postoperative complications after en bloc salvage surgery for head and neck cancer. Arch Otolaryngol Head Neck Surg. 2003;129(12):1317–21.
59. Ganly I, Patel S, Matsuo J, et al. Postoperative complications of salvage total laryngectomy. Cancer. 2005;103(10):2073–81.
60. Furuta Y, Homma A, Oridate N, et al. Surgical complications of salvage total laryngectomy following concurrent chemoradiotherapy. Int J Clin Oncol. 2008;13(6):521–7.
61. Weber RS, Berkey BA, Forastiere A, et al. Outcome of salvage total laryngectomy following organ preservation therapy. Arch Otolaryngol Neck Surg. 2003;129(1):44.
62. Lavertu P, Bonafede JP, Adelstein DJ, et al. Comparison of surgical complications after organ-preservation therapy in patients with stage III or IV squamous cell head and neck cancer. Arch Otolaryngol Head Neck Surg. 1998;124(4):401–6.
63. Klozar J, Cada Z, Koslabova E. Complications of total laryngectomy in the era of chemoradiation. Eur Arch Oto-Rhino-Laryngol. 2012;269(1):289–93.
64. Patil VM, Noronha V, Thiagarajan S, et al. Salvage surgery in head and neck cancer: does it improve outcomes? Eur J Surg Oncol J Eur Soc Surg Oncol Br Assoc Surg Oncol. 2020;46(6):1052–8.
65. Boukovalas S, Goepfert RP, Smith JM, et al. Association between postoperative complications and long-term oncologic outcomes following total laryngectomy: 10-year experience at MD Anderson Cancer Center. Cancer. 2020;126(22):4905–16.
66. Basheeth N, Gerard O, Sheahan P. Pharyngocutaneous fistula after salvage laryngectomy: impact of interval between radiotherapy and surgery, and performance of bilateral neck dissection. Head Neck. 2014;36(4):580–4.
67. Herranz J, Sarandeses A, Fernandez MF, Barro CV, Vidal JM, Gavilán J. Complications after total laryngectomy in nonradiated laryngeal and hypopharyngeal carcinomas. Otolaryngol Head Neck Surg. 2000;122(6):892–8.
68. Putten L, Bree R, Doornaert PA, et al. Salvage surgery in post-chemoradiation laryngeal and hypopharyngeal carcinoma: outcome and review. Acta Otorhinolaryngol Ital. 2015;35(3):162–72.
69. van la Parra RFD, Kon M, PPA S, Braunius WW, Pameijer FA. The prognostic value of abnormal findings on radiographic swallowing studies after total laryngectomy. Cancer Imaging. 2007;7(1):119–25.
70. White HN, Golden B, Sweeny L, Carroll WR, Magnuson JS, Rosenthal EL. Assessment and incidence of salivary leak following laryngectomy. Laryngoscope. 2012;122(8):1796–9.
71. Amin J, Ortlip TE, Cohen D, Vakharia K, Lubek JE. The utility of barium swallow studies for evaluation of pharyngocutaneous fistula after total laryngectomy. Arch Otorhinolaryngol Neck Surg. 2020;4(2):2–7.
72. Sweeny L, Golden JB, White HN, Magnuson JS, Carroll WR, Rosenthal EL. Incidence and outcomes of stricture formation postlaryngectomy. Otolaryngol - Head Neck Surg. 2012;146(3):395–402.
73. Worley ML, Graboyes EM, Blair J, et al. Factors associated with gastrostomy tube dependence following salvage total laryngectomy with microvascular free tissue transfer. Head Neck. 2019;41(4):865–70.
74. Schuman AD, Birkeland AC, Farlow RJ, Lyden T, Spector PME, Rosko AJ. Predictors of stricture and swallowing function following salvage laryngectomy. Otolaryngol Head Neck Surg. 2020; Epub ahead.

29 Management of Tracheal Tumors

Ricard Simo, Iain Nixon, and Cesare Piazza

Key Points

- PTTs are uncommon, more frequently diagnosed in the adult population, and most of them are malignant.
- Squamous cell carcinoma and adenoid cystic carcinoma represent over 60% of PTTs.
- PTTs often present late as symptoms are nonspecific (mainly shortness of breath at rest or on exertion).
- Central airway obstruction represents a life-threatening complication that requires a multidisciplinary team experienced approach.
- Surgical resection constitutes the primary treatment of choice.
- Endoscopic techniques such as transoral endoscopic laser debulking/debridement or endoluminal stenting should be considered as symptom control and palliative measures.
- Tracheal resection and reconstruction by end-to-end anastomosis has shown good results and is a viable option for these patients.
- Tracheal transplantation remains controversial as is yet to prove reproducible results.
- Radiotherapy is reserved as an adjuvant therapy after surgical resection or as a palliative local control option.
- Chemotherapy and immunotherapy are yet to be proven helpful in the management of PTTs.

R. Simo (✉)
Department of Otorhinolaryngology, Head and Neck Surgery, Guy's and St Thomas' Hospital NHS Foundation Trust, London, UK
e-mail: ricard.simo@gstt.nhs.uk

I. Nixon
Department of Otorhinolaryngology, Head and Neck Surgery, NHS Lothian, Edinburgh, UK
e-mail: iain.nixon@nhslothian.scot.nhs.uk

C. Piazza
Department of Otorhinolaryngology, Head and Neck Surgery, University of Brescia—Asst Spedali Civili Brescia, Brescia, Italy

29.1 Introduction

Primary tracheal tumors (PTTs) are extremely rare, accounting for 0.1–0.4% of all tumors [1–4]. Metastatic tumors to the trachea are even rarer. PTTs in children are mainly benign; however, in adults, they are often malignant [5]. The main presenting symptom of PTT is shortness of breath, which often delays the diagnosis, as hemoptysis and stridor are late symptoms. PTTs are commonly misdiagnosed as asthma or chronic

M. Remacle, H. E. Eckel (eds.), *Textbook of Surgery of Larynx and Trachea*,
https://doi.org/10.1007/978-3-031-09621-1_29

obstructive pulmonary disorders and patients only undergo further investigations once the tumor has advanced in size to cause airway obstruction or hemoptysis [5]. Histopathological subtype and disease staging will guide the management of PTTs. The main options include surgical resection either via an external approach or endocopically, with radiotherapy as adjuvant treatment [5–7]. Radiotherapy may also be used in the palliative setting together with endotracheal stenting or tumor debridement with laser or other modalities for symptomatic relief [8, 9]. Transoral laser excision, microdebridement, or cryotherapy can also be used as a temporary measure prior definitive treatment [9].

29.2 Epidemiology

PTTs are uncommon, and in adults, most of them are malignant. In a report by the Netherlands Cancer Registry, the incidence of PTT is 0.1 per 100.000 inhabitants per year, corresponding only to a 0.2% of all epithelial tumors of the respiratory tract [10]. However, secondary tumors from the surrounding anatomical structures such as the esophagus, thyroid, or lung are much more common. The most common histopathological type is squamous cell carcinoma (44.8%), followed by adenoid cystic carcinoma (16.3%) [11, 12].

29.3 Etiology

Several risk factors have been associated with the development of tracheal squamous cell carcinomas, and they are essentially the same as those of causing lung and laryngeal cancers (mainly smoking, exposure to inhaled hydrocarbons, and prior history of lung cancer) [13]. With regards to adenoid cystic carcinoma, to date, no predisposing factors have been identified [14].

29.4 Anatomy

The trachea is a 10–13 cm long tubular structure connecting the larynx to the carina, made up of incomplete C-shaped cartilage rings. In the young adult, 5 cm of the trachea usually lies above the suprasternal notch connecting to the cricoid cartilage superiorly [15, 16]. The internal lumen, with a diameter 1.5–2.5 cm, is lined by ciliated pseudostratified columnar epithelium. Posteriorly, the trachea is strengthened by longitudinal and transverse smooth muscles that make up the pars membranacea or party wall [5].

The blood supply to the superior half of the trachea is from the tracheo-esophageal vessels, branches from the inferior thyroid artery. The superior thyroid artery also contributes fine branches to the anterior tracheal wall via the thyroid isthmus. The subclavian, internal mammary, and innominate arteries also contribute small branches to the inferior portion of the trachea [16, 17]. The azygos and hemi azygos vessels provide venous drainage from the trachea. Lymphatic drainage from this organ is to the paratracheal and deep cervical nodes. Innervation to the trachealis muscle comes from the thoracic sympathetic plexus and the inferior ganglion of the vagus nerve. Innervation to the trachea permits for complex airway physiological functions including mucous production, airway constriction, and dilation. Reflex cough and sneezing response is triggered via the afferent vagal fibers [16].

29.5 Histopathological Tumor Types

Both benign and malignant PTTs originate either from ciliated epithelial cells, minor salivary glands, or mesenchymal components of the trachea. In adults, 90% of PTTs are malignant and the reverse is observed in the pediatric population, with the majority of PTT (80–90%) being benign. The management of pediatric laryngotracheal tumours has been already addressed in previous chapters. The predominant histological subtypes of PTT in the adult population are squamous cell carcinoma (SCC) and adenoid cystic carcinoma (AdCC), which comprise over 75% of malignant PTTs. SCC of the trachea has a male predominance and is associated with tobacco smoking. Regional metastasis to the mediastinum and lungs can occur in up to 30% of cases. AdCC has an equal sex distribution with no cor-

Table 29.1 Classification of PTTs (adapted from Subramaniam and O'Neil) [9]

Benign	Malignant
Epithelial neoplasms	
• Papilloma • Viral papillomatosis	• Squamous cell carcinoma • Adenocarcinoma • Undifferentiated carcinoma • Neuroendocrine carcinomas
Salivary gland neoplasms	
• Pleomorphic adenoma • Mucinous cystadenoma • Myoepithelioma	• Adenoid cystic carcinoma • Mucoepidermoid carcinoma • Carcinoma ex-pleomorphic adenoma
Mesenchymal neoplasms	
• Fibroma • Haemangioma • Paraganglioma • Glomus tumor • Chondroma • Leiomyoma	• Soft tissue sarcoma • Chondrosarcoma • Lymphoma

relation to history of smoking [9]. These tumors are associated with slow growth, perineural invasion, and delayed presentation of distant metastasis independently from loco-regional disease control [1, 18]. The most common histological variants of PTTs are summarized in Table 29.1.

29.6 Clinical Presentation

Early or small PPTs are asymptomatic and can be detected as incidentalomas at imaging or endoscopy performed for other reasons. Symptoms of PPTs are secondary to upper airway obstruction. With tumor growth occluding 50–75% of tracheal lumen, patients often present with stridor, usually biphasic, wheeze, shortness of breath, chronic cough due to mucosal irritation, and hemoptysis secondary to ulceration or tumor hypervascularity [2, 5] (Fig. 29.1).

Recurrent or nonresolving pneumonias should prompt clinicians to consider an underlying malignant pathology as tracheal obstruction by neoplasm as this may lead to mucus stasis and atelectasis. Large tumors extending into mediastinum or within the neck could also invade adjacent structures such as the recurrent laryngeal nerve causing paralysis [9]. Due to the nonspecific nature of these symptoms, diagnosis can be delayed as patients undergo initial investigations and management of common conditions such as chronic obstructive airway disease or asthma before malignant pathology is considered. These pathway delays will cause diagnosis of PTTs in advanced stages of disease, often necessitating more radical management. Unfortunately, this sometimes may not be possible due to the presence of regional or distant metastases. The radicality of the surgery could potentially leave the patient with a poor functional status, quality of life, and at a higher risk of disease recurrence [5, 19].

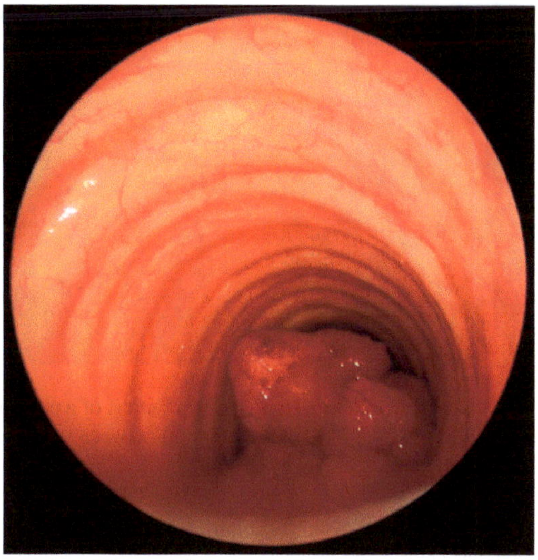

Fig. 29.1 Endoscopic view of a patient with almost complete tracheal obstruction by a squamous cell carcinoma of the cervical trachea

29.7 Evaluation and Diagnosis

As symptoms associated with PTT can be very nonspecific, with the majority of patients experiencing mainly shortness of breath, a high index of suspicion is required by clinicians investigating these patients particularly in those cases in which symptoms fail to resolve with initial medical management or in patients with high-risk profile [9, 19]. A plain X-ray chest radiograph (CXR) has and still is the most common modality used to investigate respiratory symptoms in primary

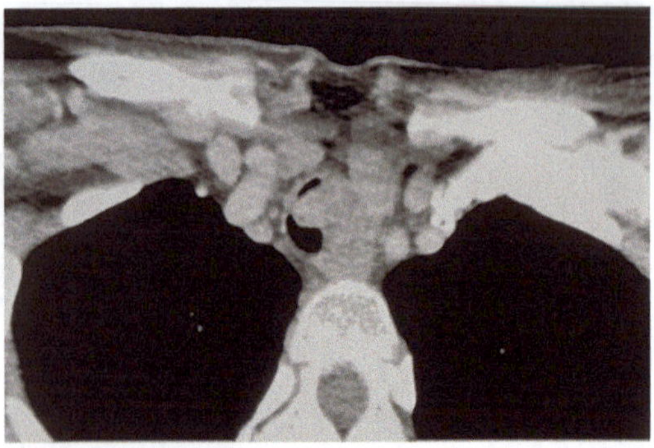

Fig. 29.2 Axial CT scan with iodine contrast of a patient presenting with an SCC at the junction between cervical and thoracic trachea

Table 29.2 TNM classification for primary tracheal carcinomas [1]

Tumour staging	Description
Tx	Tumor cannot be assessed.
T1	Tumor confined to trachea <2 cm.
T2	Tumor confined to trachea >2 cm.
T3	Tumor invades cartilage but not adjacent mediastinal structures.
T4	Tumor involves mediastinal structures.
Nodal status	**Description**
Nx	Nodal status cannot be assessed.
N0	No evidence of regional nodal involvement.
N1	Positive regional nodal disease.
Metastasis	**Description**
Mx	Distant metastasis cannot be assessed.
M0	No distant metastasis.
M1	Distant metastasis present.

care. Findings of distal airway dilation, air trapping and chronicity or recurrent nonresolving findings on serial CXRs may indicate the presence of underlying neoplastic airway pathology, prompting further investigations. A high-resolution computer tomography (CT) scan of the thorax with iodine contrast provides a rapid diagnosis with primary tumor anatomy and staging [1, 13] (Fig. 29.2).

Bronchoscopy (rigid or flexible) should be used to obtain tissue for histological diagnosis [8]. The procedure could also be therapeutic if local debridement or stenting is required. Bhattacharyya et al. [1] in 2004 proposed a Tumor Nodal Metastasis Staging for tracheal carcinomas. This classification is summarized in Table 29.2. The American Joint Committee on Cancer (AJCC) does not have a defined TNM staging specific to the trachea. However, the AJCC criteria for lung cancer stages all tracheal tumors as Stage IV.

29.8 Setting

In view of the rarity and complexity of managing PTT, these patients are best treated in centers with an experienced multidisciplinary team including anesthetists, laryngologists, head and neck, thoracic, and plastic surgeons, as well as histopathologists, radiologists, radiation, and medical oncologists [10, 20].

29.9 Management

The current practice in management of PTT with curative intent involves surgical resection with or without adjuvant radiotherapy when indicated. There have been no randomized clinical trials to validate the best treatment option for the management of PTT due to the rarity and its diverse histopathological variation [2, 10]. Selecting the optimum treatment option as in the case of any other cancer should involve a multidisciplinary team approach. These should include the consideration of factors such as patient's fitness for surgery, histopathology, and staging. In cases whereby patients present acutely with symptoms of airway obstruction, endotracheal approach with tumor debulking or airway stenting may be necessary. Restoring and retaining sufficient airway to enable adequate respiratory function is pertinent as it has a significant impact on patient's quality of life post treatment [21].

29.10 Surgery

The employed surgical technique for the management of PTT is dependent on tumor location [21]. Proximal tumors such those involving the cervical trachea and subglottis or thyroid gland may require laryngotracheal resection with or without thyroidectomy [9, 20]. Distal tumors involving the thoracic trachea may require resection of the carina and lung parenchyma [9, 12]. Combined trachea-esophageal resection may be performed if the esophagus is involved.

The operative description in this chapter focuses on surgical approach in resection of PTTs with primary anastomosis, not involving other surrounding structures. This is by far the most common clinical scenario.

The anesthetic technique of patients undergoing tracheal surgery is addressed in a previous chapter of this book.

The patient is appropriately prepared in a supine position with extension of the neck and a shoulder support to facilitate exposure of the cervical trachea. The authors prefer to utilize neuromonitoring of the recurrent laryngeal nerve to help with the identification and preservation of this nerves whenever possible.

A cervical collar incision with or without partial midline sternal split is the preferred approach for cervical tracheal tumors. A formal median sternotomy or thoracotomy may be required to approach the thoracic trachea. The need for adequate oncological margin clearance needs to be constantly balanced against reducing tension at the site of anastomosis and preserving meaningful respiratory function. The approach for malignant PTT may require regional lymph nodes to be included in the specimen; however, care is required not to compromise the segmental or lateral blood supply to the trachea [22]. Compromising tracheal vasculature could lead to necrosis of the retained segments of trachea or cause the anastomosis to break down [9]. The maximum length of trachea that is usually resected (at least in young patients) is up to 6 cm. In older people, however, a length of 4 cm of resected airway can already put the anastomosis at considerable stress, increasing the chance for anastomotic dehiscence (Piazza et al., Ann Otol Rhinol Laryngol, 2014 PMID 24944273). An infrahyoid release and a distal tracheal mobilization is often recommended to facilitate tracheal reconstruction and prevent anastomotic breakdown.

Reconstruction with an end-to-end anastomosis can be performed with traction sutures to approximate the retained proximal and distal ends of the trachea. Flexing the patient's neck, arching the chin toward the sternum, and infrahyoid muscle release can all aid in reducing dead space between the exposed ends [7]. If the surgeon is satisfied that reconstruction can be continued without excessive traction on the anastomosis site, coated absorbable 4–0 polyglactin (VICRYL) or polydioxanone (PDS) sutures can be used to complete the anastomosis passing through cartilage, beginning posteriorly, laterally, and then anteriorly at 3–4 mm apart [9]. The completed anastomosis can be checked for air leak by deflating the intubation tube cuff and irrigating the surgical field with saline solution. A fibrin sealant can be used to further strengthen the anastomosis and close small gaps to prevent minor postoperative air leakage [14, 23] (Figs. 29.3, 29.4, 29.5, 29.6, 29.7, 29.8).

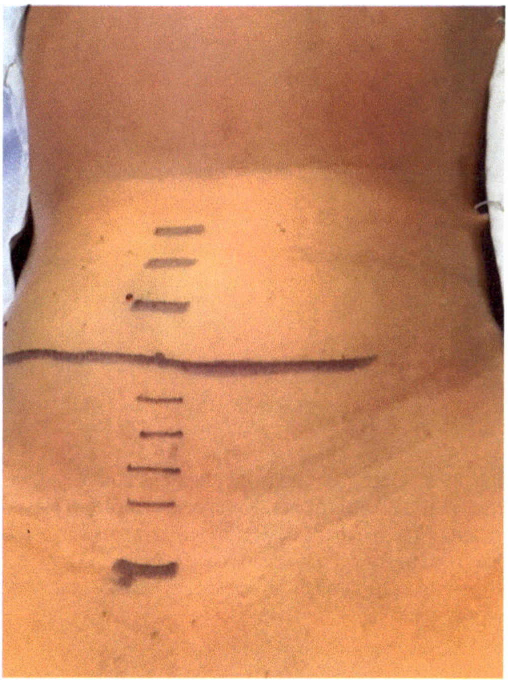

Fig. 29.3 Cervical incision for surgery in a malignant PTT

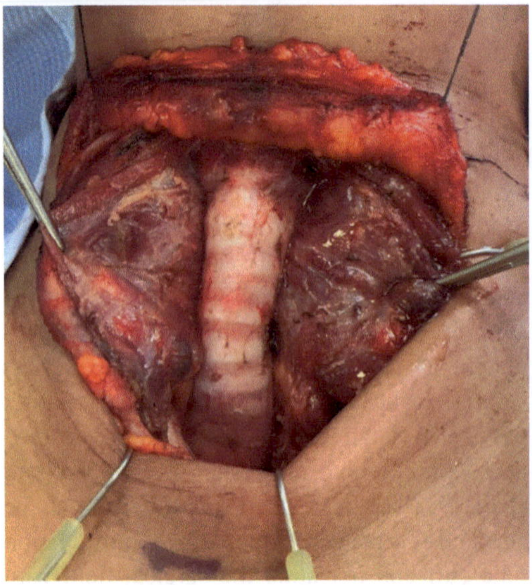

Fig. 29.4 Tracheal exposure after division of the thyroid gland isthmus. In this case, the patient had also a benign multinodular goiter

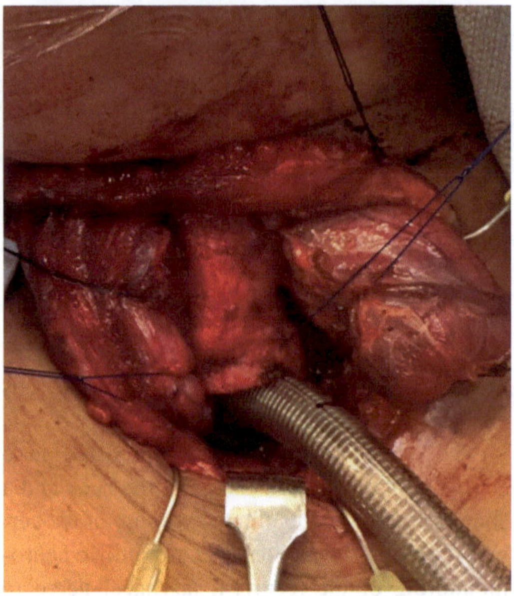

Fig. 29.6 In a manner similar to that of performing a laryngectomy, the surgeon asks the anesthetist to ensure full oxygenation of the patient, to deflate the endotracheal tube cuff, and to withdraw the tube at the level of the vocal cords. Then the inferior incision is performed and a new endotracheal tube is inserted distally as shown

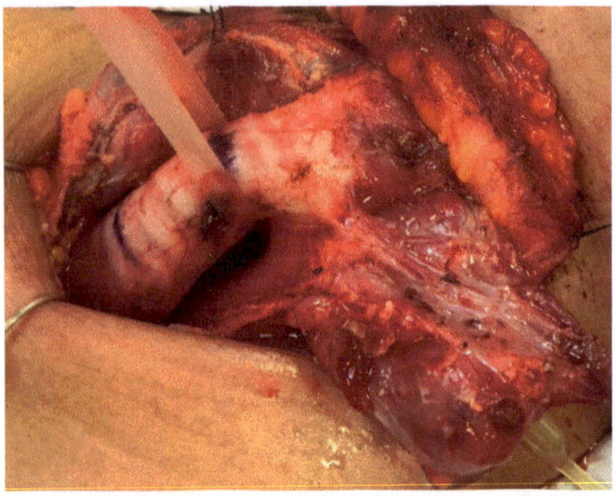

Fig. 29.5 Once the infrahyoid release is completed, the trachea is dissected from the esophagus ensuring preservation of the recurrent laryngeal nerves whenever possible. Then the resection incisions are marked and a rubber sling is passed through around the trachea to facilitate airway control

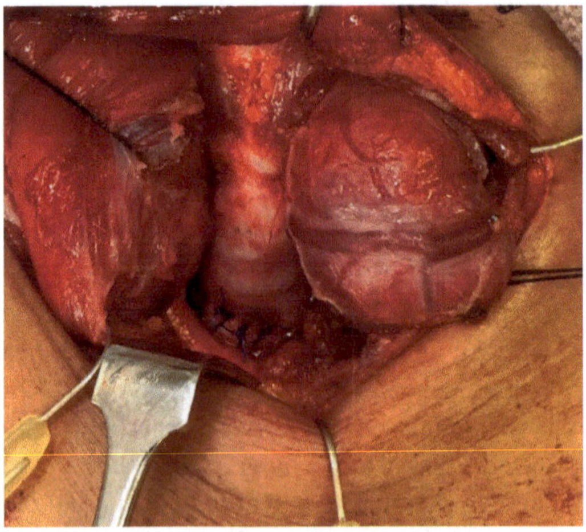

Fig. 29.7 Once the resection is completed, the original endotracheal tube is advanced and the recurrent laryngeal nerves stimulated to ensure vocal cord function. The reconstruction is completed with 2.0 Vicryl sutures with the knots exteriorly. Then the wound is irrigated with warm saline solution and Valsalva maneuver is performed to check for hemostasis and air anastomotic leaks

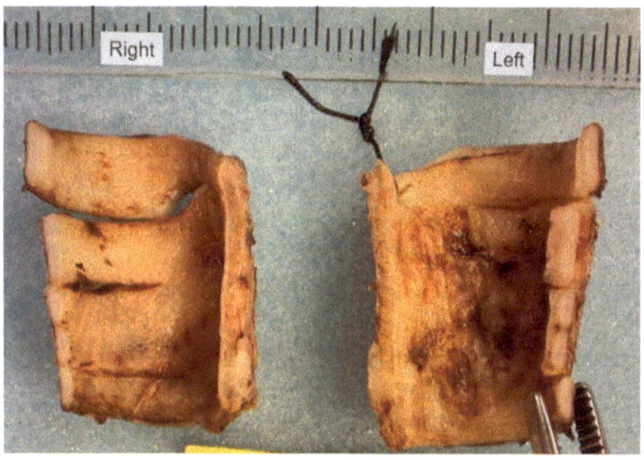

Fig. 29.8 Histopathological analysis of an SCC tracheal resection specimen

29.11 Transoral and Endotracheal Debridement

Endotracheal tumor debridement is often performed to provide symptomatic relief from airway obstruction. This may be required for control of acute tumor-associated hemorrhage. Tracheal lumen patency can be established with cold steel tumor debridement, electrocautery, or laser debulking, prior more definitive treatment [5, 8].

29.12 Endotracheal Stenting

In patients with more advanced unresectable neoplasms, palliative symptomatic airway control can be achieved with endotracheal stenting. Tracheal stents can be placed under sedation either under flexible or rigid bronchoscopy [24, 25].

29.13 Radiotherapy

Current evidence on adjuvant therapy is from outcomes based on retrospective cohort reports. Current indications for radiotherapy after surgical resection of PTTs are for cases with positive margins and intermediate- or high-grade malignant tumors [20, 25]. The observed outcomes to date are encouraging as both SCC and AdCC are radiosensitive tumors. There is a role for radiotherapy in the management of unresectable tracheal tumors or for symptoms control [5, 6]. For microscopically retained disease, 60 Gy photon radiation is administered over a period of 6–8 weeks. The dose is increased to 60–70 Gy for macroscopic residual tumor control [12, 19]. This higher dose of radiation is also used for surgically unresectable disease. Endotracheal brachytherapy has been shown to prolong survival and improve symptoms management in palliative or advanced tracheal tumors [23, 26]. There is lack of evidence on the role of combined endotracheal brachytherapy and external beam radiotherapy.

29.14 Chemotherapy

There is currently no evidence to support the use of chemotherapy in addition to surgery and radiotherapy for PTT. In the available literature, cisplatin is the most commonly used drug along with cyclophosphamide. Both these drugs have not been shown to improve overall survival or be of great help in palliation of airway symptoms [17, 25].

29.15 Immunotherapy

Immunotherapy has been tried in cases of recurrent SCC of the trachea and some case reports have showed significant response. Nivolumab has been proved to provide good response [26].

29.16 Conclusion

PTTs are rare neoplastic lesions with a wide variety of both benign and malignant tumor histotypes. Most patients with PTTs are diagnosed at an advanced stage due to the nonspecific nature of the presenting symptoms. Primary surgical resection with adjuvant radiotherapy is the main modality of treatment and offers the best outcomes for most patients. Transoral endotracheal debridement with laser, microdebridement, or cryotherapy can be used for symptom control. Radiotherapy alone can be used in patients not suitable for surgical resection and for symptom control.

References

1. Bhattacharyya N. Contemporary staging and prognosis for primary tracheal malignancies: a population-based analysis. Otolaryngol Head Neck Surg. 2004;131(5):639–42.
2. Licht PB, Friis S, Pettersson G. Tracheal cancer in Denmark: a nationwide study. Eur J Cardiothorac Surg. 2001;19(3):339–45.
3. Gelder CM, Hetzel MR. Primary tracheal tumours: a national survey. Thorax. 1993;48(7):688–92.
4. Manninen MP, Antila PJ, Pukander JS, Karma PH. Occurrence of tracheal carcinoma in Finland. Acta Otolaryngol. 1991;111(6):1162–9.
5. Macchiarini P. Primary tracheal tumours. Lancet Oncol. 2006;7(1):83–91.
6. Mathisen DJ. Primary tracheal tumor management. Surg Oncol Clin N Am. 1999;8(2):307.
7. Grillo HC, Mathisen DJ, Wain JC. Management of tumors of the trachea. Oncology (Williston Park). 1992;6(2):61–7; discussion 8, 70, 2.
8. Wood DE. Management of malignant tracheobronchial obstruction. Surg Clin North Am. 2002;82(3):621–42.
9. Subramaniam T, O'Neill JP. Management of primary tracheal tumours. J ENT Masterclass. 2017;10(1):105–8.
10. Honings J, van Dijck JA, Verhagen AF, van der Heijden HF, Marres HA. Incidence and treatment of tracheal cancer: a nationwide study in the Netherlands. Ann Surg Oncol. 2007;14(2):968–76.
11. Diaz-Mendoza J, Debiane L, Peralta AR, Simoff M. Tracheal tumors. Curr Opin Pulm Med. 2019;25(4):336–43.
12. Napieralska A, Miszczyk L, Blamek S. Tracheal cancer - treatment results, prognostic factors and incidence of other neoplasms. Radiol Oncol. 2016;50(4):409–17.
13. Honings J, Gaissert HA, van der Heijden HF, Verhagen AF, Kaanders JH, Marres HA. Clinical aspects and treatment of primary tracheal malignancies. Acta Otolaryngol. 2010;130(7):763–72.
14. Chen F, Huang M, Xu Y, Li T, Xie K, Zhang L, et al. Primary tracheal adenoid cystic carcinoma: adjuvant treatment outcome. Int J Clin Oncol. 2015;20(4):686–92.
15. Drevet G, Conti M, Deslauriers J. Surgical anatomy of the tracheobronchial tree. J Thorac Dis. 2016;8(Suppl 2):S121–9.
16. Salassa JR, Pearson BW, Payne WS. Gross and microscopical blood supply of the trachea. Ann Thorac Surg. 1977;24(2):100–7.
17. Varela P, Pio L, Brandigi E, Paraboschi I, Khen-Dunlop N, Hervieux E, et al. Tracheal and bronchial tumors. J Thorac Dis. 2016;8(12):3781–6.
18. Benissan-Messan DZ, Merritt RE, Bazan JG, D'Souza DM, Abdel-Rasoul M, Moffatt-Bruce SD, et al. National Utilization of surgery and outcomes for primary tracheal cancer in the United States. Ann Thorac Surg. 2020;110(3):1012–22.
19. Subramaniam T, Lennon P, Kinsella J, O'Neill JP. Laryngeal preservation in managing advanced tracheal adenoid cystic carcinoma. Case Rep Otolaryngol. 2015;2015:404586.
20. Webb BD, Walsh GL, Roberts DB, Sturgis EM. Primary tracheal malignant neoplasms: the University of Texas MD Anderson Cancer Center experience. J Am Coll Surg. 2006;202(2):237–46.
21. Gaafar AH, Shaaban AY, Elhadidi MS. The use of metallic expandable tracheal stents in the management of inoperable malignant tracheal obstruction. Eur Arch Otorhinolaryngol. 2012;269(1):247–53.
22. Kacker A, Huo J. Reinforcement of an end-to-end tracheal resection anastomosis with fibrin glue: a case report. Ear Nose Throat J. 2001;80(4):234–6, 8.
23. Nguyen NT, Timotin E, Hunter R, Hann C, Puksa S, Sur RK. Endotracheal brachytherapy alone: an effective palliative treatment for tracheal tumors. Brachytherapy. 2015;14(4):543–8.
24. Cheung AY. Radiotherapy for primary carcinoma of the trachea. Radiother Oncol. 1989;14(4):279–85.
25. Manninen MP, Pukander JS, Flander MK, Laippala PJ, Huhtala HS, Karma PH. Treatment of primary tracheal carcinoma in Finland in 1967-1985. Acta Oncol. 1993;32(3):277–82.
26. Arora S, Bhargava A, Singh R. Airway management for tracheal stent insertion in a patient with difficult airway. Indian J Anaesth. 2013;57(6):617–9.

Reconstruction of the Laryngeal and Pharyngeal Defects

30

Xavier León, Carmen Vega, Maria Casasayas, and Miquel Quer

Core Messages

- The elements to take into account when planning a reconstructive surgery are the extent of the defect, the general condition and comorbidities of the patient, the surgical team's experience, and the available resources.
- The optimal technique is the one that allows a one-stage reconstruction, with the lowest associated morbidity, minimizing the hospital stay, and offering an early functional recovery.
- Previous treatments with radiotherapy or chemo-radiotherapy alter tissue properties, which can hinder the healing process.
- In almost all cases of simple total laryngectomy without extension to the hypopharynx, a sufficient amount of mucosa is available to allow closure by direct suture.
- In patients undergoing an extended total laryngectomy with a partial pharyngectomy in which the direct suture of the remaining hypopharyngeal mucosa is not feasible, it is necessary the supply of tissue to achieve the reconstruction of the neo-pharynx.
- Reconstructive options in patients treated with an extended total laryngectomy with a partial pharyngectomy include the use of pedicled regional flaps such as the pectoralis major or the supraclavicular flaps, or free flaps such as the radial forearm or the anterolateral tight free flaps.
- Patients treated with a total laryngopharyngectomy require circumferential reconstruction of the pharyngeal segment. The techniques that allow this circumferential reconstruction include regional flaps such as the pectoralis major flap, fasciocutaneous flaps as the radial forearm or the anterolateral thigh

X. León (✉) · M. Casasayas · M. Quer
Otorhinolaryngology Department, Hospital de la Santa Creu i Sant Pau, Universitat Autònoma de Barcelona, Barcelona, Spain
e-mail: xleon@santpau.cat; mcasasayas@santpau.cat; mquer@santpau.cat

C. Vega
Plastic Surgery Department, Hospital de la Santa Creu i Sant Pau, Universitat Autònoma de Barcelona, Barcelona, Spain
e-mail: cvega@santpau.cat

M. Remacle, H. E. Eckel (eds.), *Textbook of Surgery of Larynx and Trachea*,
https://doi.org/10.1007/978-3-031-09621-1_30

free flaps, or visceral flaps as the jejunal or the gastro-omental free flaps.
- The reconstruction of choice in cases of laryngo-pharyngo-esophagectomy is the gastric transposition ('gastric pull-up').
- The purpose of salivary bypass tubes is to channel saliva and secretions, minimizing the exposure of suture lines to saliva contamination, and to maintain the caliber of the reconstruction of an otherwise highly collapsible neopharynx.

30.1 Introduction

The elements to take into account when planning a reconstructive strategy after laryngopharyngeal surgery are the extent of the defect created after oncological ablation, the general condition and comorbidities of the patient, the surgical team's experience, and the available resources. The ultimate goal of the reconstructive surgery is to achieve a functional restoration of the three main functions of the laryngopharyngeal segment: breathing, swallowing, and speech, minimizing postoperative morbidity and improving patient's quality of life.

The optimal technique is one that allows a one-stage reconstruction, with the lowest associated morbidity, minimizing the hospital stay, and offering an early functional recovery. Before surgery, it is necessary to perform an individualized assessment of each patient, considering the location and extent of the defect to be reconstructed, patient's characteristics and comorbidities, and previous treatments received. It is necessary to perform a nutritional assessment as well as an optimization of any existing systemic disease. In patients treated previously with radiotherapy, it is important to specifically assess the thyroid function.

Nowadays, a majority of resections of initial laryngeal or hypopharyngeal tumors are done transorally by laser or robotic platforms, usually without requiring a reconstruction time. In addition, the generalized use of preservation protocols in patients with advanced tumors has resulted in an increase of salvage surgery in previously irradiated fields. When planning surgical reconstruction, these previous treatments must be taken into account, since they can alter the healing process and favor the appearance of postoperative complications.

30.2 Classification of Laryngopharyngeal Defects

Table 30.1 shows a modified classification of laryngopharyngeal defects based on the proposal of Van der Putten et al. [1]. Type I laryngeal defects refer to the resection created after vertical hemilaryngectomy via external approach, and type II to a simple total laryngectomy. Type I hypopharyngeal defects refer to limited resections of the posterior hypopharyngeal wall (Ia) or the lateral hypopharyngeal wall (Ib), which are frequently combined with a partial supraglottic laryngectomy. Type II hypopharyngeal defect or greater imply performing an extended total laryn-

Table 30.1 Classification of pharyngolaryngeal defects

		Laryngeal defect	Hypopharyngeal defect
Larynx	I	Partial laryngectomy (hemilaryngectomy)	None
	II	Total laryngectomy	None or partial
Hypopharynx	Ia	None	Partial (posterior wall)
	Ib	Partial laryngectomy (supraglottic)	Partial (pyriform sinus)
	II	Total laryngectomy	Partial
	III	Total laryngectomy	Total circumferential
	IV	Total laryngectomy	Total circumferential + esophagectomy

gectomy with a variable resection of hypopharyngeal parts.

30.3 Type I Laryngeal Defect (Vertical Hemilaryngectomy)

After performing a vertical hemilaryngectomy involving the removal of one arytenoid, in order to avoid aspirations and improve phonation, reconstruction is needed. Many techniques have been described to reconstruct the hemilarynx, including the pedicled thyroid ala cartilaginous flaps, local rotation flaps such as the infrahyoid or the platysma flap, or free flaps such as the radial forearm free flap.

30.4 Type II Laryngeal Defect (Simple Total Laryngectomy)

In almost all cases of simple total laryngectomy without extension to the hypopharynx, a sufficient amount of mucosa is available to allow closure by direct suture. The aim is to obtain a watertight closure with the adequate approximation to avoid the vascular compromise and the excessive tension in the suture line. Suture techniques of the hypopharyngeal mucosa vary based on the surgeon's experience and preferences. Some studies have compared the results obtained with T-type, linear vertical or horizontal closures, finding few significant differences related to swallowing function or the risk of developing fistulas [2]. In a study that compared the horizontal versus vertical closure method in the surgical closure of the pharynx after total laryngectomy, Thrasyvoulou et al. [3] concluded that horizontal closure of the neopharynx was superior to vertical closure in terms of postoperative swallowing function.

In selected cases with endolaryngeal tumors, the use of mechanical stapling devices is feasible. This technique has shown similar postoperative complication rates compared to the traditional suture techniques, without compromising oncological results [4]. According to the results obtained by Gonçalves et al. [5], primary closure using mechanical stapling devices achieved a significant reduction in the percentage of pharyngocutaneous fistula compared to standard suturing techniques (7% vs 37%, $P = 0.0005$).

In cases of extended total laryngectomy with limited resection of the hypopharyngeal mucosa, a direct suture of the residual pharyngeal mucosa is sometimes feasible. According to Hui et al. [6], the minimum extension of residual pharyngeal mucosa needed to perform a primary reconstruction without swallowing difficulty is 1.5 cm relaxed and 2.5 cm stretched. Ragbir et al. [7] suggested that pharyngeal defects with more than 3.5 cm of remaining pharyngeal mucosal could be closed primarily, but defects with less than 3.5 cm require interposition of imported tissue.

When the surgeon has to decide how much mucosa will allow a direct reconstruction of the pharynx, it should take into account that previous treatments with radiotherapy or chemoradiotherapy alter tissue properties. In irradiated patients, a swollen, nonelastic, and devascularized residual hypopharyngeal mucosa hinders the possibility of primarily closure. To reduce the risk of major wound complications in patients undergoing a salvage total laryngectomy with direct closure of the hypopharynx, several authors advocate for the use of onlay flaps in order to provide a well-vascularized and nonirradiated tissue on the pharyngeal closure to reinforce the sealing of the wound. Technical options include regional flaps such as the pectoralis major myofascial flap or the supraclavicular flap, or free flaps as the radial forearm free flap or the temporoparietal fascial free flap. In a study of patients treated with a salvage total laryngectomy after radiotherapy, Gendreau-Lefèvre et al. [8] found that the elective use of an onlay pectoralis major flap reduced significantly the incidence of pharyngocutaneous fistula, which was 14% in the onlay flap group compared to 36% when only primary closure was done ($P = 0.004$). A systematic review proved a 22% decreased risk of pharyngocutaneous fistula in patients undergoing an onlay pectoralis major flap compared to primary closure [9]. Other authors have shown the utility of other onlay flaps in patients treated with a salvage laryngectomy such as the supraclavicular flap [10], the radial forearm free flap, the anterolateral thigh flap [11], or the temporoparietal fascia free flap [12].

In the cases in which an extended total laryngectomy with en-bloc resection of the prelaryngeal soft tissues and the cervical skin (squared laryngectomy) is performed, a reconstruction of the anterior neck defect is needed. The most commonly used method is the pectoralis major flap, although other regional skin flaps have also been used such as the deltopectoral, supraclavicular, or internal mammary perforator flaps, or free flaps [13].

30.5 Type Ia Hypopharyngeal Defect (Defect in the Hypopharyngeal Posterior Wall)

Little defects in the posterior wall of the hypopharynx without connection to the neck can be left to heal secondarily or can be reconstructed using split-thickness skin grafts. Most times, the best option is to let the area heal by secondary intention after fixing down the remnant edges of the mucosa to the prevertebral fascia with interrupted sutures to form a watertight seal.

30.6 Type Ib Hypopharyngeal Defect (Defect in the Hypopharyngeal Lateral Wall)

Frequently, the removal of tumors located on the lateral wall of the hypopharynx with an external approach is associated with a supraglottic laryngectomy. Small defects can usually be closed with direct suture. Occasionally, depending on the extension of the resection or previous treatments with radiotherapy, which let foresee healing problems, a reconstructive time will be indicated. For defects smaller than 3 cm, there are a variety of local flaps available, including the infrahyoid flap, the sternocleidomastoid muscle flap, or the platysma flap. For defects greater than 3 cm, it is required to provide tissue by using regional or free flaps. Regional flap options that allow to place a skin paddle in the defect include the supraclavicular flap, the submental flap, or the pectoralis major myocutaneous flap. In cases where a free flap reconstruction is preferred, a radial forearm flap or an anterolateral thigh free flap should be considered.

30.7 Type II Hypopharyngeal Defects (Total Laryngectomy with Partial Pharyngectomy)

In patients undergoing an extended total laryngectomy with a partial pharyngectomy in which the direct suture of the remaining hypopharyngeal mucosa is not feasible, it is necessary the supply of tissue to achieve the reconstruction of the neo-pharynx. Reconstructive options include the use of pedicled regional flaps such as the pectoralis major or the supraclavicular flaps, or free flaps such as the radial forearm or the anterolateral tight free flaps.

30.7.1 Regional Flaps

30.7.1.1 Pectoralis Major Myocutaneous Flap

Since its description by Ariyan in 1979 [14], the pectoralis major myocutaneous flap has been used extensively in the reconstruction of head and neck defects, including laryngopharyngectomy cases. The advantages offered by this flap compared to other pedicled flaps are its rich vascularization, which makes it a robust and reliable flap, the skin paddle that can be included, the disposal of a rotation arch that allows easy reaching of the anterior cervical region, and the primary closure of the donor-site in most occasions. The flap can be designed with a skin paddle to reconstruct hypopharyngeal defects, or as an onlay fasciomuscular flap for support in cases of salvage total laryngectomy. Compared to free flaps, one of the advantages of the pectoralis major flap is that it is a simple reconstruction technique, with reduced operative time, especially important in fragile and elderly patients, and it is a great option to consider in patients with a vessel-depleted neck. In addition, it does not require microsurgical training, which facilitates its use in centers with a small number of cancer patients or limited resources.

The main disadvantage of the pectoral flap is that, depending on the patient's constitution, it is excessively bulky, which makes it difficult to suture and adapt it to the defect. In addition, in cases where a significant portion of the base of the tongue or the lateral wall of the oropharynx is resected, the weight and downward traction of the flap can significantly limit the mobility of the residual tongue, impairing speech articulation and swallowing function.

Donor site morbidity includes cosmetic deformity altering the nipple position, impairment of upper limb motion, and restriction of chest-wall expansion. In female patients, the flap design should be placed under the breast, with a more distal skin paddle and susceptible to failure, being a suboptimal reconstructive option in most cases.

The surgical technique includes the design of the skin paddle based on an arc of rotation placed in the midpoint of the clavicle. The skin paddle is then sutured to the pharyngeal margins, using the muscular portion of the flap to reinforce the mucosal suture and protect the vascular axis, especially in the case of irradiated patients.

The reliability of the pectoralis major myocutaneous flap is very high, with an overall reduced incidence of complete flap failure, which was 0.5% in a review of 279 cases published by different authors after a partial or total laryngopharyngectomy [15]. The grouped frequency of pharyngeal cutaneous fistula was 27%, and the frequency of distal stenosis was 17%. The variables that have been related to flap necrosis are age over 70 years, female sex, overweight, and low nutritional status [16].

Several authors have analyzed the use of the pectoralis major flap in comparison with free flaps in the reconstruction of the hypopharynx. According to Shektman et al. [17], the benefits, complications, and functional outcomes of both techniques appear to be comparable. However, for van Brederode [18], free flaps result in a significantly better functional outcome and fewer recipient site complications than the pectoralis major myocutaneous flap.

Today, for most teams, the pectoralis major flap appears as a second option after free flaps for reconstruction after a partial or total laryngopharyngectomy. It should be considered as a first option in elderly patients with high comorbidities, who would not tolerate the complexity required by a free flap.

30.7.1.2 Supraclavicular Flap

The supraclavicular artery island flap, originally described by Pallua et al. [19], is a pedicled fasciocutaneous flap based on the supraclavicular vessels, which arise from the transverse cervical vessels. It allows to obtain a flap with a skin paddle designed on the ventral side of the deltoid muscle, within the angiosome of the supraclavicular vessels, with extensions up to 15 cm in length and 12 cm in width. It has been used in the reconstruction of partial defects of the pharynx [10], and tubularized, allows the reconstruction of the defect created after a total laryngopharyngectomy [20] (Fig. 30.1). Since the distance between the pharynx and the supraclavicular fossa is relatively short, the island does not need to be designed beyond the superior half of the deltoid. An advantage of the supraclavicular flap is that it is a thin and pliable flap, easily adaptable to the hypopharyngeal defect. Up to 20% of patients will not

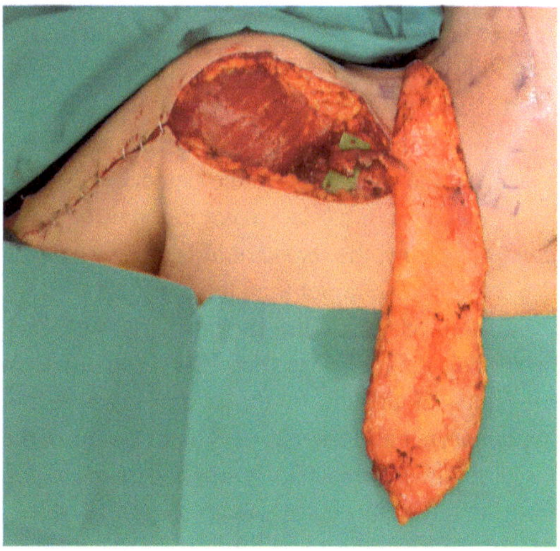

Fig. 30.1 Supraclavicular flap

have the branch of the transverse cervical artery and preoperative audible doppler will allow for assessment of this vessel as it runs over the lateral clavicle into the deltoid region [21].

It has been described as an adipofascial flap placed onlay to reinforce the hypopharyngeal suture of patients treated with a salvage total laryngectomy after radiotherapy [10].

Reiter et al. [22] compared the results of the supraclavicular flap with those obtained with the radial forearm and anterolateral thigh free flaps in patients treated with a partial or total laryngopharyngectomy. No significant differences were found between the different groups in the rate of pharyngocutaneous fistulas (supraclavicular flap 11% vs. anterolateral thigh flap14% vs. radial forearm flap 11%; $P = 0.944$), distal stenosis (supraclavicular flap 11% vs. anterolateral thigh flap14% vs. radial forearm flap 16%; $P = 0.874$), or gastric tube dependency (supraclavicular flap 28% vs. anterolateral thigh23% vs. radial forearm flap 16%; $P = 0.590$).

30.7.2 Free Flaps

30.7.2.1 Radial Forearm Free Flap

Described by Yang et al. on 1981 [23], the specific advantage of the radial flap in hypopharyngeal reconstruction compared to other free flaps such as the anterolateral tight free flap is that it is a thin and pliable flap that is easily contoured. It is an easily harvested flap with a long pedicle and an excellent caliber of the vessels. In addition, the thickness of the skin paddle matches the thickness of the pharyngoesophageal wall, which facilitates the adaptation to the defect.

In cases of total laryngectomy with partial pharyngectomy, the flap should be designed such that it is 10–20% larger than the defect itself so as to accommodate for tissue shrinkage, and then proceed to the interposition of the skin paddle on the mucosal defect. In those cases where the hypopharyngeal defect is less than 50% of the visceral lumen, this flap is applied in its patch form, while in those cases with a subtotal resection of the hypopharynx with just a residual strip of posterior hypopharyngeal mucosa, the reconstruction acquires an "omega" shape [24].

The main drawback of the radial flap is related to the morbidity of the donor area, including delays in healing due to skin graft loss, tendon exposure with stiffness, poor aesthetic outcomes, and cold intolerance of the hand because of hypovascularization. In addition, the proximity of the upper extremity to the cervical region, although it does not prevent the simultaneous work of the cervical resection and reconstruction teams, makes it more uncomfortable compared to other more distal flaps.

As a consequence of these disadvantages, many centers do not consider the radial forearm free flap as the first option in the reconstruction of the hypopharynx after a partial or total laryngopharyngectomy. The radial forearm free flap would appear as the technique of choice in obese patients, in which treatment alternatives, like regional flaps such as the pectoralis major flap or free flaps such as the anterolateral tight flap, would offer a suboptimal reconstruction.

30.7.2.2 Anterolateral Thigh Free Flap

Described by Song et al. [25] in 1984, the anterolateral thigh flap has gained popularity, becoming the reconstructive technique of choice for head and neck soft tissue defects for a large number of surgical teams due to its anatomic consistency, reliability, and plastic versatility. In the majority of patients, the anterolateral thigh donor site provides a well-vascularized, thin, and pliable tissue ideal for reconstruction of partial pharyngeal defects. Depending on the patient's constitution, the thickness of this flap can be very variable, limiting its use as a first choice technique in obese patients.

The anterolateral thigh flap can be raised as a chimeric flap with a muscular component of the vastus lateralis muscle, which can be used to protect the suture line and cover the vascular axis in patients treated with a radical neck dissection, or as a vascular bed for skin grafting in the reconstruction of skin defects [26]. Moreover, two separate skin paddles can be harvested based on independent perforating arteries or with a deepithelialized bridge of subcutaneous tissue, allowing a simultaneous reconstruction of the pharynx and cervical skin defects [27].

The main advantage of the anterolateral thigh flap lies in the low donor-site morbidity. A direct closure of the donor site is usually possible, and typically the only sequels include a vertically scar along the thigh and some thigh numbness. In addition, given the distance between the donor area and the neck, it facilitates the simultaneous work of the resection and reconstruction teams.

30.8 Type III Hypopharyngeal Defect (Total Laryngectomy with Total Pharyngectomy)

Patients treated with a total laryngopharyngectomy require circumferential reconstruction of the pharyngeal segment, which entails a higher risk of postoperative complications and long-term morbidity compared to patients with a partial resection of the pharynx. The techniques that allow this circumferential reconstruction include regional flaps such as the pectoralis major flap, as well as fasciocutaneous or visceral free flaps.

30.8.1 Regional Flaps

30.8.1.1 Pectoralis Major Myocutaneous Flap

The bulkiness of the cutaneous and muscular portions of the pectoralis major myocutaneous flap usually prevents its tubularization, or it is associated with an unacceptable frequency of fistulization and stenosis. In order to avoid these limitations, Fabian [28] proposed a technical modification involving a "horseshoe-shaped" reconstruction of the circumferential hypopharyngeal defect. It consists in suturing the lateral edges of the pectoralis major flap skin paddle directly to the prevertebral fascia, while the posterior wall is reconstructed with a skin graft placed over the prevertebral fascia. In this way, it is possible to reduce the flap thickness and obtain an adequate lumen caliber (Fig. 30.2).

The main drawback of this technique is the high percentage of fistulization, which reaches 50% of cases [29], increasing postoperative mor-

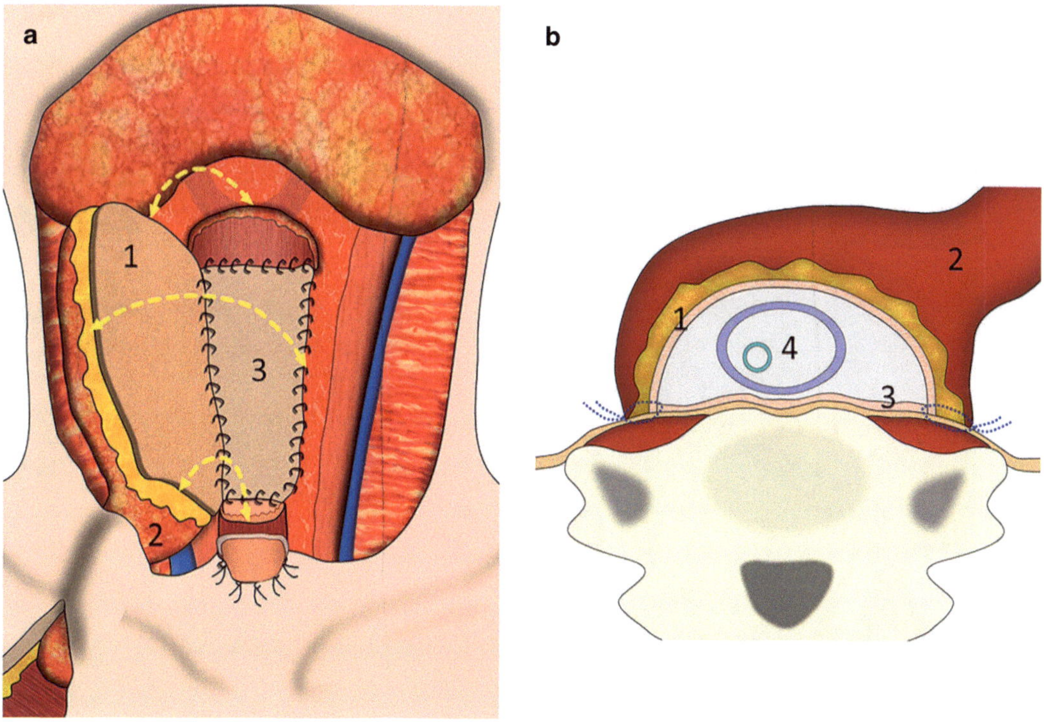

Fig. 30.2 Reconstruction of a total laryngopharyngectomy with pectoralis major myocutaneous flap. (**a**) Frontal view. (**b**) Axial section of the reconstruction. (*1* Cutaneous paddle, *2* Pectoralis major muscle, *3* Skin graft placed over the prevertebral fascia, *4* Salivary bypass tube and nasogastric tube)

bidity and duration of hospital stay in comparison with other reconstruction techniques.

As in the reconstruction of partial pharyngeal defects, this technique would be indicated in those patients with high morbidity in whom the use of free flaps is considered contraindicated.

30.8.2 Free Flaps

30.8.2.1 Radial Forearm Free Flap

One of the most commonly used options in the reconstruction of the hypopharyngeal defect after a total laryngopharyngectomy is the radial forearm free flap following the technique described in 1985 by Harii et al. [30]. This technique consists in performing a complete tubularization of the flap by vertical interrupted sutures into the inverted skin paddle, that it is anastomosed to the oropharynx superiorly and to the cervical esophagus inferiorly (Fig. 30.3). Chen et al. [31] proposed a technical modification consisting in a deepithelialization of the vertical edges with a two-layer suture as a reliable method to decrease the postoperative leakage rate (Fig. 30.4). The radial forearm flap allows to obtain a skin paddle up to 12–14 cm long, making possible the reconstruction of almost all the defects after a total laryngopharyngectomy. In order to prevent stricture formation and stenosis at the level of the flap suture with the cervical esophagus, it is important to avoid circular sutures. To break up the circumferential scar, once the posterior wall of the cervical esophagus is sutured to the prevertebral fascia, it is advisable to make a vertical incision at the anterior edge of the cervical esophagus and interpose an extension of the flap according to a lock-and-key closure (Fig. 30.5).

The use of a "horseshoe-shaped" conformation of the free fasciocutaneous flaps has been described in cases of total laryngopharyngectomy, suturing the lateral margins of the flap to the prevertebral fascia and creating two vertical suture lines in a similar way to the technique described by Fabian with the pectoralis major flap, which allows the reduction of the size of the skin island required [32].

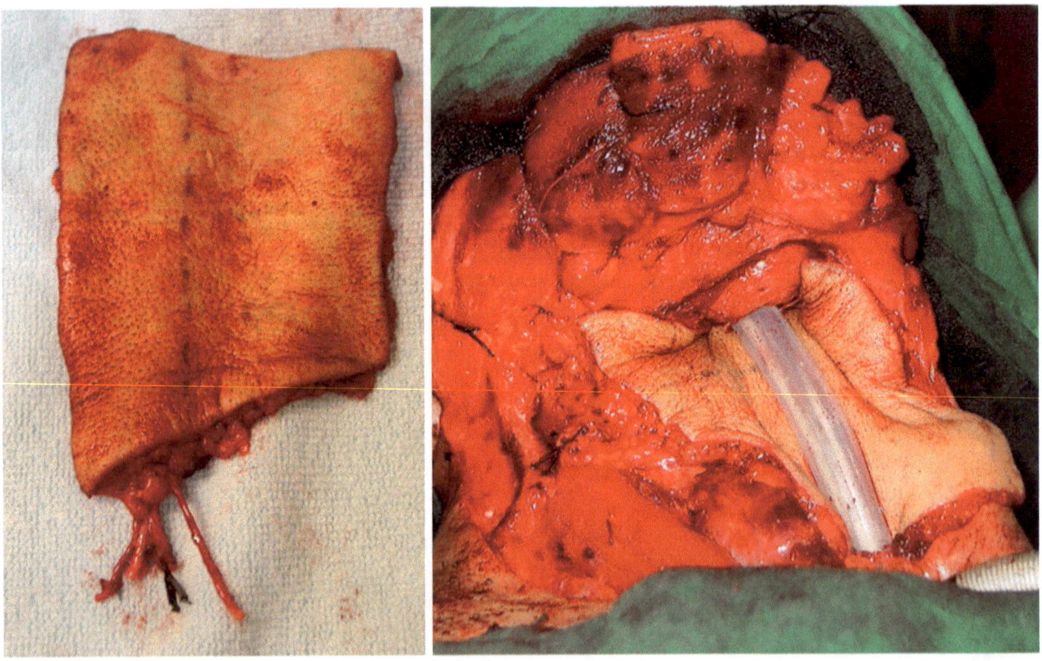

Fig. 30.3 Reconstruction of a total laryngopharyngectomy defect with a radial forearm free flap

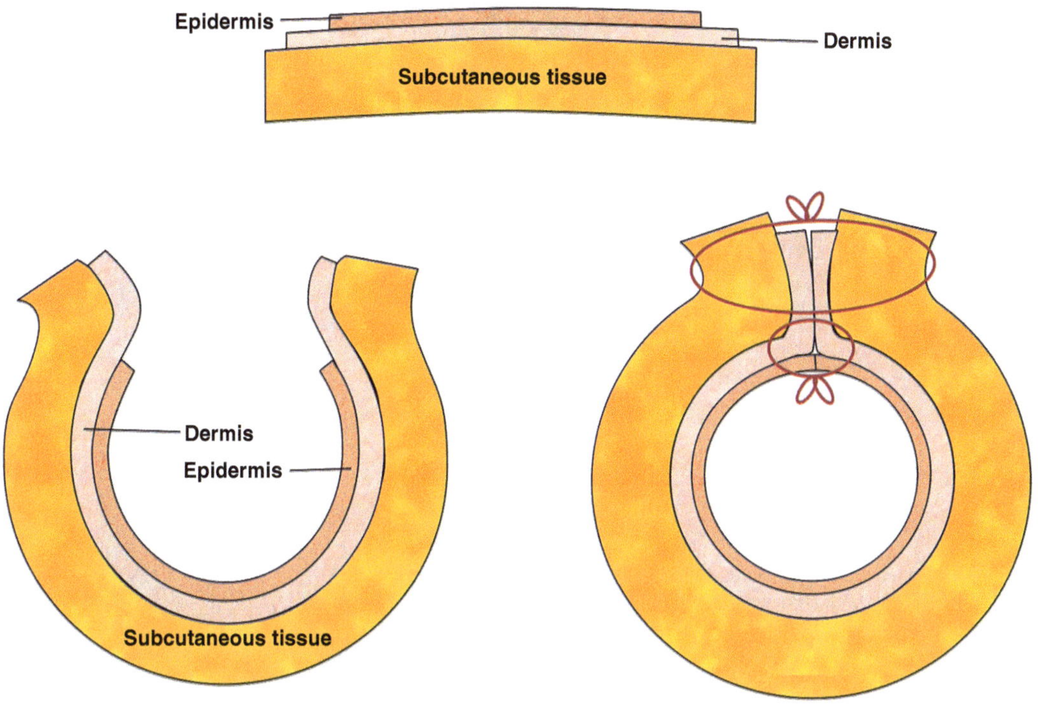

Fig. 30.4 Tubing of edge-deepithelialized skin flap with two-layered sutures. Note that deepithelialized flap edges were sutured at each other (modified of Chen et al. [31])

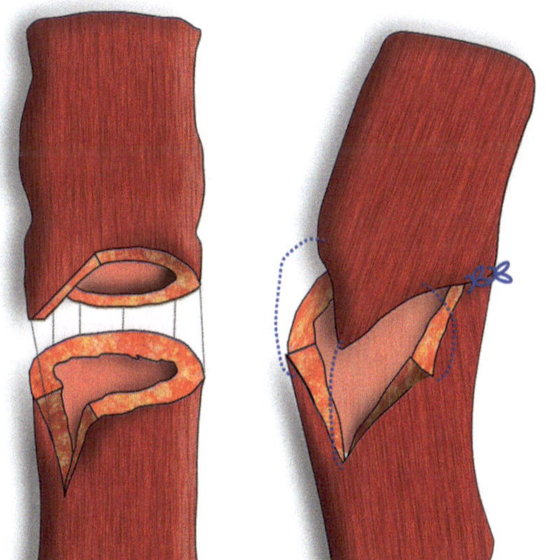

Fig. 30.5 Vertical incision at the anterior edge of the cervical esophagus and interposition of an extension of the flap to break the circumferential scar

In a review of different series of patients treated with a partial or total laryngopharyngectomy reconstructed with a radial forearm free flap, the mean incidence of pharyngocutaneous fistulas was of 20%, with a stenosis rate of 11% [15].

30.8.2.2 Anterolateral Thigh Free Flap

The anterolateral thigh flap can be tubularized in cases where a circumferential reconstruction of the hypopharynx is required, following the same technique as previously described for the radial forearm flap (Fig. 30.6). Another option is to fold the skin paddle on itself to form a conical design as proposed by Genden et al. [33]. When the thickness of the flap difficult its tubularization, an alternative consists in suturing it to the prevertebral fascia in accordance with the "horseshoe-shaped" design used in reconstructions with a pectoralis major myocutaneous flap.

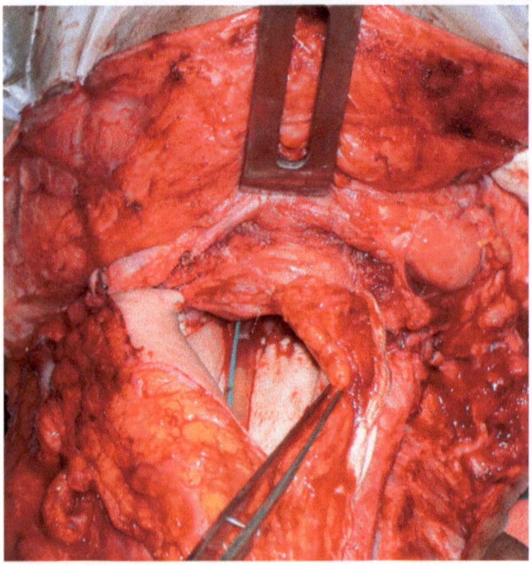

Fig. 30.6 Reconstruction of a total laryngopharyngectomy defect with a tubed anterolateral thigh free flap (courtesy of Dr. Jirky Vuola)

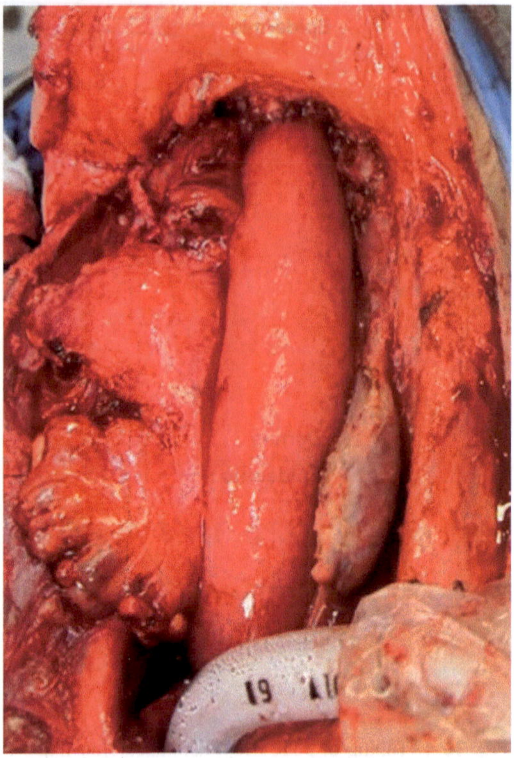

Fig. 30.7 Reconstruction of a total laryngopharyngectomy defect with a jejunal free flap (courtesy of Dr. Frederic Kolb)

The mean fistulization rate in hypopharyngeal reconstructions with anterolateral thigh flaps has been calculated at 15%, with a risk of distal stenosis of 9% [15].

Based on the results obtained, for some authors, the anterolateral thigh free flap has become the method of choice in the reconstruction of circumferential pharyngeal defects, with the exception of obese patients in which an alternative technique such as a radial forearm free flap or a visceral flaps would be indicated [34].

30.8.2.3 Jejunal Free Flap

The jejunal free flap, described by Seidenberg in 1959 [35], is the oldest reconstructive technique for circumferential pharyngeal defects still in use. From the 1980s, with the development of microsurgery, this flap gained popularity in the reconstruction of the hypopharynx and cervical esophagus (Fig. 30.7). However, throughout the last decades, it has been progressively substituted in many centers by fasciocutaneous free flaps such as the anterolateral thigh flap.

The main advantage of reconstruction with a jejunal free flap is the low percentage of fistulization compared to other reconstructive methods. However, the need for an abdominal time adds complexity to the postoperative period as well as the possibility of serious complications would justify its abandonment in favor of simpler techniques that offer similar functional results [36, 37]. Mean perioperative mortality of the jejunum free flap is 2.5%, at least four times higher than that reported using fasciocutaneous free flaps [15]. Another drawback of the jejunum free flap is that the length of the vascular pedicle is shorter than in other alternative flaps, and it has a limited tolerance to ischemia, with a consequently shorter time for microvascular anastomosis. Furthermore, swallowing can be impaired by small bowel peristalsis uncoordinated with the rest of the upper digestive tract [37]. Besides, the continued secretion of mucus from the jejunum results in a "wet" voice after voice rehabilitation with a tracheoesophageal prosthesis.

According to the results of a review including patients undergoing a laryngopharyngectomy reconstructed with a jejunal free flap, the mean frequency of fistulization was 12%, and of distal stricture 11% [15]. These results are comparable to those obtained using a fasciocutaneous flap as the anterolateral thigh flap, which have a lower morbidity and a lower risk of severe complications.

30.8.2.4 Gastro-Omental Free Flap

The gastro-omental free flap is a tubular flap that is formed from the greater curve of the stomach, which is nourished by the right gastroepiploic artery and vein, which also supplies an apron of omentum. The main advantage of this visceral flap is the possibility of having a large amount of highly vascularized tissue with wound-healing properties provided by the rich source of fibroblasts and other progenitor cells of the omentum. This tissue facilitates the local healing process, minimizing the risk of fistulization in the irradiated fields associated with salvage surgeries [38]. Additional advantages include the length of the vascular pedicle (up to 30 cm), its caliber (2–4 mm), and the plasticity and mobility of the omentum, which can be simultaneously used for draping the neopharyngeal conduit, covering exposed vessels, and filling dead spaces.

The disadvantage of this flap is the morbidity of the abdominal time surgery, with a mean percentage of donor-site complications of 13%, and a perioperative mortality of 3.2%, similar to the one reported for patients treated with a jejunal free flap [15].

30.9 Type IV Hypopharyngeal Defect (Laryngo-Pharyngo-Esophagectomy)

In those patients in whom the hypopharyngeal tumor extends to the cervical esophagus and caudally reaches the thoracic inlet, it is technically impossible to perform the distal anastomosis with a regional flap or a tubularized free flap. Furthermore, from an oncological point of view and in order to achieve satisfactory resection margins, the performance of a laryngo-pharyngo-esophagectomy is indicated in these patients.

The reconstruction of choice in cases of laryngo-pharyngo-esophagectomy is the gastric transposition ("gastric pull-up"). The main advantage of this technique is to allow the reconstruction of the digestive tract with just one suture line, using a highly vascularized tissue and without the requirement of vascular microanastomosis (Fig. 30.8). The abdominal time can be done with a laparotomy or using an endoscopic approach. The abdominal team frees the stomach keeping its irrigation from the right gastroepiploic vessels and transposes it through the posterior mediastinum to make stomach's fundus to reach the upper pharyngostome [39], or tubing the stomach by resecting the lesser curvature [40]. The main disadvantage of this technique is its morbidity and mortality, so its indication should be carefully made considering the medical history and general condition of the patient. In a meta-analysis of the results obtained from the gastric pull-up technique, Butskiy et al. [41] found a significant reduction in perioperative mortality associated with this type of procedure over time. During the studies published between 1959 and 1978, the mortality rate was 19%, while for studies published between 2002 and 2012, it was 6%. The three most common causes of death were respiratory complications (30% of deaths), complications associated to an anastomotic leak

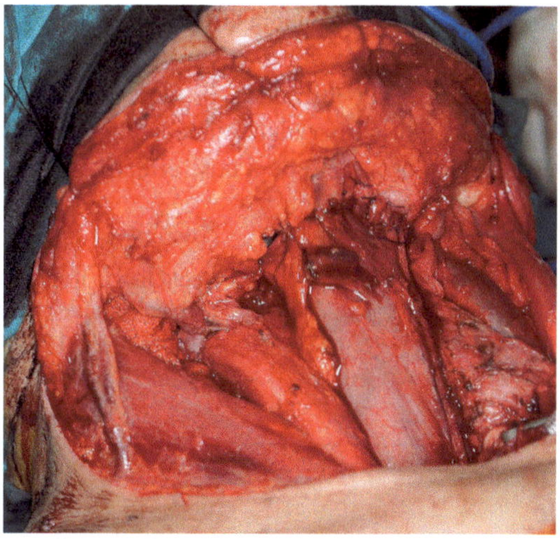

Fig. 30.8 Reconstruction of a laryngo-pharyngo-esophagectomy with a tubularized gastric pull-up

(24% of deaths), and cardiovascular complications (12% of deaths). The risk of anastomotic complications (including anastomotic leak, fistula formation, graft necrosis, and graft failure) was 16%.

In cases where, as a result of a pathology or previous abdominal surgery, it is not possible to use the stomach, a reconstructive alternative would be the use of a colonic interposition.

30.10 Salivary Bypass Tubes

The purpose of salivary bypass tubes is to channel saliva and secretions, minimizing the exposure of suture lines to saliva contamination. It also helps maintain the caliber of the reconstruction of an otherwise highly collapsible neopharynx. According to several authors, its use in patients treated with a laryngopharyngectomy, mainly in those cases reconstructed with a tubed flap, could prevent the appearance of pharyngocutaneous fistulas and stenosis [42, 43].

In our center, we systematically use salivary bypass tubes in those patients treated with a partial or total laryngopharyngectomy, which requires flaps for the reconstruction of the hypopharynx. In absence of complications, the salivary bypass tube is kept in place for a minimum period of 12 days. According to the results of a study carried out in patients treated with a laryngopharyngectomy, the salivary bypass tube achieved a faster resolution in the event of the appearance of a pharyngocutaneous fistula, and it has been proven to be a cost-effective procedure [44].

Acknowledgments The authors would like to thank Dr. Anna Holgado for her assistance in the preparation of the manuscript and Dr. Albert Pujol for the elaboration of the drawings.

References

1. van der Putten L, Spasiano R, de Bree R, Bertino G, Leemans CR, Benazzo M. Flap reconstruction of the hypopharynx: a defect orientated approach. Acta Otorhinolaryngol Ital. 2012;32(5):288–96.
2. Qureshi SS, Chaturvedi P, Pai PS, Chaukar DA, Deshpande MS, Pathak KA, et al. A prospective study of pharyngocutaneous fistulas following total laryngectomy. J Cancer Res Ther. 2005;1(1):51–6. https://doi.org/10.4103/0973-1482.16092.
3. Thrasyvoulou G, Vlastarakos PV, Thrasyvoulou M, Sismanis A. Horizontal (vs. vertical) closure of the neo-pharynx is associated with superior post-operative swallowing after total laryngectomy. Ear Nose Throat J. 2018;97(4–5):E31–5. https://doi.org/10.1177/0145561318097004-502.
4. Sansa-Perna A, Casasayas-Plass M, Rovira-Martínez C, López-Vilas M, García-Lorenzo J, Quer-Agusti M, et al. Pharyngeal closure after a total laryngectomy: mechanical versus manual technique. J Laryngol Otol. 2020;134(7):626–31. https://doi.org/10.1017/S0022215120001371. Epub 2020 Jul 29.
5. Gonçalves AJ, de Souza JA Jr, Menezes MB, Kavabata NK, Suehara AB, Lehn CN. Pharyngocutaneous fistulae following total laryngectomy comparison between manual and mechanical sutures. Eur Arch Otorhinolaryngol. 2009;266(11):1793–8. https://doi.org/10.1007/s00405-009-0945-4. Epub 2009 Mar 13.
6. Hui Y, Wei WI, Yuen PW, Lam LK, Ho WK. Primary closure of pharyngeal remnant after total laryngectomy and partial pharyngectomy: how much residual mucosa is sufficient? Laryngoscope. 1996;106(4):490–4. https://doi.org/10.1097/00005537-199604000-00018.
7. Ragbir M, Brown JS, Mehanna H. Reconstructive considerations in head and neck surgical oncology: United Kingdom National Multidisciplinary Guidelines. J Laryngol Otol. 2016;130(S2):S191–7. https://doi.org/10.1017/S0022215116000621.
8. Gendreau-Lefèvre AK, Audet N, Maltais S, Thuot F. Prophylactic pectoralis major muscle flap in prevention of pharyngocutaneous fistula in total laryngectomy after radiotherapy. Head Neck. 2015;37(9):1233–8. https://doi.org/10.1002/hed.23742. Epub 2014 Jul 24.
9. Guimarães AV, Aires FT, Dedivitis RA, Kulcsar MA, Ramos DM, Cernea CR, et al. Efficacy of pectoralis major muscle flap for pharyngocutaneous fistula prevention in salvage total laryngectomy: a systematic review. Head Neck. 2016;38(Suppl 1):E2317–21. https://doi.org/10.1002/hed.24248. Epub 2015 Nov 11.
10. Emerick KS, Herr MA, Deschler DG. Supraclavicular flap reconstruction following total laryngectomy. Laryngoscope. 2014;124(8):1777–82. https://doi.org/10.1002/lary.24530. Epub 2014 Jan 15.
11. Patel UA, Moore BA, Wax M, Rosenthal E, Sweeny L, Militsakh ON, et al. Impact of pharyngeal closure technique on fistula after salvage laryngectomy. JAMA Otolaryngol Head Neck Surg. 2013;139(11):1156–62. https://doi.org/10.1001/jamaoto.2013.2761.
12. Higgins KM, Ashford B, Erovic BM, Yoo J, Enepekides DJ. Temporoparietal fascia free flap for pharyngeal coverage after salvage total laryngectomy. Laryngoscope. 2012;122(3):523–7. https://doi.org/10.1002/lary.22477. Epub 2011 Dec 6.

13. León X, López M, García J, Casasayas M, Rovira C, Quer M. Indications and results of extended total laryngectomy with en-bloc resection of overlying cervical skin. Eur Arch Otorhinolaryngol. 2019;276(11):3179–84. https://doi.org/10.1007/s00405-019-05573-8. Epub 2019 Jul 26.
14. Ariyan S. The pectoralis major myocutaneous flap. A versatile flap for reconstruction in the head and neck. Plast Reconstr Surg. 1979;63(1):73–81. https://doi.org/10.1097/00006534-197901000-00012.
15. Piazza C, Taglietti V, Nicolai P. Reconstructive options after total laryngectomy with subtotal or circumferential hypopharyngectomy and cervical esophagectomy. Curr Opin Otolaryngol Head Neck Surg. 2012;20(2):77–88. https://doi.org/10.1097/MOO.0b013e328350a5cc.
16. Shah JP, Haribhakti V, Loree TR, Sutaria P. Complications of the pectoralis major myocutaneous flap in head and neck reconstruction. Am J Surg. 1990;160(4):352–5. https://doi.org/10.1016/s0002-9610(05)80541-0.
17. Shektman A, Silver C, Strauch B. A re-evaluation of hypopharyngeal reconstruction: pedicled flaps versus microvascular free flaps. Plast Reconstr Surg. 1997;100(7):1691–6. https://doi.org/10.1097/00006534-199712000-00007.
18. van Brederode TD, Halmos GB, Stenekes MW. Functional outcome after one-stage flap reconstruction of the hypopharynx following tumor ablation. Eur Arch Otorhinolaryngol. 2017;274(2):969–76. https://doi.org/10.1007/s00405-016-4279-8. Epub 2016 Aug 26.
19. Pallua N, Machens HG, Rennekampff O, Becker M, Berger A. The fasciocutaneous supraclavicular artery island flap for releasing postburn mentosternal contractures. Plast Reconstr Surg. 1997;99(7):1878–84; discussion 1885-6. https://doi.org/10.1097/00006534-199706000-00011.
20. Henderson MM, Chiu ES, Jaffer AS. A simple approach of tubularizing the supraclavicular flap for circumferential pharyngoesophageal defects. Plast Reconstr Surg. 2010;126(1):28e–9e. https://doi.org/10.1097/PRS.0b013e3181dab4a5.
21. Lamberty BG. The supra-clavicular axial patterned flap. Br J Plast Surg. 1979;32(3):207–12. https://doi.org/10.1016/s0007-1226(79)90033-x.
22. Reiter M, Baumeister P. Reconstruction of laryngopharyngectomy defects: comparison between the supraclavicular artery island flap, the radial forearm flap, and the anterolateral thigh flap. Microsurgery. 2019;39(4):310–5. https://doi.org/10.1002/micr.30406. Epub 2018 Dec 17.
23. Yang GF, Chen PJ, Gao YZ, Liu XY, Li J, Jiang SX, He SP. Forearm free skin flap transplantation: a report of 56 cases. 1981. Br J Plast Surg. 1997;50(3):162–5. https://doi.org/10.1016/s0007-1226(97)91363-1.
24. Disa JJ, Pusic AL, Hidalgo DA, Cordeiro PG. Microvascular reconstruction of the hypopharynx: defect classification, treatment algorithm, and functional outcome based on 165 consecutive cases. Plast Reconstr Surg. 2003;111(2):652–60; discussion 661-3. https://doi.org/10.1097/01.PRS.0000041987.53831.23.
25. Song YG, Chen GZ, Song YL. The free thigh flap: a new free flap concept based on the septocutaneous artery. Br J Plast Surg. 1984;37(2):149–59. https://doi.org/10.1016/0007-1226(84)90002-x.
26. Lawson BR, Moreno MA. Head and neck reconstruction with chimeric anterolateral thigh free flap: indications, outcomes, and technical considerations. Otolaryngol Head Neck Surg. 2016;154(1):59–65. https://doi.org/10.1177/0194599815606438. Epub 2015 Sep 24.
27. Agarwal JP, Stenson KM, Gottlieb LJ. A simplified design of a dual island fasciocutaneous free flap for simultaneous pharyngoesophageal and anterior neck reconstruction. J Reconstr Microsurg. 2006;22(2):105–12. https://doi.org/10.1055/s-2006-932504.
28. Fabian RL. Reconstruction of the laryngopharynx and cervical esophagus. Laryngoscope. 1984;94(10):1334–50. https://doi.org/10.1288/00005537-198410000-00015.
29. Casasayas M, Sansa A, García-Lorenzo J, López M, Orús C, Peláez X, et al. Pharyngocutaneous fistula after total laryngectomy: multivariate analysis of risk factors and a severity-based classification proposal. Eur Arch Otorhinolaryngol. 2019;276(1):143–51. https://doi.org/10.1007/s00405-018-5200-4. Epub 2018 Nov 13.
30. Harii K, Ebihara S, Ono I, Saito H, Terui S, Takato T. Pharyngoesophageal reconstruction using a fabricated forearm free flap. Plast Reconstr Surg. 1985;75(4):463–76. https://doi.org/10.1097/00006534-198504000-00001.
31. Chen Y, Chen H, Vranckx JJ, Schneeberger AG. Edge deepithelialization: a method to prevent leakage when tubed free skin flap is used for pharyngoesophageal reconstruction. Surgery. 2001;130(1):97–103. https://doi.org/10.1067/msy.2001.115354.
32. Varvares MA, Cheney ML, Gliklich RE, Boyd JM, Goldsmith T, Lazor J, et al. Use of the radial forearm fasciocutaneous free flap and Montgomery salivary bypass tube for pharyngoesophageal reconstruction. Head Neck. 2000;22(5):463–8. https://doi.org/10.1002/1097-0347(200008)22:5<463::aid-hed4>3.0.co;2-s.
33. Genden EM, Jacobson AS. The role of the anterolateral thigh flap for pharyngoesophageal reconstruction. Arch Otolaryngol Head Neck Surg. 2005;131(9):796–9. https://doi.org/10.1001/archotol.131.9.796.
34. Murray DJ, Gilbert RW, Vesely MJ, Novak CB, Zaitlin-Gencher S, Clark JR, et al. Functional outcomes and donor site morbidity following circumferential pharyngoesophageal reconstruction using an anterolateral thigh flap and salivary bypass tube. Head Neck. 2007;29(2):147–54. https://doi.org/10.1002/hed.20489.
35. Seidenberg B, Rosenak SS, Hurwitt ES, Som ML. Immediate reconstruction of the cervical esophagus by a revascularized isolated jejunal seg-

ment. Ann Surg. 1959;149(2):162–71. https://doi.org/10.1097/00000658-195902000-00002.
36. Yu P, Lewin JS, Reece GP, Robb GL. Comparison of clinical and functional outcomes and hospital costs following pharyngoesophageal reconstruction with the anterolateral thigh free flap versus the jejunal flap. Plast Reconstr Surg. 2006;117(3):968–74. https://doi.org/10.1097/01.prs.0000200622.13312.d3.
37. Yeh DH, Sahovaler A, Fung K. Reconstruction after salvage laryngectomy. Oral Oncol. 2017;75:22–7. https://doi.org/10.1016/j.oraloncology.2017.10.009. Epub 2017 Oct 21.
38. Bayles SW, Hayden RE. Gastro-omental free flap reconstruction of the head and neck. Arch Facial Plast Surg. 2008;10(4):255–9. https://doi.org/10.1001/archfaci.10.4.255.
39. Sasaki CT, Salzer SJ, Cahow E, Son Y, Ward B. Laryngopharyngoesophagectomy for advanced hypopharyngeal and esophageal squamous cell carcinoma: the Yale experience. Laryngoscope. 1995;105(2):160–3. https://doi.org/10.1288/00005537-199502000-00009.
40. Sallum RA, Coimbra FJ, Herman P, Montagnini AL, Machado MA. Modified pharyngogastrostomy by a stapler technique. Eur J Surg Oncol. 2006;32(5):540–3. https://doi.org/10.1016/j.ejso.2006.02.022.
41. Butskiy O, Rahmanian R, White RA, Durham S, Anderson DW, Prisman E. Revisiting the gastric pull-up for pharyngoesophageal reconstruction: a systematic review and meta-analysis of mortality and morbidity. J Surg Oncol. 2016;114(8):907–14. https://doi.org/10.1002/jso.24477. Epub 2016 Oct 24.
42. Minni A, Ralli M, Di Cianni S, Cialente F, Candelori F, Colizza A, et al. Montgomery salivary bypass tube in head and neck cancer: the experience of our otolaryngology clinic. Ear Nose Throat J. 2020:145561320961754. https://doi.org/10.1177/0145561320961754. Epub ahead of print.
43. Torrico Román P, García Nogales A, Trinidad RG. Utility of the Montgomery salivary tubes for preventing pharyngocutaneous fistula in total laryngectomy. Am J Otolaryngol. 2020;41(4):102,557. https://doi.org/10.1016/j.amjoto.2020.102557. Epub 2020 May 26.
44. León X, Quer M, Burgués J. Montgomery salivary bypass tube in the reconstruction of the hypopharynx. Cost-benefit study. Ann Otol Rhinol Laryngol. 1999;108(9):864–8. https://doi.org/10.1177/000348949910800908.

Surgery of Larynx and Trachea: Voice Restoration and Total Laryngectomy

31

Peter Kress

Key Points

- Voice prostheses are the golden standard for voice restoration after total laryngectomy.
- Successful voice restoration and tracheostoma care are essential for postlaryngectomy quality of life.
- Effective management of voice prosthesis complications is essential to prevent severe complications.
- Alternative methods for voice restoration are available for special treatment situations.

31.1 Historical Development of Voice Restoration

Total laryngectomy was pioneered by Billroth and his team in 1873. In preparation of this dangerous operation, Gussenbauer, an assistant of Billroth, developed a tracheostomy tube with a bypass valve to allow airflow into the pharynx through a surgically created shunt and thus enable voice. Unfortunately, there was a lot of aspiration and the patient died of pneumonia. Even today, talking about a total laryngectomy, the loss of speech is the most threatening aspect for the patient, beside the permanent tracheostomy [1, 2]. And leakage?—It is still the most dangerous aspect of modern voice restoration!

Since the days of Billroth and Gussenbauer, many ways of voice restoration have been developed and most of them failed. All the surgical methods to create a shunt between trachea and pharynx for example the "Staffiery plasty" or the "Hagen laryngoplasty" disappeared over the years, as they were difficult to create, tended to leak or caused a bad smell during phonation.

Parallel to the experience with surgical methods for voice restoration, several groups of Head and Neck Surgeons and SLPs around the world tried to develop a prosthetic device for speech after total laryngectomy [3, 4]. The first commercially available voice prosthesis for placement in a tracheosesophageal puncture inside the tracheostomy was the Blom-Singer® Duckbill prosthesis in 1978 (Fig. 31.1).

The surgical method to produce a tracheoesophageal puncture (TEP) was simple and the voice quality with the voice prosthesis was superior to esophageal speech and electro-larynx [5]. Therefore, using a voice prosthesis to restore speech after laryngectomy became the golden standard over the last 40 years [6–8].

P. Kress (✉)
Department of ENT & Head and Neck Surgery, Kinikum Mutterhaus der Borromäerinnen, Trier, Rhineland Palatinate, Germany
e-mail: peter.kress@mutterhaus.de

M. Remacle, H. E. Eckel (eds.), *Textbook of Surgery of Larynx and Trachea*,
https://doi.org/10.1007/978-3-031-09621-1_31

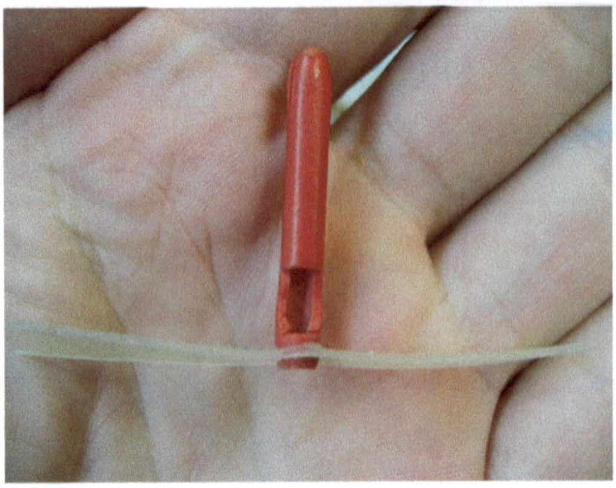

Fig. 31.1 Experimental prototype of a Blom-Singer® Duckbill voice prosthesis handmade from a red rubber bladder catheter and a silicon flange (before 1978)

31.2 Technical and Physiological Aspects of Voice Restoration with Voice Prostheses

Forty years of voice restoration with voice prostheses also meant 40 years of development. Voice prostheses from several manufacturers, in different sizes, materials, and diameters with different valve types and coatings, came onto the market – and most of them disappeared again. Today two manufacturers produce 99% of all voice prostheses (see Table 31.1). Silicone is the typical material for voice prostheses. It is widely used for implants, has proven to be very well tolerated in the human body, and there are few known allergies.

Every voice prosthesis has a shaft housing the valve and flanges on the esophageal and tracheal ending to secure the prosthesis in the TEP. The outer shaft diameter is traditionally given in French Gauge (1 mm $\approx$ 3 Fr). The shaft length is measured between the flanges and given in millimeter. Typical shaft lengths range from 4 to 10 mm.

In 2019, an industry standard for voice prostheses was published to define important technical aspects like the airflow resistance, the opening pressure of the valve, and the result of a leak test (ISO DIS 21917). The standard also regulates marking, sizing, labelling, biocompatibility, safety, and quality aspects [9].

In the beginning of voice prostheses, the patient was supposed to remove the prosthesis from the TEP for daily cleaning. After cleaning, the patient must be skilled enough to reinsert the prosthesis into the TEP and secure its retention strap with an adhesive tape. This required very skillful patients and voice prostheses with a small diameter and little flanges for easy removal and insertion. To prevent accidental displacement, these prostheses have a permanent retention strap to secure them to the skin above the tracheostomy. They are called “nonindwelling” voice prostheses and are still available today. They allow very cost-effective voice restoration as the daily cleaning prevents biofilm development. Therefore, nonindwelling voice prostheses have a longer service life than “indwelling” voice prostheses. Due to the skills needed, many patients were not able to change their voice prosthesis by themselves and there was a need for a prosthesis that was changed by a health professional and left in the TEP as long as it worked. These prostheses are called “indwelling” voice prostheses. They have larger flanges to secure them in the TEP without an additional retention strap (Fig. 31.2). The larger flanges require a tool for the placement of the prosthesis. In the beginning, these prostheses were inserted retrograde via the mouth. That is a very safe way to insert a voice prosthesis and to make sure the esophageal flange is definitely placed in the esophagus, but it is very unpleasant for the patient. Modern placement tools allow the placement of the voice prosthesis anterograde through the tracheostomy, but it is still very important to ensure that the esophageal flange is completely placed in the esophagus! Today, indwelling voice prostheses have largely replaced nonindwelling voice prostheses in industrial countries [10].

The inner diameters of the shaft and the valve are the major factors for the airflow resistance during speech (see Fig. 31.6). Today all voice prostheses have flap valves that open into the esophagus. Flap valves have proven to be supe-

Table 31.1 Overview of the most common voice prostheses, their specifics, indications, available lengths, and sizes

Product name	Manufacturer	Specifics	Indication	Diameters	Available lengths
Provox® Vega™	Atos medical	Indwelling Silicon flap valve in a fluoroplastic housing, defined opening pressure	Standard + primary intraoperative placement + secondary placement (puncture set)	17 Fr 20 Fr 22,5 Fr	4 mm 6 mm 8 mm 10 mm 12,5 mm 15 mm
Provox® ActiValve®	Atos medical	Indwelling Magnetic valve in fluoroplastic housing, 3 strengths (light, strong, extra strong)	Underpressure Biofilm Only in selected patients	22,5 Fr	4 mm 6 mm 8 mm 10 mm 12,5 mm
Provox® XtraSeal™	Atos medical	Indwelling, large esophageal flange, silicon flap valve in a fluoroplastic housing	Leakage around standard prosthesis	17 Fr 20 Fr 22,5 Fr	4 mm 6 mm 8 mm 10 mm 12,5 mm 15 mm
Provox® 2	Atos medical	Indwelling Silicon valve	Standard	22,5 Fr	4,5 mm 6 mm 8 mm 10 mm 12,5 mm 15 mm
Provox® NID™	Atos medical	Nonindwelling	Standard	17 Fr 20 Fr	6 mm 8 mm 10 mm 12 mm 14 mm 18 mm

(continued)

Table 31.1 (continued)

Product name	Manufacturer	Specifics	Indication	Diameters	Available lengths
Blom-Singer® CLASSIC™	Inhealth technologies®	Indwelling Silicone flap valve	Standard + primary intraoperative placement + secondary placement (puncture set)	16 Fr 20 Fr	4 mm 5 mm 6 mm 7 mm 8 mm 9 mm 10 mm 12 mm 14 mm 16 mm 18 mm 20 mm
Blom-Singer® ADVANTAGE® Hard Valve Assembly	Inhealth Technologies®	Indwelling Flap valve Silicone with silver oxide Titanium ring	Standard/Biofilm	20 Fr	4 mm 6 mm 8 mm 10 mm 12 mm
Blom-Singer® ADVANTAGE® Soft Valve Assembly	Inhealth Technologies®	Indwelling Flap valve Silicone with silver oxide	Standard/Biofilm	16 Fr 20 Fr	4 mm 6 mm 8 mm 10 mm 12 mm 14 mm
Blom-Singer® Duckbill	Inhealth Technologies®	Nonindwelling Slit valve	Standard Under-pressure	16 Fr	8 mm 10 mm 12 mm 14 mm 18 mm

Blom-Singer® Low Pressure	Inhealth Technologies®	Nonindwelling Flap valve Large range of available lengths	Standard	16 Fr 20 Fr	4 mm 6 mm 8 mm 10 mm 12 mm 14 mm 18 mm 20 mm 22 mm 25 mm 28 mm (16 Fr)
Blom-Singer® Increased Resistance	Inhealth Technologies®	Indwelling reinforced flap valve	Under-pressure	16 Fr 20 Fr	6 mm 8 mm 10 mm 12 mm
Blom-Singer® Large Esophageal Flange	Inhealth Technologies®	Indwelling Silicone flap valve, large flange on esophageal side	Leakage around standard prosthesis	16 Fr 20 Fr	4 mm 5 mm 6 mm 7 mm 8 mm 10 mm 12 mm 14 mm
Blom-Singer® Large Esophageal Flange & Tracheal Flanges	Inhealth Technologies®	Indwelling Silicone flap valve, large flange on both sides	Leakage around standard prosthesis	16 Fr 20 Fr	4 mm 6 mm 8 mm 10 mm 12 mm 14 mm
Blom-Singer® Large Esophageal Flange/ increased Resistance	Inhealth Technologies®	Indwelling reinforced flap valve, large flange on esophageal side	Leakage around standard prosthesis + underpressure	16 Fr 20 Fr	4 mm 6 mm 8 mm

(continued)

Table 31.1 (continued)

Product name	Manufacturer	Specifics	Indication	Diameters	Available lengths
Blom-Singer® Dual Valve™	Inhealth Technologies®	Indwelling 2 silicon flap valves with silver oxide	Underpressure + Biofilm	20 Fr	6 mm 8 mm 10 mm 12 mm 14 mm
Blom-Singer® Dual Valve™ Large Flange	Inhealth Technologies®	Indwelling 2 silicon flap valves with silver oxide Large flange on both sides	Underpressure + Biofilm + Leakage around prosthesis	20 Fr	6 mm 8 mm 10 mm 12 mm 14 mm

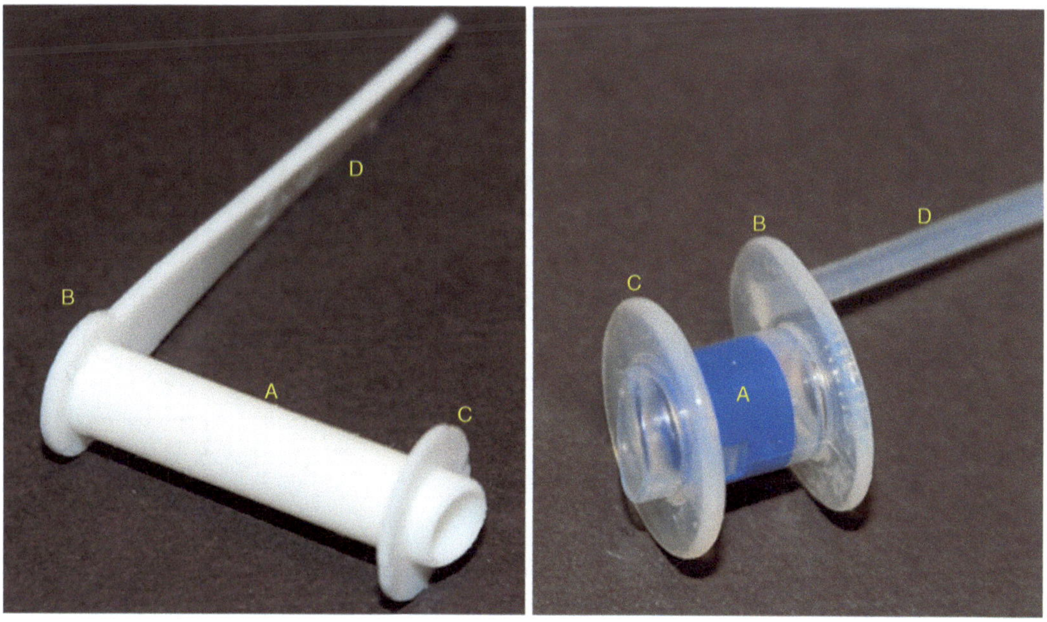

Fig. 31.2 (Left) nonindwelling voice prosthesis Blom-Singer® Low Pressure, (right) indwelling voice prosthesis Provox® Vega™, A = shaft, B = tracheal flange, C = esophageal flange, D = retention strap

rior to other valve types. They have a low profile and do not push into the esophagus mucosa. They have low opening pressures and can be cleaned with a brush or rinsed with a syringe. The biggest disadvantage of the flap valve in a voice prosthesis is the fact that it is not completely resistant to underpressure in the esophagus. This leads to unintended openings of the flap valve if the pressure in the esophagus is lower than the pressure in the trachea. During inspiration the negative pressure in the thoracic cavity also includes the thoracic part of the esophagus. In roughly two-thirds of all laryngectomized patients, CT scans show a voice prosthesis positioned in the upper thoracic cavity (Fig. 31.3).

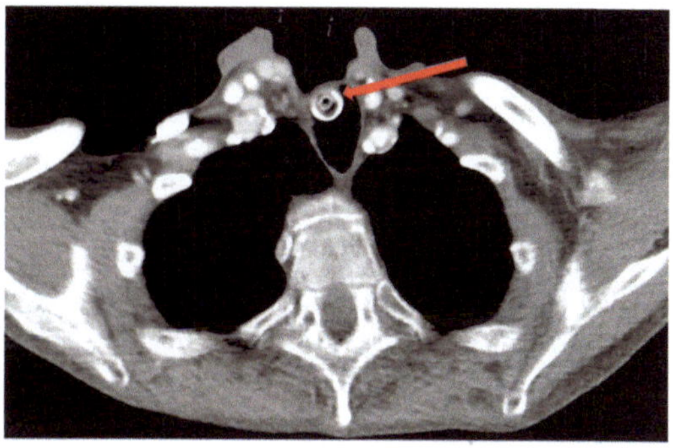

Fig. 31.3 CT Scan of the typical location of a voice prosthesis (arrow) in the upper thorax. The esophagus behind the prosthesis is extended due to underpressure during inspiration!

This means the voice prosthesis is exposed to the alternating pressures during respiration. If the valve opening pressure (see Fig. 31.4) is lower than the underpressure during inspiration, it will open. These unintended openings can happen during calm respiration or during forced inspiration and are visible on inspection with an endoscope.

For the flap valve, they cause a lot of stress leading to material fatigue and early valve failure. The typical clinical situation is a voice prosthesis leaking through the valve after 30–50 days, corresponding to roughly one million breathing cycles, without visible biofilm (Fig. 31.5).

If a flap valve is fully opened, the airflow resistance is dependent on the inner diameter of the shaft. Therefore, voice prostheses with large diameters were introduced in order to allow easy speech. On the other hand, voice prosthe-

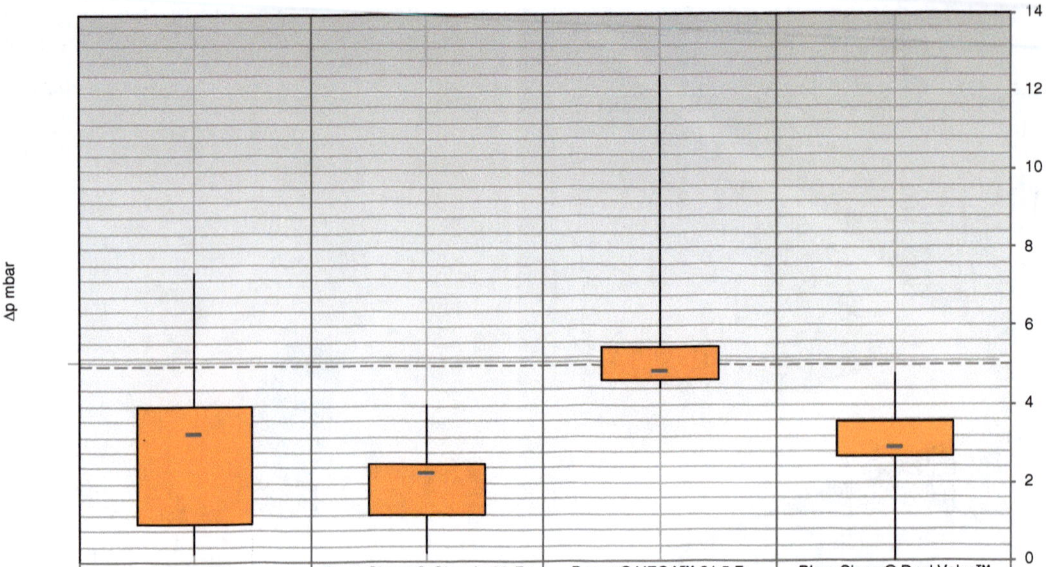

	Provox® 2	Blom-Singer® Classic 20 Fr	Provox® VEGA™ 21.5 Fr	Blom-Singer® Dual Valve™
q1	0,975	1,2	4,625	2,675
max	7,4	4,03	12,4	4,8
min	0,2	0,2	4,4	0
q3	4	2,5	5,45	3,55
– median	3,25	2,25	4,85	2,9

Fig. 31.4 Example for valve opening pressures of voice prostheses ($n = 10$ each)

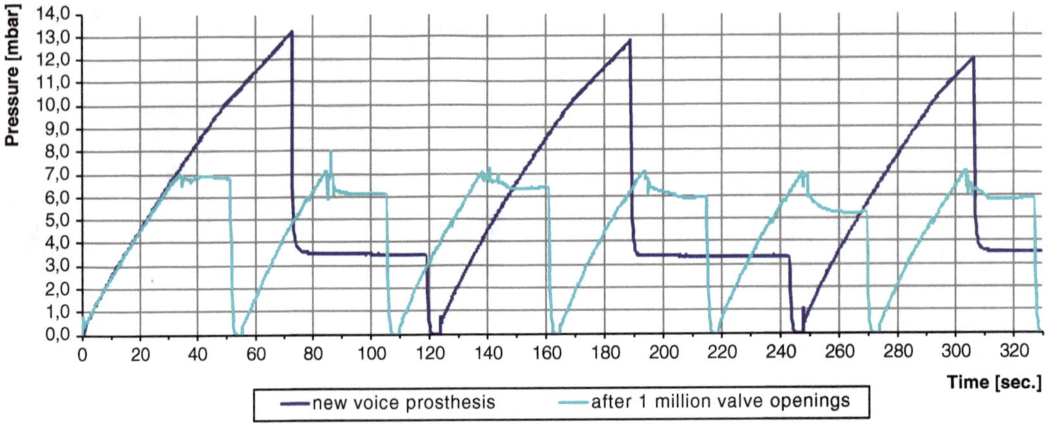

Fig. 31.5 Material fatigue of a voice prosthesis shown with a cycle test with one million openings. The opening pressure drops significantly

ses with a large diameter cause bigger trauma to the TEP and are believed to lead to a higher rate of TEP complications and leakage around the voice prosthesis [11]. Scientific lab tests at the University of Esslingen showed that diameters of 20 Fr–21,5 Fr have good airflow characteristics and their clinical use showed acceptable rates of TEP problems (see Fig. 31.6).

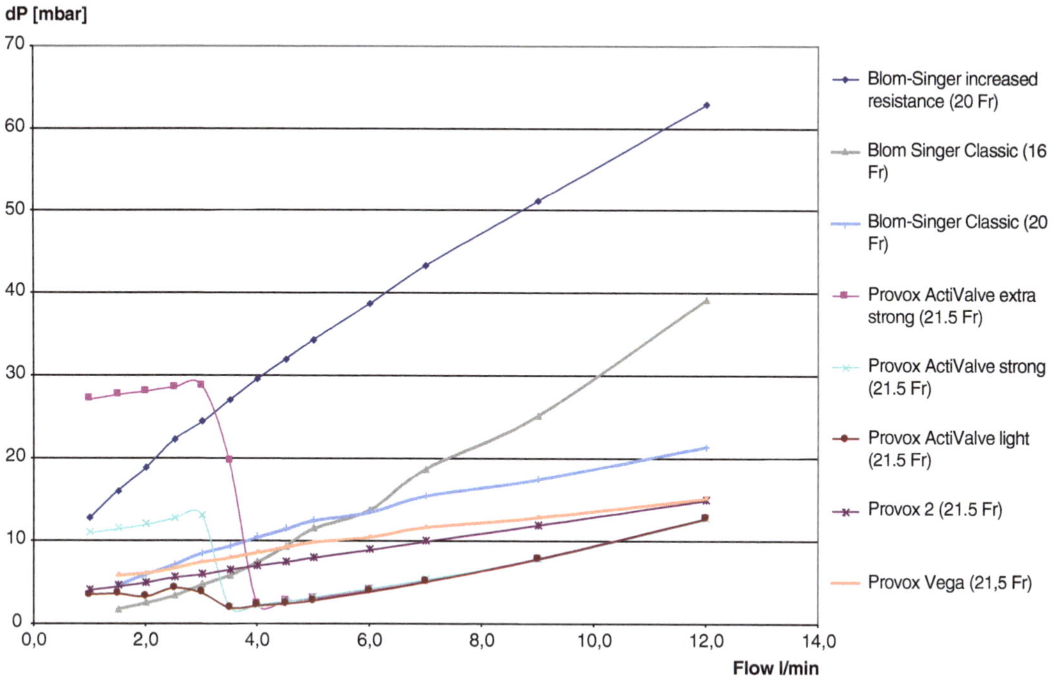

Fig. 31.6 Comparison of airflow resistance of voice prostheses with 10 mm shaft length depending on valve type and diameter

31.3 Surgical Procedures Required for Successful Utilization of a Voice Prosthesis

In the beginning of voice restoration with voice prostheses, the placement of a voice prosthesis happened as a secondary procedure many months after the laryngectomy when the wound had healed and chemo-radiation was completed. Roughly half of the patients could not speak with a voice prosthesis as no myotomy had been performed during the laryngectomy and a secondary myotomy was a dangerous procedure. This led to the idea of primary placement of the voice prosthesis during the initial laryngectomy, which allows a precise myotomy exactly to the TEP and a neurectomy of the plexus pharyngis adapted to the resection and reconstruction of the pharynx [12, 13]. Success rates for primary voice restoration today range between 90% and 95% and patients can speak 7–10 days after surgery. This enormous improvement in the early quality of life has made primary placement of a voice prostheses the golden standard. Today a secondary placement may be necessary, for example, if large resections of the pharynx and esophagus have to be reconstructed and the voice prostheses would go through a free flap.

Successful primary voice restoration with a voice prosthesis is dependent on 6 critical surgical procedures: the tracheostomy, the pharynx closure, the tracheoesophageal puncture (TEP), the myotomy of the constrictor muscle, and the neurectomy of the pharyngeal plexus.

During a laryngectomy, a permanent and terminal tracheostomy is created. Size and shape of the tracheostomy are very important for the later use of tracheostomy accessories like heat and moisture exchangers (HMEs), tracheostomy tubes, and tracheostomy valves and have a large impact on the quality of life of a laryngectomee. The neck around the tracheostomy should have a flat profile to allow the use of adhesive tracheostomy housings. In some cases, an incision in the lower part of the sternocleidomastoid muscle can help to flatten the neck profile. The size of the tracheostomy should be roughly the size of the end link of the middle finger of the patient to allow digital occlusion. A larger tracheostomy is difficult to occlude for speaking, a smaller one can shrink and cause breathing problems without a tracheostomy tube. To create a stable and good-sized tracheostomy, a complete tracheal ring should be sutured into a separate skin incision caudal of the surgical incision for the laryngectomy.

After a stable tracheostomy is created, the tracheoesophageal puncture (TEP) is performed. The location of the puncture is of utmost importance. A puncture deep in the trachea will cause severe problems in the later course of voice restoration. Closing it is difficult and every changing procedure of the voice prosthesis becomes a challenge! The perfect location is 7 mm below the dorsal sutures of the tracheostomy exactly in the midline. Once the voice prosthesis is in place, a lateral myotomy and a neurectomy of the plexus pharyngis has to be performed to make sure that airflow into the upper pharynx is possible. If a circular ring of pharynx muscles above the TEP remains functionally intact, airflow from the voice prosthesis upward can be blocked by reflex pharynx constriction. The patient cannot speak with the voice prosthesis although the pharyngeal passage for food is wide and swallowing is fine. In literature that problem is named "hypertonicity" or "constrictor muscle spasm" and it can be treated with Botox injections into the constrictor muscle. To avoid the problem of a pharyngeal spasm, which is nothing else than the original reflex to prevent retrograde flow into the pharynx, the pharynx muscle has to be paralyzed from the base of the tongue to the TEP on one side. The other side should be left intact to help swallowing. The most reliable way to achieve that is a combination of a lateral myotomy and a same sided neurectomy of the plexus pharyngis. Each method alone has inferior results. A lateral myotomy does not affect the stability of the TEP, leaves one side of pharynx muscles intact, and covers the area from the TEP to the pharynx resection. The neurectomy of the pharyngeal plexus covers the area from the pharyngeal resection to the tonsillar region [14–18].

Pharyngeal strictures are a typical complication after laryngectomy [19–21]. They affect swallowing and voice restoration. Strictures are typically located right above the voice prosthesis causing problems with leakage around the voice prosthesis as the high pressures during swallowing cannot be sealed by the flanges of the voice prosthesis. To avoid pharyngeal stenosis, a basic rule should be kept in mind when the pharynx is closed: To create a circular pharynx with a diameter of 1 cm the remaining strip of pharynx mucosa after resection has to be at least 4 cm wide ($2r\pi$ + suture)! If ever this is not the case, the pharynx should be reconstructed with a flap [22–26].

31.4 Management of Voice Prostheses and Their Complications

Standard voice prostheses have a limited service life of 90–100 days in industrial countries with full reimbursement of the costs. The most frequent reason for a replacement of the voice prosthesis is leakage through the valve. In developing countries and countries where patients have to travel a long way to see a health professional, leakage through the valve is tolerated a long time and the recorded lifetimes of voice prostheses are significantly longer. Leakage through the valve is usually caused by biofilm growing on the closing surfaces, leaving the valve unable to fully close [27–29]. Biofilm needs several weeks to grow and can be reduced by brushing and rinsing the prosthesis and good oral hygiene [30–32]. As biofilm is a complicated structure of bacteria, fungi, and matrix proteins, it is not effective to treat it with antibiotics or antimycotics (Fig. 31.7).

If one type of voice prostheses fails to reach the expected service life of 90–100 days several times in one patient, the use of a special prosthesis should be considered [33]. There are special prostheses with an increased resistance against biofilm, for underpressure-related problems and for the combinations of the both (see Table 31.1). The effectiveness of special prostheses differs a lot between individual patients and cannot be predicted very well. By far the longest service life of more than 1 year in many patients is achieved with the Provox® ActiValve® prosthesis,

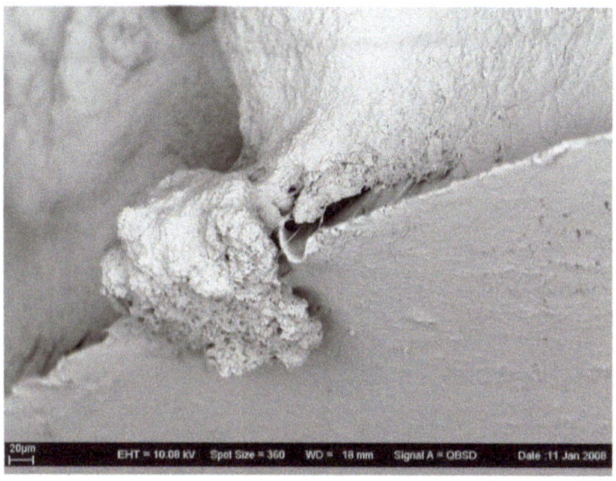

Fig. 31.7 Electron microscopic image of a biofilm growing over the closing surface of the valve of a voice prosthesis. Copyright Hochschule Esslingen

which has a magnetic valve made from biofilm resistant fluoroplastic [34]. If voice prostheses stay in the patient longer than a year, the risk of TEP problems increases as the shaft of the voice prosthesis is colonized by biofilm. The biofilm can lead to an infection of the surrounding tissues of the TEP. A good range for the intended service life of a voice prostheses is 3 months up to one year.

If a voice prosthesis leaks without visible biofilm, material fatigue of the valve due to "underpressure" is the most common reason. It can reliably be detected with an endoscope placed in front of the valve during inspiration. Some of these patients complain of a gastric air-filling during heavy physical work. Several voice prostheses with reinforced valves are available and can be very helpful. If patients with underpressure-related problems use a high resistance HME, the underpressure-related problems increase, as inspiration through the HME causes higher underpressure!

Problems with the length of the shaft of the voice prosthesis are common, as the TEP can shrink, for example, after the puncture and it can develop a swelling during infections. As a consequence, the indwelling prosthesis becomes too long or too short. If the prosthesis is too long, the flanges no longer fix it in place and it can move in the TEP (see Fig. 31.8). This can cause a discreet leakage. If a tracheostomy tube is inserted, it is important to make sure that the prosthesis is not

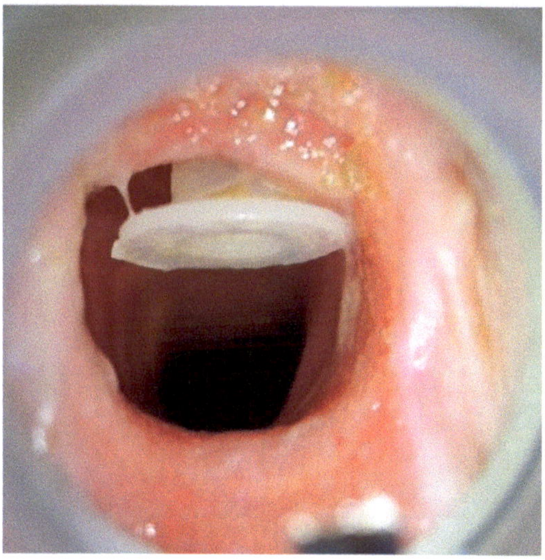

Fig. 31.8 If the voice prosthesis is too long, it can move in the TEP

dislocated by hooking the distal opening of the tube to the tracheal flange of the prosthesis. If the shaft is 2–4 mm long, it is recommended to change to a shorter prosthesis.

Much more dangerous is a voice prosthesis with a shaft that is too short, especially in indwelling devices. The flanges cause pressure on the tissue in the TEP leading to necrosis and shunt failure. This situation has to be recognized immediately and patients should be trained to check for the signs of a "too short prosthesis." Typically, there is some pain around the prosthesis, some swelling, a very tight fit, and white tissues with reduced blood flow below the flanges (see Fig. 31.9).

If the prosthesis is replaced by a longer one, the problem can be solved with little effort. If the too short prosthesis stays in place, a necrosis of the TEP develops and leakage around the prosthesis occurs.

Leakage around the voice prosthesis is a problem of the TEP! There are two types of leaking TEPs: the "dilated and atrophic" TEP and the "infected and necrotic" TEP. If an infection of the TEP with necrosis and leakage around the prosthesis has occurred, the infected voice prosthesis is removed and replaced by a clean new one with sufficient shaft length. Sometimes it is helpful to use a voice prosthesis with an enlarged flange to

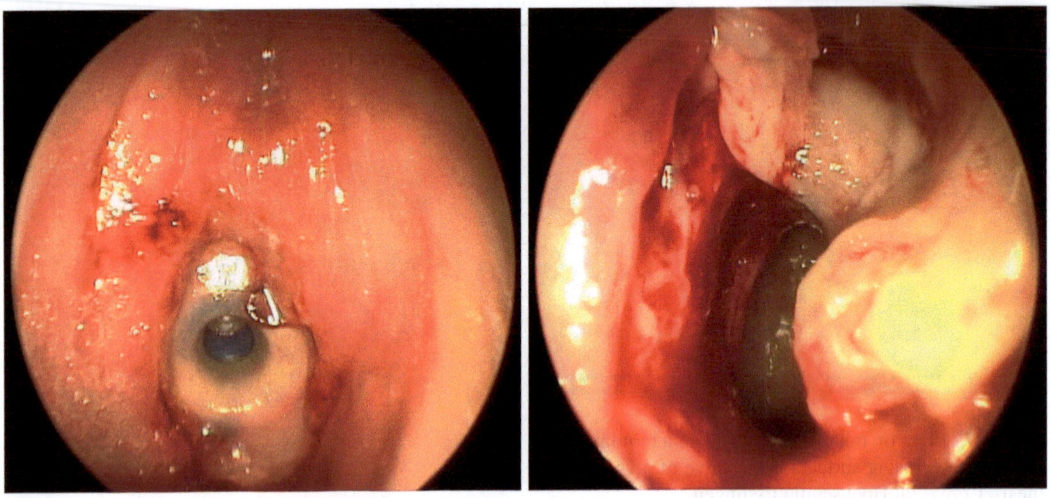

Fig. 31.9 Too short voice prosthesis before removal (left), necrosis of the TEP tissues after removal of a too short voice prosthesis (right)

cover the infected tissues and protect them from saliva and gastric fluids, which facilitates healing [35].

A dilated and atrophic TEP develops over a longer period. Tissues around the voice prosthesis become thinner and thinner, which finally leads to leakage around even the shortest prostheses. To manage the problem, a voice prosthesis with enlarged flanges and a perfect fit is most effective. Surgical methods to stabilize the TEP like sutures, injections of fillers, and autologous fat help only for a short time. Patients with a dilatated and atrophic shunt should be checked for systemic diseases like diabetes, hypothyroidism, and tumor recurrence. Treatment of these conditions helps the TEP tissues a lot. If the TEP cannot be sealed at all, the TEP has to be closed surgically by interposition of fascia, tracheal resection, or a flap interposition [36].

31.5 Changing a Voice Prosthesis

Indwelling voice prostheses are changed by a health professional in a professional setup with sufficient light, a suction, a dilator for the TEP, and some basic surgical tools. The patient should be in a sitting position and tracheostomy tubes and housings should be removed to allow good visibility and access to the voice prosthesis. Prior to removing the voice prosthesis, the shaft length is checked by pulling lightly on the tracheal flange with a pair of forceps. If there is 2 mm or less movement of the shaft, the same length can be used. If there is more than 2 mm of shaft movement, a shorter prosthesis should be considered.

In order to remove the prosthesis, the patient is asked to swallow and open the moth to prevent swallowing and aspiration during the extraction of the prosthesis. Now the prosthesis is removed by clamping the tracheal flange with a locking anatomical clamp and a short and unhesitant pull on the flange. The removed prosthesis is checked to be complete and a dilator is placed in the TEP to prevent aspiration. If necessary, the shaft length can be measured with a measuring tool. The new prosthesis is loaded into the specific placement tool. Then the patient is again asked to swallow and open the mouth before the dilator is removed and the prosthesis is placed. It is very important to make sure the esophageal flange is placed completely in the esophagus. Therefore, it needs to be checked if the prosthesis rotates freely, the valve opens and closes again, there is no leakage during swallowing, and the prosthesis stays in the TEP if a little traction is applied. In cases where the placement is difficult, and the checks above mentioned are inconclusive, an endoscopy through the prosthesis or through the pharynx is mandatory to rule out misplacement before the retention strap is cut off.

31.6 Speaking Problems with a Voice Prosthesis

Dealing with speaking problems, it is essential to know if speaking was ever possible after placement of the voice prosthesis. If speaking was easy in be beginning and became more and more difficult over a period of time, there might be a developing pharyngeal stricture or the TEP tissues are growing over the voice prosthesis. Both conditions are easily checked by endoscopy. A pharyngeal stricture is accompanied with increasing swallowing problems and can be treated with balloon dilatation or pharynx reconstruction. A voice prosthesis that is overgrown by shunt mucosa, either on the tracheal or esophageal side, is replaced by a longer prosthesis to cover the tissues with the flanges.

If the passage for air from the tracheal side of the prosthesis is clear up to the mouth, and speaking is still not possible, a pharyngeal spasm can be suspected. It is then very important to check the patient's occlusion of the tracheostomy during phonation. Some patients compress the tracheostomy site with a lot of pressure to force a seal. This compressing of the pharynx can imitate a pharyngeal spasm. If speech does not work with a tracheostomy valve or the light occluding touch of the health professional, a video fluoroscopy of the pharynx can show the pharyngeal spasm that blocks the stream of air into the mouth (see Fig. 31.10).

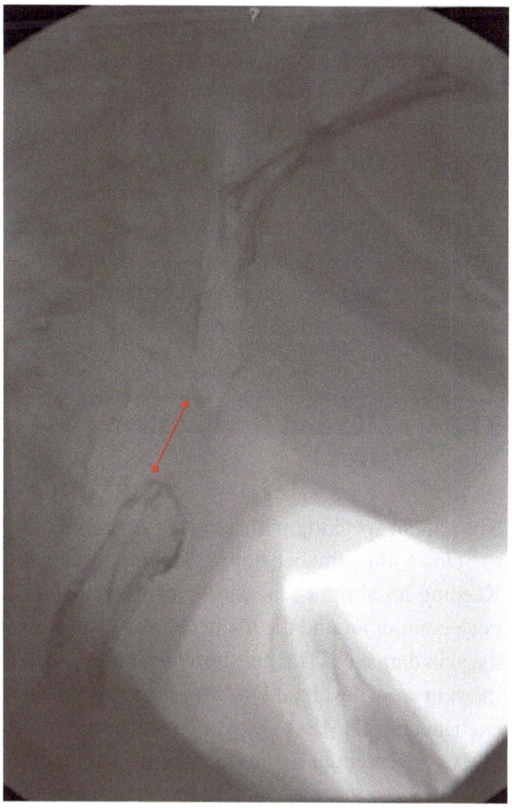

Fig. 31.10 Lateral video-fluoroscopy of the contrasted pharynx during phonation. The red line shows the constricted pharyngeal segment in a patient with a pharyngeal spasm

During a lateral projection, the patient is asked to swallow a contrasting liquid. The typical finding during swallowing is a wide pharynx. Now the patient is asked to phonate. The pharynx below the constricting area is filled with air and a closed pharynx above can be detected. A still image of that situation is used to measure the distance from the voice prosthesis to the contracting part of the pharynx. The length of the contracting area is measured for later Botox injection. If the clinical symptoms are not completely clear, for example, if a pharynx stenosis is coexistent, a test injection with lidocaine can be performed. If the pharynx can be relaxed with lidocaine and the patient can speak, the pharynx spasm has been proofed. For the transdermal Botox injection, the constricting area of the pharynx is marked on the skin medial of the carotid artery. With an EMG-controlled needle, the pharynx muscles are detected and 100 IU Botox A or an equivalent are placed over the length of the stricture [37, 38]. The effect is expected after 5–7 days and lasts forever in one-third of the patients. Some patients need repeated injections.

31.7 Gastroesophageal Reflux

Symptoms associated with gastroesophageal reflux are frequently reported by laryngectomized patients, which is not surprising as the upper esophagus sphincter is surgically compromised in many cases. In recent literature, gastroesophageal reflux was made responsible for a variety of voice prosthesis problems, including TEP problems and early leakage through the prosthesis. In daily practice, treating these patients for reflux for the rest of their lives has to be balanced against the side effects of the drugs used for it. Only in some patients, gastroesophageal reflux and voice-prosthesis-related problems are more than a coincidence [39–41].

31.8 HMEs and Tracheostomy Valves

The patient speaking with a voice prosthesis needs to close the tracheostomy during phonation. Keeping an airtight seal can be challenging if the neck contour around the tracheostomy is uneven or the skin damaged. Tracheostomy housings glued to the skin were developed to carry heat and moisture exchangers (HMEs) or tracheostomy valves. HMEs are essential for laryngectomized patients as they filter the inspired air, add to tracheal and lung humidity, and reduce symptoms like coughing, mucus production, and fatigue [42–44]. Tracheostomy valves allow hands-free speech [45], which is often very important for patients who are still working their job. In laryngectomized patients, it is important to use a tracheostomy valve with a cough valve and an expiration function!

31.9 Alternatives to Voice Prostheses

Esophageal speech has been the method of choice for voice restoration after total laryngectomy before the voice prosthesis in a TEP was developed. For esophageal speech, the patient has to learn to swallow or suck in some air into the esophagus, retain the air for a moment, and release it similar to gulping. The resulting vibrations are formed in the pharynx and mouth for speech. Most patients need weeks with a speech and language pathologist to learn this demanding technique. Some patients cannot learn esophageal speech at all, for example, if the upper esophagus has been resected and the upper sphincter cannot willingly be controlled. The big advantage of esophageal speech is, that patients need not depend on medical devices and the repeated service of a health professional to speak. Anyhow esophageal speech allows only short sentences and changing between breathing and speaking is tiresome. If the voice prosthesis fails, esophageal speech is rarely an option, as there should be a surgically relaxed upper esophagus sphincter and pharynx, which does not allow retention of air in the esophagus. In this situation, the use of an electro-larynx should be considered [46–48].

The electro-larynx devices have a vibrating coupler that is connected to the neck tissues in order to generate vibration of the pharyngeal mucosa and air. The resulting sound is formed in the mouth and allows to communicate. Most electro-larynx devices have only one frequency making the sound of electro-larynx speech kind of "robot like" and difficult to understand for people that are unaccustomed to the sound. To couple the vibrating head of the device to the neck, the tissues have to be stable and a little flexible. In patients with massive edema and fibrosis, it may be difficult and painful to connect to the tissues and find a spot that vibrates. Anyhow if a short time solution for speech is needed, a TEP is too dangerous to perform, lifetime is limited, or the medical situation is difficult, the electro-larynx is a reliable and safe fallback option [49, 50].

If all the other options fail or in times between procedures, a communication tablet computer or cellphone app can be used to communicate. These devices allow to type-write questions and thoughts in advance and show to nursing personnel or family. Some of these devices can "speak" written text and even translate it.

References

1. Ackerstaff AH, Hilgers FJ, Aaronson NK, Balm AJ. Communication, functional disorders and lifestyle changes after total laryngectomy. Clin Otolaryngol Allied Sci. 1994;19(4):295–300. https://doi.org/10.1111/j.1365-2273.1994.tb01234.x.
2. Hilgers FJ, Ackerstaff AH, Aaronson NK, Schouwenburg PF, Van Zandwijk N. Physical and psychosocial consequences of total laryngectomy. Clin Otolaryngol Allied Sci. 1990;15(5):421–5. https://doi.org/10.1111/j.1365-2273.1990.tb00494.x.
3. Mozolewski E. Surgical rehabilitation of **voice** and speech following laryngectomy. Otolaryngol Pol. 1972;26(6):653–61.
4. Singer MI, Blom ED. Medical techniques for voice restoration after total laryngectomy. CA Cancer J Clin. 1990;40(3):166–73. https://doi.org/10.3322/canjclin.40.3.166.
5. van Sluis KE, van der Molen L, van Son RJJH, Hilgers FJM, Bhairosing PA, den Brekel v. Objective and subjective voice outcomes after total laryngectomy: a systematic review. MWM Eur Arch Otorhinolaryngol. 2018;275(1):11–26. https://doi.org/10.1007/s00405-017-4790-6. Epub 2017 Oct 31.
6. Deschler DG, Gray ST. Tracheoesophageal speech following laryngopharyngectomy and pharyngeal reconstruction. Otolaryngol Clin N Am. 2004;37(3):567–83.
7. Mendelsohn M, Morris M, Gallagher R. A comparative study of speech after total laryngectomy and total laryngopharyngectomy. Arch Otolaryngol Head Neck Surg. 1993;119(5):508–10.
8. Balm AJ, van den Brekel MW, Tan IB, Hilgers FJ., The indwelling voice prosthesis for speech rehabilitation after total laryngectomy: a safe approach., Otolaryngol Pol 2011;65(6):402–409. doi: https://doi.org/10.1016/S0030-6657(11)70731-4
9. ISO/DIS 21917 Anesthetic and respiratory equipment—Voice prostheses.
10. Petersen JF, Lansaat L, Timmermans AJ, van der Noort V, Hilgers FJM, van den Brekel MWM. Postlaryngectomy prosthetic voice rehabilitation outcomes in a consecutive cohort of 232 patients over a 13-year period. Head Neck. 2019;41(3):623–31. https://doi.org/10.1002/hed.25364. Epub 2019 Jan 7.
11. Blom ED. Some comments on the escalation of tracheoesophageal voice prosthesis dimensions. Arch Otolaryngol Head Neck Surg. 2003;129(4):500–2. https://doi.org/10.1001/archotol.129.4.500-b.
12. Luu K, Chang BA, Valenzuela D, Anderson D. Primary versus secondary tracheoesophageal puncture for voice rehabilitation in laryngectomy patients: a systematic review. Clin Otolaryngol. 2018;43(5):1250–9. https://doi.org/10.1111/coa.13138. Epub 2018 May 31.
13. Guttman D, Mizrachi A, Hadar T, Bachar G, Hamzani Y, Marx S, Shvero J. Post-laryngectomy voice rehabilitation: comparison of primary and secondary tracheoesophageal puncture. Isr Med Assoc J. 2013;15(9):497–9.
14. Singer MI, Blom ED. Selective myotomy for voice restoration after total laryngectomy. Arch Otolaryngol. 1981;107(11):670–3. https://doi.org/10.1001/archotol.1981.00790470018005.
15. Bayles SW, Deschler DG. Operative prevention and management of voice-limiting pharyngoesophageal spasm. Otolaryngol Clin N Am. 2004;37(3):547–58. https://doi.org/10.1016/j.otc.2004.01.005.
16. Medina JE, Reiner SA. Pharyngeal myotomy for voice restoration: a midline approach. Laryngoscope. 1990;100(3):309–12. https://doi.org/10.1288/00005537-199003000-00019.
17. Deschler DG, Doherty ET, Reed CG, Hayden RE, Singer MI. Prevention of pharyngoesophageal spasm after laryngectomy with a half-muscle closure technique. Ann Otol Rhinol Laryngol. 2000;109(5):514–8. https://doi.org/10.1177/000348940010900513.
18. Blom ED, Pauloski BR, Hamaker RC. Functional outcome after surgery for prevention of pharyngospasms in tracheoesophageal speakers. Part I: speech characteristics. Laryngoscope. 1995;105(10):1093–103. https://doi.org/10.1288/00005537-199510000-00016.
19. Hanasono MM, Lin D, Wax MK, Rosenthal EL. Closure of laryngectomy defects in the age of chemoradiation therapy. Head Neck. 2012;34(4):580–8.
20. Richmon JD, Samji HA, Deschler DG. National laryngopharyngectomy and reconstructive surgery survey. Laryngoscope. 2009;119(8):1472–8.
21. Sweeny L, Golden JB, White HN, Magnuson JS, Carroll WR, Rosenthal EL. Incidence and outcomes of stricture formation postlaryngectomy. Otolaryngol Head Neck Surg. 2012;146(3):395–402.
22. Lewin JS, Barringer DA, May AH, et al. Functional outcomes after circumferential pharyngoesophageal reconstruction. Laryngoscope. 2005(115, 7):1266–71.
23. Lewin JS, Barringer DA, May AH, et al. Functional outcomes after laryngopharyngectomy with anterolateral thigh flap reconstruction. Head Neck. 2006;28(2):142–9.
24. Yu P, Hanasono MM, Skoracki RJ, et al. Pharyngoesophageal reconstruction with the anterolateral thigh flap after total laryngopharyngectomy. Cancer. 2010;116(7):1718–24.
25. Deschler DG, Doherty ET, Reed CG, Singer MI. Quantitative and qualitative analysis of tracheoesophageal voice after pectoralis major flap reconstruction of the neopharynx. Otolaryngol Head Neck Surg. 1998;118(6):771–6.

26. Sinclair CF, Rosenthal EL, McColloch NL, et al. Primary versus delayed tracheoesophageal puncture for laryngopharyngectomy with free flap reconstruction. Laryngoscope. 2011;121(7):1436–40.
27. Leonhard M, Schneider-Stickler B. Voice prostheses, microbial colonization and biofilm formation. Adv Exp Med Biol. 2015;830:123–36. https://doi.org/10.1007/978-3-319-11038-7_8.
28. Somogyi-Ganss E, Chambers MS, Lewin JS, Tarrand JJ, Hutcheson KA. Biofilm on the tracheoesophageal voice prosthesis: considerations for oral decontamination. Eur Arch Otorhinolaryngol. 2017;274(1):405–13. https://doi.org/10.1007/s00405-016-4193-0. Epub 2016 Jul 11.
29. Free RH, Van der Mei HC, Dijk F, Van Weissenbruch R, Busscher HJ, Albers FW. Biofilm formation on voice prostheses: influence of dairy products in vitro. Acta Otolaryngol. 2000;120(1):92–9. https://doi.org/10.1080/000164800760370918.
30. Galli J, Calo L, Meucci D, Giuliani M, Lucidi D, Paludetti G, Torelli R, Sanguinetti M, Parrilla C. Biofilm in voice prosthesis: a prospective cohort study and laboratory tests using sonication and SEM analysis. Clin Otolaryngol. 2018;43(5):1260–5. https://doi.org/10.1111/coa.13141. Epub 2018 Jun 6.
31. Talpaert MJ, Balfour A, Stevens S, Baker M, Muhlschlegel FA, Gourlay CW. Candida biofilm formation on voice prostheses. J Med Microbiol. 2015;64(Pt 3):199–208. https://doi.org/10.1099/jmm.0.078717-0. Epub 2014 Aug 8.
32. Leonhard M, Zatorska B, Tan Y, Moser D, Schneider-Stickler B. In vitro biofilm growth on modern voice prostheses. Head Neck. 2018;40(4):763–9. https://doi.org/10.1002/hed.25053. Epub 2017 Dec 29.
33. Kress P, Schäfer P, Schwerdtfeger FP, Rösler S. Are modern voice prostheses better? A lifetime comparison of 749 voiceprostheses. Eur Arch Otorhinolaryngol. 2014;271(1):133–40. https://doi.org/10.1007/s00405-013-2611-0. Epub 2013 Jun 29.
34. Hilgers FJ, Ackerstaff AH, Balm AJ, Van den Brekel MW, Bing Tan I, Persson JO. A new problem-solving indwelling voice prosthesis, eliminating the need for frequent Candida- and "underpressure"-related replacements: Provox ActiValve. Acta Otolaryngol. 2003;123(8):972–9. https://doi.org/10.1080/00016480310015371.
35. Kress P, Schäfer P, Schwerdtfeger FP. The custom-fit voice prosthesis, for treatment of periprothetic leakage after tracheoesophageal voice restoration. Laryngorhinootologie. 2006;85(7):496–500. https://doi.org/10.1055/s-2006-925081. Epub 2006 Feb 21.
36. Hutcheson KA, Sturgis EM, Lewin JS. Early risk factors for enlargement of the tracheoesophageal puncture after total laryngectomy: nodal metastasis and extent of surgery. Arch Otolaryngol Head Neck Surg. 2012;138(9):833–9.
37. Hamaker RC, Blom ED. Botulinum neurotoxin for pharyngeal constrictor muscle spasm in tracheoesophageal voice restoration. Laryngoscope. 2003;113(9):1479–82. https://doi.org/10.1097/00005537-200309000-00010.
38. Ramachandran K, Arunachalam PS, Hurren A, Marsh RL, Samuel PR. Botulinum toxin injection for failed tracheo-oesophageal voice in laryngectomees: the Sunderland experience. J Laryngol Otol. 2003;117(7):544–8. https://doi.org/10.1258/002221503322112978.
39. Lorenz KJ, Ehrhart T, Grieser L, Maier H. Coincidence of fistula enlargement and supra-oesophageal reflux in patients after laryngectomy and prosthetic voice restoration. HNO. 2009;57(12):1253–61. https://doi.org/10.1007/s00106-009-1956-6.
40. Lorenz KJ, Kraft K, Graf F, Pröpper C, Steinestel K. Role of reflux-induced epithelial-mesenchymal transition in periprosthetic leakage after prosthetic voice rehabilitation. Head Neck. 2015;37(4):530–6. https://doi.org/10.1002/hed.23622. Epub 2014 Apr 9.
41. Cocuzza S, Bonfiglio M, Chiaramonte R, Serra AJ. Relationship between radiotherapy and gastroesophageal reflux disease in causing tracheoesophageal voice rehabilitation failure. Voice. 2014;28(2):245–9. https://doi.org/10.1016/j.jvoice.2013.08.008. Epub 2013 Oct 2.
42. Lorenz KJ, Maier H. Pulmonary rehabilitation after total laryngectomy using a heat and moisture exchanger (HME). Laryngorhinootologie. 2009;88(8):513–22. https://doi.org/10.1055/s-0029-1225619. Epub 2009 Jul 30.
43. Zuur JK, Muller SH, de Jongh FH, van Zandwijk N, Hilgers FJ. The physiological rationale of heat and moisture exchangers in post-laryngectomy pulmonary rehabilitation: a review. Eur Arch Otorhinolaryngol. 2006;263(1):1–8. https://doi.org/10.1007/s00405-005-0969-3. Epub 2005 Jul 7.
44. Bień S, Okła S, van As-Brooks CJ, Ackerstaff AH. The effect of a heat and moisture exchanger (Provox HME) on pulmonary protection after total laryngectomy: a randomized controlled study. Eur Arch Otorhinolaryngol. 2010;267(3):429–35. https://doi.org/10.1007/s00405-009-1018-4.
45. Hilgers FJ, Ackerstaff AH, Van As CJ, Balm AJ, Van den Brekel MW, Tan IB. Development and clinical assessment of a heat and moisture exchanger with a multi-magnet automatic tracheostoma valve (Provox FreeHands HME) for vocal and pulmonary rehabilitation after total laryngectomy. Acta Otolaryngol. 2003;123(1):91–9. https://doi.org/10.1080/00365540 21000028083.
46. Hashiba M, Sugai Y, Izumi T, Ino S, Ifukube T. Development of a wearable electro-larynx for laryngectomees and its evaluation. Annu Int Conf IEEE Eng Med Biol Soc. 2007;2007:5267–70. https://doi.org/10.1109/IEMBS.2007.4353530.
47. Globlek D, Stajner-Katusic S, Musura M, Horga D, Liker M. Comparison of alaryngeal voice and speech. Logoped Phoniatr Vocol. 2004;29(2):87–91. https://doi.org/10.1080/14015430410033218.

48. Green G, Hults M. Preferences for three types of alaryngeal speech. J Speech Hear Disord. 1982;47(2):141–5. https://doi.org/10.1044/jshd.4702.141.
49. Cox SR, Doyle PC. The influence of electrolarynx use on postlaryngectomy voice-related quality of life. Otolaryngol Head Neck Surg. 2014;150(6):1005–9. https://doi.org/10.1177/0194599814524704. Epub 2014 Feb 21
50. Kaye R, Tang CG, Sinclair CF. The electrolarynx: voice restoration after total laryngectomy. Med Devices (Auckl). 2017;10:133–40. https://doi.org/10.2147/MDER.S133225. eCollection 2017.

Da Vinci Robotic Surgery for Laryngeal Cancers

32

Abie H. Mendelsohn and Georges Lawson

Key Points

- With robotic head and neck surgery being established as a minimally invasive approach for successful treatment for oropharyngeal benign and malignant lesions, evidence is growing in support of the surgical treatment for laryngeal conditions.
- Technologic advances such as the Single Port (SP) robotic surgical system improve an already reliable surgical option for supraglottic cancers.
- Robotic surgery offers improved visualization, instrumentation, and dexterity as compared with direct laryngoscopic and microscopic approaches to the laryngeal subsites.
- Early experience, described herein, for transoral robotic hypopharyngectomy utilizing the SP system, shows promise toward avoiding the morbidity of open surgical approaches to this recessed region of the larynx.

32.1 Introduction

Robotic-assisted surgery continues to act as one of the fastest growing areas of Head and Neck surgery. As technology continues to improve, the reach of transoral robotic surgery (TORS) for pharyngeal and laryngeal tumors continues to expand. While the earliest clinical trials had focused mainly on oropharyngeal tumors, [1] the reach and access of robotic instruments and visualization has allowed the application of TORS beyond the oropharynx and into the larynx. This chapter will review the specifics of robotic-assisted surgery for the larynx and airway, describe clinical applications, and comment on future applications for robotic surgery of the larynx and airway.

A. H. Mendelsohn (✉)
Department of Head & Neck Surgery, David Geffen School of Medicine at UCLA, Los Angeles, CA, USA

G. Lawson
Otolaryngology, Head and Neck Surgery Department, Louvain University Hospital of Mont-Godinne, Yvoir, Belgium
e-mail: Georges.Lawson@uclouvain.be

M. Remacle, H. E. Eckel (eds.), *Textbook of Surgery of Larynx and Trachea*,
https://doi.org/10.1007/978-3-031-09621-1_32

32.2 The da Vinci Robotic Surgical System

After a decade of TORS, the da Vinci robotic surgical system (Intuitive Surgical, Sunnyvale, California, USA) is the primary technology utilized. This chapter will therefore will focus solely on the da Vinci systems, though motivated readers are encouraged to become familiar with alternative platforms such as Flex Robotic System (MedRobotics, Raynham, Massachusetts, USA) as well as emerging robotic surgical systems such as the Enos system (Titan Medical, Toronto, Canada).

Initial FDA approval of TORS in 2009 was provided with the "*S*" generation of the da Vinci. Since that time, the newer da Vinci models (*Si, Xi*) have become the workhorses for robotic-assisted surgeries. Most recently, the single port "*SP*" model has been approved for TORS use and has begun to show tremendous improvement in access. Figure 32.1 displays a side-by-side visual comparison of the newer surgical models. Additionally, many of the system factors important to TORS performance are compared in Table 32.1.

The traditional systems (non-SP) provide four independent robotic arms, anatomic narrowing

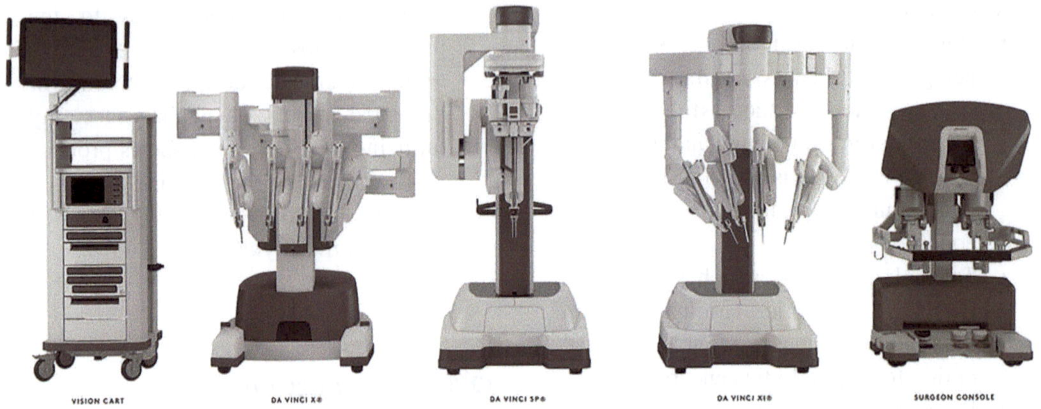

Fig. 32.1 da Vinci Robotic Surgical Models. The currently available surgical systems are demonstrated, including the two multiarmed models of the X and Xi compared with the single arm SP system. *[Permission is given to use these materials in their entire unmodified form. Permission is not granted if these materials are modified in any way. Images must be reproduced in high resolution. Reproduced images should be accompanied by the following copyright notice: ©2021 Intuitive Surgical, Inc.]*

Table 32.1 Comparative chart of da Vinci Surgical System Models

	Si	X	Xi	SP
New system available to purchase in 2021	No	Yes	Yes	Yes
Number of instruments (TORS)	2	2	2	3
Endoscope factors	8.5 mm outer diameter; rigid	8 mm outer diameter; rigid	8 mm outer diameter; rigid	9 mm oblong diameter; flexible
Instrument factors	5 mm outer diameter; flexible wristing	8 mm outer diameter; jointed wristing	8 mm outer diameter; jointed wristing	7 mm outer diameter; flexible elbow and wristing
Maximal camera angulation	30°	30°	30°	28°
Advanced energy instruments (vessel sealer, harmonic scalpel)	Yes	Yes	Yes	No
Near-infrared (NIR) imaging	Yes	Yes	Yes	No
Boom rotation	No	No	Yes	Yes
Bedside cart footprint	Limited	Limited	Expanded	Expanded

currently restricts TORS to the use of three arms. The central arm is equipped with the robotic endoscope that contains two visual channels along with multiple light apertures. With the limited access to the larynx, the 8.5 mm endoscope is recommended to improve operative spacing. Endoscopes are also available with a straight (0-degree) view or with an angled (30-degree) view. This angled endoscope can be quite useful when reaching anterior areas of the larynx. The endoscope can be positioned with the angled view anteriorly (up-looking) or posteriorly (down-looking). However, as with endoscopic sinus surgery, use of angled endoscopes can alter the expected position of anatomic landmarks and should be used with caution.

The arms on each side of the central endoscope are equipped with robotic instruments. With well over 30 types of instrument designs, identifying the exact optimal device can sometimes be laborious. Instruments are broadly categorized by their diameter and by their function. The first generation of robotic instruments maintained 8 mm outer diameter, which included a right-angled jointed instrument. However, newer instruments now maintain a smaller 5 mm outer diameter. The 5 mm instruments are recommended within the tight spacing of the pharynx and larynx. The newer 5 mm instruments are also designed with a wristed joint to allow for improved reach and dexterity.

The instrument function can be categorized as either *cutting* or *retracting*. Given the specialized tissue of the larynx and airway, the cutting energy options need to be reviewed. The most common cutting energy instrument is the Bovie monopolar cautery, which can be delivered by either a spatula or hooked tip. TORS is typically carried out with the use of the spatula tip. Bipolar cautery instruments were previously only available in 8 mm diameter, but 5 mm bipolar cautery forceps have recently been made available for clinical use. Bipolar will likely become adapted within TORS procedures as clinical experience collects.

Harmonic scalpel (Ethicon Endo-Surgery, Inc., Cincinnati, Ohio, USA) robotic instrument is available in both 8 mm and 5 mm diameters; however, complexity in energy delivery has prevented the harmonic scalpel from obtaining the same degree of wristed angulation that is typical of the robotic instrument. As such, its description has to date been limited to blood vessel control within cervical compartment surgeries. With improved degrees of motion, the harmonic scalpel will likely have a larger role in laryngeal TORS, specifically endoscopic ligation of the superior laryngeal artery.

Laser integrated instruments make up the last group of cutting instruments. *Intuitive Surgical* only offers the thulium laser fiber delivery as an integrated robotic instrument. While a positive experience with the thulium laser in the larynx and pharynx has been described, [2, 3] popular use is still limited. This underutilization may be related to relative unfamiliarity with the thulium wavelength or perhaps from the capital requirement of purchasing a new thulium laser system in addition to the robotic system. Third party laser adapters have allowed for the conversion of standard retracting instruments into robotic-assisted CO_2 laser delivery systems. Specifically, *Lumenis Inc.* (Yokneam, Israel) producing the *FiberLase Robotic Drop-in Guide* and *OmniGuide Inc* (Cambridge, Massachusetts, USA) producing the *FlexGuide Ultra* provide CO_2 fiber delivery instruments. Overall, both systems provide a flexible fiber guide that is fitted for robotic graspers (recommended instrument is the 5 mm needle driver) as seen in Fig. 32.2. The fiber can be delivered and removed as needed throughout each procedure. On a practical level, both systems offer individual differences that can be considered when comparing the laser system.

The most distinct difference between the *Omniguide* and *FiberLase* by *Lumenis* is the laser energy dispersion. Energy dispersion is seen when the laser spot widens as the tip of the fiber is moved away from the target. The energy dispersion reduces the final laser power density, or cutting efficiency. However, the energy dispersion also helps coagulate small diameter (~1 mm) blood vessels. *OmniGuide* laser energy typically has a wider field of energy dispersion than the *FiberLase*. This increased dispersion can be seen as an advantage for either system depending on surgeon preference. A more dispersed energy beam will

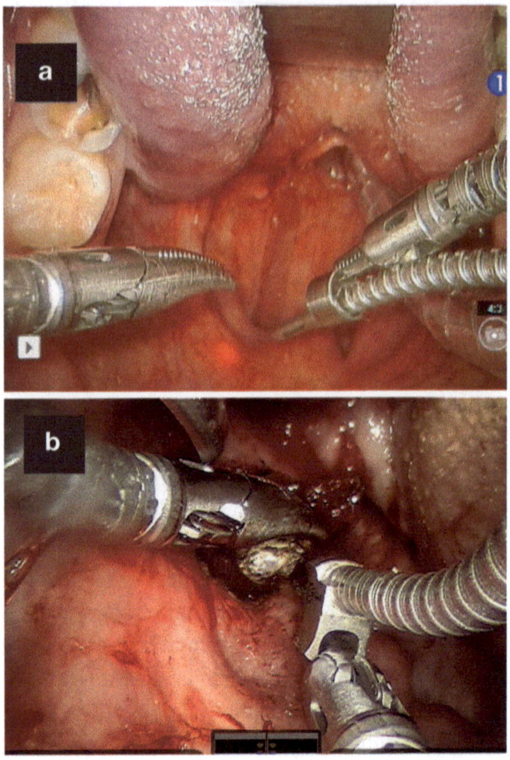

Fig. 32.2 CO_2 Laser fiber guides adaptable with TORS instrumentation. (**a**) demonstrates the FiberLase guide for the Lumenis laser fiber and (**b**) demonstrates the FlexGuide guide for the Omniguide laser fiber. A key difference seen is the aiming beam of the Lumenis system

coagulate more effectively, while a more focused energy beam will offer a more precise incision line. Another difference between the two fiber laser systems is that the FiberLase provides a HeNe aiming beam, similar to standard articulated armed CO_2 delivery systems. Both robotic-assisted CO_2 laser systems have been reported with good early clinical experience [4, 5]. Table 32.2 reviews the general advantages and disadvantages of the available cutting instruments.

32.3 TORS Versus Microsuspension Laryngoscopy

A TORS approach for laryngeal and airway surgery is the next iteration to the more traditional endoscopic approach of microsuspension Direct Laryngoscopy (mDL). mDL can be performed either through a rigid laryngoscope or with the use of similar distending bivalved, or bladed,

Table 32.2 Summary of strengths and limitations of TORS cutting instrumentation

	Width of incision	Thermal damage	Blood vessel coagulation
Flexible fiber CO_2 laser	++++	++	+
Thulium laser	++	+++	++
Electrocautery	+	++++	+++
Harmonic scalpel	+	++++	++++
Cold knife	++++	–	–

retractors, which are also utilized for TORS exposure. Oncologic resection, particularly in the glottis, has been performed successfully with either laser or cold knife mucosal incisions, whereas electrocautery is typically the mainstay for TORS incisional work.

Despite the considerable differences between the microscope-assisted visualization of mDL and the endoscopic-assisted visualization of TORS providing many to favor one approach over the other, all laryngeal surgeons must be well versed regarding the strict indications/contraindications applicable to both transoral approaches. Specifically, potential mDL and TORS patients must

- Maintain overall health to undergo the strains of general anesthesia.
- Tolerate cervical spinal extension without pain or discomfort (assessed preoperatively).
- Demonstrate unrestricted mandibular excursion.
- When malignancy is present, the tumor must be amenable to endoscopic resection. Specifically, regarding laryngeal cancer, a fixed arytenoid motion should be considered a strong contraindication.
- Tolerate some level of swallow dysfunction, particularly when consideration of endoscopic supraglottic laryngectomy or hypopharyngectomy.

Surgical risks are fairly similar comparing mDL and TORS. Preoperative discussion of risk for both approaches should include possible chipped teeth, lacerated lip, tongue numbness, taste alterations, need for parental feeding, airway swelling, or bleeding.

Overall, it is the authors' experience that when both approaches can be safely offered, TORS offers tremendous advantage over the mDL approach. The high-definition wide-angle endoscope of the robotic system offers a superior visualization of the operative field. As demonstrated in Fig. 32.3, TORS offers wide-field visualization of the entire operative field while still being able to magnify the area of interest. The difference in field of view can be minimal in the case of lesions confined to the glottis, yet larger lesions, which extend beyond the anatomic boundaries of the glottis, typically exceed the view of standard direct laryngoscopes. The robotic visualization is also enhanced by a three-dimensional (3D) display, which is superior to that of binocular display of the operative microscopes. Adjusting the operative view is also improved with the robotic system. The surgeon-controlled endoscope movement (by way of the console foot pedal) can rapidly recenter the surgical view without effort or disruption to the surgical momentum, which is in contrast to the surgical disruption required for microscope readjustments.

TORS also provides improvement in surgical dexterity. With degrees of freedom at the instrument wrist, angled surgical motion can achieve improved direction of retraction and cutting over that of the static directionality of long-handled mDL instruments. Additionally, the long-handled mDL instruments enhance physiologic hand tremor. However, the movement scaling of the robotic system provides a tremor-free surgical action along with graded motion. Finally, the placement of the cutting instrument in the field of surgery (as in the spatula bovie arms) provides a two-handed surgical experience. In contrast, when an articulated-arm laser system is used, one hand is required for beam aiming, leaving only one surgical instrument in the surgical field.

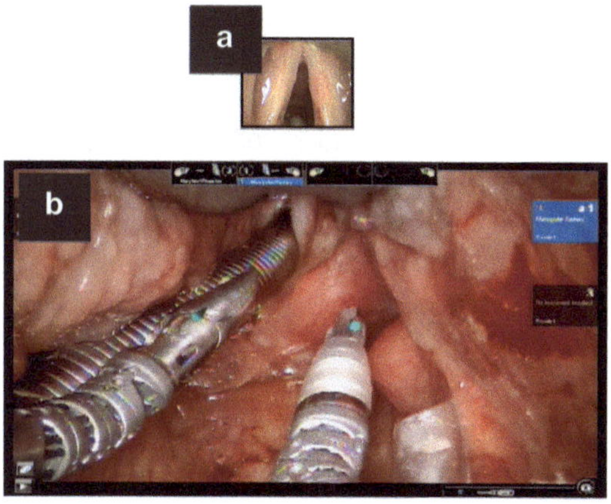

Fig. 32.3 Comparative views of (**a**) Microsuspension Direct Laryngoscopy (mDL) and (**b**) Transoral Robotic Surgery (TORS). The vocal folds are held at a consistent relative size; however, the field outside the area of focus is dramatically enhanced with the use of the robotic system

Laryngeal TORS approach also adds improvement with education and training of future surgeons. mDL procedures can prove to be challenging to observe with frequent microscope adjustments and limited field of view. In comparison, the wide-field view of TORS will typically provide an improved observing experience for students and surgeons-in-training. The robotic systems generally can provide an additional layer of improved training with the dual console. Surgeons-in-training can observe the surgical procedures from the exact perspective of the operative surgeon. The observing personnel can also move the surgical controls along with the surgery as a "rehearsal." When the nonoperating console moves the surgical controls, visual markers are displayed across the digital displays as blue pointers, as shown in Fig. 32.3b. Once sufficient experience is acquired, operative control of the robotic instruments may be alternated between the two consoles, between the two surgeons, so that initial surgical experiences may be provided in a controlled manner. Finally, the computer-based simulator of the robotic system allows for standardized skills training and objective trainee metrics. In all, the transition from mDL to TORS approach when appropriate may allow for improved training of the next generation of laryngeal surgeons.

32.4 Single Port "SP" da Vinci System

In 2020, TORS received a major system upgrade with the SP system release along with FDA approval for TORS clinical use. This approval was based on mostly the early clinical trials by Chan et al. including the Phase I trial published in 2017, [6] which was followed quickly by the prospective phase II clinical trial published in 2019 [7]. The results of these trials were summarized by Holsinger et al. in 2019, [8] which combined the results of these two important trials. None of the 47 patients included in the 2 trials required conversion from the SP TORS approach, neither to non-SP robotic systems, mDL, nor open approaches. There were no intraoperative complications or device-related serious adverse events. The SP TORS operative experience and postoperative course matched those factors, which have been well documented over the past decade utilizing multiport surgical systems, including an acceptable level of blood loss, oncologic margin clearance, tracheostomy placement, postsurgical swallowing function, and postoperative hemorrhage. These three publications provided the data for the FDA to conclude that SP driven TORS surgical procedures would be safe, and since this time, there has been a steady increase in SP surgeon experience worldwide.

However, apart from safety and equivalency trials, it is very unlikely that the literature will be able to prove superiority of the newest SP system as compared with the standard multiport da Vinci systems. Whereas the SP demonstrates some clear advantages over the multiport systems, there are also a few challenges. Advantages of the SP system include a third robotic surgical instrument able to fit into the oral cavity while the arms of the multiport limit the surgeons to only two instruments. The SP camera and instruments, as demonstrated in Fig. 32.4, have increased flexibility with the design incorporating two points of mobility (termed the wrist and elbow). This flexibility provides much more reliable access into the laryngeal subsites, and with patients with optimal mouth opening, this system can operate even beyond the larynx to reach the cervical esophagus. The SP's single port measures 2.5 cm in diameter, which presents both an opportunity to focus patient oral cavity retraction at the point of the dentition, yet also limits the surgeons' traditional retraction strategy with bladed pharyngoscopes (i.e., LARS or FK-WO) expanding the diameter of the oropharyngeal airway. Additionally, with the instruments and camera sharing a common insertion site, there is more risk of camera and instrument collisions. This is of particular importance given the recent prospective data showing multiport TORS surgical skill is directly correlated to the avoidance instrument collisions, as illustrated in Fig. 32.5 [9]. How SP system TORS surgical performance is affected by such instrument collisions needs further investigation.

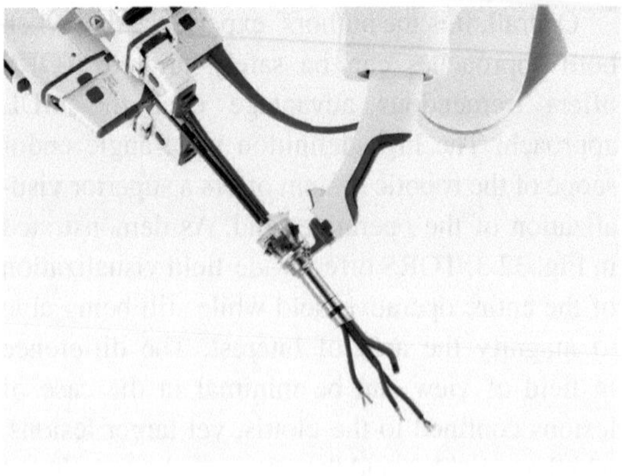

Fig. 32.4 The Single Port (SP) da Vinci system is the latest generation approved for TORS, which provides 3 flexible surgical instruments combined with a flexible endoscope, which are inserted through a single 2.5 cm diameter cannula

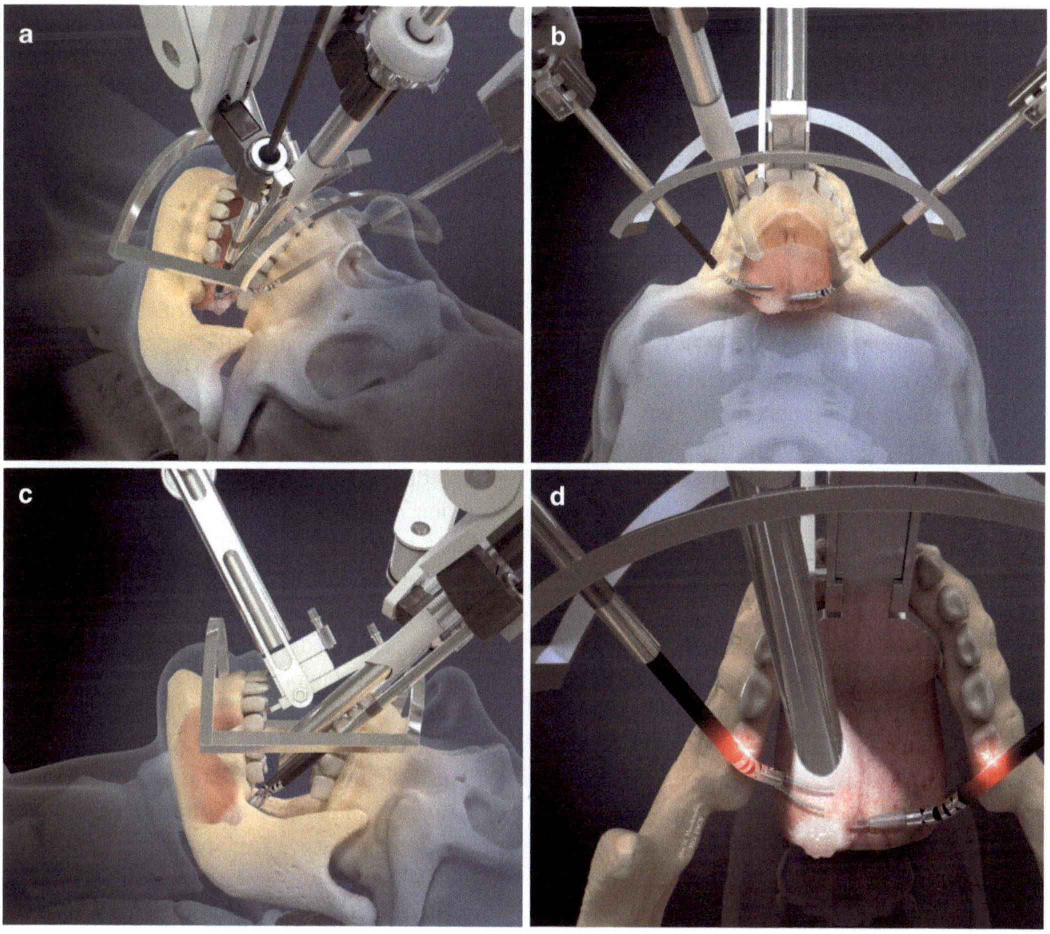

Fig. 32.5 Computer graphic renderings of TORS "out-of-field" anatomic collisions. Panels (**a**, **b**, and **c**) show standard TORS endoscope and instrument setup for a left base of tongue tumor resection. As the instruments are manipulated for tumor resection, panel (**d**) illustrates instrument shaft collisions along the mandibular molars bilaterally. Red highlighting dramatizing effects are illustrated to accentuate their position outside of the robotic endoscopic field of view. The field of view is illustrated in panel (**d**) by the cone of light emanating from the endoscope aperture

32.5 Clinical Applications

From the technical advantages, a number of robotic-assisted surgical approaches have been adapted to the larynx and airway. This chapter will now discuss more frequently described applications. The surgical approaches described require extensive training. Endoscopic laryngeal and airway surgery experience will also clearly enhance the transition to endoscopic robotic surgery. An "inside-out" understating of laryngeal neurovascular anatomy, which is critical in avoiding major surgical complications [10]. These approaches also require specialized head and neck training for the robotic system concentrating on transoral exposure and transoral placement of instrumentation to access the larynx and airway [11]. Additionally, robotic surgery programs should allow surgeons the appropriate time to progress through the expected learning curve [12] and should plan cases more proximal in the head and neck, such as the palatine tonsillar fossa, reserving laryngeal robotic surgery for only the experienced robotic surgeon.

32.6 TORS Supraglottic Laryngectomy

For many tumors of the supraglottis, primary surgical resection may offer an excellent treatment option. While the most common malignancy of the supraglottis is squamous cell carcinoma, surgical resection can also be commonly recommended for other tumors of the supraglottis such as nerve sheath tumors, [13] paragangliomas, [14] and carcinoid tumors [15].

Operative Technique

The operative technique for TORS supraglottic laryngectomy parallels the techniques for endoscopic CO_2 laser supraglottic laryngectomy [16]. Large variations in technique are required based on the anatomic location and extent of tumor progression. With the large body of work with endoscopic laser–assisted supraglottic laryngectomy, TORS surgical excision of supraglottic laryngeal cancers is therefore similarly described according to the classification scheme of the European Laryngological Society (ELS) (see Fig. 32.6) [17]. The Exposure is obtained utilizing the operative pharyngoscope of choice. The authors use the Laryngeal Advanced Retraction System (LARS) pharyngoscope. Resections limited to the suprahyoid epiglottis can be exposed with a tongue blade fitted to retract the oropharyngeal tongue. The remaining resections including deeper portions of the supraglottis, such as the aryepiglottic fold or false vocal folds, should be first exposed with a laryngeal (long, narrow width) tongue blade fitted at the petiole. With this configuration, the posterior-most boundaries may be incised first before blood can obscure the dependent portions of the operative field. If needed, the epiglottis can then be released from retraction with minor adjustments to the pharyngoscope for epiglottic or vallecular incisions. Figure 32.7 displays the surgical steps of a TORS Supraglottic Laryngectomy.

A "Limited Excision" (type I) supraglottic laryngectomy entails excision of small superficial tumors on the free border of the epiglottis, the aryepiglottic fold, the arytenoids, or the ventricular fold or any other part of the supraglottis. In cases of small and superficial T1 tumors of the laryngeal surface of the epiglottis located above the hyoid bone, the resection includes half of the suprahyoid epiglottis. This procedure is a "Limited Medial" supraglottic laryngectomy without resection of the preepiglottic space (type IIa).

"Medial" supraglottic laryngectomy without resection of the preepiglottic space (type IIb) should be applied for T1 tumors of the laryngeal surface of the epiglottis extending below the hyoid bone. In these cases, a total epiglottectomy is performed. The incision line goes through the preepiglottic space without its complete excision. The pharyngoepiglottic, aryepiglottic, and ventricular folds are preserved.

The resection of T1 or T2 tumors extending to the petiole of the epiglottis must include the preepiglottic space. This procedure is the "Medial supraglottic laryngectomy with Resection of the Preepiglottic Space" (type IIIa). The incision is guided along the vallecula until the hyoid bone is reached. The incision line moves caudally from the hyoid bone toward the thyrohyoid membrane until the upper border of the thyroid cartilage is exposed. From this point, the whole entity of the preepiglottic space is removed along the inner surface of the lamina of the thyroid cartilage together with the epiglottis, toward the anterior commissure of the vocal folds.

T1-T2 tumors of the infrahyoid epiglottis extending to the ventricular fold can be resected with the same technique (type IIIb). The ventricular folds can be completely dissected from the thyroid cartilage along the inner surface toward the ventricle of Morgagni.

In cases of tumors of the aryepitglottic fold (also known as marginal tumors) with possible extension to the ventricular folds, the resection includes the free edge of the epiglottis, the three folds' region, and the ventricular fold. This procedure is the "Lateral" supraglottic laryngectomy (type IVa).

The "Lateral supraglottic laryngectomy with Arytenoid Resection" (type IVb) was proposed in case of extension to the mobile arytenoids; the arytenoid is included in the resection. The resection may include the inner or medial and anterior part of the pyriform sinus.

As much as possible en bloc resections should be performed. The specimen is examined, but frozen sections are typically taken from the laryngeal margins after tumor resection. Tracheostomy is not a recommended portion of this surgery. Cervical nodal basins also require intervention, either through selective neck dissections or through sentinel lymph node biopsy [18]. The details of these procedures are beyond the scope of this chapter but should be part of the surgical plan. The authors routinely perform the neck surgeries during the same anesthetic administration as the robotic-assisted resection.

Postoperative care includes intravenous steroid, or steroid nebulization, for 8–10 days, preventive antibiotics for three to four days, and proton pump inhibitors until the healing is completed. Oral intake with a pureed diet is resumed the day after surgery under speech therapist guidance.

The authors' previously published experience with TORS supraglottic laryngectomy currently described 18 patients who underwent robotic-assisted surgical resection as illustrated in Fig. 32.8 [19]. There were no (0%) tracheostomies performed at any point during treatment. Overall, patients required an average of 4.5 days for safe swallow for solids and 5.5 days for safe swallow for thin liquids. Female gender, advanced pathologic T-stage (III/IV), simultaneous neck dissection, and temporary postoperative vocal fold hypomobility were associated with significant delays in return of swallow function. There were no gastrostomies tubes placed at any point during treatment. Over a 2-year follow-up period, there were no local recurrences leading to a local control rate of 100%. Three (16.7%) patients developed regional recurrences. Four

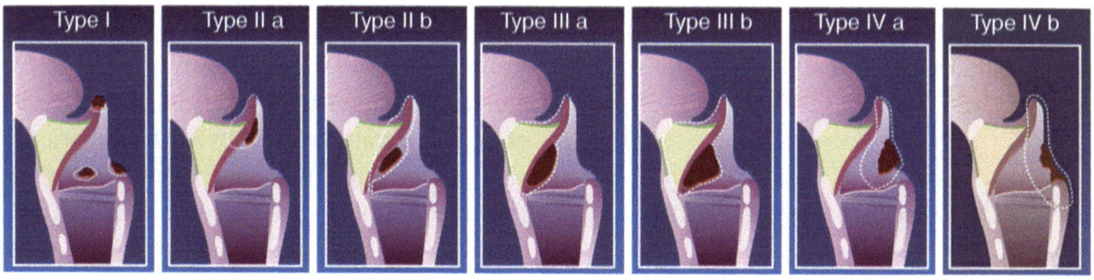

Fig. 32.6 The European Laryngological Society (ELS) Classification for Supraglottic Laryngectomy [17]. Limited excision (Type I) entails excision of small superficial tumors on the free border of the epiglottis, the aryepiglottic fold, the arytenoid or the ventricular fold, or any other part of the supraglottis. Medial supraglottic laryngectomy with partial resection of the preepiglottic space (Type II), the resection includes half of the suprahyoid epiglottis (Type IIa). For tumors extending below the hyoid bone, a total epiglottectomy is performed (Type IIb). Medial supraglottic laryngectomy with resection of the preepiglottic space (Type III), with tumors extending to the petiole of the epiglottis and must include the preepiglottic space (Type IIIa). Tumors of the infrahyoid epiglottis extending to the ventricular fold can readily be resected (Type IIIb). Lateral supraglottic laryngectomy (Type IV), with the resection includes the free edge of the epiglottis, the threefolds' region, and the ventricular fold (Type IVa). In case of extension to the mobile arytenoid, the arytenoid is included in the resection (Type IVb)

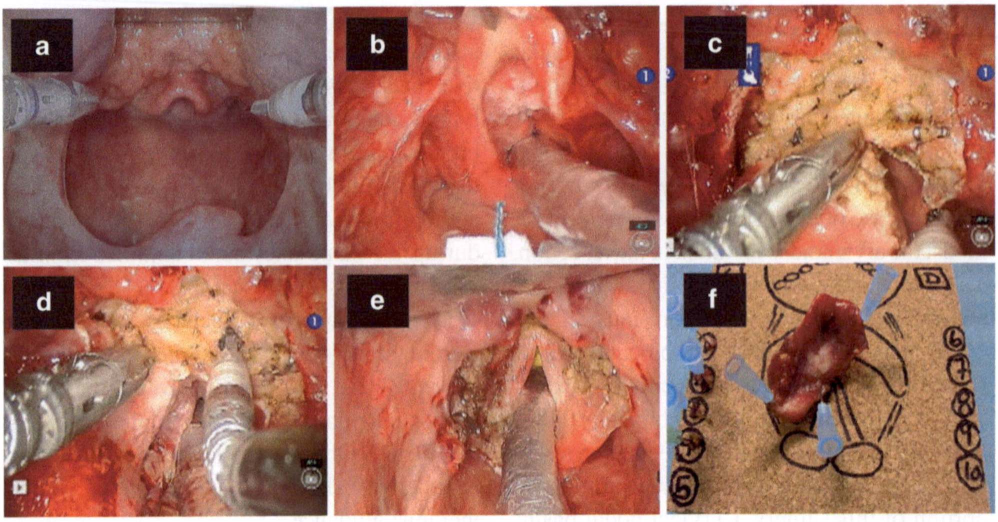

Fig. 32.7 TORS Supraglottic laryngectomy. The procedure begins with retraction of the oropharyngeal tongue and insertion of the robotic instruments (**a**). Following this, the resection proceed from posterior to anterior. The posterior cuts are made under visualization in a bloodless field (**b**). Laterally, along the pharyngoepiglottic fold, the superior laryngeal artery is dissected and surgically controlled, in this view a titanium hemo-clip has been applied (**c**). The incision is then carried anteriorly to include as much of the pre-epiglottic space fat as oncologically indicated (**d**). The postresection larynx typically demonstrates minimal edema at this point, and if so, no tracheostomy is required (**e**). The tumor is oriented for pathologic analysis with margin assessment. The use of pathologic corkboard and 25-G needles provides reliable tumor fixation without the need for inking (**f**)

(22.2%) developed distant metastases. Only overall cancer stage IV was found to be significantly associated with the development of distant metastasis. Two patients died during the follow-up period (cardiopulmonary failure), leading to a 2-year overall survival of 88.9%. The authors' positive experience with TORS supraglottic laryngectomy has been confirmed with several studies demonstrating good functional and oncologic outcomes [20–23].

32.7 TORS Glottic Cordectomy

Despite the major advances in approach and access brought by the SP da Vinci system, it remains the opinion of the authors that in its current state robotic surgery does not match the advantages of CO_2 laser microsurgery. With glottic surgery confined to the laryngeal introitus, the ability to quickly adjust the robotic endoscope plays less of a role as compared to more involved surgery of the supraglottic larynx. The advantages of robotic-assisted surgery over traditional endoscopic surgery including visualization, surgeon tremor filtration, and improved surgical dexterity are all not acutely required as compared with standard mDL experience.

In the past several years, there have been several reports of TORS glottic surgery [24, 25]. Robotic vocal fold cordectomy for glottic carcinoma has demonstrated successful achievement of negative margins; however, the experience is also complicated with infrequent feeding tube and tracheostomy tube placement [25], which is typically not seen with mDL CO_2 laser cordectomy. However, in this largest series of TORS for glottic cancer, a higher rate of synechia formation is seen likely due to either cautery thermal effect or inadvertent mucosal injury away from the intended mucosal incision sites. As such, TORS can be combined with flexible fiber CO_2 delivery to improve the critical thermal damage, which Bovie cautery transmits within the specialized

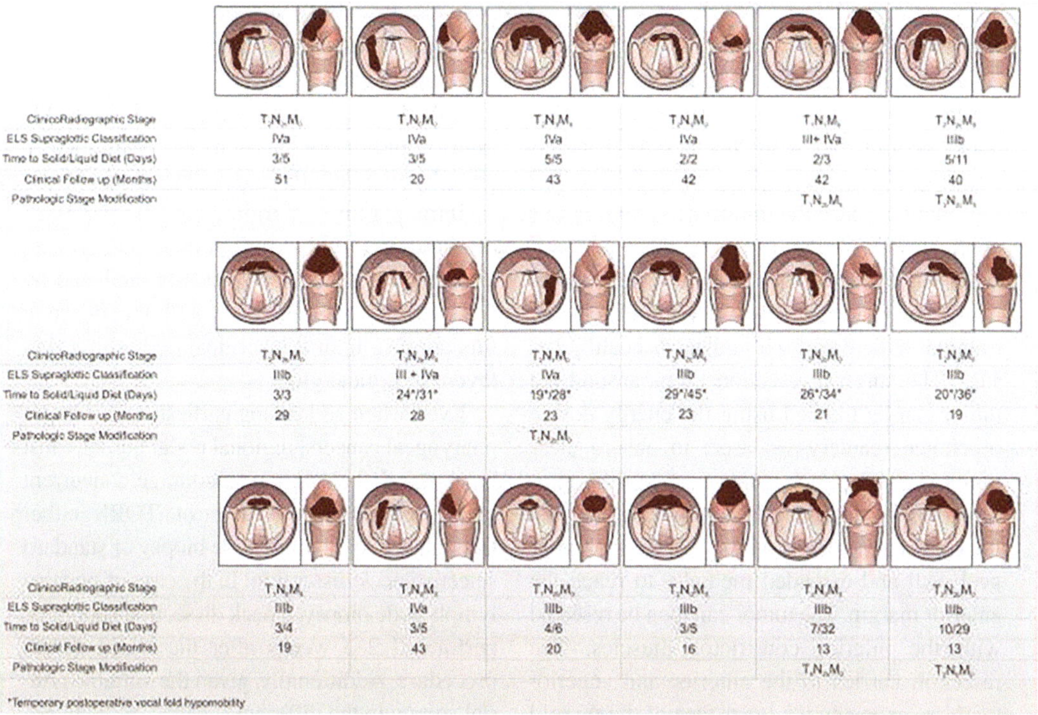

Fig. 32.8 Clinical and Tumor Classification of TORS Supraglottic laryngectomy from the Authors' published experience. Each tumor extent is illustrated along with dotted line borders of surgical resection. For each case, presenting clinical stage is listed along with the European Laryngologic Society (ELS) classification of supraglottic laryngectomy. Functional outcome of diet is listed separately for solid and liquid diet advancement

tissue of the glottis [26]. However, until further experience with TORS CO_2 laser glottic surgery can be shared, it is unclear how this combined robotic and laser approach offers a noticeable improvement from standard microscopic laser glottic surgery.

32.8 TORS Hypopharyngectomy

There are to date less than a handful of papers describing the TORS hypopharyngectomy experience [27–30]. With the presentation of resectable hypopharyngeal cancers being less common than primary glottic or supraglottic cancers, it is likely that this subsite of laryngeal cancers will see the slowest growth in the TORS experience. Overall, the early experience shows oncologic control rates in-line with both open surgical hypopharyngectomy as well as nonsurgical therapy of radiation with or without chemotherapy. Patients should be counselled regarding the likely 10–15% likelihood for temporary tracheostomy tube placement as well as the average 5–7 days wait until oral feeding can be safely resumed. Risks of postoperative hemorrhage, need for adjuvant therapy, as well as possible salvage laryngectomy. Nonetheless, it is the authors' opinion that TORS hypopharyngectomy appears to be able to supplant open and mDL laser endoscopic approaches as the primary surgical modality in the treatment of early staged hypopharyngeal cancers.

Operative Technique

The authors' TORS Hypopharyngectomy described in Fig. 32.9 utilizes a multiport da Vinci system, but with the increased access and dexterity of the single port system, the SP will likely replace the multiport system in this application.

TORS hypopharyngectomy starts by mobilizing the lesion to assess its limits and the eventual adherences with adjacent healthy tissues. The surgical resection limits around the tumor can be marked using the energy device of choice (cautery vs laser) to ensure clear tumor margins. Once mapped, as in the supraglottic technique, it is important that the first incision was achieved on the posterior pharyngeal wall and extended medially to reach the anterior margin. The tumor can then be resected with the inferior constrictor muscles. The resection carries to the anterior and superior margins, exposing the inner face of the thyroid cartilage. Thyroid cartilage perichondrium can be resected if indicated. Care is taken throughout the soft tissue dissection for both arterial and venous vessels lager than 3 mm and, if identified, are surgically ligated. Finally, the inferior and lateral incisions are performed to complete the initially mapped incision.

Intraoperative margins can be assessed after tumor resection in four quadrants as well as along the deep aspect, ideally analyzed by fresh frozen sections. Many authors choose at this point to treat the surgical bed with a thin layer of surgical glue.

Even when addressing earliest staged hypopharyngeal cancers, regional nodal burden must be assessed. The authors encourage concurrent nodal surgery at the time of TORS either through sentinel lymph node biopsy or standard selective neck dissection. In the case of positive lymph-node biopsy, a neck dissection should be performed 2–3 weeks after the initial TORS procedure. Additionally, given the variable arterial supply to the different subsites of the hypopharynx, cervical surgical preventive vascular ligation is generally not indicated.

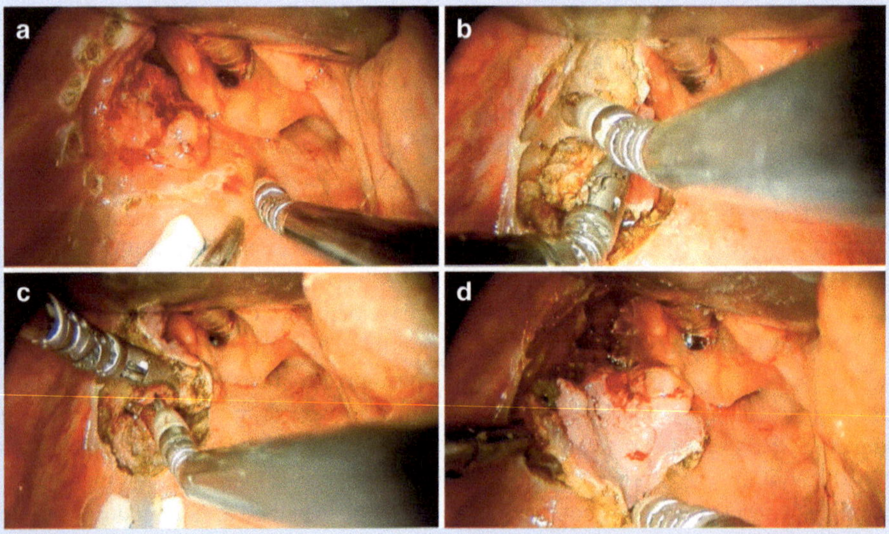

Fig. 32.9 TORS Hypopharyngectomy. The procedure begins with exposure of the hypopharynx, in this case, a left lateral pyriform sinus cancer (**a**). Exposure of the hypopharynx is generally improved with the pharyngoscope blade retracting the endotracheal tube anteriorly and thereby suspending the larynx away from the posterior pharyngeal wall. The mucosal incisions are marked out, ideally maintaining 1 cm free margin when possible. The tumor is then dissected along its deep aspect, always resecting the inferior constrictor muscles and exposing the inner aspect of the thyroid cartilage (**b**). Blood vessels should be surgically controlled, here with a titanium hemoclip (**c**). Care should proceed once the tumor is released in order to preserve correct anatomic orientation for accurate margin assessment (**d**) Additionally, limited tumor manipulation reduces the risks for "floaters" of carcinoma transplanted onto otherwise normal tissue

32.9 TORS Total Laryngectomy

The authors introduced total laryngectomy as a new TORS technique designed to decrease treatment-related morbidities and to increase post-operative quality of life [31]. Shortly following, several case reports were published with additional experience with this technique [32, 33]. The common motivation from these reports was to provide a minimally invasive approach, which could potentially improve healing and to speed recovery time following total laryngectomy.

Operative Technique

The procedure begins with a standard tracheostomy skin incision, approximately 4 cm in length, midway between the cricoid cartilage and the sternal notch. After the superior subplatysmal skin flap is raised, the strap muscles are divided along the midline raphe to expose the trachea and cricoid cartilages. A thyroid isthmusectomy is performed, and the lateral lobes are dissected off of the lateral tracheal walls. A complete transection of the trachea is placed at the third tracheal space with rising posterior tracheal mucosal cuts. Inferior stomal stitches are placed to secure the caudal trachea. The 4-cm skin incision allows ample visualization to dissect around the remaining rostral trachea and cricoid cartilage, which includes sectioning bilateral recurrent laryngeal nerves. At this point, heavy braided sutures are placed around the lateral walls of the rostral trachea and are threaded atraumatically through glottis for intraoral retraction. The stoma site is then covered with sterile drapes to minimize contamination from the transoral portion.

Initial placement of the LARS pharyngoscope uses the intraoral retractor blade retracting the epiglottis at the petiole. After optimal visualization is obtained, the initial incision is positioned along the superior-most aspect of the arytenoid mucosa. With the dissector forceps holding the postcricoid mucosa posteriorly, the Bovie separates this mucosal layer from the underlying cricoid cartilage. Subsequently, the epiglottis is then released from retraction, and the vallecula incision is made along lingual surface of the epiglottis in the direction toward the superior border of thyroid cartilage. Extending the vallecular incision laterally and posteriorly, the superior laryngeal vessels are encountered as they course through the thyrohyoid membrane. Multiple clips are placed on the vessels and divided. Dissection is continued caudally until the thyroid cartilage is encountered. Keeping the hyoid bone retracted underneath the intraoral retractor blade, the thyrohyoid membrane is transected. The instruments are directed along the external thyroid cartilage perichondrium. As progress continues inferiorly, tension will be required on the previously placed inferior tracheal retraction sutures. These sutures will give a rostral pull to the inferior portion of the laryngeal skeleton, as well as allowing for lateral deflection of the specimen to improve visualization. Dissection continues caudally until the larynx is freed from its attachments. The larynx is then delivered orally.

The pharyngotomy is closed endoscopically by approximating the pharyngeal mucosa to the base of tongue with 3–0 braided absorbable sutures placed with the use of the 5-mm robotic needle holder and dissecting forceps. In our experience, given the extensive mucosal preservation, the pharyngotomy can be closed in a horizontal orientation. Following a watertight closure, fibrin glue is placed over the incision transorally. At this time, optional steps of salivary bypass tube placement or primary tracheal-esophageal prosthesis placement may be performed in a typical manner depending on surgeon preference. Intraoral retraction is released.

With the skin flap in superior retraction, the pharyngotomy may be bolstered with placed sutures along the cervical aspect of tongue base musculature. The strap muscles are reapproximated over the pharyngotomy site. A small suction drain is placed superior to the stoma site. The superior skin flap is released, and the superior stomaplasty is performed using braided absorbable suture. At the conclusion of the procedure, the endotracheal tube is replaced with a standard laryngectomy tube.

More than a demonstration of technologic capacity, the application of TORS for total laryngectomy was proposed to address two specific surgical concerns of standard open approach for total laryngectomy. The first is the standard open pharyngotomy. The incision lines of open laryngectomy, even with optimal pyriform sinus mucosal preservation, results in pharyngotomy defects of considerable size. Some authors have proposed closing the large pharyngotomy defects in a "T" pattern as opposed to the more conventional linear closure [34]. Conventional practice continues with linear pharyngotomy closures; however, the risk of psuedodiverticula formation and postlaryngectomy dysphagia remains [35]. The endoscopic TORS approach allows for substantial reduction in pharyngotomy size with maximal mucosa-sparing incisions. In fact, the pharyngotomy is closed in a completely horizontal linear orientation. The initial experience of the authors has not identified psuedodiverticula or persistent dysphagia; however, additional cases and longer follow-up is required to make conclusions comparing swallowing outcomes between surgical approaches.

The second motivating factor to transition laryngectomy to TORS is to improve the formation of pharyngocutaneous fistulae. Fistula formation is the most common major complication following total laryngectomy [36]. Most commonly seen in postradiated larynges, fistula formation is thought to be secondary to decreased blood supply, tissue necrosis, and subsequent pharyngeal suture line breakdown. Along with prolonged hospitalizations with IV antibiotics, fistula contents can ultimately track laterally in the neck to the carotid sheath and artery. The infected salivary contents weaken the arterial wall, risking psuedoaneurysm formation and carotid rupture [37]. The TORS approach targets this potential complication in two ways. First, the limited pharyngotomy closure reduces the area of sutured mucosa at risk for breakdown. Secondly, without lateral surgical dissection of an open approach, fascial barriers remain intact between the neopharynx and the carotid sheath following the perilaryngeal dissection of TORS. The elimination of natural drainage paths between the pharyngeal suture line and carotid artery targets the lethal laryngectomy complication of carotid rupture. Though TORS laryngectomy patients in the several clinical reports have experienced fistula formation, this patient population is comprised of extremely poor laryngeal tissue quality with diffuse fibrosis from high-dose chemoradiotherapy. Fistula contents following the midline dissection path maintain a medial drainage path, away from the lateral neck contents supporting the surgical proposal.

The first clinical reports of TORS total laryngectomy has demonstrated feasibility and safety. For oncologic indications, TORS total laryngectomy has also demonstrated clear pathologic margins. While the initial outcomes are promising following TORS, long-term follow-up and additional case series are needed to understand the benefits of this minimally invasive approach.

32.10 Conclusions

Cancers of the larynx are frequently amenable to primary surgical resection, which can decrease the level of radiation, with or without chemotherapy, and at times serve as single modality therapy. We have seen tremendous advantages over the past decade with the adoption of the da Vinci robotic system toward this goal, namely, with the popularization of TORS Supraglottic laryngectomy. Expanding fields include TORS hypopharngectomy and TORS total laryngectomy, for which additional experience will be able to define the precise advantages over nonsurgical therapy and alternative surgical approaches. As we see a growth of the number of approved robotic surgical systems and advanced miniaturization of available technology, we should also see a growth of primary glottic cancer resections performed with robotic assistance.

References

1. Weinstein GS, O'Malley BW Jr, Snyder W, Sherman E, Quon H. Transoral robotic surgery: radical tonsillectomy. Arch Otolaryngol Head Neck Surg. 2007;133(12):1220–6.
2. Benazzo M, Canzi P, Occhini A. Transoral robotic surgery with laser for head and neck cancers: a fea-

sibility study. ORL J Otorhinolaryngol Relat Spec. 2012;74(3):124–8.
3. Van Abel KM, Moore EJ, Carlson ML, Davidson JA, Garcia JJ, Olsen SM, Olsen KD. Transoral robotic surgery using the thulium:YAG laser: a prospective study. Arch Otolaryngol Head Neck Surg. 2012;138(2):158–66.
4. Desai SC, Sung CK, Jang DW, Genden EM. Transoral robotic surgery using a carbon dioxide flexible laser for tumors of the upper aerodigestive tract. Laryngoscope. 2008;118(12):2187–9.
5. Remacle M, Matar N, Lawson G, Bachy V, Delos M, Nollevaux MC. Combining a new CO2 laser wave guide with transoral robotic surgery: a feasibility study on four patients with malignant tumors. Eur Arch Otorhinolaryngol. 2012;269(7):1833–7.
6. Chan JYK, Wong EWY, Tsang RK, Holsinger FC, Tong MCF, Chiu PWY, Ng SSM. Early results of a safety and feasibility clinical trial of a novel single-port flexible robot for transoral robotic surgery. Eur Arch Otorhinolaryngol. 2017;274(11):3993–6.
7. Chan JYK, Tsang RK, Holsinger FC, Tong MCF, Ng CWK, Chiu PWY, Ng SSM, Wong EWY. Prospective clinical trial to evaluate safety and feasibility of using a single port flexible robotic system for transoral head and neck surgery. Oral Oncol. 2019;94:101–5.
8. Holsinger FC, Magnuson JS, Weinstein GS, Chan JYK, Starmer HM, Tsang RKY, Wong EWY, Rassekh CH, Bedi N, Hong SSY, Orosco R, O'Malley BW Jr, Moore EJ. A next-generation single-port robotic surgical system for transoral robotic surgery: results from prospective nonrandomized clinical trials. JAMA Otolaryngol Head Neck Surg. 2019;145(11):1027–34.
9. Mendelsohn AH, Kim C, Song J, Singh A, Le T, Abiri A, Berke GS, Geoghegan R. Transoral robotic surgical proficiency via real-time tactile collision awareness system. Laryngoscope. 2020;130(Suppl 6):S1–S17.
10. Goyal N, Yoo F, Setabutr D, Goldenberg D. Surgical anatomy of the supraglottic larynx using the da Vinci robot. Head Neck. 2014;36(8):1126–31.
11. De Virgilio A, Park YM, Kim WS, Baek SJ, Kim SH. How to optimize laryngeal and hypopharyngeal exposure in transoral robotic surgery. Auris Nasus Larynx. 2013;40(3):312–9.
12. Lawson G, Matar N, Remacle M, Jamart J, Bachy V. Transoral robotic surgery for the management of head and neck tumors: learning curve. Eur Arch Otorhinolaryngol. 2011;268(12):1795–801.
13. Kayhan FT, Kaya KH, Yilmazbayhan ED. Transoral robotic approach for schwannoma of the larynx. J Craniofac Surg. 2011;22(3):1000–2.
14. Tülin Kayhan F, Hakan Kaya K, Altıntas A, Fırat P, Sayin I. First successful transoral robotic resection of a laryngeal paraganglioma. J Otolaryngol Head Neck Surg. 2012;41(6):E54–7.
15. Muderris T, Bercin S, Sevil E, Acar B, Kiris M. Transoral robotic surgery for atypical carcinoid tumor of the larynx. J Craniofac Surg. 2013;24(6):1996–9.
16. Remacle M, Lawson G, Hantzakos A, Jamart J. Endoscopic partial supraglottic laryngectomies: techniques and results. Otolaryngol Head Neck Surg. 2009;141(3):374–81.
17. Remacle M, Hantzakos A, Eckel H, Evrard AS, Bradley PJ, Chevalier D, Djukic V, de Vincentiis M, Friedrich G, Olofsson J, Peretti G, Quer M, Werner J. Endoscopic supraglottic laryngectomy: a proposal for a classification by the working committee on nomenclature. Eur Laryngol Soc Eur Arch Otorhinolaryngol. 2009;266(7):993–8.
18. Lawson G, Matar N, Nollevaux MC, Jamart J, Krug B, Delos M, Remacle M, Borght TV. Reliability of sentinel node technique in the treatment of N0 supraglottic laryngeal cancer. Laryngoscope. 2010;120(11):2213–7.
19. Mendelsohn AH, Remacle M, Van Der Vorst S, Bachy V, Lawson G. Outcomes following transoral robotic surgery: supraglottic laryngectomy. Laryngoscope. 2013;123(1):208–14.
20. Park YM, Kim WS, Byeon HK, Lee SY, Kim SH. Surgical techniques and treatment outcomes of transoral robotic supraglottic partial laryngectomy. Laryngoscope. 2013;123(3):670–7.
21. Ozer E, Alvarez B, Kakarala K, Durmus K, Teknos TN, Carrau RL. Clinical outcomes of transoral robotic supraglottic laryngectomy. Head Neck. 2013;35(8):1158–61.
22. Olsen SM, Moore EJ, Koch CA, Price DL, Kasperbauer JL, Olsen KD. Transoral robotic surgery for supraglottic squamous cell carcinoma. Am J Otolaryngol. 2012;33(4):379–84.
23. Hans S, Chekkoury-Idrissi Y, Circiu MP, Distinguin L, Crevier-Buchman L, Lechien JR. Surgical, oncological, and functional outcomes of transoral robotic supraglottic laryngectomy. Laryngoscope. 2020; https://doi.org/10.1002/lary.28926. [Epub ahead of print.]
24. Lallemant B, Chambon G, Garrel R, Kacha S, Rupp D, Galy-Bernadoy C, Chapuis H, Lallemant JG, Pham HT. Transoral robotic surgery for the treatment of T1-T2 carcinoma of the larynx: preliminary study. Laryngoscope. 2013;123(10):2485–90.
25. Kayhan FT, Koc AK, Erdim I. Oncological outcomes of early glottic carcinoma treated with transoral robotic surgery. Auris Nasus Larynx. 2019;46(2):285–93.
26. Blanco RG, Ha PK, Califano JA, Saunders JM. Transoral robotic surgery of the vocal cord. J Laparoendosc Adv Surg Tech A. 2011;21(2):157–9.
27. Hassid S, Van der Vorst S, Delahaut G, Ambroise J, Lawson G. Transoral robotic surgery hypopharyngectomy (TORSH): feasibility and outcomes. Eur Arch Otorhinolaryngol. 2020;277(10):2883–92.
28. Mazerolle P, Philouze P, Garrel R, Aubry K, Morinière S, El Bedoui S, Ton Van J, Ferron C, Malard O, Jegoux F, Berard E, Vergez S. Oncological and functional outcomes of trans-oral robotic surgery for pyriform sinus carcinoma: a French GETTEC group study. Oral Oncol. 2018;86:165–70.
29. Dziegielewski PT, Kang SY, Ozer E. Transoral robotic surgery (TORS) for laryngeal and hypopharyngeal cancers. J Surg Oncol. 2015;112(7):702–6.

30. Wang CC, Liu SA, Wu SH, Wang CP, Liang KL, Jiang RS, Lin JC. Transoral robotic surgery for early T classification hypopharyngeal cancer. Head Neck. 2016;38(6):857–62.
31. Lawson G, Mendelsohn AH, Van Der Vorst S, Bachy V, Remacle M. Transoral robotic surgery total laryngectomy. Laryngoscope. 2013;123(1):193–6.
32. Smith RV, Schiff BA, Sarta C, Hans S, Brasnu D. Transoral robotic total laryngectomy. Laryngoscope. 2013;123(3):678–82.
33. Dowthwaite S, Nichols AC, Yoo J, Smith RV, Dhaliwal S, Basmaji J, Franklin JH, Fung K. Transoral robotic total laryngectomy: report of 3 cases. Head Neck. 2013;35(11):E338–42.
34. Davis RK, Vincent ME, Shapshay SM, Strong MS. The anatomy and complications of "T" versus vertical closure of the hypopharynx after laryngectomy. Laryngoscope. 1982;92:16.
35. Deschler DG, Blevins NH, Ellison DE. Postlaryngectomy dysphagia caused by an anterior neopharyngeal diverticulum. Otolaryngol Head Neck Surg. 1996;115(1):167–9.
36. Ganly I, Patel S, Matsuo J, Singh B, Kraus D, Boyle J, Wong R, Lee N, Pfister DG, Shaha A, Shah J. Postoperative complications of salvage total laryngectomy. Cancer. 2005;103(10):2073–81.
37. Weber RS, Berkey BA, Forastiere A, Cooper J, Maor M, Goepfert H, Morrison W, Glisson B, Trotti A, Ridge JA, Chao KS, Peters G, Lee DJ, Leaf A, Ensley J. Outcome of salvage total laryngectomy following organ preservation therapy: the Radiation Therapy Oncology Group trial 91-11. Arch Otolaryngol Head Neck Surg. 2003;129(1):44–9.

Robotic Surgery: FLEX System

33

Stephan Lang, Timon Hussain,
and Stefan Mattheis

Key Messages

- The Flex Robotic System was developed specifically for head and neck surgery and provided access to difficult-to-reach regions of the pharynx and larynx with excellent intraoperative visualization.
- Analyses of oncologic outcomes after Flex surgery showed encouraging results with high rates of local tumor control.

The Flex Robotic System (Medrobotics Corporation, Raynham, MA) was commercially available between 2014 and 2020 and was developed specifically for transoral pharyngeal and laryngeal surgery. The computer-assisted flexible endoscope has a built-in chip on tip 3D 1080P reusable camera at the distal end of the scope. The system provides two accessory channels, one on each side of the flexible scope for the insertion of flexible instruments, allowing the surgeon to grasp and resect tissue. The Flex instruments articulate 85 degrees in any direction, providing a wide range of access within the cavity. All regions of the pharynx and larynx can be reached with the system [1, 2]. Unlike other robotic systems in head and neck surgery, the instruments are operated via a hands-on approach, allowing for direct tactile feedback for the surgeon. While the Flex Robotic System is currently no longer commercially available, its functional principles provided a promising addition to the head and neck surgeon's portfolio.

33.1 Retractors

To sufficiently expose the anatomical region of interest, different types of retractors have been introduced for the use in TORS. Most commonly, the Feyh-Kastenbauer–Weinstein-O'Malley (FK–WO) retractor, the Flex retractor (Fig. 33.1) [3], the Dingman Mouth retractor, the Crow Davis mouth gag, and the Laryngeal Advanced Retractor System (LARS) are used. While shorter blades are preferred for the oropharynx and base of tongue, longer blades are inserted to expose the supraglottic and glottic level. Most commonly, to improve the exposure of the supraglottic region, the tip of the spatula is placed into the vallecula, thereby elevating the epiglottis and the larynx from the posterior pharyngeal wall. If lesions extend to the postcricoid region, the tip of the spatula may be placed under the epiglottis;

S. Lang (✉) · T. Hussain · S. Mattheis
Department of Otorhinolaryngology, Head and Neck Surgery, University Hospital Essen, University of Duisburg-Essen, Essen, Germany
e-mail: Stephan.Lang@uk-essen.de; Timon.Hussain@uk-essen.de; Stefan.Mattheis@uk-essen.de

M. Remacle, H. E. Eckel (eds.), *Textbook of Surgery of Larynx and Trachea*,
https://doi.org/10.1007/978-3-031-09621-1_33

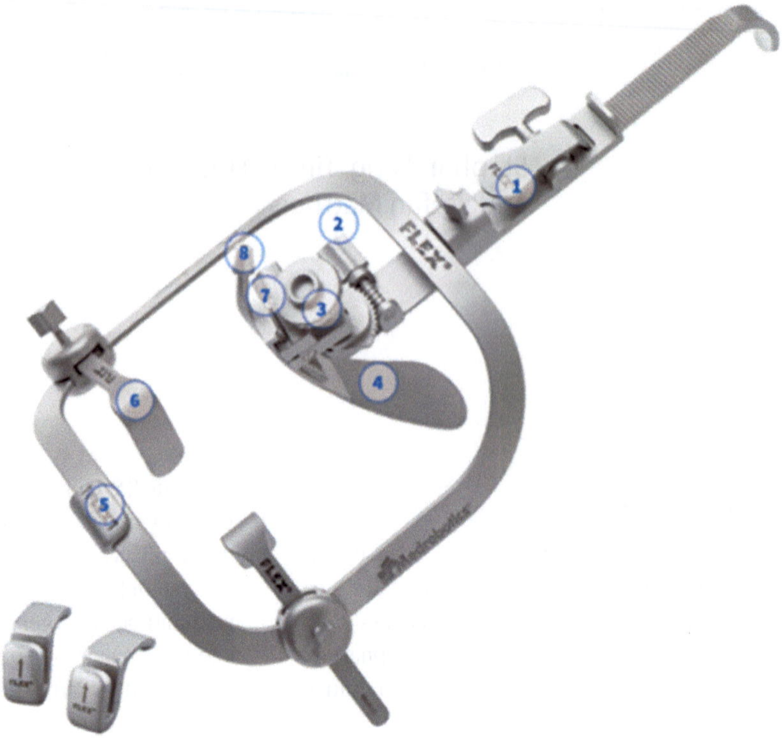

Fig. 33.1 Flex retractor. Elements of the device: *1* Jaw spreader, *2* Adjustable axial blade, *3* Adjustable tongue blade, *4* Blades are loaded and unloaded from the top, *5* Tooth brace, *6* Adjustable cheek retraction, *7* Adjustable tongue blade insertion, *8* Smoke evacuation

similarly, longer and more curved blades can be placed under the epiglottis to reach the glottis. The Flex and the Crow Davis retractors provide blades with an integrated suction for smoke evacuation during surgery. In addition, the Flex and FK-WO retractors allow the surgeon to adjust the insertion depth as well as the blade angle. The Flex retractor uniquely incorporates the possibility to rotate the tongue blade axially.

33.2 Instruments

Different types of instruments are available for tissue resection in transoral surgery, ranging from cold steel cutting scissors to monopolar or laser devices. Advantages of cold steel instruments include the absence of any thermal damage to the tissue. This is relevant for both healthy tissues as well as the excised tissue for the analysis of surgical margins by the pathologist. Monopolar cutting devices offer excellent cutting ability with few tissue type restrictions, including cartilage. However, thermal damage is considerable and complicates the tissue assessment by the pathologist. Most commonly, lasers are used for tissue resection, particularly for malignant tumors. While providing hemostasis, the zone of carbonization is reduced to minimum, particularly for pulsed CO_2-lasers.

33.3 Applications I: Benign Lesions

TORS with flexible robotic systems such as the Flex system may be advantageous for the surgeon to improve the intraoperative visualization of various benign lesions of the pharynx, such as cysts, benign tumors such as fibromas, chondromas, or papillomas, Reinke's edema, and vascular malformations. Depending on the localization of the tumor, different spatula can be used to optimize the visualization and accessibility of the lesion. For example, to expose supraglottic tumors, the tip of the spatula is placed in the vallecula, thereby elevating the epiglottis and the larynx from the posterior pharyngeal wall. To expose the posterior cricoid region, the spatula is placed under the epiglottis. The Flex retractor may also be used to expose vascular malformations of the pharynx for intralesional sclerotherapy. The superior three-dimensional visualization of the lesion enables a highly accurate application of the sclerosant, such as Bleomycin, Sodium Tetradecyl Sulfate, or OK-432.

33.4 Applications II: Malignant Tumors

TORS can be similarly valuable to improve visualization and exposure of tumors located in difficult-to-reach regions of the pharynx and larynx, such as the lower parts of the oropharynx, hypopharynx, and supraglottis, and potentially facilitate *en-bloc* resection. Transoral microsurgery (TLM) limits the surgeon to a straight line of view, oftentimes resulting in a piecemeal resection of the tumor. While generally accepted as a sound resection technique, evaluation of the surgical margin by the pathologist is substantially limited.

Retrospective analyses comparing the resection of supraglottic carcinomas via TLM and TORS with the Flex system have shown encouraging results [4, 5]. Tumor visualization with the Flex system was excellent (Fig. 33.2), resulting in high rates of local tumor control. Results compared favorably to TLM.

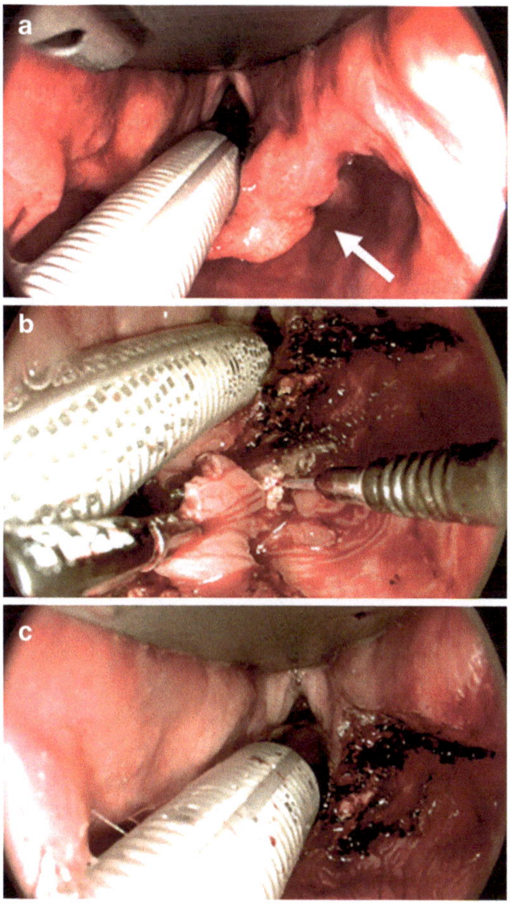

Fig. 33.2 Excellent visualization of a supraglottic laryngeal cancer of the right aryepiglottic fold with the FLEX system. (**a**) Three-dimensional intraoperative view of the tumor prior to resection. (**b**) Tumor resection with a flexible laser fiber. (**c**) View of the tumor site after resection

33.5 Conclusion and Outlook

During its time, the Flex Robotic System was shown to be a valuable addition to existing technologies for the transoral resection of benign and malignant tumors of the pharynx and larynx. Oncologic outcomes of supraglottic tumor resections in particular were highly encouraging. Based on these results, establishing novel flexible robotic systems in head and neck surgery in the future has to be considered worthwhile.

References

1. Mattheis S, Hasskamp P, Holtmann L, Schafer C, Geisthoff U, Dominas N, Lang S. Flex Robotic System in transoral robotic surgery: The first 40 patients. Head Neck. 2017;39(3):471–5.
2. Lang S, Mattheis S, Hasskamp P, Lawson G, Guldner C, Mandapathil M, Schuler P, Hoffmann T, Scheithauer M, Remacle M. A European multicenter study evaluating the flex robotic system in transoral robotic surgery. Laryngoscope. 2017;127(2):391–5.
3. Hasskamp P, Lang S, Holtmann L, Stuck BA, Mattheis S. First use of a new retractor in transoral robotic surgery (TORS). Eur Arch Otorhinolaryngol. 2016;273(7):1913–7.
4. Hussain T, Lang S, Hasskamp P, Holtmann L, Hoing B, Mattheis S. The Flex robotic system compared to transoral laser microsurgery for the resection of supraglottic carcinomas: first results and preliminary oncologic outcomes. Eur Arch Otorhinolaryngol. 2020;277(3):917–24.
5. Mattheis S, Lang S, Holtmann L, Hasskamp P, Hussain T. Transoral resection of supraglottic laryngeal tumors with the Flex Robotic System. HNO. 2020;68:662–5.

34 Surgery for Swallowing Disorders

Zao M. Yang and Gregory N. Postma

Key Points

- A thorough history and physical, endoscopic examination of the larynx, esophagoscopy, fluoroscopic radiography, and high-resolution manometry are essential tools for evaluation of patients with dysphagia.
- True vocal fold augmentation can be valuable in aspirating patients with glottic incompetence.
- In cases of retractable aspiration with an afunctional larynx, narrow-field total laryngectomy is a viable option.
- Balloon dilation and cricopharyngeus myotomy improve dysphagia secondary to cricopharyngeus muscle dysfunction. Careful patient selection for treatment using CP Botox is advised, as some patients experience transient worsening of symptoms.
- Gastroesophageal reflux disease is common and can contribute to dysphagia.
- Esophageal webs, strictures, and stenosis can be treated with esophageal dilation, and complete esophageal stenosis can be treated with an antegrade-retrograde rendezvous technique.
- Open and endoscopic repair techniques for Zenker's diverticulum are efficacious.
- Killian-Jamieson diverticula warrant open surgical diverticulectomy with careful dissection and preservation of the recurrent laryngeal nerve.
- Motility disorders are diagnosed with high-resolution manometry and categorized using the Chicago Classification v3.0.

Z. M. Yang (✉) · G. N. Postma
Department of Otolaryngology—Head and Neck Surgery, University of Texas Health San Antonio, San Antonio, TX, USA

Department of Otolaryngology—Head & Neck Surgery, Medical College of Georgia at Augusta University, Augusta, GA, USA
e-mail: yangz1@uthscsa.edu

34.1 Introduction

Dysphagia describes the *symptom* of difficulty swallowing and is not a diagnosis. Dysphagia can be caused by a variety of heterogenous disorders and diseases. Swallowing is a complex mechanism that can be disrupted by pathology along the swallowing tract, including the oral cavity, pharynx, larynx, and esophagus. Dysphagia is frequently multifactorial in etiology. It has a profound impact on quality of life and is increasing in prevalence, with up to 20% of the general population experiencing symptoms [1]. Eating is an integral part of human culture, and patients

M. Remacle, H. E. Eckel (eds.), *Textbook of Surgery of Larynx and Trachea*,
https://doi.org/10.1007/978-3-031-09621-1_34

with dysphagia experience decreased quality of life and social isolation [2] in addition to the morbidity and mortality that occurs with malnutrition and aspiration. Age-related changes to swallowing function and cognitive comorbidities that impact swallowing make dysphagia and its sequelae of particular importance in the elderly, especially as the proportion of older people in the global population continues to grow. The total health-care cost associated with dysphagia has been estimated at over $500 million in the United States alone [3].

Otolaryngologists play a valuable role in the assessment and management of dysphagia. A team-based approach in conjunction with speech language pathology, gastroenterology, gastrointestinal surgery, radiology, and neurology can offer multiple modalities of treatment for a variety of pathologies of the proximal swallowing tract. Although clinical management of dysphagia can be intimidating, many patients can experience safer and more efficacious swallowing with a systematic evaluation and guided nonsurgical and surgical interventions.

34.2 Evaluation of Dysphagia

Obtaining a thorough history of patients with dysphagia is vital. Symptoms of dysphagia range in severity, and it should be specified whether symptoms occur with solids, liquids, or both. A sensation of incomplete deglutition, foreign body sensation, or food getting "stuck" after swallowing solid food can indicate an obstructive process. The patient's subjective feeling of the level of obstruction is poorly specific, as previous studies have demonstrated that only half of patients can accurately localize the level of obstructive pathology [4, 5]. Many patients who perceive their level of obstruction to be above the clavicles frequently have pathology located more distal in the thoracic esophagus. Presence and degree of weight loss can be used as a corollary of dysphagia severity, or can increase the provider's suspicion for head and neck or esophageal malignancy, especially with a concomitant history of significant tobacco abuse, unilateral otalgia, or odynophagia. Isolated liquid dysphagia potentially indicates aspiration, especially in the presence of coughing after drinking or prior episodes of pneumonia. Diverticula, diseases of motility, and severe obstructive pathology can present with a variety of symptoms of solid and liquid dysphagia. Regurgitation of partially digested or undigested food can occur with reflux, diverticula, and dysmotility. Chest pain with swallowing can occur with spastic esophageal motility disorders. Prior head and neck malignancy, treatment with radiation therapy, or previous head and neck or spine surgeries should also be noted.

A full head and neck physical exam should be performed, with targeted examination of the lower cranial nerves. Weakness of the tongue and pharyngeal musculature can impact the oral and pharyngeal phases of swallowing, and disorders of the vagus nerve can have a profound impact on multiple components of swallowing. The neck should be examined for sequelae of prior radiation therapy, including soft tissue lymphedema or fibrosis, which can impact swallowing.

Flexible endoscopic examination of the pharynx and larynx should be performed on initial evaluation. The nasopharynx should be assessed for strength and symmetry of palatal elevation and for presence of velopharyngeal insufficiency. The pharyngeal squeeze maneuver can be used to assess contractility of the oropharynx [6]. Pooling of secretions within the vallecula, pyriform sinuses, or the post cricoid region can be indicative of pathology and should be noted. Hypomobility or immobility of the true vocal folds and glottic incompetence can contribute to aspiration. The presence of poor laryngeal sensation or a patulous pharyngoesophageal segment (PES) should be noted if present. A simultaneous flexible endoscopic evaluation of swallowing (FEES) can be performed when suspicious of aspiration, though in severe cases, obvious aspiration of oral secretions can be seen on transnasal fiber-optic laryngoscopy [7].

Radiographic evaluation of dysphagia includes the esophagram (barium swallow) and the modified barium swallow study (MBSS), which is also known as a videofluoroscopic swallow study (VFSS). During an esophagram, the patient ingests a radio-opaque liquid under fluoroscopy, which allows for assessment of pathology, including cricopharyngeus muscle dysfunction (CPMD), strictures, stenoses, webs, reflux, hernias, masses, diverticula, and motility disorders. A 13 mm barium tablet is a helpful adjunct for identification of the level of obstruction. The esophagram is the study of choice when evaluating patients with symptoms specific for solid foods or with obstructive symptoms. The MBSS is a fluoroscopic exam performed in conjunction with speech language pathology that examines the function of the oral and pharyngeal phases of swallowing, and utilizes ingestion of different bolus consistencies and volumes to evaluate for laryngeal penetration and aspiration. It is particularly useful for patients following a stroke or with a neurologic etiology of dysphagia. An MBSS should also include an esophageal sweep to screen for esophageal pathology [8].

Esophageal endoscopy can be performed in the operating room with intravenous sedation or general anesthesia, or in an office setting with transnasal esophagoscopy (TNE). Benefits of TNE include a favorable safety profile, with less than 3% of patients experiencing epistaxis and 0.3% of patients experiencing a vasovagal episode [9], and equal diagnostic accuracy when compared to conventional sedated endoscopy [10]. Indications for esophagoscopy include examination for dysphagia, reflux and its sequela including Barrett's metaplasia, evaluation and removal of esophageal foreign bodies, biopsy of lesions and masses or the esophagus, endoscopically guided nasogastric tube placement, and screening and follow-up exams for head and neck cancer.

TNE is performed using a flexible endoscope with a 2 mm working channel and suction and insufflation/irrigation valves. Topical anesthesia and decongestion of the nasal cavity are instrumental for patient tolerance of the procedure. The endoscope is hovered above the larynx in the oropharynx to minimize stimulation, and the patient is instructed to initiate a "hard swallow" as the tip of the endoscope is advanced postcricoid into the esophagus. Examination of the proximal and mid esophagus is deferred until the endoscope is withdrawn. The lower esophageal sphincter (LES) and Z-line are examined for mucosal changes indicative of esophagitis and Barrett's metaplasia. The gastric fundus is evaluated and retroflexion is performed to examine the gastric cardia and visualize if a hiatal hernia is present (Fig. 34.1). Air is suctioned from the stomach prior to withdrawal of the endoscope into the esophagus in order to minimize discomfort, bloating, and nausea. As the endoscope is withdrawn, the esophageal mucosa is carefully evaluated for pathology. Biopsies are indicated for suspicious lesions or masses or if eosinophilic esophagitis is suspected.

High-resolution manometry (HRM) is a vital diagnostic tool in patients with nonobstructive dysphagia. The study is performed using a catheter with pressure sensors at 36–40 points at 1 cm intervals along the length of catheter. The tip of the catheter is passed transnasally through the pharynx and esophagus into the stomach. There are multiple sensors at each point to calculate an average pressure at their respective anatomic locations. The patient is guided through a series of swallows with the catheter in place. This information is then used to determine strength and coordination of pharyngeal and esophageal contraction, clinical significance of a cricopharyngeal bar, and disorders of esophageal motility.

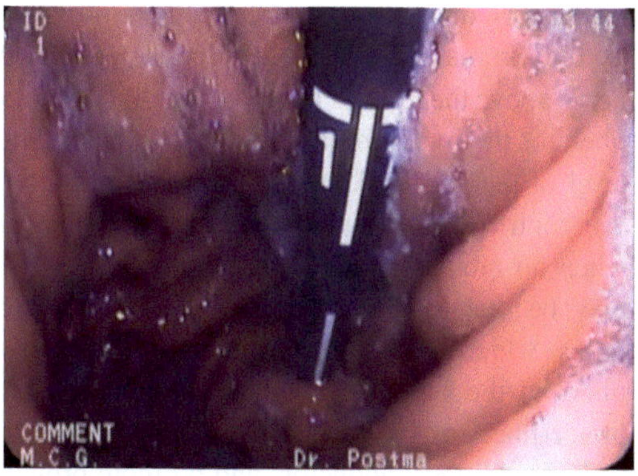

Fig. 34.1 Retroflexion maneuver performed during TNE demonstrates a hiatal hernia. The tip of the TNE scope is articulated 180 degrees to visualize itself as it enters the stomach across the EGJ. The diaphragmatic contraction onto the stomach is located at the inferior aspect of the hiatal hernia

HRM can frequently elucidate an etiology for a patient's symptoms even after negative radiographic evaluation or endoscopy. HRM is also utilized in preoperative evaluation for antireflux surgery.

Gastroesophageal reflux disease (GERD) can present with dysphagia, and patients with a suspected diagnosis of GERD who fail empiric treatment with a proton pump inhibitor (PPI) may additionally benefit from esophageal pH testing to confirm diagnosis. This is typically done on an ambulatory basis, and reflux events are typically measured over 24–48 h. Concomitant impedance testing can be performed to evaluate nonacid reflux events.

34.3 Management of Dysphagia

34.3.1 Aspiration

Although penetration and aspiration can occur in 11.4–15% and 0.6–3% respectively of patients with "normal" swallowing function [11, 12], aspiration pneumonia is a sequela of aspiration that is associated with high morbidity and mortality, particularly in the aging population. Protective mechanisms of the larynx against aspiration include inversion of the epiglottis over the laryngeal vestibule, medialization of the TVF and FVF, and hyolaryngeal elevation.

Sensory innervation of the larynx is provided by the internal branch of the superior laryngeal nerve above the level of the glottis and by sensory fibers of the recurrent laryngeal nerve below the level of the glottis. Aberrant laryngeal sensation can contribute to dysphagia and aspiration even when no motor deficits are identified [13]. This may be due to loss of the laryngeal adductor reflex, which occurs with stimulation of sensory fibers of the superior laryngeal nerve to trigger motor fibers of the recurrent laryngeal nerve to activate laryngeal adductors and promote protection against aspiration. Patients with an absent laryngeal adductor reflux are almost 7 times more likely to develop aspiration pneumonia [14], and when combined with poor pharyngeal squeeze, aspiration risk is particularly high [15].

Failure of aspiration to trigger a cough reflex in the setting of poor laryngeal sensation is known as silent aspiration. In a series of 400 inpatients with dysphagia, 28% were found to have silent aspiration [16]. Risk factors for silent aspiration include neurologic diseases such as developmental delay, stroke [17], and traumatic brain injury [18]. Patients with silent aspiration may be at higher risk of developing aspiration pneumonia when compared to patients with overt aspiration [17].

Incomplete glottic closure can contribute to dysphagia and aspiration via failure of the glottic barrier when swallowing. In a study of Parkinson's patients, degree of TVF atrophy as a marker of glottic incompetence was correlated with severity of aspiration [19]. This effect has also been demonstrated in patients with unilateral TVF immobility. Dysphagia in this patient population has been reported in 55.6–69% with an associated 20–50% rate of aspiration [20]. Medialization procedures including injection augmentation and medialization laryngoplasty in patients with unilateral TVF immobility have been demonstrated to improve dysphagia in some patients. Early intervention with injection augmentation in patients with acute-onset TVF immobility may decrease the risk of aspiration pneumonia [21]. Incomplete glottic closure can also result in inability to produce a strong cough, as forced expiration against a closed glottis generates the pressure differential required to expel aspirated material upon glottic opening. Patients with glottic incompetence in the setting of TVF immobility have been shown to have a stronger cough with increased peak airflow after undergoing injection augmentation [22].

Management of TVF paralysis in the setting of a high-vagal injury can be particularly challenging [23], given that these patients frequently have multifactorial dysphagia including poor palatal elevation and pharyngeal contraction (Fig. 34.2), decreased laryngopharyngeal sensation, CPMD, and esophageal dysmotility due to loss of vagal innervation at multiple levels in the pharynx, larynx, and esophagus. In these patients, consideration of ipsilateral pyriform

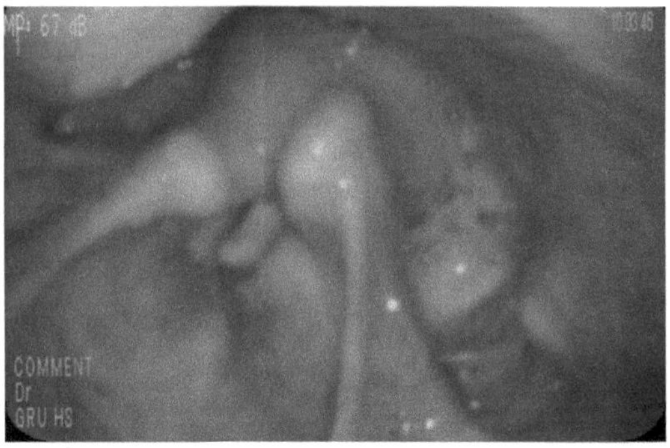

Fig. 34.2 A patient with a left-sided high-vagal nerve paralysis demonstrates paralysis of the left hemi-larynx with asymmetric pooling of secretions in the left pyriform and significantly reduced pharyngeal contraction during a pharyngeal squeeze maneuver

sinus ablation and concomitant CP myotomy may be warranted in addition to TVF medialization procedures.

In aspirating patients with concomitant CPMD, CP dilation or myotomy may have some benefit in improving symptoms by promoting passage of the food bolus into the esophagus rather than the larynx. This effect is amplified with the addition of laryngeal suspension [24], wherein permanent suture is used to statically elevate the larynx anteriorly and superiorly, in order to suspend it in a more favorable location under the tongue base and epiglottis. The anterior and upward displacement of the hyolaryngeal complex simultaneously creates a force vector promoting the passive opening of the PES.

Patients who are unable to safely maintain their nutritional requirements by PO intake alone in spite of therapeutic and surgical management may need supplementation with enteral feeding, and patients with severe aspiration with all consistencies may require enteral feeding as a primary nutritional source. Despite this, pneumonia remains the leading cause of death in patients who are G-tube dependent secondary to aspiration [25]. In cases of retractable aspiration with an afunctional larynx, narrow-field total laryngectomy is a viable option. Functional laryngectomies have high rates of complication (32–56%) including pharyngocutaneous fistula. However, long-term outcomes of laryngectomy in the management of end-stage dysphagia have shown improved dysphagia symptoms as well as decreased G-tube dependence, aspiration, and rates of aspiration pneumonia [26, 27].

34.3.2 Cricopharyngeus Muscle Dysfunction (CPMD)

Disorders of the cricopharyngeus (CP) muscle are heterogenous and can contribute to dysphagia. The pathophysiology for this spectrum of disorders stems from incomplete relaxation or failure of relaxation of the CP [28] or from the obstructive physical protrusion of the CP muscle into the esophageal lumen [29]. Various nomenclature includes CP bar and CP achalasia. The CP muscle can frequently be identified on fluoroscopic imaging, and although the presence of a CP bar has been demonstrated to decrease opening of the UES, this has not been correlated with an increase in bolus transit time [30]. Additionally, manometric studies have demonstrated normal UES relaxation and motility across the PES in some patients with CP bars [31]. Therefore, presence of a CP bar on imaging is not necessarily diagnostic of CPMD, and the size of the CP bar should be taken into account with considering surgical intervention. HRM findings can be considered in borderline or questionable cases, as a finding of increased basal resting pressure or failure of relaxation of the UES may be predictive of success with dilation or myotomy.

Surgical options for treatment of CPMD include dilation, Botox [32], and CP myotomy. Endoscopic dilation procedures of the CP muscle can be performed in a sitting position in a clinic setting or in a procedural suite with IV sedation using a TNE endoscope [33]. The esophagus is intubated with the endoscope and a guidewire is passed into the esophagus and left in place as the endoscope is withdrawn. An esophageal balloon is then passed over the guidewire while being visualized using the endoscope, which is reintroduced through the nose, to the level of obstruction at the CP muscle and slowly inflated (Fig. 34.3). After inflation to the desired size, the guidewire, balloon, and endoscope are removed from the patient.

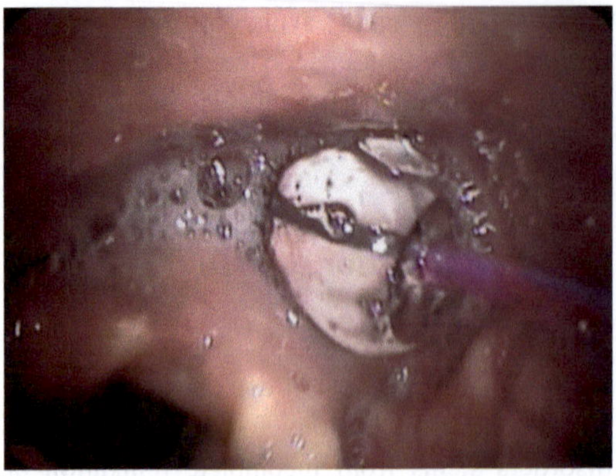

Fig. 34.3 Balloon dilation is performed at the PES in an unsedated, awake patient in an office setting with visualization using a TNE scope

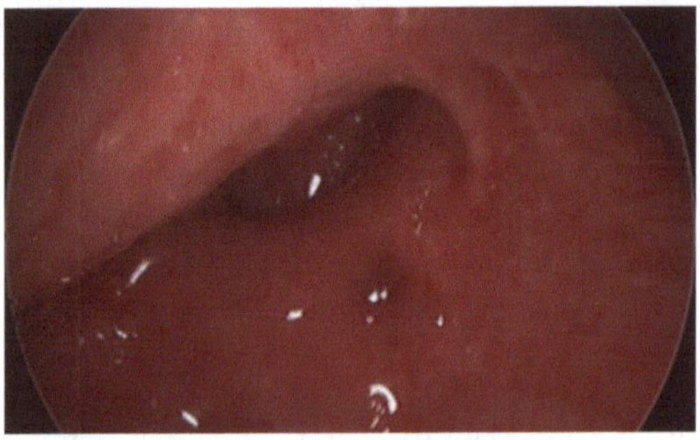

Fig. 34.4 A right-sided web at the PES is demonstrated on rigid endoscopic examination of the hypopharynx. This web arises from the anterior mucosa of the postcricoid hypopharynx and connects to the mucosa above the CP muscle

CP dilation can also be performed intraoperatively while supine with the assistance of general anesthesia. A suspended laryngoscope can be passed into the postcricoid hypopharynx to facilitate exposure of the esophageal introitus and to visualize the CP muscle, as well as examine for hypopharyngeal and proximal esophageal webs and strictures (Fig. 34.4). An esophageal balloon can then be passed to the level of the CP under visualization with a rigid Hopkins telescope and inflated for dilation. Large diameter dilation is safe and may be of increased efficacy [34, 35]. Effects of CP dilation are typically temporary, and patients may require repeat procedures.

CP Botox treatment similarly utilizes a laryngoscope to expose the CP with injection of Botox into the muscle. Botox, also known as Onabotulinum A, is a derivative of Botulinum toxin that temporarily prevents presynaptic release of acetylcholine at the neuromuscular junction, which causes a flaccid paralysis of the targeted musculature, thereby decreasing the CP tension that can occur in CPMD. Reported doses vary widely but average about 40 units [36]. Caution is advised when using a low concentration or high volume injection, as postinjection diffusion of CP Botox has been reported to cause true vocal fold paralysis [37] and pharyngeal weakness. Additionally, a substantial proportion of patients experience transient worsening of dysphagia [36]. This is thought to be secondary to the obstructive protrusion of the CP into the esophageal lumen that can occur in roughly 29% of elderly patients even when under complete relaxation [29], highlighting the heterogenous etiologies of CPMD. Careful patient selection for treatment using CP Botox is therefore advised.

A systematic review by Kocdor, et al. demonstrated efficacy of dilation, Botox, and CP myotomy in CPMD, although Botox may be beneficial in a lower percentage of patients [38]. The effects of dilation and Botox are frequently temporary, with a significant proportion of patients requiring repeat procedures and ultimately definitive treatment with CP myotomy. CP myotomy is the initial treatment of choice for certain diseases associated with CPMD, such as oculopharyngeal muscular dystrophy [39]. CP myotomy can be performed endoscopically with a laser or open. Endoscopic CP myotomy is the preferred method when the muscle can be exposed transorally, and studies suggest a higher success rate with endoscopic treatment (84% vs 71%) and a lower rate of complications (2% vs 11%) [38], while simultaneously minimizing risk of injury to the recurrent laryngeal nerve. In this procedure, a Weerda or Dohlman diverticuloscope is used to visualize the CP muscle, with a flange of the diverticuloscope on either side of the muscle causing distension of the CP (Fig. 34.5). The mucosa overlying the mucosa and muscle fibers are then divided using the laser down to the layer of the buccopharyngeal fascia (Fig. 34.6).

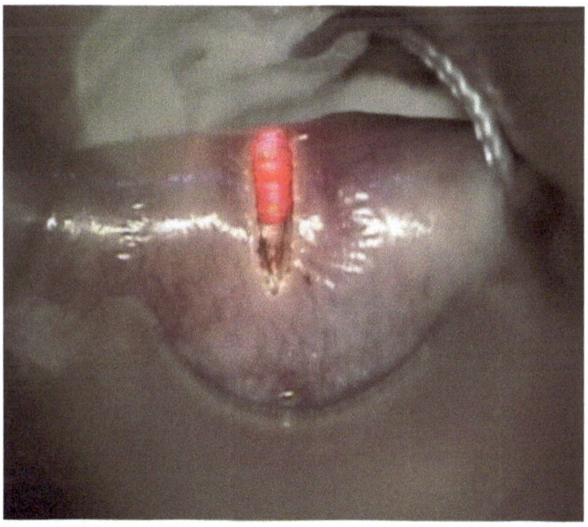

Fig. 34.5 The CP muscle is placed under tension using a Weerda diverticuloscope and endoscopically divided using a CO_2 laser attached via a micromanipulator to an operating microscope

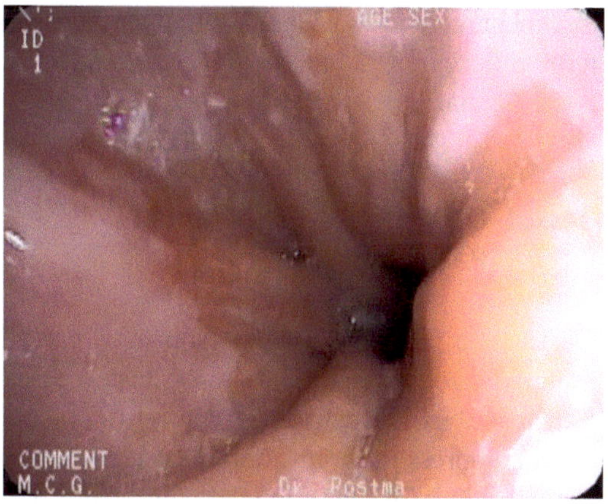

Fig. 34.7 An irregular Z-line located at the LES is visualized during TNE and may be indicative of Barrett's esophagus, which describes metaplastic changes to the distal esophageal mucosa that occur with chronic exposure to acid

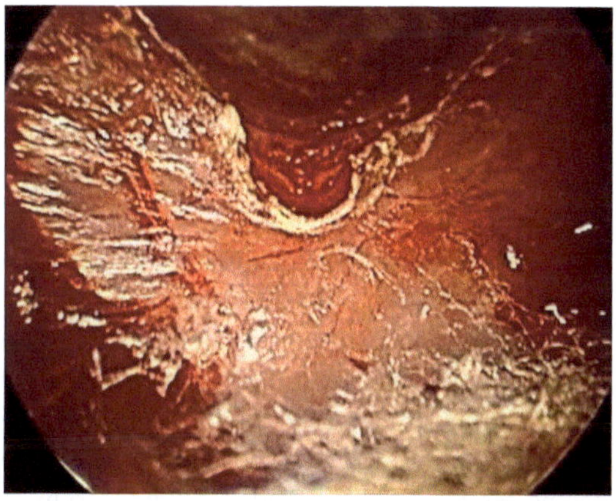

Fig. 34.6 The buccopharyngeal fascia marks the deep plane encountered during endoscopic CP myotomy and can be identified by its wispy, white appearance

34.3.3 Gastroesophageal Reflux Disease (GERD)

GERD is estimated to occur in up to 30% of the population in Western countries [40]: 28–37% of patients with GERD experience dysphagia, and severity of reflux is correlated with severity of dysphagia [41, 42]. Pathophysiology of GERD stems from impaired function of the LES. The LES is comprised of smooth muscle that is contracted at rest to prevent retrograde reflux of stomach contents into the esophagus, and is tethered to the diaphragmatic crura at the esophageal hiatus via the phrenoesophageal ligament. Tonicity and contraction of the diaphragmatic crura also contribute to the intraluminal pressure at the LES [43].

Incompetence of the LES contributes to reflux, and GERD can result from transient LES relaxation (TLESR), intraluminal hypotension at the LES, or hiatal hernia, which occurs with translocation of the LES from the esophageal hiatus of the diaphragm. Chronic acid exposure in the esophagus can result in Barrett's esophagus (Fig. 34.7), which describes metaplasia of the distal esophagus from stratified squamous epithelium to simple columnar epithelium and is a precursor to esophageal adenocarcinoma.

Although symptoms of heartburn and regurgitation can be persistent in up to one-third of patients despite PPI therapy [44], dysphagia secondary to reflux improves in up to 80% of patients treated with a PPI [42, 45]. Patients with GERD refractory to medical therapy warrant referral to gastrointestinal surgery and gastroenterology specialists for consideration of intervention. Fundoplication has documented efficacy in improving reflux and even dysphagia in the setting of LES incompetence or hiatal hernia [46]. Other procedures, including LINX magnetic sphincter augmentation, transoral incisionless fundoplication, and Stretta radiofrequency treatment, can be considered, although the long-term efficacy of some of these procedures is controversial.

34.3.4 Obstructive Esophageal Pathology

Obstructive pathology of the esophagus can be grouped into extrinsic and intrinsic etiologies. Extrinsic obstructive disorders result from esophageal compression from external structures such as vasculature (dysphagia lusoria, dysphagia aortica), cervical spine exostoses or hardware, or thyroid goiter, and treatment if indicated is typically targeted to the underlying pathology, not the esophagus. Intrinsic obstructive esophageal disorders include webs, strictures, stenosis, and masses.

Webs occur in the postcricoid hypopharynx and cervical esophagus at the PES and may be associated with age, having been identified in 68% in a cadaveric study [47]. Webs can be associated with Plummer Vinson syndrome, which is additionally characterized by iron-deficiency anemia, glossitis, and angular cheilitis. Flexible endoscopic examination is limited by the natural luminal collapse of the PES. Webs can be identified on lateral and oblique views on an esophagram as a ledge or shelf along the anterior or anterolateral lumen, although they can frequently be missed, as fluoroscopic diagnosis requires adequate resolution and sufficient distension of the PES in correspondence with timing of the imaging sequence (Fig. 34.8). Accurate diagnosis therefore relies on intraoperative distension of the postcricoid region.

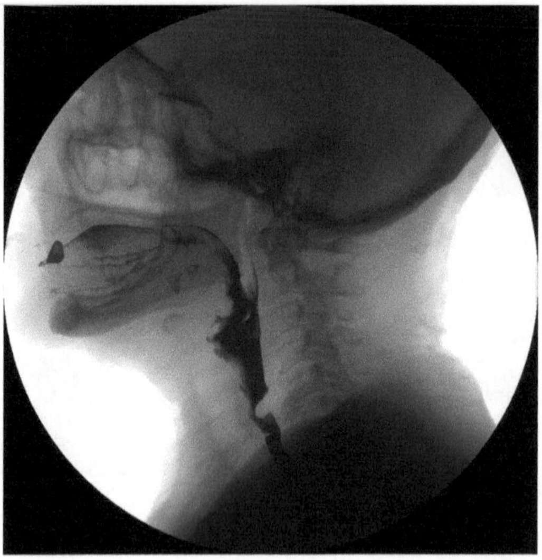

Fig. 34.8 An esophageal web can be seen on this lateral fluoroscopic image along the anterior wall of the esophageal lumen inferior to the CP muscle

Noncongenital stenotic diseases of the esophagus (stricture, stenosis) can develop as a result of inflammation, mucosal injury, or scar and can be iatrogenic. Contraction during tissue healing can result in segments of narrowing of the esophageal lumen. Esophageal strictures and stenosis can develop from prior treatment with radiation therapy and represent a prominent component of dysphagia in otolaryngologic patients with head and neck cancer. These injuries can also result from reflux, caustic ingestion, eosinophilic esophagitis, or prior esophageal surgery. A segmental narrowing of the esophageal lumen on esophagram with inability of a 13 mm barium tablet to pass is indicative of a stenotic process (Fig. 34.9).

Webs, strictures, and stenosis are treated with esophageal dilation with or without intralesional steroid injection. Esophageal dilation while in a supine position under anesthesia can be tailored to the level of obstruction and difficulty of bypassing the obstructed area. A suspended laryngoscope can be passed into the postcricoid hypopharynx to facilitate exposure of the esophageal introitus and to visualize the CP muscle, as well as examine for webs. If the desired focus of dilation is distal to the PES, a flexible esophagoscope can then be passed through the suspended laryngoscope to perform simultaneous endoscopy and endoscopic dilation. A guidewire can be used if the obstructive segment is difficult to pass with the endoscope. If a guidewire is placed, an esophageal balloon or Savory dilators are then passed over the wire for dilation. Maloney dilators can be passed blindly or through a suspended laryngoscope, although the size of the laryngoscope will limit the size of dilation. If greater dilation is required, then the dilator can be passed parallel and adjacent to the laryngoscope into the esophagus (Fig. 34.10). Dilation using

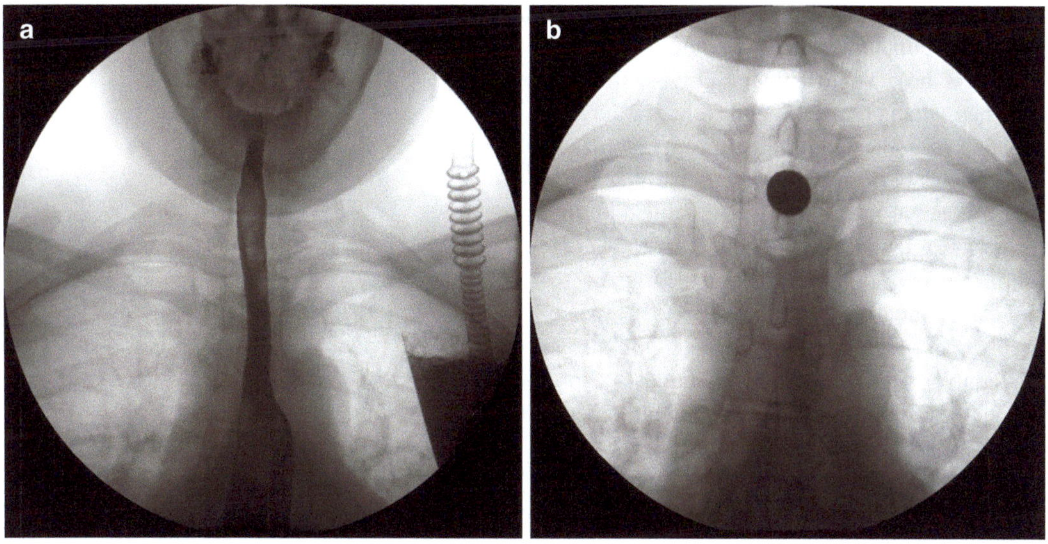

Fig. 34.9 Anterior-posterior sequences on a barium esophagram show no obvious stenosis with liquid barium (**a**). The same patient shows obstruction of a 13 mm barium tablet at the thoracic inlet, indicating an obstructive process at this level of the esophagus (**b**)

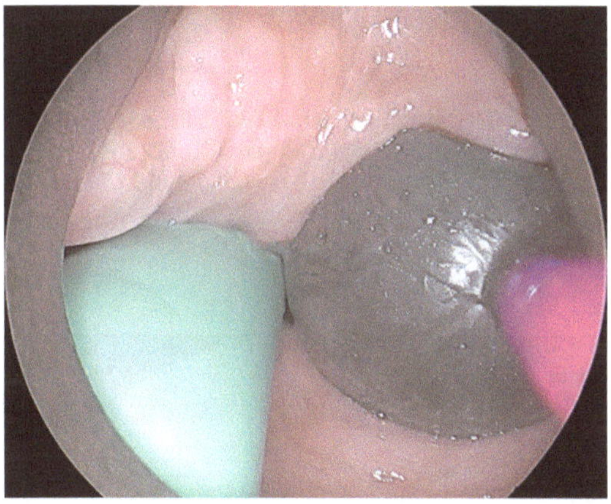

Fig. 34.10 Esophageal superdilation can be performed with a simultaneous Maloney dilator and a parallel balloon to achieve a greater caliber of dilation than with a 20 mm balloon alone

Maloney or Savory dilators can be more dangerous for the patient, given that the dilation is not visualized by endoscopy and can result in significantly more trauma due to the shearing forces applied during this method of dilation, as opposed to radial forces with balloon dilation. Balloon dilation is associated with less pain than serial bougie dilation [48].

In the setting of complete esophageal stenosis, an antegrade-retrograde rendezvous technique can be used for recanalization [49]. In this procedure, a flexible endoscope or rigid esophagoscope is introduced antegrade transorally and a separate endoscope is advanced through an existing G-tube site retrograde through the stomach into the esophagus to visualize the proximal and distal ends of the stenosis respectively. Intraoperative fluoroscopy and transillumination using the endoscopes can be used to estimate the length and course of stenosis. The stenotic tract can then be dissected and catheterized with a guidewire. Dilation is cautiously performed over the guidewire as previously described. Conservative initial dilation followed by scheduled serial dilations to increase diameters is advised to minimize the risk of perforation. Stenting the recanalized lumen until the next procedure can be performed with a nasogastric tube, and the G-tube is replaced after removal of the retrograde endoscope.

Benign esophageal masses are rare, with a prevalence of less than 1% [50]. They are frequently asymptomatic, but symptomatic patients have complaints ranging from dysphagia secondary to intraluminal mass effect to regurgitation of a pedunculated mass. Pathology of benign masses is broad and includes polyps, lipomas, myomas, hemangiomas, and others. Surgical excision is indicated for symptomatic masses and can be performed endoscopically or open with a variety of techniques depending on tumor location and size. Malignant masses of the esophagus are more common than benign masses and can be identified on evaluation as a cause of dysphagia. Esophageal adenocarcinoma is related to GERD and Barrett's metaplasia as previously described, and is increasing in incidence in Western countries. Incidence of esophageal squamous cell carcinoma has extreme geographic variability and is associated with alcohol and tobacco abuse [51].

34.3.5 Diverticular Diseases

Hypopharyngeal diverticula develop in anatomic areas of weakness and are relatively uncommon. The diverticular relationship to the CP and its orientation on fluoroscopic imaging are vital for accurate diagnosis, which impacts the recommended management. Cervical diverticula include Zenker's diverticula (ZD), Killian-Jamieson diverticula (KJD), and Laimer diverticula (LD) (Fig. 34.11).

An overwhelming majority of hypopharyngeal diverticula are ZD. ZD are pulsion pseudodiverticula, which occur in an area of muscular dehiscence known as Killian's triangle, defined superiorly by the oblique fibers of the thyropharyngeus component of the inferior constrictor and inferiorly by the transverse fibers of the CP muscle. ZD therefore appear on radiography to be *superior* and posterior to the CP (Fig. 34.12). ZD are more common on the left.

Surgical treatment is recommended with ZD and can be performed via an endoscopic or cervical approach. Data comparing these two techniques have been controversial and inconsistent, and to date, there is a paucity of large-scale prospective data comparing the repair options. Meta-analyses have demonstrated the efficacy of both techniques for improving dysphagia [52]. Advantages of the endoscopic approach include

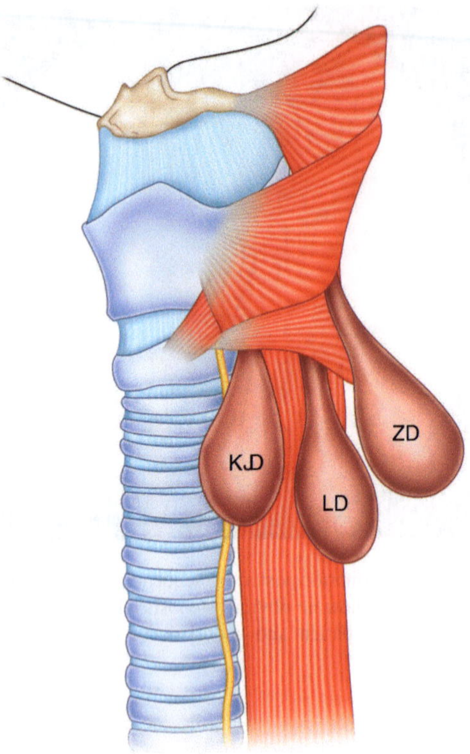

Fig. 34.11 Schematic figure showing the relationship of various cervical diverticula to the CP. ZD are posterior diverticula located superior to the CP muscle. LD are posterior diverticula inferior to the CP muscle. KJD are anterolaterally located inferior to the CP and are intimately associated with the RLN

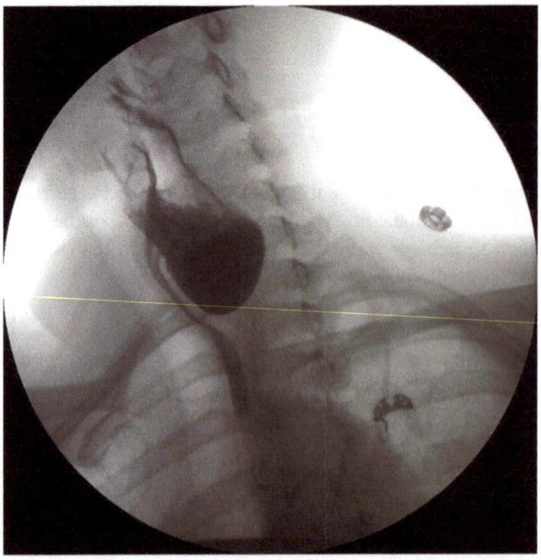

Fig. 34.12 A lateral fluoroscopic image on an esophagram demonstrates liquid barium collecting within a posterior cervical diverticulum located superior to the CP muscle, consistent with a ZD

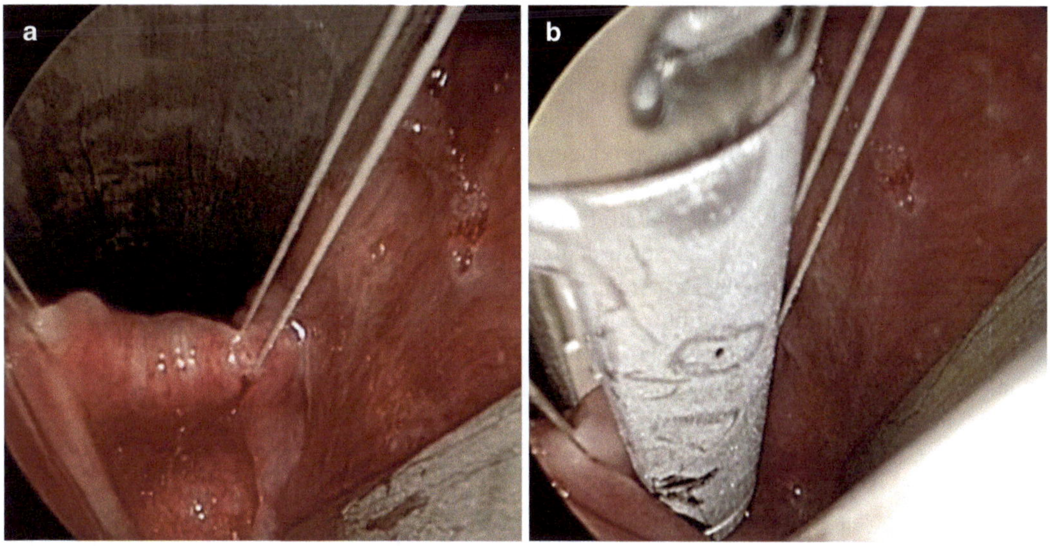

Fig. 34.13 Vicryl retraction sutures are placed in the lateral aspects of the CP muscle, which forms the wall separating the esophageal lumen anteriorly and the ZD posteriorly (**a**). These can be used to provide countertraction for stapling during endoscopic repair of ZD (**b**)

lack of a skin incision, shorter surgical time, minimal risk of injury to the recurrent laryngeal nerve, and fewer serious complications. Disadvantages include potential inability to expose the diverticulum, which occurs in 5% of patients [53], and potential for dental injury. A systematic review by Verdonck suggests a lower recurrence rate with open repair (2.8% vs. 3.9%) [54]. Patient functional status, medical comorbidities, patient age, and size if diverticulum should be considered when determining surgical approach.

Endoscopic surgical treatment for ZD is performed using a Weerda or Dohlman diverticuloscope to expose the diverticulum. The anterior flange is placed into the esophagus and the posterior flange is placed into the diverticular pouch and distended in order to place tension on the CP muscle, which runs within the wall separating the esophagus and the pouch. Several methods have been described to perform the CP myotomy. Both CO_2 laser and stapler have documented efficacy and safety in treating ZD. The CO_2 laser is used to incise or ablate the septum and CP down to the layer of the buccopharyngeal fascia and has the advantage of a complete myotomy, whereas the myotomy with the endoscopic stapler is limited by the lack of staples at the distal tip of the device. Suture retraction of the diverticular septum proximally into the stapler can be beneficial, particularly for small diverticula (Fig. 34.13). Patients who have undergone successful endoscopic surgical management of ZD may still have evidence of a remnant diverticulum on fluoroscopic swallowing evaluations despite symptomatic control [55].

KJD are pulsion pseudo-diverticula that occur *inferior* to the CP near its insertion to the cricoid cartilage in an area of anterolateral esophageal weakness. This is adjacent to the course of the recurrent laryngeal nerve (RLN) as it enters the larynx near the cricothyroid joint, and as a result KJD are intimately related to the RLN. KJD are much more common on the left side (76.1%), but can occur on the right (16.4%) or rarely bilaterally (7.5%) [56]. Although endoscopic management of KJD has been reported, open resection with careful identification and dissection of the RLN is recommended due to the intimate relationship of the medial diverticular wall and the RLN.

LD are exceedingly rare, with documentation limited to case reports. Laimer's triangle occurs near midline in the posterior cervical esophagus inferior to the CP and superior to the confluence of the longitudinal muscle fibers of the esophagus. As a result, only circular esophageal muscle fibers are present in Laimer's triangle, producing an area of relative weakness. LD are reported to be enclosed in esophageal muscle and are therefore considered to be true diverticula. Development of LD is thought to be related to underlying esophageal dysmotility, although questions regarding pathogenesis and optimal management are limited by its rarity. Most authors advocate for open surgical diverticulectomy [57].

Open repair of cervical diverticula begins with endoscopic exposure of the diverticulum to confirm the type of diverticulum and to pack the pouch for identification and manual feedback during dissection. An endoscope can then be passed into the esophagus for palpation and endoluminal visualization during the case. A skin incision is made within a prominent skin crease, typically favoring the left side. Subplatysmal skin flaps are elevated. The approach to the diverticulum can be performed medial or lateral to the strap muscles. A medial approach is performed with division of the strap musculature at the midline raphe with elevation of the straps off larynx and thyroid gland. This approach favors anterolateral diverticula due to the increased rotational retraction of the larynx required for exposure of posteriorly-oriented diverticula. For the lateral approach, the omohyoid muscle is identified at the medial border of the sternocleidomastoid and dissected medially to the lateral border of the strap musculature. Dissection then proceeds medial to the carotid and lateral to the strap muscles until reaching the retropharyngeal space between the buccopharyngeal fascia and the prevertebral fascia. The vertebral bodies can be palpated posteriorly. At this point the pouch is dissected with identification and careful dissection of the RLN in KJD. After dissection of the diverticular pouch, the packing is withdrawn from the mouth and a stapler is positioned across the mouth of the pouch to separate it from the esophagus. The previously placed endoscope can be used to confirm that there is not significant impingement of the esophageal lumen adjacent to the staple line prior to firing (Fig. 34.14). After diverticulectomy, the esophagus can be insufflated through the endoscope to check for a leak [58]. Simultaneous open CP myotomy is imperative for ZD due to its role in pathogenesis, while the role of CP myotomy in KJD is not clearly delineated.

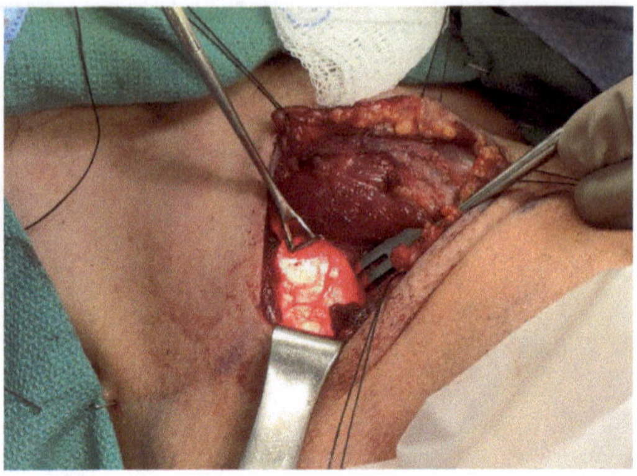

Fig. 34.14 Transillumination from the TNE scope can be used to delineate a cervical diverticulum from adjacent soft tissue attachments during open repair

34.3.6 Motility Disorders

Motility disorders are diagnosed with HRM using the Chicago Classification v3.0, and are categorized into three groups: (1) disorders that impact outflow of the esophagogastric junction (EGJ); (2) major disorders of peristalsis; (3) minor disorders of peristalsis. Findings on HRM can be used to make diagnoses of achalasia, outflow obstruction of the esophagogastric junction, diffuse esophageal spasm, jackhammer esophagus, absent peristalsis, ineffective esophageal motility, and fragmented peristalsis [59]. Management of these disorders includes medical and surgical treatments, and warrants referral to gastrointestinal surgery and gastroenterology specialists.

Take-Home Messages

- Dysphagia is a symptom that can be caused by a variety of heterogenous disorders and diseases, and is frequently multifactorial.
- Otolaryngologists play a valuable role in a multispecialty, team-based approach to dysphagia evaluation and treatment.

34.4 Multiple Choice Questions

1. A 39-year-old male presents to clinic with worsening dysphagia over the past 6 months. He states that when he swallows solid foods, he feels a sensation of food getting stuck in his throat. His symptoms are very bothersome, and he avoids certain foods for this reason but has not lost any weight. Denies tobacco use. Physical exam and transnasal flexible laryngoscopy are unremarkable. What is the best next step in evaluation?

   (a) Modified barium swallow
   (b) **Barium esophagram**
   (c) High-resolution manometry
   (d) Esophageal pH testing

2. A 76-year-old female is admitted to the intensive care unit after thoracic surgery. Postoperatively she complains of dysphonia and "choking" on liquids. She is found to have paralysis of the left true vocal fold with a sizable glottic gap on phonation. What is the best next step in management?

   (a) Observation
   (b) Modification of diet with thickener
   (c) **Injection augmentation**
   (d) Consultation for G-tube

3. A 54-year-old female with solid-food dysphagia secondary to cricopharyngeus muscle dysfunction responded well to previous balloon dilation of the upper esophageal sphincter. Her symptoms have recurred. Which treatment option would provide the lowest chance of needing another procedure in the future?

   (a) Additional treatment is contraindicated
   (b) Balloon dilation
   (c) Botox injection
   (d) **Cricopharyngeal myotomy**

4. A 61-year-old male presents with dysphagia and regurgitation of undigested foods and pills. On fluoroscopic radiography, he is found to have a cervical diverticulum inferior to the cricopharyngeus muscle. What is the most likely diagnosis?

   (a) Zenker's diverticulum
   (b) **Killian-Jamieson diverticulum**
   (c) Laimer diverticulum
   (d) Traction diverticulum

References

1. Cho SY, Choung RS, Saito YA, et al. Prevalence and risk factors for dysphagia: a USA community study. Neurogastroenterol Motil. 2015;27:212–9.
2. Jones E, Speyer R, Kertscher B, et al. Health-related quality of life and oropharyngeal dysphagia: a systematic review. Dysphagia. 2018;33:141–72.
3. Altman KW, Yu GP, Schaefer SD. Consequence of dysphagia in the hospitalized patient: impact on prognosis and hospital resources. Arch Otolaryngol Head Neck Surg. 2010;136:784–9.
4. Ashraf HH, Palmer J, Dalton HR, et al. Can patients determine the level of their dysphagia? World J Gastroenterol. 2017;23:1038–43.
5. Wilcox CM, Alexander LN, Clark WS. Localization of an obstructing esophageal lesion. Is the patient accurate? Dig Dis Sci. 1995;40:2192–6.
6. Bastian RW. The videoendoscopic swallowing study: an alternative and partner to the videofluoroscopic swallowing study. Dysphagia. 1993;8:359–67.
7. Hiss SG, Postma GN. Fiberoptic endoscopic evaluation of swallowing. Laryngoscope. 2003; 113:1386–93.
8. Belafsky PC, Kuhn MA. The clinician's guide to swallowing fluoroscopy. New York: Springer; 2014.
9. Postma GN, Cohen JT, Belafsky PC, et al. Transnasal esophagoscopy: revisited (over 700 consecutive cases). Laryngoscope. 2005;115:321–3.
10. Jobe BA, Hunter JG, Chang EY, et al. Office-based unsedated small-caliber endoscopy is equivalent to conventional sedated endoscopy in screening and surveillance for Barrett's esophagus: a randomized and blinded comparison. Am J Gastroenterol. 2006;101:2693–703.
11. Allen JE, White CJ, Leonard RJ, Belafsky PC. Prevalence of penetration and aspiration on videofluoroscopy in normal individuals without dysphagia. Otolaryngol Head Neck Surg. 2010;142:208–13.
12. Butler SG, Stuart A, Markley L, Rees C. Penetration and aspiration in healthy older adults as assessed during endoscopic evaluation of swallowing. Ann Otol Rhinol Laryngol. 2009;118:190–8.
13. Santoso LF, Kim DY, Paydarfar D. Sensory dysphagia: a case series and proposed classification of an

under recognized swallowing disorder. Head Neck. 2019;41:E71–8.
14. Kaneoka A, Pisegna JM, Inokuchi H, et al. Relationship between laryngeal sensory deficits, aspiration, and pneumonia in patients with dysphagia. Dysphagia. 2018;33:192–9.
15. Aviv JE, Spitzer J, Cohen M, et al. Laryngeal adductor reflex and pharyngeal squeeze as predictors of laryngeal penetration and aspiration. Laryngoscope. 2002;112:338–41.
16. Leder SB, Sasaki CT, Burrell MI. Fiberoptic endoscopic evaluation of dysphagia to identify silent aspiration. Dysphagia. 1998;13:19–21.
17. Holas MA, DePippo KL, Reding MJ. Aspiration and relative risk of medical complications following stroke. Arch Neurol. 1994;51:1051–3.
18. Leder SB. Fiberoptic endoscopic evaluation of swallowing in patients with acute traumatic brain injury. J Head Trauma Rehabil. 1999;14:448–53.
19. Yiu Y, Curtis JA, Perry SE, Troche MS. Relationship of vocal fold atrophy to swallowing safety and cough function in Parkinson's disease. Laryngoscope. 2020;130:303–8.
20. Zhou D, Jafri M, Husain I. Identifying the prevalence of dysphagia among patients diagnosed with unilateral vocal fold immobility. Otolaryngol Head Neck Surg. 2019;160:955–64.
21. Bhattacharyya N, Batirel H, Swanson SJ. Improved outcomes with early vocal fold medialization for vocal fold paralysis after thoracic surgery. Auris Nasus Larynx. 2003;30:71–5.
22. Dion GR, Achlatis E, Teng S, et al. Changes in peak airflow measurement during maximal cough after vocal fold augmentation in patients with glottic insufficiency. JAMA Otolaryngol Head Neck Surg. 2017;143:1141–5.
23. Reder L, Bertelsen C, Angajala V, et al. Hospitalized patients with new-onset vocal fold immobility warrant inpatient injection laryngoplasty. Laryngoscope. 2020;
24. Kos MP, David EF, Aalders IJ, et al. Long-term results of laryngeal suspension and upper esophageal sphincter myotomy as treatment for life-threatening aspiration. Ann Otol Rhinol Laryngol. 2008;117:574–80.
25. Tomioka H, Yamashita S, Mamesaya N, Kaneko M. Percutaneous endoscopic gastrostomy for aspiration pneumonia: a 10-year single-center experience. Respir Investig. 2017;55:203–11.
26. Theunissen EA, Timmermans AJ, Zuur CL, et al. Total laryngectomy for a dysfunctional larynx after (chemo)radiotherapy. Arch Otolaryngol Head Neck Surg. 2012;138:548–55.
27. Topf MC, Magana LC, Salmon K, et al. Safety and efficacy of functional laryngectomy for end-stage dysphagia. Laryngoscope. 2018;128:597–602.
28. Sivarao DV, Goyal RK. Functional anatomy and physiology of the upper esophageal sphincter. Am J Med. 2000;108(Suppl 4a):27S–37S.
29. Leaper M, Zhang M, Dawes PJ. An anatomical protrusion exists on the posterior hypopharyngeal wall in some elderly cadavers. Dysphagia. 2005;20:8–14.
30. Leonard R, Kendall K, McKenzie S. UES opening and cricopharyngeal bar in nondysphagic elderly and nonelderly adults. Dysphagia. 2004;19:182–91.
31. Dantas RO, Cook IJ, Dodds WJ, et al. Biomechanics of cricopharyngeal bars. Gastroenterology. 1990;99:1269–74.
32. Schneider I, Thumfart WF, Pototschnig C, Eckel HE. Treatment of dysfunction of the cricopharyngeal muscle with botulinum a toxin: introduction of a new, noninvasive method. Ann Otol Rhinol Laryngol. 1994;103:31–5.
33. Rees CJ, Fordham T, Belafsky PC. Transnasal balloon dilation of the esophagus. Arch Otolaryngol Head Neck Surg. 2009;135:781–3.
34. Clary MS, Daniero JJ, Keith SW, et al. Efficacy of large-diameter dilatation in cricopharyngeal dysfunction. Laryngoscope. 2011;121:2521–5.
35. Randall DR, Evangelista LM, Kuhn MA, Belafsky PC. Improved symptomatic, functional, and fluoroscopic outcomes following serial "series of three" double-balloon dilation for cricopharyngeus muscle dysfunction. J Otolaryngol Head Neck Surg. 2018;47:35.
36. Kelly EA, Koszewski IJ, Jaradeh SS, et al. Botulinum toxin injection for the treatment of upper esophageal sphincter dysfunction. Ann Otol Rhinol Laryngol. 2013;122:100–8.
37. Kim MS, Kim GW, Rho YS, et al. Office-based electromyography-guided botulinum toxin injection to the cricopharyngeus muscle: optimal patient selection and technique. Ann Otol Rhinol Laryngol. 2017;126:349–56.
38. Kocdor P, Siegel ER, Tulunay-Ugur OE. Cricopharyngeal dysfunction: a systematic review comparing outcomes of dilatation, botulinum toxin injection, and myotomy. Laryngoscope. 2016;126:135–41.
39. Perie S, Eymard B, Laccourreye L, et al. Dysphagia in oculopharyngeal muscular dystrophy: a series of 22 French cases. Neuromuscul Disord. 1997;7(Suppl 1):S96–9.
40. El-Serag HB, Petersen NJ, Carter J, et al. Gastroesophageal reflux among different racial groups in the United States. Gastroenterology. 2004;126:1692–9.
41. Bollschweiler E, Knoppe K, Wolfgarten E, Holscher AH. Prevalence of dysphagia in patients with gastroesophageal reflux in Germany. Dysphagia. 2008;23:172–6.
42. Vakil NB, Traxler B, Levine D. Dysphagia in patients with erosive esophagitis: prevalence, severity, and response to proton pump inhibitor treatment. Clin Gastroenterol Hepatol. 2004;2:665–8.
43. Hershcovici T, Mashimo H, Fass R. The lower esophageal sphincter. Neurogastroenterol Motil. 2011;23:819–30.
44. El-Serag H, Becher A, Jones R. Systematic review: persistent reflux symptoms on proton pump inhibitor therapy in primary care and community studies. Aliment Pharmacol Ther. 2010;32:720–37.
45. Oda K, Iwakiri R, Hara M, et al. Dysphagia associated with gastroesophageal reflux disease is

improved by proton pump inhibitor. Dig Dis Sci. 2005;50:1921–6.
46. Wetscher GJ, Glaser K, Gadenstaetter M, et al. The effect of medical therapy and antireflux surgery on dysphagia in patients with gastroesophageal reflux disease without esophageal stricture. Am J Surg. 1999;177:189–92.
47. Mehdizadeh OB, Wickwire P, Said M, Belafsky PC. The prevalence of cricopharyngeal webs in elderly cadavers. Laryngoscope. 2019;129:63–6.
48. Josino IR, Madruga-Neto AC, Ribeiro IB, et al. Endoscopic dilation with bougies versus balloon dilation in esophageal benign strictures: systematic review and meta-analysis. Gastroenterol Res Pract. 2018;2018:5874870.
49. Maple JT, Petersen BT, Baron TH, et al. Endoscopic management of radiation-induced complete upper esophageal obstruction with an antegrade-retrograde rendezvous technique. Gastrointest Endosc. 2006;64:822–8.
50. Choong CK, Meyers BF. Benign esophageal tumors: introduction, incidence, classification, and clinical features. Semin Thorac Cardiovasc Surg. 2003;15:3–8.
51. Codipilly DC, Qin Y, Dawsey SM, et al. Screening for esophageal squamous cell carcinoma: recent advances. Gastrointest Endosc. 2018;88:413–26.
52. Howell RJ, Giliberto JP, Harmon J, et al. Open versus endoscopic surgery of Zenker's diverticula: a systematic review and meta-analysis. Dysphagia. 2019;34:930–8.
53. Crawley B, Dehom S, Tamares S, et al. Adverse events after rigid and flexible endoscopic repair of Zenker's diverticula: a systematic review and meta-analysis. Otolaryngol Head Neck Surg. 2019;161:388–400.
54. Verdonck J, Morton RP. Systematic review on treatment of Zenker's diverticulum. Eur Arch Otorhinolaryngol. 2015;272:3095–107.
55. Allen J, Blair D, Miles A. Assessment of videofluoroscopic swallow study findings before and after cricopharyngeal myotomy. Head Neck. 2017;39:1869–75.
56. Haddad N, Agarwal P, Levi JR, et al. Presentation and management of Killian Jamieson diverticulum: a comprehensive literature review. Ann Otol Rhinol Laryngol. 2020;129:394–400.
57. Johnson CM, Postma GN. Not all pharyngeal pouches are created equal: management of "non-zenker" hypopharyngeal diverticula. Oper Tech Otolayngol Head Neck Surg. 2016;27:80–5.
58. Howell RJ, Edelmayer LW, Postma GN. The utility of flexible esophagoscopy during open hypopharyngeal (Zenker's) diverticulum surgery. Laryngoscope. 2019;
59. Kahrilas PJ, Bredenoord AJ, Fox M, et al. The Chicago classification of esophageal motility disorders, v3.0. Neurogastroenterol Motil. 2015;27:160–74.

35 Preoperative and Postoperative Speech Therapy

Lise Crevier-Buchman, Aude Julien-Laferriere, and Gregoire Viallate de Pemille

Key Points

The two main principles of voice, speech, and swallowing management are as follows:

i. **A direct therapeutic,** which corresponds to the treatment of the organ, its pathology, or the consequences of treatments to re-educate or adapt the phonatory, respiratory, and swallowing functions.
ii. **An indirect therapeutic,** which corresponds to a global care of the person in his/her environment, that is, the Quality of Life dimension.

The aim is to help the patient to be an actor in his or her own care and to participate in rehabilitation.

The role of Speech Language Therapist (SLT) varies according to the specificities of the pathologies

i. **Benign functional lesions** related to the use of phonation that is not adapted to its environment, vocal misuse or overuse, or congenital and scarring lesions will be treated by speech therapy and phonosurgery, with the aim of restoring voice quality and an efficient phonatory function that is adapted to the individual,
ii. **Cancerous lesions** require radical surgical and/or adjuvant therapy, that is, chemoradiotherapy (CRT) with phonatory, swallowing, and quality of life consequences. The goal is no longer just to treat the tumor but to ensure the most physiological functional recovery of swallowing, breathing, and phonation. The SLT helps motivate patients to reorganize and reinvest in their life projects with the caregiver

The **organic and physiological assessment** of laryngeal functions such as voice production and deglutition should be a prerequisite when taking care of laryngeal pathologies and the consequences of their treatment. This information should be shared within the ENT/SLT team

L. Crevier-Buchman (✉) · A. Julien-Laferriere
G. Viallate de Pemille
Voice, Speech, Swallowing Lab, Laryngology - Head & Neck Surgery Department (ENT), Hôpital Foch, Paris-Saclay University, Suresnes, Phonetics & Phonology Lab, LPP, CNRS-UMR7018, Univ. Sorbonne-Nouvelle, Paris, France
e-mail: l.crevier-buchman@hopital-foch.com; a.julien-laferriere@hopital-foch.com; g.vialatte-de-pemille@hopital-foch.com

M. Remacle, H. E. Eckel (eds.), *Textbook of Surgery of Larynx and Trachea*, https://doi.org/10.1007/978-3-031-09621-1_35

ENTs and SLTs need to work as a **team** for the patient's benefit and dialog should be maintained throughout the rehabilitation program in order to optimize functional progress and maintain the patient's confidence in the team that takes care of them.

The patients' **self-assessment** is important to take into consideration, in order to best support them and meet their expectations.

35.1 Place of the Speech Language Therapist in the care pathway

Whatever the laryngeal pathology, the laryngeal-tracheal and cervical region (i) is the place of vocal production, (ii) corresponds to the upper part of the respiratory tract, and (iii) has a protective role for the lower airway during swallowing. Any pathology and/or its treatment can modify the three main functions of the larynx and be a source of handicap that can even be life threatening.

Changes in voice and speech can affect oral communication, individual identity, and social interaction, thereby disrupting and altering quality of life. If we refer to the principles dictated by the WHO: "Today, disability is understood to arise from the interaction between a person's health condition or impairment and the multitude of influencing factors in their environment." https://www.who.int/health-topics/disability#tab=tab_1

"It is a complex phenomenon resulting from the interaction between a person's bodily characteristics and the characteristics of the society in which he or she lives." https://www.who.int/topics/disabilities/fr/

Head and Neck cancer has the particularity of modifying the Quality of Life (QoL) of relationship and can bring into play the vital prognosis: aesthetics, speaking, breathing, eating, and drinking.

The Speech Language Therapist (SLT) has a role to play in informing, preparing, and accompanying the patient for the most adequate possible functional restitution and contributes to the success of the treatment, whatever its nature.

However, while a country is fortunate to have developed a health-care system that allows access to SLT care, there are still disparities in the presence and availability of SLTs (geographical distribution and skills) as well as in their graduate and postgraduate training. For more details about SLT in European Union: https://cplol.eu/

The role of the SLT will depend (i) locally: on the lesion, benign or cancerous, its location, its extent, the proposed therapies, and their consequences, and (ii) globally: on the patient himself or herself in his or her environment [1].

The main principles of voice, speech, and swallowing management are based on (i) a direct therapeutic approach with a synergistic use of the resonators (the articulators, an optimized resonance), the vibrator (the vocal folds, the quality of their phonatory contact, modified structures or other structures in case of surgery), and the source of energy (the respiratory system), and (ii) an indirect therapeutic approach adapted to the social, professional, and personal vocal requirements and the environmental constraints specific to each patient [2].

35.1.1 Voice and Swallowing Assessment as a Starting Point for Patient's Management

The organic and physiological assessment of laryngeal functions such as voice production and deglutition should be a prerequisite when taking care of laryngeal pathologies and the consequences of their treatment. This information should be shared within the ENT/SLT team

Assessment aims at

- Understanding and quantifying the symptoms,
- Establishing a diagnosis
- Determining treatment method and explaining treatment plan
- Monitoring and follow-up of outcomes
- Quantifying the effect of treatment

Depending on the country and on the health-care system, we can find important disparities in medical settings, availability of material as well as the use of validated translation for questionnaires and screening tests.

35.1.1.1 Voice and Speech Assessment

Numerous evaluation methods exist, corresponding to a strong tendency to quantify the vocal function. However, at present, there are very few standardized protocols other than the recommendations for a Basic protocol published by the ELS phoniatric committee in 2001 [3]. However, the desire to harmonize our practices is emerging as with the new ASHA recommendations [4].

Interviewing the Patient, Self-Evaluation Questionnaires/Scales

The first step of assessment is by listening to the patient describing the complaints and the symptoms that are the main reason why the patient seeks a treatment.

It can be done by filling the patient's self-evaluation questionnaire and scale to evaluate

- the quality of life, the functional impairment such as with the Voice Handicap Index (VHI) [5] or the Speech Handicap Index (SHI) [6], as well as Voice-related quality of life (V-RQOL) [7]
- diagnosis-oriented scales like Voice Symptom Scale (VoiSS) [8]

Self-assessment also provides an objective dimension to meet the patient's demands according to his or her complaints and makes it possible to monitor progress during the course of treatment.
Notably, these self-evaluation questionnaires add no time to the consultation, as the patient can do it in the waiting room.

Quantitative Subjective Perceptual Assessment

The perceptual assessment is a simple method describing what we hear. The most used scale for dysphonic voices is the GRBAS [9], and for substitute voices after partial or total laryngectomy, the IINFVo [10].

Acoustic Parameters for Objective Measures

To measure acoustic parameters, it is necessary to record the patient's voice to keep a voice sample for pre- and postoperative reference and follow-up. It is advisable to record one vowel, most often the vowel /a/, and a sample of speech or reading of a short text [11].

The most frequently used acoustic parameters to describe

- Voice quality are the Fundamental Frequency (f0), perturbation parameters such as Jitter and Shimmer and Harmonic to Noise Ratio (NHR)
- Maximum Phonation Time (MPT), a simple physiologic and aerodynamic measure

Multidimensional measures have been developed, such as

- Multidimensional Voice Profile (MDVP, Kay Elemetrics)
- Acoustic Voice Quality Index (AVQI) [12]
- Voice Range Profile (VRP) [13] giving a wider view of the patient's voice range

Laryngeal Imaging: Examining Laryngeal Anatomy and Function

The objective is to determine the origin of the pathology and monitor the results of the treatment. Complementary techniques can be used:

- Nasofibroscopy video to explore the vocal tract, place of acoustic resonances with the velopharynx, the base of the tongue, and the laryngeal tube as a whole.

  Special attention will be paid to mobility and sensitivity, synchronization, and coordination of movements during physiologic behavior like breathing, coughing, and phonation. This examination also makes it possible to observe abnormal muscle tension and to note hyper- or hypocompensation by abnormal contraction of muscular structures.
- Stroboscopic light examination (with a flexible nasopharyngoscope or a rigid endoscope) provides valuable insight into the vibratory

component of the mucous membrane of the vocal folds:

- In a context of dysphonia with benign lesions, this examination allows the analysis of glottic closure asymmetries, muscle tensions, vibratory pattern, and mucosal ondulation and impairments.
- In a context of laryngeal cancer, it allows, on the one hand, to explore the dynamics of the glottic vibrator modified by the tumor (mucosal rigidity of the vocal folds due to the deep invasion of the tumor [14, 15]) and, on the other hand, to evaluate the functioning of the neovibrator after partial laryngectomies [16].

35.1.1.2 Swallowing Assessment

Swallowing disorders can have an impact not only on the quality of life, but also on the nutritional status of the patient as they can lead to denutrition as well as to a pulmonary status that can be life threatening. They most often occur after external laryngeal surgery.

The main objective is to have an initial organic and functional inventory that will guide the SLT and allow to monitor the rehabilitation of the swallowing function [17].

Some studies have shown that patients with head & Neck cancer can significantly improve their swallowing if they are treated early, hence the interest of an early postoperative assessment [18, 19].

Interview and Self-Evaluation Questionnaires and Scales

The questionnaires and tests such as

- Deglutition Handicap Index (DHI) [20],
- Swallowing-Quality of Life (SWAL-QoL) [21],
- Eating Assessment Tool (EAT-10) [22], and
- other bed-side screening tests

allow one to

- collect the patient's feel about the eating situation, his/her apprehensions, and obstacles,
- describe food and nutritional behavior,
- roughly detect disturbances or risk situations,
- bring a dimension of objective to be reached: in order to answer to the patient's demand, on one hand, and, on the other hand, to ensure pulmonary safety and nutritional and vital balance.

These tests are of growing interest to include quality of life in the results of therapeutic management.

Here again, it adds no time to the consultation, the patient can fill the questionnaire in the waiting room.

Swallowing Imaging: Examining Pharyngo-Laryngeal Anatomy and Function

The aims are

- To determine the mechanisms of oropharyngeal dysphagia, with particular attention to mobility and sensitivity, synchronization, and coordination of pharyngo-laryngeal movements
- To guide the SLT in swallowing rehabilitation (when the SLT does not carry it out themselves, depending on country's legislation and clinical training)
- To follow the evolution of the swallowing resumption and its functional improvement

Eating testing, where possible, can be carried out by two techniques depending on the equipment available:

- Radiographic evaluation of swallowing (video fluoroscopy/Modified Barium Swallow VFS/MBSS) [23]. This technique has the advantage of allowing the visualization and quantification of the path of the bolus, the penetration/aspiration, and the timing of the swallowing process.
- Fibro-endoscopic evaluation of swallowing (FEES), carried out with a nasofibroscope and video recording, allows to see the efficiency of muscle contractions during propulsion and peristalsis and to identify stasis and penetration/aspiration situations.

Scales have been developed to quantify the risk and severity in the swallowing process adapted for head and neck cancer patients [24].

This entire voice and swallowing assessment benefits from the collaboration and the complementarity between SLT and ENT. Some assessments are done mostly by one or the other (SLT or ENT).

Table 35.1 presents a quick overview of the most frequently used scales and instrumentations for voice and swallowing evaluation, done by ENT and/or SLT

35.1.2 General Goals of the SLT

The collaboration between the SLT and the ENT surgeon contributes to the patient's sense of confidence in the team that cares for him or her and consistency in care: the patient is not just taken in for surgery and then dropped off on his or her own on discharge.

The SLT can participate in announcements, providing information to reinforce the patient's understanding of and adherence to the diagnosis and its management.

General principles of voice, speech, and swallowing rehabilitation are beginning to be published [4, 19], depending on the pathologies and their treatment, but there is still a great deal of variation, with most often flexibility and adaptation of the tools to each patient, which makes it difficult to systematize a rehabilitation protocol [25].

We present here a general point of view of the two main axis of management of voice and swallowing, in the context of both benign and malignant laryngeal pathologies. Details and specificities will be discussed with each group of pathology and their treatment.

Table 35.1 Presents a quick overview of the most frequently used scales and instrumentations for voice and swallowing evaluation, done by ENT and/or SLT

	Voice disorders	Swallowing disorders	Who?
Self-administered questionnaires	VHI, V-RQOL, VOISS Specific questionnaires (TVQ, S-VHI, etc.)	SWAL-QoL DHI EAT-10	ENT = SLT
Non-invasive measurements and tests	Auditory-perceptual assessment of voice GRBAS (Hirano) Specific scales (IINFVo for substitute voice)		SLT ≥ ENT
Non-invasive measures and tests	Analytical and behavioral observation of voice and speech production (posture, respiration, oral-peripheral examination)	Dynamic and analytical assessment (motion, strength, sensitivity of the different structures involved in swallowing)	
	Aerodynamic and acoustic measurements (MPT for minimal assessment)	Swallowing screening tests and mealtime observations	
Instrumental imaging assessment	Laryngeal imaging: videolaryngoendoscopy and videolaryngostroboscopy	Radiographic evaluation of swallowing: VFS / MBSS Fibro-endoscopic evaluation of swallowing FEES	ENT ≫ SLT Depending on country legislation and clinical training regarding instrumental swallowing examination

VHI Voice handicap Index, *V-RQOL* Voice-related quality of Life, *VOISS* Voice Symptom Scale, *S-VHI* Singing Voice Handicap Index, *TVQ* Transsexual voice Questionnaire, *SWAL-QOL* Swallowing Quality of Life, *DHI* Dysphagia Handicap Index, *EAT10* Eating Assessment Tool, *GRBAS* Grade-Roughness-Breathiness-Asthenia-Strained, *IINFVo* Impression-intelligbility-Noise-Fluency-Voicing, *MPT* Maximum Phonation Time

- Indirect therapy, which corresponds to a global care of the person in his/her environment, that is, the Quality of Life dimension (QoL). This management makes it possible to support and convince the patient and his/her entourage, helping him/her to understand what is wrong (pathology, vocal use), what will be modified by the treatment, and what it is proposed to do.
- direct therapy, which corresponds to the treatment of the organ, its pathology, or the consequences of treatments to reeducate or adapt the phonatory, respiratory, and swallowing functions. it will also improve qol.

35.1.2.1 Indirect Therapy, Holistic and Behavioral

In this aspect of care, the patient and his/her quality of life are central, and the patient's expectations and objectives must be in line with what is being proposed. The aim is to help the patient to be an actor in his or her own care and to participate in rehabilitation (Table 35.2).

Table 35.2 General principles of indirect therapy applied to voice and swallowing disorders

	Voice disorders	Swallowing disorders
Patient information	• Anatomy and normal physiology • Modified anatomy (if that is the case) and physiopathology	
Environmental factors and management	Vocal hygiene: • Vocal misuse and overuse management: acoustic features (room organization, amplification, etc.), voice rest, compensations, etc. • Hydration and laryngopharyngeal reflux (LPR) diet	• Meal settings • Texture adaptation • Patient installation • Nutritional and pulmonary health education (warning signs monitoring)
Patient support and counseling	• Impact of stress and anxiety on voice production and ideas on how to reduce them • Support regarding self-image and vocal identity	• Patient and caregiver counseling (patient and caregiver burden)
	• Motivational issues: SLT attendance, adaptation, and rehabilitation compliance	

35.1.2.2 Direct Therapy, Organic and Functional

In this aspect of care, the aim is to restore the most effective possible functionality to the structures modified by pathology or surgery, whether by improving the vibratory quality of the tissues at the glottic level and epithelial mobilization or by compensating and/or adapting the musculo-mucosal structures.

The SLT finds its place to orient, guide, and optimize the most functional compensation/adaptation possible, reduce primary or secondary muscle tension, achieve or accelerating the most natural and safe recovery possible (Table 35.3).

35.1.2.3 Global Management

The balance between the 2 direct and indirect approaches contributes to the therapeutic progress of any laryngeal pathology and its treatment [26].

Increasing lifespan/survival must be synonymous with preserving physical, functional, social and emotional, or psychological quality of life. The patient's point of view (self-assessment) is important to take into consideration, in order to best support him/her and meet his/her expectations.

The earliest possible treatment, before bad habits or reactive depression set in, is a guarantee of the most balanced rehabilitation possible, without forgetting to include caregivers [19].

This management is optimized by the multidisciplinary approach and especially by the complementary nature of the ENT-SLT collaboration [27].

Table 35.3 General principles of direct therapy applied to voice and swallowing disorders

	Voice disorders	Swallowing disorders
Analytical training	• Direct manipulation • Targeted exploration (breathing/posture/glottal closure/vocal tract-articulators)	• Oral motor exercises – Motion – Resistance • Other targeted exercises • Electrical stimulation
Functional training: involves actual swallowing or voice/speech production	• Flow phonation • Resonant voice therapy • Etc.	• Targeted maneuvers (effortful swallowing and other manoeuvers targeting pharyngeal constriction, laryngeal elevation, etc.) • Oral sensory stimulation
	• Transfer to speech • Conversation training therapy ©	• Posture and maneuver compensation—training (multiple, supraglottic swallowing, etc.; chin-tuck, head rotation, etc.)

35.1.2.4 SLT's Role According to the Specificities of the Pathologies

Depending on the pathologies, the speech therapist's role presents particularities that will help to better target the objectives of management.

- Benign functional lesions related to the use of phonation that is not adapted to its environment, vocal misuse or overuse, or congenital and scarring lesions will be treated by speech therapy and phonosurgery, with the aim of restoring voice quality and an efficient phonatory function that is adapted to the individual [28].
- Cancerous lesions require radical surgical and/or chemoradiotherapy (CRT) treatment with phonatory, swallowing, and quality of life consequences that will be optimized and adapted with the guidance of the speech therapist.

35.2 Benign Pathologies of the Larynx with Surgery Limited to the Glottis

The context of benign lesions of the vocal folds informs the management of restoring the functioning of the laryngeal vibrator either by speech therapy and/or phonosurgery, the aim of which is not to remove a tumor but to restore the vibratory function of the vocal folds [2, 29].

Speech therapy

Direct and indirect speech therapy management contributes greatly to the treatment of the origin of the exudative lesion according to the context of use and vocal behavior, socio-professional and lifestyle constraints, as well as to the improvement of vocal quality with resonator/vibrator +/– respiration at the same time, this is notably the challenge of “resonant voice therapy,” for example.

Phonosurgery

The goal of phonosurgery is to restore the functional anatomy of the vocal fold. The results will be all the more convincing as it is performed outside of any emergency with a postoperative period of vocal rest, the duration of which is subject to debate.

35.2.1 Exudative Lesions of Reinke's Space, Phonotraumatic Vocal Hyperfunction

We include in “exudative lesions of Reinke's space” all nodules, polyps, and oedemas as Hantzakos et al. (2000) have described them [30].

Voice abuse, muscle tension dysphonia, and phonotrauma as well as environmental factors (e.g., a rich diet contributing to increase in laryngopharyngeal reflux (LPR) can be depicted as the origin of most of these lesions [31]).

In all these different cases, indication of phonosurgery and SLT (both indirect and direct voice therapy in different proportions depending on patient history and complaint) can be discussed.

On an indicative basis,

- Nodules tend to be the result of chronic vocal abuse. The more recent they are, the more easily they tend to yield to voice therapy, both indirect (in order to reduce vocal overuse and constraints as well as to avoid aggravating factors), and direct (so that the patient recovers functional voice use and reduces chronic microphonotrauma).
- Polyps tend be caused by acute phonotrauma, which can occur in patients who are unaware of more or less chronic vocal misuse and/or overuse.
- Reinke's edemas are typical of more or less heavy smoker patients for whom indirect therapy could play a key role in reducing aggravating factors.
- The same can be said about mixed etiology intermediate lesions: there exists most probably an irritating factor (whether it is LPR, repeated microphonotrauma, airborne irritants, etc.) or several, and either or both indirect and/or direct voice therapy can play a key role in long-term recovery.

Because of the etiology of these lesions, voice therapy has a prominent place in the treatment of the patients affected by them [32].

The complementarity of surgery and voice therapy benefits the patient by both increasing rapidity and durability of the results.

Nevertheless, each solution presents pros and cons, which should always be balanced with the patient's needs and wishes. For example, a singing teacher with two young children at home may be a bit more in a hurry for results than someone who tends to be quiet most of the time. A preschool teacher will need long-term reliable vocal results with as less relapse as possible. A performing singer will be very sensitive to the slightest vocal fold scaring. Some other patients will come to the ENT's office only to be reassured that their dysphonia isn't caused by a malignant lesion and are not affected by it even if it is severe.

For each individual case, different options and SLT-phonosurgery association can be considered (Table 35.4).

Table 35.4 Treatment options for exudative lesions of Reinke's space

	Pros	Cons
SLT only	Treats the origin of the lesion (vocal abuse, muscle tension dysphonia, and environmental issues). Noninvasive, no surgery-related risks (scaring, etc.).	Results can be long to obtain and are variable. Time and energy consuming (and with a financial cost depending on the country and health-care system), motivational issues.
Surgery only	Rapidly obtained results. Breaks the vicious circle of vocal strain (vocal abuse => lesion => compensatory muscle tension dysphonia => lesion worsens, etc.). Less time and energy consuming than SLT.	Surgery-related risks (scaring, etc.). Risk of relapse given that vocal misuse and/or overuse aren't tackled.
Surgery + pre- and postoperative SLT	Rapidly obtained results. Reduced risk of relapse (the origin of the lesion is treated with SLT), and maximized healing by early epithelial mobilization. SLT is facilitated by the resection of the lesion.	Surgery-related risks (scaring, etc.). Time and energy consuming when it comes to SLT.
Neither (the "do nothing" option)	Should be considered insofar as the lesion does not represent a life-threatening emergency (certainty that the lesion is benign and entails no breathing difficulties) and if the felt vocal handicap is low. No time and energy cost. No surgery-related risk.	Lesion and vocal function could worsen over time.

These surgeries only extremely rarely account for an emergency, although the degree of urgency can be different depending on the patient's vocal use and felt vocal handicap (e.g., teachers, singers might need rapid results more than a retired clerk).

The timing of voice therapy, if combined with surgery, could consist (depending on patient's history) in a few sessions (or one intensive session):

- Before the surgery: indirect therapy mostly with physiological and pathological explanations, aggravating factors control, vocal hygiene, but also may concern voice rest after the surgery. Basic notions of functional voice use and detection of signs of vocal abuse can also be addressed [33].
- After the surgery and vocal rest, the resumption of voice production can be accompanied by the SLT as soon as tissue healing and the direct therapy really starts [34, 35].
- In other cases, direct therapy will have already been partly or widely covered before the surgery.
- Timing will also be dictated by the patient's constraints and needs [2, 3].

35.2.2 Cyst, Sulcus, Scar

Regarding epidermoid cysts, mucosal bridges, sulci (which can be considered as a continuum [36] and vocal fold scars [37], we have to think differently.

The etiology of the first group of lesions is congenital, and scars are usually due to previous vocal fold surgery. Vocal abuse and phonotrauma, as well as external factors such as diet-induced LPR or airborne chemicals are not the cause of these lesions.

Compensatory vocal abuse is frequently observed in these patients and environmental factors can aggravate the situation. Indirect and direct voice therapy will therefore not tackle the cause of these lesions but help the patient to cope with their laryngeal situation.

Surgical treatments haven't always proven to be effective, especially when it comes to sulci and vocal fold scars, where adding a scar to a scar even risks aggravating the situation.

However, successful interventions in the case of cysts can be of great help to the patient.

Once again, voice therapy and surgery have to be carefully considered and can be complementary, always depending on the context, the patient's needs, wishes, and constraints.

Indirect vocal therapy and vocal hygiene counseling (with SLT) can play a key role in these cases and are complementary to surgical treatment (Table 35.5).

The timing is similar to what has been described above for the inflammatory lesions.

Nevertheless, what can differ is that since surgical outcomes are more variable,

- SLT can be a first-line treatment with cysts, sulci, and scars to improve vocal function.
- Surgery might be attempted as a second-line treatment considering the risks [38].

If not, immediate postsurgical voice therapy will be most important in order to reduce the aggravation of scaring as much as possible and help the healing process, by limiting inflammatory factors (vocal abuse, LPR, etc.) and inducing gentle vocal fold epithelial mobilization (similarly to what cicatricial massages would do externally).

- In scar tissue, some hope could come from new developing treatment with stem cell injection but there again, voice therapy will still be an important complement to direct and indirect care [39].

35.2.3 Unilateral Vocal Fold Immobility

There are several effective ways to surgically intervene in a larynx that presents unilateral vocal fold immobility. The outcomes are known to be

Table 35.5 Treatment options for congenital and scar lesions

	Pros	Cons
SLT only	Noninvasive, no surgery-related risks (aggravation of scaring, etc.), no noxious secondary effects Reduces additional vocal abuse and phonotrauma	Results can be long to obtain and are variable. Time and energy consuming (and with a financial cost depending on the country and health-care system), motivational issues.
Surgery only	Less time and energy consuming than SLT Can be effective with cysts > mucosal bridges > sulci and scars	Discussed effectiveness of surgical treatment of VF scars, major risk of aggravation.
Surgery + pre- and postoperative SLT	Reduced risk of additional phonotrauma and external aggravating factors that would jeopardize healthy VF healing Epithelial mobilization in early postoperative period to maximize healing Possible positive outcome of surgery additionally to reducing vocal effort and increasing vocal effectiveness	Remaining specific surgery related risks (scaring, etc.). Time and energy consuming when it comes to SLT.
Neither (the "do nothing" option)	Should be considered if the felt vocal handicap is low No time and energy cost No surgery-related risk	Risk of secondary lesions (exudative lesions of Reinke's space as described above) due to compensatory muscle tension.

very positive, depending on laryngeal configuration and patient profile. The surgery can be very adaptative (in office, with local or general anesthesia, injecting a product or placing an implant etc.). The object of this chapter is not to discuss the different techniques that can be used.

With such surgical efficacy, one could question the need for complementary SLT.

- For one thing, some patients would like to avoid surgery as much as possible and voice therapy can prove to be effective in compensating a unilaterally paralyzed larynx.
- Additionally, even though the paralyzed vocal fold has been medialized, there persists a laryngeal asymmetry, especially regarding vocal fold tonicity [40]. This can lead to malfunctioning compensatory vocal behavior, which surgery cannot fix.
- By the time the patient consults an ENT, the patient might already have developed dysfunctional compensatory vocal habits (using supraglottal constriction), which also leads to vocal abuse, vocal fatigue, discomfort, and lack of vocal efficacy.

The SLT can also access and rehabilitate swallowing, which can also be impaired when it comes to unilateral vocal fold immobility. It is not always the case and, here again, options should be considered on a case-by-case basis (Table 35.6).

Perioperative SLT timing depends, as usual on the patient's history.

- Indirect therapy makes sense mostly when it comes to providing physiological and pathological explanations, and environment adaptation (amplification, etc.), and voice rest additionally to other vocal hygiene advice, since patients with unilateral immobility tend to be more sensitive to vocal fatigue. That can be dispensed ahead of surgery.
- Direct therapy can be tackled before surgery if hyperfunctional compensations have set in, but makes most sense with the new medialized laryngeal configuration.

Swallowing assessment and rehabilitation are a priority compared to voice therapy because of the pulmonary and nutritional risks involved.

Table 35.6 Treatment options for unilateral vocal fold immobility

	Pros	Cons
SLT only	Helps prevent or deconstruct effortful vocal compensation Noninvasive Assessment and rehabilitation of swallowing if needed	Results can be long to obtain and are variable. Time and energy consuming (and with a financial cost depending on the country and health-care system), motivational issues.
Surgery only	Rapidly obtained results Variety of effective options with good prognosis Less time and energy consuming than SLT	Minimal surgical risks. Risk of compensatory vocal straining.
Surgery + pre- and postoperative SLT	Rapidly obtained results Reduced risk of compensatory vocal straining Assessment and rehabilitation of swallowing if needed	Minimal surgery-related risks. Time and energy consuming when it comes to SLT.
Neither (the "do nothing" option)	Can be considered if there is no swallowing-related threat and if felt vocal handicap is low No time and energy cost No surgery-related risk	Hyperfunctional compensation could increase over time.

35.3 Laryngeal Cancer and General Principles for SLTs

In this chapter, we will not discuss voice changes after total laryngectomy or "alaryngeal substitute voice." Communication modalities, the characteristics of this alaryngeal voice, and the modes of its management are presented in another chapter.

The surgical treatment of cancerous lesions of the larynx will be responsible for anatomical and functional changes due to the surgery; it is no longer a phonosurgery that respects the vocal function, but the treatment of a tumor in a context of cancer – a possibly life-threatening disease.

35.3.1 Collaboration for a Better Quality of Life

The place of the speech therapist and their close collaboration with the surgeon contributes to the success of the treatment in Head & Neck cancerology. The goal is no longer just to treat the tumor but to ensure the most physiological functional recovery of swallowing, breathing and phonation, and prevention of nutritional and pulmonary consequences of oro-pharyngeal dysphagia, thus improving the quality of life and the survival of patients. SLTs are integrated into the multidisciplinary team recommended in the Cancer and Public Health plans that now exist in some European countries.

https://ec.europa.eu/health/non_communicable_diseases/cancer_fr

35.3.2 Cancer Disease and Life Plans

In the therapeutic project, in addition to the technical dimension that is essential to ensure the effectiveness of a protective sphincter of the respiratory tract and a laryngeal neo-vibrator, these interventions are carried out in the context of a cancerous disease with all its emotional implications, a dimension that cannot be neglected and which may sometimes require the intervention of other professionals.

The patient must be involved in the therapeutic process and have a participatory attitude, which largely determines the success of this rehabilitation. The SLT helps motivate patients to reorganize and reinvest in their life projects [41, 42].

35.3.3 Caregiver Involvement

The therapeutic rehabilitation project will be considered if possible, in the preoperative period and in the presence of the spouse, a family member, or an outside helper. Indeed, the caregiver's support is one of the guarantees of the success of this rehabilitation, which will last long. The family collaboration will facilitate the resumption of swallowing by making the caregiver aware of the hygiene-dietary rules. For the voice, they will encourage the patient to complete daily exercises as well as local care. The caregiver's participation in the rehabilitation sessions also helps address the need to accept the patient's changed vocal characteristics [43].

35.3.4 Associated Treatments

Chemoradiotherapy does not preclude further rehabilitation, but it can delay vocal and swallowing progress because of general and local consequences such as induced dysphagia or trismus. During this period, emphasis will be placed on regular and short oro-facial muscle exercises as well as training breathing and relaxation exercises to relieve the pain of radiotherapy. It will be done at the patient's own pace, avoiding long and tiring trips [44].

35.4 Voice, Speech, and Swallowing Assessment in the Context of Laryngeal Cancer

The assessment of voice and swallowing is performed as soon as possible when local healing is satisfactory, generally before the end of the first postoperative week.

The clinical and physical examination is the same for the voice production, speech articulation, and swallowing functions and begins with a motor and sensitive exploration of the oro-facial regions and the lips, tongue cheeks, and velum. The patient's ability to perform voluntary and reflex gestures (coughing, throat clearing, gag reflex, and automatic saliva swallowing) is evaluated.

The instrumental assessment will be used to determine the general guidelines for the most efficient management and will guide the treatment plan.

The goal of the SLT will be to involve the patient and encourage them to take charge of their own care.

Management will include the direct rehabilitation of the organ and of the phonatory, respiratory, and swallowing functions, as well as the indirect therapy of the cancerous disease and its consequences on the patient's quality of life.

35.4.1 Voice and Speech Assessment and Management

The voices produced are called "neoglottic substitute voices" following glottic surgery, or "neolaryngeal substitute voices" after modification of the laryngeal tube (supracricoidal partial laryngectomies with reconstruction).

35.4.1.1 Perceptual and Self-Evaluation of Voice

Perceptual evaluation with the specific GRBAS [9]/IINFVo scales [10] as well as self-evaluations (VHI) [5] contributes to establish a vocal profile as a benchmark of evolution and recovery of speech components and patient satisfaction.

35.4.1.2 Acoustic Evaluation

The acoustic assessment may be questionable due to the dysphonia, sometimes too severe to have an analyzable acoustic signal; however, it is necessary to record the voice to have a starting point of vocal characteristics and to follow the evolution.

The main alterations will concern the following:

- The pitch of the voice (fundamental frequency f0) as well as the amplitude/modulation of the voice
- The intensity, which is always decreased
- The voice quality with hoarseness or breathiness, due to asymmetry and glottic incompetence

Vocal fatigue remains for a long time, as well as a decrease in speaking duration related to an alteration of the glottic closure.

35.4.1.3 Laryngeal Imaging

The functional assessment of the patient's phonatory behavior with videostroboscopic examination allows to evaluate the following:

- The mechanisms of closure and laryngeal vibration. The examination will provide information on the remaining structures, their possible mobilization toward the creation of a neoglottis, the compensations that are put in place, the quality of the mucous membrane, the tissues and their elasticity, and the fibrous transformations linked to healing.

This assessment will be repeated to monitor the evolution of recovery and to avoid deviant compensations such as behaviors with over- or undercompensations that can increase the tight or breathy quality of the voice as well as vocal effort.

35.4.1.4 The SLT's Treatment Plan

In the preoperative period or in the postoperative period, the SLT will explain what are the anatomical structures involved in normal phonation and those he/she will have to use after the surgical modifications, using simple diagrams.

The patient's motivation in relation to their voice is a determining factor in the speed of vocal recovery. A patient who is working, or is involved in a community or social activity, will generally invest more time and energy in rehabilitation than a patient living alone, unemployed or retired. He/she will be more motivated and ready to invest in this long relearning process.

Direct Therapy

The aim is to obtain a good neoglottic closure that will ensure that the expiratory breath restarts as the aerodynamic source for a vibrating neoglottis, to reintroduce the dynamics of phonation [16].

- Sphincteric function: the first step to recreate an efficient laryngeal sphincter for airway protection requires significant muscle contractions. Over time, the degree of effort will then be less strong to set up a laryngeal vibrator for phonation.
- Vibrating function: neoglottic vibration requires the use of adapted phonetic production to promote the recovery of voicing and speech articulation [45]. This step is accompanied by the discovery of new vibratory sensations and a voice that is not always aesthetic, effective or adaptable at first. Faced with this new voice which is often lower and hoarser than the previous laryngeal voice, some patients settle down to using a whispered voice. It is not to be encouraged, because it is tiring and inefficient, or even in functional opposition to the vibrating neoglottis.
- Resonant function: the oro-pharyngeal resonance cavities are useful for speech articulation; therefore, they should not be neglected as they will compensate for the lack of intensity by increasing intelligibility and slowing down the phonatory flow.

All these structures can only function harmoniously and synergistically if they are relaxed.

Relaxation may be proposed in the care of these patients. It will also have a role to decrease the stress felt by most cancer patients. The goal is to teach them to gain better control of their physical and emotional body.

Indirect Therapy

- Rehabilitation plays an important role in getting over the loss of the previous voice by rehabilitating the mutilated organ and helping the patient regain vocal function in harmony with their personality, an essential step in the acceptance of the new voice.
- The role of the SLT, in addition to providing technical support, will be to guide the patient in the personal work of becoming aware of their new voicing skills.
- Rehabilitation is often long, and requires the patient's commitment and willingness to regain a verbal mode of communication.

35.4.2 Swallowing Assessment and Management

External partial laryngectomies can affect the swallowing function by the following methods:

- Modifying the upper airway
- Decreasing the efficiency of the laryngeal sphincter
- Sacrificing the nerves involved in motor function and pharyngolaryngeal sensitivity

Consequently, the bolus localization and the protective reflex of the respiratory tract will be diminished or delayed.

The detection and management of dysphagia must be early as it can be life-threatening.

35.4.2.1 The Organic and Functional Assessment

The assessment will include the motor units as well as the sensitivity of the pharyngeal-laryngeal region; it will be a support to guide the management performed by the SLT and monitor the patient's evolution on that point.

- The patient's interview collects functional signs such as meal duration, respiratory signs, weight changes, asthenia, fever, altered general condition.
- The swallowing screening and self-assessment scales contribute to the initial assessment and are benchmarks of progress.
- Videofibroscopic exploration of the swallowing phases:

This examination allows to detect sphincter closure insufficiencies, laryngeal ascension defects, aspiration-penetration mechanisms, blockage, and stasis sites and will guide adaptations such as facilitation or protective postures of the respiratory tract.

- Identifying difficulties related to the texture, volume, and consistency of the bolus will allow dietary advice to be given and meals to be adapted to the patient's abilities.
- Liquids are the most difficult consistencies with high risk of penetration because of weak laryngeal closure. Thick drinks to fluid liquids will be the last to be reintroduced [46].

35.4.2.2 The SLT's Treatment Plan

The double support with the direct and indirect therapy management, optimizes functional results and quality of life.

Direct Therapy

- The work of the sphincter functions will be done during the postoperative resting phase of the aerodigestive tube that can last from a few days to three weeks, depending on the type of surgery. Usually, a gastrostomy (or a nasogastric tube depending on the importance and duration of the expected difficulties in refeeding) is put in place at the end of the surgical procedure. The SLT is going to make the most of the rest phase period to work on the motor units involved in swallowing e.g., work on the strength and amplitude of the oral-lingual and mandibular muscle contractions…
- The work of breathing, coughing, throat clearing (larynx and tongue base) and spitting will help to tone up the laryngeal sphincter and to react efficiently in case of penetration
- The work of the laryngeal sphincter will participate in the restoration of swallowing apnea, which is difficult to achieve because the laryngeal sphincter is less efficient.
- The work of cervico-cephalic postures will be explained. They allow to reinforce the levels of laryngeal closure in order to reduce laryngeal penetrations. The patient should tilt the head forward, with the chin close to the sternum. It is sometimes associated with a rotation of the head on the operated side in vertical partial surgeries or supracricoid surgeries with preservation of a single arytenoid (rotation on the side of the missing arytenoid). These postures facilitate the protection of the respiratory tract, increase the opening of the remaining piriform sinus to receive the food bolus, and promote the ascent of the larynx and the backward movement of the base of the tongue.

Indirect Therapy

- Dental condition and oral hygiene contribute to the proper preparation of the bolus and the

smooth swallowing process. The SLT will participate in this education, which helps to limit the risk of infection and pain.
- Food textures will be carefully selected as it will contribute to the success of the initial re-feeding, as well as the nutritional balance and gradual diversification of the diet according to functional progress. A European standardization (IDDSI) of the nomenclature of textures is also underway for a better classification and recommendation of possible types of food [47, 48].
- Stimulation of the pleasure of tasting by learning how to vary textures and tastes as soon as possible and according to the evolution of the patient's capacities and desires.
- Manage more general complications such as those of chemoradiotherapy, infections, psychological distress...that can delay the swallowing recovery process and expose to increased risk of penetration.
- The SLT also has a vigilance role, thanks to weekly visits that allow them to be on the front line to observe any regression or stagnation of learning, or alteration in general condition, and in such events must refer the patient to their doctor.

35.5 SLT Specific Management for Endoscopic or External Laryngeal Surgery

The role of the SLT will depend on the degree of disruption of laryngeal function resulting from

- different surgeries for lesions of the glottic and supraglottic level and
- on the surgical procedures, namely, endoscopic transoral microsurgery and external surgery.

The timing will be adapted to the postoperative state and the spontaneous rehabilitation capacities of the patients. Obtaining optimal functional results of swallowing, breathing, and phonation requires the earliest possible postoperative intervention of the SLT.

The laryngeal sphincter mechanisms that will be mobilized to restore efficient phonation and safe swallowing will involve, to varying degrees, the 3 laryngeal levels, glottic, supra-glottic (ventricular folds), and aryepiglottic folds with the arytenoids.

The role of the SLT will be to guide and dose the compensatory efforts in order not to fall into excess, which is just as harmful as insufficiency.

35.5.1 Transoral Surgery

Endoscopic surgery has the advantage of being targeted, not very extensive, limiting anatomical changes and with simpler and faster post-operative outcomes than external surgery.

35.5.1.1 Glottic Carcinoma

The removal of a variable part of the vocal fold will affect the voice quality.

According to the type of cordectomy [49].

- For cordectomy types I and II, the rehabilitation is similar to that of benign vocal fold lesion's surgeries and the **SLT's** work aims at improving the quality of closure of the vocal folds and the vibration of the vocal fold mucosa, with softening of the scar area. Vocal recovery is satisfactory within 1–3 months post-operatively [50, 51]
- For cordectomy types III to VI, muscle resection varies according to the type of cordectomy, with a residual notch in the excision bed of the vocal fold being more or less extensive. This leaves fibrous scar tissue with a defect in the closure of the glottis, which can vary from case to case [52].

SLT Goals

Glottic inefficiency with breathy voice will be compensated by recruiting neighboring structures such as the contralateral vocal fold and sometimes ventricular fold, in order to obtain an efficient closure. However, speech therapy will be cautious not to develop harmful effortful behavior (discomfort and degraded sound). Rehabilitation is similar to that of unilateral laryngeal paralysis mentioned previously.

Timing

Direct therapy often begins around Day 15 to avoid reactive forcing behavior to postoperative dysphonia and to insist on respiration exercises. The delay of healing of the vocal fold usually imposes a delay of 1 month before being able to obtain satisfactory sounds for the vocal training itself.

Vocal Results

Dysphonia can be characterized by various degrees of breathiness with reduced intensity and pitch modulations, and a shortening of the phonatory duration. The glottic effort of compensation can sometimes give a hoarse component to the voice.

35.5.1.2 Supraglottic Carcinoma

Supraglottic laryngeal surgery (supraglottic laryngectomy) for limited lesions can be performed by laser (transoral laser surgery) or robot-assisted (transoral robotic surgery, TORS) [53].

Voice Rehabilitation

These surgeries are rarely responsible for severe dysphonia, at most a change in resonance. Postoperative radiotherapy may contribute to aggravate the dysphonia due to oedemas and stiffness of the pharyngo-laryngeal mucous membranes. The SLT will intervene according to the degree of voice disability expressed by the patient.

Swallowing Rehabilitation

The primary concern after supraglottic endoscopic surgery is the swallowing function, which will need to be carefully assessed at an early stage [54–56].

- Oro-facial mobilization: the treatment can begin gently with the work of the oro-facial mobilisation from Day4/Day5, especially for the tongue that has been sometimes traumatized by the robotic setting and the base of the tongue which sometimes enters the surgical field.
- Then the work of muscular reinforcement on the peristalsis and pharyngeal emptying (pharyngeal constrictors and tongue base backward movement) to maximize the protection of the respiratory tract.
- The reintroduction of food will be done first with soft solid, smooth and homogeneous textures (IDDSI 3_4) by adapting the respiratory tract protection postures and/or manoeuvres and then diversification by introducing liquids last.
- Patients can start eating soft food between Day1 and Day3.

35.5.2 External Surgery

Rehabilitation will be undertaken as soon as possible, to the extent permitted by the patient's condition, that is, before the end of the first postoperative week.

If a tracheotomy is necessary, it will not delay the rehabilitation process of the upper airway by using a fenestrated cannula with a phonation valve (or by plugging the cannula manually), even intermittently during speech therapy sessions. This early stimulation will allow sensitive stimulation of the remaining pharyngeal-laryngeal structures, and neural reappropriation facilitating the restoration of laryngeal function and protection of the respiratory tract (throat clearing, coughing, spitting).

For phonation, the presence of the tracheotomy cannula does not interfere with articulatory or respiratory exercises or the beginning of the vibration of the glottic sphincter.

As soon as the wound heals, the instrumental swallowing assessment will allow to establish the functional prognosis and to evaluate the modalities of swallowing management according to anatomical and dynamic data [57].

35.5.2.1 Glottic Carcinoma

For external surgery, we will not go into the details of the different surgical techniques, but will focus on the main components of the resections and the anatomical and functional modifications.

Vertical Partial Laryngectomy

Phonation is modified by a median leak between the healthy vocal fold and the excised vocal fold responsible for a breathy voice with vibrator asymmetry.

SLT's Goal

- The exercises proposed to compensate the lack of symmetry of the vibrator will be laryngeal manipulations, of the "forced adduction exercises" type, more or less associated with laryngeal vibration exercises, to recreate a phonatory valve.
- The SLT will be careful not to switch to overcompensation and overtightening, which would be detrimental to voice quality.
- It will also be necessary to improve pneumophonatory control, because glottic leakage is responsible for shortness of breath in phonation. This shortness of breath leads to fatigue when speaking, and the patient prefers to reduce their speaking time, gradually leading the patient to isolate himself or herself.

Vocal Results

The vocal recovery results in a breathy voice, sometimes hoarse.

The lack of intensity remains the main complaint [58, 59].

The swallowing function is not modified and is resumed within 48 h.

Supracricoid Partial Laryngectomy with Cricohyoidoepiglottopexy (CHEP)

Horizontal supracricoid partial laryngectomies with reconstruction are the most mutilating partial procedures for voice and swallowing. The entire glottic space has been removed, leaving only one or two mobile arytenoids posteriorly and part of the suprahyoid epiglottis (CHEP) anteriorly.

SLT's Goal

- For voicing, the neoglottic closure is obtained by placing the arytenoids against each other inward and forward toward the epiglottis.
- In order to have the arytenoids to vibrate, a sufficient neoglottic occlusion to provide an obstacle to the passage of expiratory air is required. These arytenoids must therefore tilt sufficiently forward to come into contact with the remaining epiglottis (rigid structure, with a lower vibratory potential). This tilting will be obtained, at the beginning, at the cost of an effort against resistance, an effort to be reduced during later rehabilitation. The pull-back movement of the tongue base will also need to be developed. An important work of reorganization of the muscular activities of the remaining pharyngo-laryngeal structures will be necessary to obtain this neoglottic sphincter.
- The rehabilitation process leads to a change in the functional orientation of the preserved laryngeal structures, which needs time to reorient themselves [45].

Vocal Results

Vocal recovery is done according to a well-defined chronology over time:

- A period of 1–3 months will be marked by a whispered voice due to the absence of closure of the neoglottis. The spontaneous horizontal movement of the arytenoids toward each other must be completed by learning and automating the forward tilt as well as the backward movement of the tongue base. Forced adduction exercises and holding the breath will improve with the better closure of the neoglottis.
- Over the next three months, the neoglottis will settle with a very hoarse, low, and irregular sound. It is then a question of working on the reduction of the effort for the vibration and the lengthening of the duration of the vibrations, obtained by a greater flexibility and relaxation of the structures in contact.
- During the first year, voicing will improve with a reduction in parasitic noise and improved regularity of the sound signal.
- The progress, although very slow, will continue during the second postoperative year with a slight improvement in the possibilities of modulating the pitch of the voice, which remains low, with low intensity and conservation of a hoarse timbre.

This notion of a two-year delay to stabilize vocal progress should not be lost sight of, as it allows the patient to be motivated throughout this rehabilitation. Speech therapy may be interrupted to allow patients to integrate and automate the newly acquired skills. This also avoids the fatigue of long treatment [60–62].

Swallowing Results

- An enteral feeding will be kept at least 10–14 days postoperatively and has the advantage of ensuring nutritional intake while giving time for the pharyngeal and laryngeal structures to adapt.
- The first trials will be done around Day14 with smooth and thick textures (IDDSI 4). Gradually, the textures will be thickened and then fluidized, but the liquids will remain thickened for a certain time while adapting to the patient's progress.
- A regular check-up every 3 months by video fibroscopy will allow to follow the functional evolution of the neoglottis.

Swallowing rehabilitation and phonation rehabilitation are carried out together in this type of surgery. Exercises that improve swallowing also improve voice and vice versa, since in both cases, it is necessary to recreate a neoglottic sphincter. Phonation requires a laryngeal sphincter that is less tight than for swallowing, allowing the vibration of the arytenoid mucosa and the aryepiglottic folds; the conservation of 2 mobile arytenoids is more favorable for obtaining this sphincter [63].

35.5.2.2 Supraglottic Carcinoma

Supraglottic Laryngectomy

As for endoscopic procedure, supraglottic external laryngeal surgery is rarely responsible for severe dysphonia, the functional concern will be the swallowing function, which will need to be evaluated early. The patient will have postoperatively a tracheotomy and nasogastric probe for about 10 days.

SLT's Goal

- The SLT will focus the management to restore the efficiency of the laryngeal sphincter to improve breathing, coughing, and swallowing.
- The training will consist in encouraging the backward movement of the tongue base, toning the laryngeal sphincter and working on the apnea and the elevation of the larynx.
- To compensate for the deficit of the laryngeal rim, muscular reinforcement for peristalsis and pharyngeal emptying (pharyngeal constrictors and backward placement of the tongue base) will be proposed to maximize the protection of the respiratory tract.
- The use of a protective posture of the respiratory tract will most often be necessary, with an anterior flexion of the head.

Supracricoid Partial Laryngectomy with Cricohyoidopexy (CHP)

This surgical technique is one of the most extensive partial laryngectomies.

It has almost the same postsurgery evolution as CHEP and the same phonation and swallowing SLT management.

The entire glottic space has been removed, only one or two mobile arytenoids remain backward and the tongue base forward, to create a speaking and swallowing sphincter.

SLT's Goal

- In phonation, the glottic closure is obtained by placing the arytenoids against each other inwardly and forwardly toward the base of the tongue.
- These arytenoids must therefore tilt sufficiently forward to come into contact with the base of the tongue, which has a flexible structure with a certain vibratory capacity for phonation.
- The acoustic characteristics are close to those of CHEP.

35.6 Conclusions

In the case of benign lesions, the SLT provides information on the mechanisms of installation and maintenance of the lesions with awareness of phonatory behavior, voice hygiene, and environmental requirements. It will guide the patient toward the most effective adaptation to their needs.

The management of glottic lesion and vocal function (direct therapy) as well as environmental arrangement and understanding of the vocal pathology and its implications (indirect therapy) are the key to success for long-term lasting voice recovery.

In the case of laryngeal cancer, preoperatively, the SLT should help the patient in understanding the treatment plan proposed by the surgeon and the consequences on voice and swallowing. The information on the prospects of functional outcomes, recovery, adaptation, and compensation should help for better involvement and motivation.

The collaboration between the surgeon and the SLT, throughout the management, aims at optimizing functional results and restoring the best physiological phonation and swallowing possible. Regular check-ups allow for a re-evaluation of progress and the adaptation of rehabilitation techniques.

The management of laryngeal cancer can no longer be conceived without the functional support including a Quality of Life dimension and the role of the SLT is paramount.

Strong recommendations emerge to encourage the implementation of consultation with the SLT, prior to surgery, and to maintain close collaboration with the surgeon throughout the management.

References

1. Le Borgne WDL, Donahue EN. Voice therapy as primary treatment of vocal fold pathology. Otolaryngol Clin North Am. 2019;52(4):649–56. https://doi.org/10.1016/j.otc.2019.03.009.
2. White AC, Carding P. Pre- and postoperative voice therapy for benign vocal fold lesions: factors influencing a complex intervention. J Voice. 2020; https://doi.org/10.1016/j.jvoice.2020.04.004.
3. Dejonckere P, Bradley P, Clemente P, Cornut G, Crevier-Buchman L, Friedrich G, Van De Heyning P, Remacle M, Woisard V. A basic protocol for functional assessment of voice pathology. Eur Arch Otorhinolaryngol. 2001;258:77–82.
4. Patel RR, Awan SN, Barkmeier-Kraemer J, Courey M, Deliyski D, Eadie T, Paul D, Švec JG, Hillman R. Recommended protocols for instrumental assessment of voice: American Speech-Language-Hearing Association Expert Panel to develop a protocol for instrumental assessment of vocal function. AJSLP. 2018;27:887–905. https://doi.org/10.1044/2018_AJSLP-17-0009.
5. Jacobson H, Jonhson A, Grywalski C, Ilbergleit A, Jacobson G, Michael S, Benninger B. The Voice Handicap Index (VHI): development and validation. Am J Speech Lang Pathol. 1997;6:66–70.
6. Rinkel R, Verdonck-De Leeuw I, Van Reij J, Aaronson K, Leemans R. Speech Handicap Index in patients with oral and pharyngeal cancer: better understanding of patients' complaints. Head Neck. 2008;30:868–74.
7. Hogikyan N, Sethuraman G. Validation of an instrument to measure voice-related quality of life (V-RQOL). J Voice. 1999;13:557–69.
8. Deary I, Wilson J, Carding P, Mac Kenzie K. VoiSS: a patient derived voice symptom scale. J Psychosom Res. 2003;54:483–9.
9. De Bodt MS, Wuyts FL, Van de Heyning PH, ChristopheCroux. Test-retest study of the GRBAS scale: Influence of experience and professional background on perceptual rating of voice quality. J. Voice. 1997;11(1):74–80.
10. Moerman M, Martens JP, Crevier-Buchman L, Dejonckere P, Woisard V. The INFVo perceptual rating scale for substitution voicing: development and reliability. Eur Arch Otolaryngol. 2006;263:435–9.
11. Maryn Y, Corthals P, Van Cauwenberge P, Roy N, De Bodt M. Toward improved ecological validity in the acoustic measurement of overall voice quality: combining continuous speech and sustained vowels. J Voice. 2010;24(5):540–55.
12. Maryn Y, De Bodt M, Roy N. The Acoustic Voice Quality Index: toward improved treatment outcomes assessment in voice disorders. J Commun Disord. 2010;43:161–74.
13. Heylen L, Wuyts FL, Mertens F, De Bodt M, Van de Heyning PH. Normative voice range profiles of male and female professional voice users. J Voice. 2002;16(1):1–7. https://doi.org/10.1016/S0892-1997(02)00065-6).
14. Mehum CS, Rosenberg T, Groentved AM, Dyrvig AK, Godballe C. Can videostroboscopy predict early glottic cancer? A systematic review and meta-analysis. Laryngoscope. 2016;126:2079–84.
15. van Balkum M, Buijs B, Donselaar EJ, Erkelens DCA, Goulin Lippi Fernandes E, Wegner I, et al. Systematic review of the diagnostic value of laryngeal stroboscopy in excluding early glottic carcinoma. Clin Otolaryngol. 2017;42:123–30.
16. Crevier-Buchman L, Brihaye S, Tessier C. La voix après chirurgie partielle du Larynx. Bruxelles: Ed De Boeck Superieur; 2003.
17. Logemann JA. Approaches to management of disordered swallowing. Bailliere's Clin Gastroenterol. 1991;5(2). ISBN: 0-7020-1530-X

18. Crary MA, Carnaby GD. Adoption into clinical practice of two therapies to manage swallowing disorders: exercise-based swallowing rehabilitation and electrical stimulation. Curr Opin Otolaryngol Head Neck Surg. 2014;22(3):172–80. https://doi.org/10.1097/MOO.0000000000000055.
19. Clarke P, Radford K, Coffey M, Stewart M. Speech and swallow rehabilitation in head and neck cancer: United Kingdom National Multidisciplinary Guidelines. J Laryngol Otol. 2016;130(Suppl. S2):S176–80. https://doi.org/10.1017/S0022215116000608).
20. Fleming SM, Weaver AW. Index of dysphagia: A tool for identifying deglutition problems. Dysphagia. 1987;1(4):206–8.
21. Rinkel RN, Verdonck-de Leeuw IM, Langendijk JA, van Reij EJ, Aaronson NK, Leemans CR. The psychometric and clinical validity of the SWAL-QOL questionnaire in evaluating swallowing problems experienced by patients with oral and oropharyngeal cancer. Oral Oncol. 2009;45(8):e67–71. https://doi.org/10.1016/j.oraloncology.2009.03.003.
22. Belafsky PC, Mouadeb DA, Rees CJ, Pryor JC, Postma GN, Allen J, Leonard RJ. Validity and reliability of the Eating Assessment Tool (EAT-10). Ann Otol Rhinol Laryngol. 2008;117(12):919–24.
23. Brady S, Donzelli J. The Modified Barium Swallow and the Functional Endoscopic Evaluation of Swallowing. Otolaryngol Clin N Am. 2013;46(6):1009–22.
24. Pizzorni N, Crosetti E, Santambrogio E, de Cillis G, Bertolin A, Rizzotto G, Fantini M, Succo G, Schindler A. The penetration-aspiration scale: adaptation to open partial laryngectomy and reliability analysis. Dysphagia. 2019;2019(35):261–71.
25. Van Stan JH, Roy N, Awan S, Stemple J, Hillman RE. A taxonomy of voice therapy. AJSLP. 2015;24:101–25. https://doi.org/10.1044/2015_AJSLP-14-0030.
26. Gartner-Schmidt JL, Roth DF, Zullo TG, Rosen CA. Quantifying component parts of indirect and direct voice therapy related to different voice disorders. J Voice. 2012;27(2):210–6.
27. Ouyoung LM, Swanson MS, Villegas BC, Damodar D, Kokot N, Sinha UK. Voice therapy outcomes for patients with head and neck cancer. Head Neck. 2016;38(Suppl 1):E1810–3. https://doi.org/10.1002/hed.24322. Epub 2015 Dec 22.
28. Friedrich G, Remacle M, Birchall M, Marie J-P, Arens C. Defining phonosurgery: A proposal for classification and nomenclature by the Phonosurgery Committee of the European Laryngological Society (ELS). Eur Arch Otorhinolaryngol. 2007;264:1191–200.
29. White A. Management of benign vocal fold lesions: current perspectives on the role for voice therapy. Curr Opin Otolaryngol Head Neck Surg. 2019;27(3):185–90. https://doi.org/10.1097/MOO.0000000000000536.
30. Hantzakos A, Remacle M, Dikkers FG, Degols J-C, Delos M, Friedrich G, Giovanni A, Rasmussen N. Exudative lesions of Reinke's space: a terminology proposal. Eur Arch OtoRhinoLaryngol. 2009;266(6):869–78. https://doi.org/10.1007/s00405-008-0863-x.
31. Crevier Buchman L, Mattei A, Giovanni A. Forçage vocal. EMC Oto-Rhino-Laryngol. 2019:1–14, Article 20-752-B-10.
32. Zhuge P, You H, Wang H, Zhang Y, Huanle D. An analysis of the effects of voice therapy on patients with early vocal fold polyps. J Voice. 2016;30(6):698–704. https://doi.org/10.1016/j.jvoice.2015.08.013.
33. Tang SS, Thibeault SL. Timing of voice therapy: a primary investigation of voice outcomes for surgical benign vocal fold lesion patients. J Voice. 2017;31(1):129.e1–7. https://doi.org/10.1016/j.jvoice.2015.12.005.
34. Ishikawa K, Thibeault S. Voice rest versus exercise: a review of the literature. J Voice. 2010;24(4):379–87.
35. Kaneko M, Shiromoto O, Fujiu-Kurachi M, Kishimoto Y, Tateya I, Hirano S. Optimal duration for voice rest after vocal fold surgery: randomized controlled clinical study. J Voice. 2017;31(1):97–103. https://doi.org/10.1016/j.jvoice.2016.02.009.
36. Bouchayer M, Cornut G, Witzig E, Loire R, Roch JB, Bastian RW. Epidermoid cysts, sulci, and mucosal bridges of the true vocal cord: a report of 157 cases. Laryngoscope. 1985;95(9 Pt 1):1087–94.
37. Hantzakos A, Dikkers FG, Giovanni A, Benninger MS, Remacle M, Sjögren EV, et al. Vocal fold scars: a common classification proposal by the American Laryngological Association and European Laryngological Society. Eur Arch Otorhinolaryngol. 2019;276(8):2289–92.
38. Tibbetts KM, Dominguez LM, Blake Simpson C. Impact of perioperative voice therapy on outcomes in the surgical management of vocal fold cysts. J Voice. 2018;32(3):347–51. https://doi.org/10.1016/j.jvoice.2017.06.004).
39. Hertegård S, Nagubothu SR, Malmström E, LeBlanc K. Treatment of vocal fold scarring with autologous bone marrow-derived human mesenchymal stromal cells-first phase I/II human clinical study. Stem Cell Res Ther. 2020;11(1):128.
40. Bakhsh Z, Crevier-Buchman L. Stroboscopic assessment of unilateral vocal fold paralysis: a systematic review. Eur Arch Oto-Rhino-Laryngol. 2019;276(9):2377–87. https://doi.org/10.1007/s00405-019-05562-x.
41. Hebel F, Mantsopoulos K, Bohr C. Assessing quality of life in patients after partial laryngectomy. Hippokratia. 2014;18:156–61.
42. Teo I, Fronczyk KM, Guindani M, Vannucci M, Ulfers SS, Hanasono MM, et al. Salient body image concerns of patients with cancer undergoing head and neck reconstruction. Head Neck. 2016;38:1035–42.
43. Longacre ML, Ridge JA, Burtness BA, Galloway TJ, Fang CY. Psychological functioning of caregivers for head and neck cancer patients. Oral Oncol. 2012;48(1):18–25. https://doi.org/10.1016/j.oraloncology.2011.11.012.

44. Carroll WR, Locher JL, Canon CL, Bohannon IA, McColloch NL, Magnuson JS. Pretreatment swallowing exercices improve swallowing function after chemoradiation. Laryngoscope. 2008;118:39–43.
45. Schindler A, Pizzorni N, Mozzanica F, Fantini M, Ginocchio D, Bertolin A, et al. Functional outcomes after supracricoid laryngectomy: what do we not know and what do we need to know ? Eur Arch Otorhinolaryngol. 2016;273:3459–75.
46. Lewin JS, Hutcheson KA, Barringer DA, May AH, Roberts DB, Holsinger FC, et al. Functional analysis of swallowing outcomes after supracricoid partial laryngectomy. Head Neck. 2008;30:559–66.
47. Cichero JA, Lam P, Steel CM, Hanson B, Chen J, Dantsa RO, et al. Development of international terminology and definitions for texture-modified foods and thickened fluids used in dysphagia management: the IDDSI Framwork. Dysphagia. 2017;32:293–314.
48. Steele C, Namasivayam-MacDonald AM, Guida BT, Cichero J, Janice Duivestein B, Hanson PL, Riquelme L. Creation and initial validation of the international dysphagia diet standardisation initiative functional diet scale. Arch Phys Med Rehabil. 2018;99(5):934–44.
49. Remacle M, Van Haverbeke C, Eckel H, Bradley P, Chevalier D, Djukic V, de Vicentiis M, Friedrich G, Olofsson J, Peretti G, Quer M, Werner J. Proposal for revision of the European Laryngological Society classification of endoscopic cordectomies. Eur Arch Otorhinolaryngol. 2007;264:499–504. https://doi.org/10.1007/s00405-007-0279-z.
50. Vilaseca I, Huerta P, Blanch JL, Fernández-Planas AM, Jiménez C, Bernal-Sprekelsen M. Voice quality after CO2 laser cordectomy-what can we really expect? Head Neck. 2008;30(1):43–9. https://doi.org/10.1002/hed.20659.
51. Crevier-Buchman L, Colomb I, Hans S, Vaissière J, Brasnu D. Evolution of voice assessment and quality of life after endoscopic laser cordectomy. Rev Laryngol Otol Rhinol (Bord). 2007;128(5):315–20.
52. Schindler A, Palonta F, Preti G, Ottaviani F, Schindler O, Cavalot AL. Voice quality after carbon dioxide laser and conventional surgery for T1A glottic carcinoma. J Voice. 2004;18(4):545–50.
53. Mendelson AH, Remacle M, Van der Vorst S, Bachy V, Lawson G. Outcomes following transoral robotic surgery: supraglottic laryngectomy. Laryngoscope. 2013;123:208–14.
54. Peretti G, Piazza C, Cattaneo A, De Benedetto L, Martin E, Nicolai P. Comparison of functional outcomes after endoscopic versus open neck supraglottic laryngectomies. Ann Ottol Rhinol Laryngol. 2006;115:827–32.
55. Hans S, Chekkouri Idrissi Y, Distinguin L, Circiu M, Crevier Buchman L, Lechien J. Surgical, oncological and functional outcomes of transoral robotic supraglottic laryngectomy. Laryngoscope. 2020; https://doi.org/10.1002/lary.28926.
56. Achim V, Bolognone RK, Palmer AD, Graville DJ, Light TJ, Li R, Gross N, Andersen PE, Clayburgh D. Long-term functional and quality-of-life outcomes after transoral robotic surgery in patients with oropharyngeal cancer. JAMA Otolaryngol Head Neck Surg. 2018;144(1):18–27. https://doi.org/10.1001/jamaoto.2017.1790.
57. Alicandri-Ciufelli M, Piccini A, Grammatica A, Chiesi A, Bergamini G, Luppi MP, et al. Voice and swallowing after partial laryngectomy: factors influencing outcome. Head Neck. 2013;35:214–9.
58. Biacabe B, Crevier-Buchman L, Hans S, Laccourreye O, Brasnu D. Vocal function after vertical partial laryngectomy with glottic reconstruction by false vocal flap: durational and frequency measures. Laryngoscope. 1999;109:698–704.
59. Biacabe B, Crevier-Buchman L, Hans S, Laccourreye O, Brasnu D. Phonatory mechanisms after vertical partial laryngectomy with glottic reconstruction by false vocal cord. Ann Otol Rhinol Laryngol. 2001;110:935–40.
60. Laccourreye O, Crevier-Buchman L, Weinstein G, Biacabe B, Laccourreye H, Brasnu D. Duration and frequency characteristics of speech and voice following supracricoid partial laryngectomy. Ann Otol Rhinol Laryngol. 1995;104:516–21.
61. Crevier-Buchman L, Laccourreye O, Weinstein G, Garcia D, Jouffre V, Brasnu D. Evolution of voice and speech following supracricoid partial Laryngectomy. J Laryngol Otol. 1995;109:410–3.
62. Laccourreye O, Crevier-Buchman L, Weinstein G, Jouffre V, Laccourreye H, Brasnu D. Acoustic parameters and speech analysis after supracricoid hemilaryngopharyngectomy. Laryngoscope. 1995;105:1223–6.
63. Crevier-Buchman L, Brihaye S, Tessier C. La deglutition après chirurgie partielle du larynx. Bruxelles: Ed. Boeck Superieur; 1998.

Correction to: Transoral Approach for Early Laryngeal Cancers

Cesare Piazza, Hans Edmund Eckel, Marc Remacle,
Pamela Dela Cruz, Giorgio Peretti,
and Claudio Sampieri

Correction to:
Chapter 24 in: M. Remacle, H. E. Eckel (eds.), *Textbook of Surgery of Larynx and Trachea,* https://doi.org/10.1007/978-3-031-09621-1_24

The last name of Pamela Dela Cruz was unfortunately published as P. D. Cruz instead of P. Dela Cruz. This error has now been corrected.

The updated original version of this chapter can be found at
https://doi.org/10.1007/978-3-031-09621-1_24

M. Remacle, H. E. Eckel (eds.), *Textbook of Surgery of Larynx and Trachea*,
https://doi.org/10.1007/978-3-031-09621-1_36

MIX
Papier aus verantwortungsvollen Quellen
Paper from responsible sources
FSC® C105338

If you have any concerns about our products,
you can contact us on
ProductSafety@springernature.com

In case Publisher is established outside the EU,
the EU authorized representative is:
Springer Nature Customer Service Center GmbH
Europaplatz 3, 69115 Heidelberg, Germany

Printed by Libri Plureos GmbH
in Hamburg, Germany